AF126780

TEXTBOOK OF
PRACTICAL PHYSIOLOGY

As per the Revised NMC CBME–2024 Curriculum

SIXTH EDITION

G K Pal

MBBS, MD (Physiology), PhD, DSc, D.Sc. (Hon.causa)
BNYT (Naturopathy and Yoga Therapy), MD (Alt. Medicine), MD (Yoga), MABMS, FRSB (London), FABMS, FABAP, FSAB, FIABS, FEFI, FAPI
Professor (Senior Scale), Jawaharlal Institute of Postgraduate Medical Education and Research (JIPMER), Puducherry
Former Ex Director, AIIMS, Patna; Former Dean, JIPMER (Karaikal), Puducherry
Former Registrar (Academic), JIPMER, Puducherry
Former Dean, Faculty of Medicine, Pondicherry University, Puducherry
Honorary Professor, Sri Aurobindo International Center of Education, Sri Aurobindo Ashram, Pondicherry
Executive Editor, International Journal of Clinical and Experimental Physiology
General Secretary, Association of Physiologists of India (ASSOPI)
President, Federation of Indian Physiological Societies (FIPS)
Architect of DM Course in Clinical and Interventional Physiology in India (established it at AIIMS, Patna)

Pravati Pal

MBBS, MD (Physiology), BNYT, MD (Alt. Medicine), MABMS
Professor (Senior Scale), Department of Physiology
Jawaharlal Institute of Postgraduate Medical Education and Research (JIPMER), Puduchery

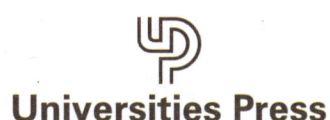
Universities Press

All rights reserved. No part of this book may be (i) modified, reproduced or utilised in any form, or by any means, electronic or mechanical, including photocopying, recording or by any information storage and retrieval system, in any form of binding or cover other than in which it is published, without permission in writing from the publisher; or (ii) used or reproduced in any manner for the purpose of training, development or operation of artificial intelligence (AI) technologies and systems, including generative AI technologies, without permission in writing from the copyright holder.

Textbook of Practical Physiology (Sixth Edition)

UNIVERSITIES PRESS (INDIA) PRIVATE LIMITED

Registered Office
3-6-747/1/A & 3-6-754/1, Himayatnagar, Hyderabad 500 029, Telangana, India
info@universitiespress.com; www.universitiespress.com

Distributed by
Orient Blackswan Private Limited

Registered Office
3-6-752 Himayatnagar, Hyderabad 500 029, Telangana, India

Other Offices
Bengaluru / Chennai / Guwahati / Hyderabad
Kolkata / Mumbai / New Delhi / Noida / Patna

© Universities Press (India) Private Limited 2001, 2005, 2010, 2016, 2020, 2026
First published 2001
Reprinted 2003, 2004
Second edition 2005
Reprinted 2006, 2007, 2008, 2009
Third edition 2010
Reprinted 2010 (Twice), 2011 (Twice), 2012, 2013, 2014, 2015
Fourth edition 2016
Reprinted 2017, 2018, 2019
Fifth edition 2020
Reprinted 2021, 2022, 2023, 2024 (Twice)
Sixth edition 2026

ISBN 978-93-49750-18-0

Cover and book design
© Universities Press (India) Private Limited 2001, 2005, 2010, 2016, 2020, 2026

Cover image source:
All product and company names are trademarks™ or registered® trademarks of their respective holders.
Use of them does not imply any affiliation with or endorsement by them.

Typeset in Life BT 10/12.5 pt *by*
Ogai Technologies, Chennai 600 032

Illustrations by
Pranchand K Verma
Amalgamation Graphics

Printed in India at
Rasi Graphics Pvt Ltd, Chennai 600 014

Published by
Universities Press (India) Private Limited
3-6-747/1/A & 3-6-754/1 Himayatnagar, Hyderabad 500 029, Telangana, India

502266

Care has been taken to confirm the accuracy of the information presented in this book. The authors and the publisher, however, cannot accept any responsibility for errors or omissions or for consequences from the application of the information in this book and make no warranty, express or implied, with respect to its contents.

Contents

The manifestation of the Supramental upon earth is no more a promise but a living fact, a reality.
It is at work here, and a day will come when the most blind, the most unconscious,
even the most unwilling shall be obliged to recognise it.

– The Mother (of Sri Aurobindo Ashram)

Acknowledgements

We are delighted to see the timely publication and release of the sixth edition of Textbook of Practical Physiology. The book has been thoroughly revised and updated as per the revised NMC CBME – 2024 guidelines to align the teaching and training of physiology with an objectivised, clinically-focused, and skill-based integrated curriculum. Given my significant administrative responsibilities at AIIMS, Patna, and the subsequent academic and research responsibilities Dr Pravati Pal and I had at JIPMER, Puducherry, the task of revising the textbook initially appeared quite daunting. However, with constant inspiration and growing demand from our readers, along with the unwavering encouragement of Mr Madhu Reddy, Director, Universities Press and President, Orient Blackswan Pvt. Ltd., we were able to complete the task smoothly and meaningfully. We express our sincere and heartfelt appreciation to Mr Madhu Reddy for his sincere support in seeing the book through to completion and for giving it a fresh, contemporary design and appeal. We are deeply thankful to Dr Astha Sawhney, Senior Development Editor, Medical Publishing, Universities Press, for conceptualising such an attractive layout for the book, providing invaluable inputs during the revision process, and overseeing of the work on this edition at every stage. We must sincerely acknowledge the profound, scrupulous, and sincere contribution of Ms Malini Gopalakrishnan, Senior Editor, Universities Press, who worked tirelessly and meticulously with us throughout the process of preparing the manuscript for this new edition. We sincerely thank her for getting this book ready within such a tight timeline. We also thank Mr Thomas Rajesh, Senior Vice President (Publishing – STMM), Universities Press for his timely assistance in the preparation of this book.

We sincerely thank our faculty colleagues—Prof. S. Velkumary, Prof. Y. Dhanalakshmi, Dr B. M. Naik, Dr S. Karthik, Dr N. Prabhu, Dr K. Saranya, Dr R. Rajalakshmi—and all our senior and junior residents and postgraduates for their constant support in this endeavour.

We are grateful to our friends from Sri Aurobindo Ashram, Pondicherry—the late Mr Narayan Mahapatra, Mr Chandramani, Ms Sujata Kar, and Mr Vasanth—for volunteering to act as subjects of our clinical examinations. Words cannot express our sincere appreciation for our caring children Dr Auroprakash Pal and Dr Auroprajna Pal, our devoted sisters Dr Nivedita Nanda and Ms Sabita Nanda, our fondly son-in-law Dr Dhirendra Kumar and affectionate sweet grand-daughter Aditi Ray (Rani *bete*), the loving members of our family who have been inexhaustible sources of inspiration and support to us throughout. We are forever indebted to our parents: the late Shri Mrutyunjay Pal, Smt. Malati Mani Pal, the late Dr Atratran Nanda, and the late Mrs Anupama Nanda, for instilling in us the values of discipline and dedication. It is to their wisdom and guidance that we owe our place in society and our successes. We will always be grateful to all our former teachers for imparting to us the knowledge that we are sharing with our readers today.

We are ever indebted to the infinite grace of Sri-Maa, the Divine Mother, and Sri Aurobindo, the Divine Master, for showering on us their immense blessings and unfathomable protection, which have guided our progress and helped us achieve the best in life.

G K Pal
Pravati Pal
Email: gkpalphysiology@gmail.com

All can be done if God-touch is there.

— **Sri Aurobindo** (in SAVITRI)

Preface to the Sixth Edition

Textbook of Practical Physiology has been greatly appreciated by students, residents, members of faculty, laboratory technical officers, and practicing physicians in India and abroad. The feedback and inputs from our readers reveal that this book is regarded the most valuable and reliable textbook of practical physiology for about two and a half decades. The popularity of this book can be attributed to the fact that it fulfils all the requirements of students and teachers—imparting detailed knowledge of techniques, helping to develop practical skills, and guiding their application in physiology and medicine, ultimately supporting the journey toward becoming a competent physician.

It has always been our aim to provide medical students with a book that is up-to-date in all aspects of applied and clinical physiology and to equip them with the requisite knowledge and skills in these areas. With the introduction of the revised curriculum prescribed by the Medical Council of India (MCI), 2019, followed by the National Medical Commission (NMC) Competency-Based Medical Education (CBME) 2021 and the revised NMC CBME – 2024, there is a clear shift towards an evidence-based, objective-oriented, clinically-focussed, and skill-based, integrated curriculum. Particularly notable are the new directives for 'Early Clinical Exposure (ECE)'—starting from the first year and allowing students to learn through real patient interactions and continuous assessments that use logbooks, OSPE (Objective Structured Practical Examination)/OSCE (Objective Structured Clinical Examination), and structured practical training and evaluation conducted throughout the year at regular intervals instead of a single final practical exam. This marks a paradigm shift in the practical teaching, training, and assessment of undergraduate medical students in India.

We take pride in noting that this *Textbook of Practical Physiology* was the first book on the subject to introduce learning objectives, objectivised structured methodology, and organised assessments. The inclusion of OSPE as part of practical assessment was first introduced in this textbook in its inaugural edition in 2001. At the time, this was an innovative initiative aligned with the medical education and training guidelines of NTTC, JIPMER.

Various sections of this sixth edition of *Textbook of Practical Physiology*—including those on hematology, human experiments, and clinical physiology—have been thoroughly revised as per the revised NMC CBME – 2024. The edition has also been fortified with new chapters on assessment of body composition, basal metabolism and obesity, energy cost of work, bicycle ergometry, demonstration of arterial pulse tracing, carotid sinus reflex, venous blood flow, venous pressure, and triple response, demonstration of H reflex, demonstration of physiologic blind spots, stereoscopic vision, dominance of the eye, subjective visual sensation, mechanical stimulation of the eye, demonstration of near point, near response and range of accommodation, demonstration of Purkinje–Sanson images, ultrasonography as a pregnancy diagnostic test, and demonstration of masking of sound and localisation of sound. A major highlight of this edition is the enhanced *VIVA* section in each practical chapter, where answers to all questions are now provided with precise references to the corresponding page, paragraph, heading, subheading, figure, and table. The number of viva questions and answers has nearly doubled in every chapter. Another special feature of this edition is the incorporation of a new section—Section V: Graphs, Charts, Calculation and Problem-Solving Questions—which includes three new chapters to further facilitate the understanding of intricate but important concepts, clinical applications, problem-based learning, and analytical interpretation of various physiological measurements (calculations). Several new flowcharts, figures, and tables have been added to simplify the perception of applied and clinical concepts.

This book is specially designed for step-by-step learning through practicals and experiments, which are vital to medical students seeking to develop expertise in clinical medicine. Many illustrations have been meticulously revised, redrawn, and re-represented to facilitate the assimilation of various techniques. Several new colour photographs have been added across the book to demonstrate the advancements in methodologies in practical physiology. We are confident that the new, contemporary four-colour design and thoroughly edited, revised, and updated sixth edition of this book will appeal to students and aid in reading and retention.

With the introduction of the D.M. Course in *Clinical and Interventional Physiology* (CIP) in July 2023—an initiative I was instrumental in conceptualising and establishing at AIIMS, Patna, during my tenure as the head of the institute—the standing of the subject 'Physiology' has increased enormously within medical science. This transformation positions the subject as a fully clinical discipline with the interventional provision of HRV biofeedback therapy, deep-brain stimulation (DBS) therapy, vagus nerve stimulation (VNS) therapy, intra-operative neuro-monitoring and intervention (IONMI), yoga therapy, exercise therapy, respiratory biofeedback therapy, and many more. With CIP now recognised as a super-specialisation subject in Physiology, we are sure many new practicals of interventional physiology will be added to future editions of this book. We firmly believe that soon physiologists will be among the top-rated clinical physicians and clinical researchers.

It is our strong belief that the sixth edition of the *Textbook of Practical Physiology* is now a comprehensive practical textbook on the subject for undergraduate and postgraduate students of physiology and medicine. We trust that our readers will find this new edition of the book fulfilling of all their requirements of contemporary knowledge and skills in practical physiology. As always, we welcome further suggestions and constructive feedback to help us continue refining and perfecting this work.

G K Pal
Pravati Pal
Email: gkpalphysiology@gmail.com

A drop of practice is better than an ocean of theories, advices and good resolutions.

—The Mother

Preface to the First Edition

This textbook of practical physiology covers all the aspects of the practicals in the subject. The authors hope that it will fulfil the needs of the medical student.

We have tried our best to provide high quality material in a precise and comprehensive form. Every effort has been made to incorporate all the aspects of practical physiology. Till now, students used to come to practical classes with a manual and a theory book. The manual helps them learn the techniques to perform the practical, and the theory book helps them understand the practical. Often, the theory books do not cover all the theoretical aspects of the practical. Therefore, in this book, we have made a sincere effort to provide the essential underlying principles of practical physiology, to help the student perform various practicals, and to learn and apply the knowledge of practical physiology in clinical medicine. This book is therefore meant to be a complete textbook of practical physiology.

The Medical Council of India (MCI) has recently suggested significant changes in the first MBBS curriculum. It has recommended an increase in the number of human practicals, reduction in experimental practicals, and more applied and clinically oriented teaching to provide an objective-oriented learning. In view of this, more than seventy per cent of this book contains human practicals, and experimental physiology has been described in a very compact (but essentially useful) form. Each practical in the book contains learning objectives, theoretical aspects of the practical, details of clinical-oriented discussion and possible viva voce questions with answers. The unique feature of this book is the introduction of objective structured practical examination (OSPE). The 'General Introduction' describes OSPE and suggests how best the book could be used.

A book of this kind may be complete but is not perfect. Indeed, we visualise the book as a project in evolution that should be able to accommodate the constructive criticism and suggestions, and the fast-changing concepts and needs of the science. We welcome the reader's views and suggestions, to make future editions of the book as useful to the students as the current edition.

G K Pal
Pravati Pal

Special Features of This Book

Education is the process that brings about desirable changes in the behaviour of the learner in the form of acquisition of knowledge, proficiency in skills and development of attitudes. Knowledge and skill should grow simultaneously and harmoniously. Knowledge without skill is useless and skill without knowledge is dangerous. Therefore, to become a good physician, a medical student should have knowledge, skill and proper attitude.

Physiology is a vast subject. Knowledge of physiology is used in all branches of medicine, from biochemistry and pharmacology to gynecology and medicine. **A good physician is a good physiologist and a true physiologist is the best physician**. Knowledge of practical physiology is applied in clinical medicine to understand the pathophysiology of the disease, to explain the clinical manifestation of the disease, to provide the physiological basis of the diagnosis and treatment of the disease, and to assess the prognosis. In this book, we have tried to explain the clinical significance of the practicals, in addition to detailed descriptions of various physiological aspects of the topics. *This introduction will help you extract maximum benefit from the book.*

Each topic of this book has most of these sections: **learning objectives, introduction, methods (including observation and result), discussion, OSPE and viva**.

Learning objectives

Objectives are to a student (or teacher) what blueprints are to an architect. Learning objectives give the student an idea of the desired competence in the form of acquisition of knowledge and skill. Unless these competencies are clearly stated, it cannot be known whether they are properly acquired. Objectives help the students organise their efforts to obtain the desired knowledge and skill. Therefore, each topic, whether theory or practical, must have learning objectives. The objectives should be relevant, unequivocal, observable, measurable and feasible.

A set of 'Learning Objectives' has been given at the beginning of each topic. The student should go through these objectives before performing the practical. The objectives are intended to inform the students what they must know and what is desirable for them to know. Accordingly, the learning objectives are divided into two categories. The first set of MUST KNOW objectives provides what students must learn *(the minimum that they should learn)* by performing that practical and the second set of DESIRABLE TO KNOW objectives describes what they may know *(it is better to learn this too, though it is not mandatory)*. In the latest recommendation by the Medical Council of India, it has been emphasised that teaching should be clinically based with clearly outlined objectives of what students must know and what is desirable for them to know. For physiology practicals, the students should read the objectives *before* starting the practical and should again look at them *after* completing the practical, to assess whether they have achieved the required skill and knowledge. The objectives that are described in this book are basic in nature. The teacher can modify these objectives according to the needs and the instructions of the university teaching curriculum.

Introduction

It is desirable that the students have a basic knowledge of the topic before they perform the practical. It helps them understand the scientific basis and the importance of the practical. Every effort has been made to give a clear and concise theoretical explanation in this section. It introduces the topic and describes the important points of the methods. Therefore, the students should read this before they perform a practical.

Methods

Under "Methods", a detailed description has been given of the different methodologies that are used widely in different laboratories. Each method contains four to five sub-sections—Principle, Requirements, Procedure, Precautions, Observation and Result. A brief description of the **"Principle"** of the method is given at the beginning. In **"Requirements"**, the equipment and chemicals required to perform the test are listed and a brief description is given about the important equipment and chemicals. A short description is also given about the *use* of the equipment. In **"Procedure"**, a detailed and stepwise description of how to perform the practical is given. Important steps are followed by a **"Note"**, which describes the significance of that particular step. A list of important **"Precautions"** are given following the procedure. The methods that are usually not used but are important from the examination point of view (likely to be asked in the viva voce) are described briefly. A practical, unless done properly following the proper procedure and precautions, is likely to yield erroneous results. Therefore, the student should read and understand the procedure and precautions thoroughly before performing the practical.

Discussion

"Discussion" gives details of the physiological and clinical significance of the practical. Only points that are pertinent to the practical have been included. Discussion of the result, merits and demerits of different methods, and practical implications of a specific test should be undertaken by the teacher only after the student has completed the practical and got the result. Therefore, the student should not read this section before performing the practical. However, *there must be discussion at the end of the practical* because only after a thorough and complete discussion does one gain complete practical knowledge.

OSPE

OSPE stands for **objective structured practical examination**. In this, a small but important component of the practical is evaluated in a stepwise manner as prefixed and described in the checklist. This is an objective method of assessment, where specific competencies are tested. In clinical examinations, it is called **OSCE**. This is a new concept of evaluation of the practical or clinical skill of medical students. Teachers have always been concerned about the reliability and uniformity of assessment of students. Traditionally, in examinations, students perform the practical and the examiner assesses their practical knowledge (not the skill) after they have already performed the test. The examiners do not evaluate the skill of the students, as they do not observe them while performing the practical. Therefore, the skill aspect of the practical, which is the most important aspect, remains under-evaluated. The skill improves and gradually attains perfection only when a practical is performed and evaluated with **specific structured objectives**. Therefore, at present, OSPE is the best way to determine the skill of the students, as it is transparent, reliable, valid and objective. OSPE is designed to overcome the deficiencies of conventional practical examinations. Since each practical is broken down into smaller components and each component has prescribed steps, a **greater degree of objectivity** is achieved. Marks are allotted for each component and for each step.

In OSPE, the students are required to perform an important component of the practical within a specified time. The examiners keep a checklist (the steps of OSPE) with them and observe whether the examinee performs the test in the proper sequence as described. The examiners *do not ask anything,* they only observe the stepwise performance by the student and enter marks against the corrected steps (for a detailed procedure on conducting the OSPE, see "Methodology of OSPE"). In this book, under OSPE, we have given a stepwise description (this serves as the checklist for the teacher) of all important practicals. Therefore, the student should practice the methods carefully as described under OSPE. It should be introduced in all medical colleges to bring about **uniformity, objectivity, validity, transparency and reliability in the evaluation** of the practical skill of the students.

Viva

The questions that are usually asked in viva voce are described under 'Viva'. This book includes a **total of about 1,300 viva questions**, each **accompanied by a corresponding answer**—a unique and valuable feature. For questions with answers available within the chapters, we have provided the **exact page number, along with the relevant heading and subheading**, to help students locate the information quickly and easily. Where answers are not directly found in the main text, **comprehensive explanations have been provided** to aid understanding of the underlying concepts. Additionally, **new questions** have been included to cover **topics introduced in the revised syllabus**. Therefore, students must read all the questions and answers in the viva section, otherwise they may miss some important points.

General Laboratory Instructions

A medical laboratory is the workshop that provides the knowledge and experience to develop practical skills and attitudes. To achieve this, the working atmosphere in the laboratory should be congenial to the teachers and students. For smooth and harmonious conduct of laboratory work, cooperation from the technical staff, attendants, students and teachers is of utmost importance.

Instructions for students

Desire to learn, dedication to study, sincerity and cooperation in work, and a caring attitude are essential qualities in a medical student. The student should keep in mind the following:

1. Wear a clean and well-ironed white coat and good-looking shining shoes while working in the laboratory. Wear your official ID card, making sure that it is visible to others.
2. Bring the necessary equipment for hematology (disposable lancets, etc.), amphibian or experimental (dissecting instruments) and human practicals (stethoscope, knee hammer, etc.).
3. Have a basic theoretical knowledge of the concerned practical (the practical of that day). For this, read the introduction to each topic, before attending the instruction of the demonstrator or before performing the practical.
4. Pay due attention to the demonstration of the practical given by the instructor or teacher.
5. Check to see if the apparatus is working properly before starting the experiment.
6. Do not disturb the instruments that are not assigned to you or are not required for the practical.
7. For any technical assistance, take help from the appointed technician or the instructor without disturbing other students.
8. Handle the apparatus gently and carry out the experiment without damaging it.
9. Perform the practical step-by-step following the proper procedure and precautions. For this, refer to the method described for each practical.
10. After obtaining the observation, discuss with the teacher about the accuracy of the result, and about the physiological and clinical utility of the practical. For this, read the discussion section given under each topic.
11. Enter the observation and result in your practical record, and note the physiological and pathological variation in the parameters and also write the answers to the questions given.
12. After completing the practical, check whether you have achieved the minimum knowledge and skill prescribed. For this, refer to the list of learning objectives given for that practical.
13. Get the practical record checked by the teacher regularly.
14. Return the apparatus to the laboratory staff before leaving the laboratory.
15. Keep the practical record and book in good condition.

Instructions for demonstrators

A medical educator has a dual ethical obligation: to produce competent health professionals for the society, and to improve the standard of the student under care. Teachers of practical physiology have two important roles to play. First, they should familiarise themselves with the objectives (both essential and desirable objectives) and select what the student should learn, and second, they should help facilitate the learning of the student. Teachers (demonstrators) should:

1. Wear a white coat while taking practical classes for the students.
2. Give proper direction to the students to follow the laboratory discipline.
3. Practise, read and understand the practical, before taking classes for the students.
4. Do the demonstration confidently and clearly, without confusion.
5. Emphasise and explain the important steps of the practical.
6. Pay equal attention to all the students.
7. Not be seen sitting idle in the laboratory.
8. Encourage students to express their difficulties without fear.
9. Try to detect and solve the individual practical problems of the students.
10. Explain the physiological and clinical importance of the practical.
11. Check and evaluate the practical record of the students regularly.
12. Give feedback to the students for their improvement.

Methodology of OSPE

Conducting OSPE needs proper planning and organisation. **Planning for OSPE** includes setting down valid, appropriate and important questions, and preparing an accurate checklist suitable for evaluating the student's performance. **Organisation** includes arrangement of stations that contain all the materials required to perform the test and motivated subjects (if clinical practicals), and trained manpower to regulate the movement of the students during the practical.

OSPE can be used for evaluating performance in class examinations as well as in the final examination. During the examination, the students move around a number of stations spending a specific amount of time (3 to 5 minutes) in each. In each station they perform a specific practical within the stipulated time and then move to the next station in response to an auditory signal (say, ringing of a bell). In the final examination, since there are usually four examiners (two internal and two external), four OSPE stations can be kept. When students perform the OSPE, examiners sit beside each of them with the checklist, observe their performance, and grade them accordingly in the checklist. The examiners must carefully check each and every step of the practical without disturbing the candidate; they are just active observers and should not interfere in any way with the performance of the candidate. They are not supposed to ask any questions nor are they expected to respond to any query from the student.

It is better to have **non-skill stations between the OSPE (skill) stations**. Ideally, the non-skill stations should have the question related to the previous skill station, so that it reinforces the skill and knowledge of the student. For example, if the skill station has asked for the student to elicit a tendon jerk, the non-skill station can have any one of the following questions:

1. Draw a reflex arc.
2. List the five important differences between upper and lower motor neuron paralysis.
3. Name two conditions each in which the tendon reflexes are i) exaggerated and ii) depressed.

Likewise, the questions can be framed according to the previous skill stations. In university examinations, eight stations (four skill and four non-skill) can be kept. The examiners evaluate the skill station on the spot and non-skill stations afterwards. This can replace conventional spotting-type examination (students write the answer according to the spotter given). After the OSPE is over, the student can perform the long and short practicals as they usually do in the university examination. Ideally, as per MCI recommendations, twenty students (not more than 25) should be evaluated for practical examination per day. In OSPE, the twenty students in eight stations (four skill and four non-skill) spending four minutes at each will not take more than 90 minutes. If the examination starts at 8.30 am, OSPE can be completed by 10.00 am and the remaining three hours can be used for other practicals and practical viva examination; the theory viva can be conducted in the afternoon. For routine class examinations, more stations (10–20) can be set up to include the maximum number of practicals. This may be done easily with the help of the junior teaching staff of the department. The students should be exposed to the OSPE at least two or three times before the final examination. OSPE should carry a weightage of 30–50 per cent of the total marks allotted for the practical.

Before the OSPE is conducted, it must be ensured that all the equipment (instrument, solution, gauze, cotton, spirit, etc.) is available in the station according to the question given. As only 3 to 5 minutes are given to each student, the students should not spend time searching for the equipment. It should also be ensured that as soon as the indication is given (ringing a bell), the student moves immediately to the next station. The OSPE questions too should be prepared in such a way that the student should be able to perform the practical (both in the skill and non-skill stations) within the stipulated time. For this, the question for **OSPE should contain only an important component of the practical**, not the whole of the practical. One of the problems in conducting OSPE, especially hematology practicals, is to supply adequate material during the examination. For example, if the question is 'Dilute the blood for total RBC count', adequate number of pipettes should be supplied, otherwise, a laboratory attendant should help throughout the examination to wash the used pipettes. Similarly in human practicals, the main problem would be to provide cooperative and motivated subjects. This will need to be planned in advance.

How to make a checklist

Question: *Examine the radial pulse of the subject and report your finding.*

Student number	1	2	3	4	5	6	7	8	9	10 20	
Criteria of OSPE											**Group score**
1. Stands on the right side ...											
2. Places three middle fingers ...											
3. Counts for 1 min											
4. Checks the condition of the ...											
5. Compares with opposite side ...											
6. Checks for radio-femoral delay											
7. Reports properly											
Individual score											

Advantages of OSPE

1. Uniform evaluation of performance of all the students.
2. Methodical assessment of skill.
3. No examiner bias.
4. Evaluation is more transparent.
5. Evaluation is valid and reliable.
6. All the students are given the same practical and are allowed the same duration of time. Therefore, there is no candidate bias.
7. Provides direct feedback to the student as well as to the teacher. The students get feedback on a mistake in a particular step (feedback is given after the practical, usually in a group). If many students make the same error in a particular step of OSPE, it indicates that the step was probably not properly demonstrated or emphasised by the teacher.
8. Junior examiners can also be appointed.

Competency Mapping Table
As per the revised NMC CBME – 2024 curriculum

No.	Competency The student will be able to:	Domain (K/S/A /C)	Level (K/KH/ SH/P)	Core (Y/N)	Suggested T/L Method	Suggested Assessment Method	Chapter (Ch.) and Page Number
Topic 2: Hematology							
PY2.11	Estimate Hb, RBC, TLC, DLC, blood groups, BT/CT, and RBC indices	S	SH	Y	DOAPs	Practical/ OSPE /Viva voce	**Hb**: Ch. 3, Page 10 **RBC**: Ch. 7, Page 42 **TLC**: Ch. 9, Page 53 **DLC**: Ch. 10 & 11, Pages 61, 71 **Blood groups**: Ch. 15, Page 90 **BT/CT**: Ch. 17, Page 102 **RBC indices**: Ch. 8, Page 50
PY2.12	Describe the test to measure erythrocyte sedimentation rate (ESR), osmotic fragility, hematocrit, and interpret its findings	K	KH	Y	Demonst-ration	Written/Viva voce/OSPE	**ESR**: Ch. 14, Page 83 **Osmotic fragility**: Ch. 16, Page 98 **Hematocrit**: Ch. 4, Page 20
PY2.13	Describe the steps for reticulocyte and platelet count	K	KH	Y	Demonst-ration	Written/Viva voce	**Reticulocyte count**: Ch. 19, Page 119 **Platelet count**: Ch. 18, Page 113
Topic 3: Nerve and Muscle Physiology							
PY3.11	Perform ergography and calculate the work done by a skeletal muscle	S	SH	Y	DOAPs	Practical/ OSPE /Viva voce	Ch. 34, Page 228
PY3.12	Observe with computer-assisted learning: i) amphibian nerve–muscle experiments and ii) amphibian cardiac experiments	S	SH	Y	DOAPs	Practical/ OSPE /Viva voce	i) **Amphibian NM experiments**: Ch. 59–67, Pages 433–459 ii) **Cardiac experiments**: Ch. 68–73, Pages 460–477
Topic 4: Gastrointestinal Physiology							
PY4.12	Obtain relevant history and conduct correct general and clinical examination of the abdomen in a normal volunteer or simulated environment	S, A, C	SH	Y	DOAPs (Simulation or real-life setting)	Skill assessment/ Viva voce/ OSCE	Ch. 55, Page 365
Topic 5: Cardiovascular Physiology							
PY5.14	Record blood pressure and pulse at rest and in different grades of exercise and postures in a volunteer or simulated environment	S	SH	Y	DOAPs (Simulation or real-life setting)	Practical/ OSPE /Viva voce	**Pulse**: Ch. 27, Page 174 **BP**: Ch. 28, Page 185 **Posture**: Ch. 29, Page 199 **Exercise**: Ch. 30, Page 203
PY5.15	Record and interpret a normal ECG in a volunteer or simulated environment	S	SH	Y	DOAPs (Simulation or real-life setting)	Practical/ OSPE /Viva voce	Ch. 26, Page 162
PY5.16	Obtain relevant history and conduct general and clinical examination of the cardiovascular system in a normal volunteer or simulated environment	S, A, C	SH	Y	DOAPs	Skill assessment/ Viva voce/ OSCE	Ch. 54, Page 353
Topic 6: Respiratory Physiology							
PY6.10	Perform spirometry and interpret the findings (digital/manual)	S	P	Y	DOAPs	Skill assessment/ Viva voce/ OSCE	Ch. 21, Page 127 Ch. 22, Page 132 Ch. 23, Page 136
PY6.11	Describe the principles and methods of artificial respiration	S	SH	Y	DOAPs	Practical/ OSPE /Viva voce	Ch. 24, Page 150
PY6.12	Obtain relevant history and conduct correct general and clinical examination of the respiratory system in a normal volunteer or simulated environment	S, A, C	SH	Y	DOAPs	Practical/ OSPE /Viva voce	Ch. 53, Page 339

No.	Competency The student will be able to:	Domain (K/S/A /C)	Level (K/KH/ SH/P)	Core (Y/N)	Suggested T/L Method	Suggested Assessment Method	Chapter (Ch.) and Page Number
PY6.13	Demonstrate the correct technique to perform the measurement of peak expiratory flow rate in a normal volunteer or simulated environment	S	SH	Y	DOAPs	Practical/ OSPE /Viva voce	Ch. 23, Page 142
Topic 9: Reproductive Physiology							
PY9.3	Describe the functional anatomy of the male reproductive system, functions of the testis, spermatogenesis and discuss the functions and regulations of testosterone hormone	K	KH	Y	LGT SGT	OSPE/Viva voce	**Semen analysis**: Ch. 49, Page 318
PY9.6	Enumerate male and female contraceptive methods, rationale of its prescription, side effects and its advantages & disadvantages	K	KH	Y	LGT, SGT, ECE, SDL	Written/Viva voce	Ch. 51, Page 325
PY9.8	Discuss the physiological basis of various pregnancy tests	K	KH	Y	LGT, SGT	Written/Viva voce	Ch. 50, Page 321
Topic 10: Central Nervous System Physiology							
PY10.19	Obtain relevant history and conduct correct general and clinical examination of the nervous system: Higher functions, sensory system, motor system, reflexes in a normal volunteer or simulated environment	S	SH	Y	DOAPs	Skill assessment/ Viva voce/ OSCE	**Higher functions**: Ch. 56, Page 373 **Sensory system**: Ch. 57, Page 391 **Motor system & reflexes**: Ch. 58, Page 405
PY10.20	Obtain relevant history and conduct correct general and clinical examination of the cranial nerves in a normal volunteer or simulated environment	S	P	Y	DOAPs	OSCE/Viva voce	Ch. 56, Page 373
Topic 11: Special Senses							
PY11.1	Describe and discuss the physiology of smell and its applied aspects	K	KH	Y	LGT, SGT	Written /Viva voce	Ch. 48, Page 315
PY11.2	Describe and discuss the physiology of taste sensation and its applied aspects	K	KH	Y	LGT, SGT	Written /Viva voce	Ch. 48, Page 313
PY11.4	Discuss the physiology of hearing, pathophysiology of deafness and hearing tests	K	KH	Y	LGT, SGT	Written /Viva voce	Ch. 47, Page 304
PY11.5	Discuss the functional anatomy of the eye, visual pathway, light and pupillary reflex and clinical implication of lesions in the visual pathway	K	HK	Y	LGT, SGT	Written /Viva voce	Ch. 44, Page 288
PY11.6	Discuss the physiology of image formation, refractive errors and physiological principles of its management	K, S	P	Y	LGT, SGT, ECE	Written /Viva voce	Ch. 44 and 45, Page 288, 300
PY11.7	Discuss physiology of vision including colour vision and colour blindness	K	KH	Y	LGT, SGT, Flipped classroom	Written /Viva voce	Ch. 46, 301
Topic 12: Special Senses							
PY12.7	Discuss the concept and criteria for the diagnosis of brain death and its implications	K	KH	Y	Small group teaching	Practical/ OSPE /Viva voce	**EEG, brain death**: Ch. 36, Page 243
PY12.9	Obtain history and perform general examination in the volunteer/simulated environment	S	SH	Y	DOAPs	Skill assessment/ Viva voce/ OSCE	Ch. 52, Page 329
PY12.10	Demonstrate basic life support in a simulated environment	S	SH	Y	DOAPs (Simulation or real-life setting	Skill assessment/ Viva voce/ OSCE	Ch. 24, Page 151

1 | Introduction to Hematology

Learning Objectives

After studying this chapter, you will be able to (MUST KNOW):
1. Define hematology.
2. List the components of blood.
3. Explain the functions of each component.
4. Name the routine hematologic tests.

5. List the sources of specimens used in a hematology laboratory.

You may also be able to (DESIRABLE TO KNOW):
1. Describe the appearance of a blood specimen after centrifugation.
2. Explain the significance of the buffy coat.

INTRODUCTION

Hematology is defined as the branch of science that deals with the study of blood. The word 'hematology' is derived from the Greek words *haima*, meaning blood, and *logos*, meaning study. It is primarily concerned with the study of the formed elements of blood.

Blood is defined as the *liquid connective tissue that fills the heart and the blood vessels*. The total volume of blood in an adult weighing 70 kg is about 5.5 litres, which is about 8 per cent of the body weight. About 45 per cent of this volume is composed of formed elements. Plasma constitutes about 5 per cent of the body weight.

BLOOD COMPONENTS AND THEIR FUNCTIONS

Blood has two major components: cells and fluid (plasma).

The Cellular Component

The cellular component consists of red blood cells (erythrocytes), white blood cells (leucocytes), and platelets (thrombocytes). The thrombocytes are the smallest (2–4 μm) of these; the erythrocytes are medium-sized (7–8 μm); and the leucocytes are the largest of all the cells with a wide range of sizes (8–20 μm). Red blood cells constitute the highest number of formed elements in circulation (4.5–6 million/mm^3 of blood) followed by platelets (1.5–4 lakhs/mm^3 of blood) and leucocytes (4–11 thousand/mm^3 of blood).

The key function of **erythrocytes** is the *transport of gases,* i.e., they carry oxygen from the lungs to the tissues and carbon dioxide from the tissues to the lungs. **Leucocytes** assist in the *defence processes* of the body. **Thrombocytes** assist in stoppage of bleeding (*hemostasis*).

The development of blood cells is called **hemopoiesis**. In post-natal life (after birth), hemopoiesis occurs in the bone marrow.

The Fluid Component

The fluid component of the blood is known as **plasma** and consists of a soluble protein called **fibrinogen**. During the process of coagulation of blood, fibrinogen is removed from plasma as fibrin, and the clear fluid left behind is called **serum**. Therefore, when plasma is required for diagnostic tests, the blood specimen collected should not be allowed to clot.

Plasma

Plasma is the principal medium for the transportation of materials from one part of the body to another through the blood vessels. It carries various substances including nutrients, metabolites, waste products, hormones, and chemicals. Plasma contains **clotting factors** that participate in blood coagulation.

Serum

Serum contains **most of the chemicals present** in the plasma *except fibrinogen and some clotting factors*. Therefore, many investigations like estimations of glucose, proteins and lipids are performed on serum, which is collected by clotting blood.

HEMATOLOGIC TESTS

Several hematologic tests such as the estimation of hemoglobin, total RBC count, total leucocyte count, ESR, and differential count of leucocytes are performed regularly as part of the initial laboratory investigations conducted for every patient. Many of these tests are considered routine and can be performed by a technician with limited training. Routine hematological investigations are performed mainly to study the patient's ability to fight diseases, to aid in the diagnosis of diseases, and to assess the prognosis of the disease.

Performing hematologic tests accurately **requires adequate skill and experience**, especially with respect to using the required instruments. In recent years, especially in advanced laboratories, many of these tests have been automated. Nevertheless, in medical college laboratories, tests are performed chiefly by manual techniques to help students understand the principles and methods involved.

A student should acquire enough knowledge about the formed elements of blood and their enumeration and characteristics to perform and analyse these tests accurately. They should, therefore, be aware of the formation, structure, and functions of blood cells, the basic principle of their quantitative determination, the use and care of equipment, the preparation of reagents, and the calculation and interpretation of results.

Specimens

Blood samples for hematologic study are usually obtained by **finger puncture** (capillary blood) or **venipuncture** (venous blood). An arterial blood sample is usually not needed for hematology practical examinations in Physiology.

Capillary blood

Capillary blood can be used with good results for **morphologic studies in hematology**. It is obtained from the **fingertip, earlobe,** heel, or big toe. *In newborns and infants*, blood is usually obtained **by heel puncture** because there is limited blood supply in the fingertips and because drawing blood by venipuncture would deplete too much blood. *In adults*, the **tip of any of the middle three fingers** is punctured to obtain a sample.

Venous blood

Capillary blood is not always suitable for hematological tests, particularly when a large volume is required for investigations. In such cases, venous blood is preferred for accurate investigations.

To ensure usability, **coagulation must be prevented**, as clotted blood cannot be used. To prevent clot formation, the blood sample should be gently mixed by repeated inversion immediately after collection. Even a tiny clot in the specimen can compromise test results.

For most hematologic studies, **EDTA (ethylenediamine tetra-acetic acid)** is the anticoagulant of choice, as it preserves the morphology of cellular elements. Blood must be mixed with anticoagulant immediately after collection to effectively prevent clotting.

If refrigerated at 4°C, white cell count, microhematocrit, platelet count, and sedimentation rate measurements remain reliable for up to 24 hours after collection in EDTA.

■ Appearance

When blood is properly drawn and preserved, plasma retains its natural colour—a very light yellow or straw-like hue. However, in certain disease states or due to improper handling, the colour of plasma may be altered.

Two types of blood samples are unsuitable for hematologic investigations:

1. **Clotted samples**
2. **Hemolysed samples** (caused by errors during collection or handling)

When blood is collected, anticoagulated, and then allowed to settle or undergo centrifugation, it separates into *three distinct layers* (Fig. 1.1):

1. **Bottom layer** – Packed red blood cells (packed cell volume), comprising 43–47% of the total blood volume.

2. **Middle layer (buffy coat)** – A thin whitish layer consisting of leucocytes and platelets, accounting for about 1% of the total volume. This layer is crucial for detecting abnormal cells such as LE cells in systemic lupus erythematosus (SLE) and atypical mononuclear cells in malignant conditions. Buffy coat smears are also useful for identifying bacteria, fungi, and parasites within circulating leucocytes.

3. **Top layer** – This layer is made up of plasma, a colloidal liquid that makes up 52–57% of the total blood volume.

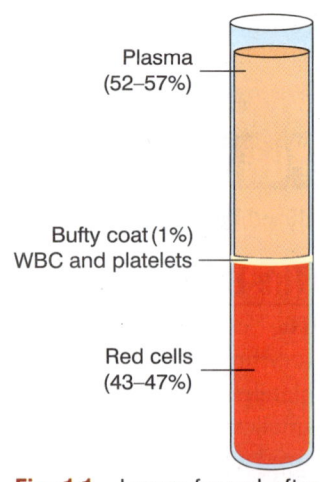

Fig. 1.1 Layers formed after centrifugation of a normal blood sample. Note the packed cell volume (red cells) is about 45%.

Plasma (52–57%)

Bufy coat (1%)
WBC and platelets

Red cells (43–47%)

VIVA

1. *Define blood and name its components.* (Ans. Refer to page 1, under the headings 'Introduction' and 'Blood components and their functions'.)
2. *What are the formed elements of blood, their normal counts, and their primary functions?* (Ans. Refer to Page 1, under the heading 'Blood components and their functions'.)
3. *What is the difference between plasma and serum?* (Ans. Refer to Page 1, under the heading 'Blood components and their functions'.)
4. *How is serum prepared in the laboratory?*
    (Ans. Blood is drawn into a tube without anticoagulant, allowed to clot, and then centrifuged. The liquid part that separates from the cells and the clot is the serum.)

5. *What is the purpose of performing routine hematologic tests?* (Ans. Refer to pages 1 and 2, under the heading 'Hematologic tests'.)
6. *What are the types of specimens collected for hematologic tests?* (Ans. Refer to page 2, under the heading 'Specimens'.)
7. *Why are the middle three fingers preferred for skin puncture?*
    (Ans. The venous bursa of the middle three fingers is limited to the hand, whereas those of the thumb and little finger are continuous with that of the limb. Drawing blood from the middle three fingers is a preventative measure to limit any infection that might occur to the hand.)
8. *Why is venipuncture not used for collecting blood samples in newborns and infants?* (Ans. Refer to page 2, under the heading 'Specimens' and the subheading 'Capillary blood'.)
9. *Which is the ideal site for collecting blood in newborns and infants and why?*
    (Ans. The ideal method of collecting blood from infants is by performing a heel puncture, as blood supply to fingertips is limited in infants and children.)
10. *Why is EDTA commonly preferred for collecting venous blood?*
    (Ans. EDTA preserves the morphology of cellular elements.)
11. *What is a buffy coat and what is its significance?* (Ans. Refer to page 2, against the bullet point titled 'Middle layer (buffy coat)'.)
12. *Why should blood be properly mixed with anticoagulants immediately after collection?*
    (Ans. To ensure proper anticoagulation.)
13. *What types of blood samples are unsuitable for hematologic tests and why?*
    (Ans. Clotted and hemolysed samples are unsuitable for hematologic tests. It is difficult to obtain plasma from a clotted sample; smears cannot be prepared from such samples either. A hemolysed sample will not yield cells and serum.)

2 | Collection of Blood Samples

Learning Objectives

After completing this practical, you will be able to (MUST KNOW):

1. List the general precautions to be observed while collecting blood.
2. List the methods of collecting a blood sample.
3. Collect peripheral blood by the finger prick method.
4. List the precautions observed while collecting blood by the finger prick method.
5. Name the specific uses of commonly used anticoagulants in hematological procedures.

You may also be able to (DESIRABLE TO KNOW):

1. Collect blood by the venipuncture method.
2. List the precautions applied while performing the venipuncture method.
3. List the steps of collecting blood by the earlobe puncture and heel puncture methods.
4. Explain the mechanism of action and uses of various anticoagulants.

INTRODUCTION

Blood is one of the most common specimens used in laboratory determinations. **Venous blood** is preferred for most hematological examinations.

Peripheral samples (capillary blood) can be used satisfactorily for most purposes if a free flow of blood is obtained. However, this procedure should be avoided in patients who are possible carriers of transmissible diseases. Capillary blood is commonly used for hemoglobin estimation, cell counts, blood grouping, bleeding and clotting time determination, and other investigations that use less blood, whereas venous blood is preferred for comprehensive hematological investigations.

General Precautions

All aseptic procedures are followed for blood collection. The word **asepsis** refers to the state of being free from contamination by any infective organism. Because of the increasing risks of fatal transmissible diseases, the following precautions must be taken while collecting a blood sample from a patient:

1. Care must be taken to prevent injuries while handling syringes and needles.
2. Only **disposable or sterilised lancets** or needles should be used. Before blood collection, the fingertip should be sterilised using cotton or a piece of gauze touched with alcohol.
3. The operator must always wear **disposable plastic/ rubber gloves.** This is especially important if the subject is uncooperative or if the operator has any cuts, abrasions, or skin breaks on their hands.
4. The specimen containers (such as bottles and bags) must be checked to ensure that there is **no leakage.**

METHODS OF COLLECTION

For physiology practicals, blood is often collected by pricking the tip of the finger. Therefore, the collection of peripheral blood by the **finger puncture method** (with details of steps and precautions) is described comprehensively in this chapter.

Principle

The two types of blood generally used for clinical laboratory tests are **peripheral (capillary) blood** and **venous blood.** For hematologic investigations that require small quantities of blood, the specimen is obtained from the capillary bed by puncturing the skin. The tip of the finger is the most common site for puncture. For larger quantities of blood, a puncture is made directly into a vein (**phlebotomy**) using a sterile syringe-and-needle collection system.

Collection of Capillary (Peripheral) Blood

Capillary blood is often used for bedside investigations but is likely to yield erroneous results if it is not collected properly. Therefore, it **should only be used when it is not possible to obtain venous blood.** A free flow of blood is essential to the proper collection of peripheral blood, and only gentle squeezing is permissible. Ideally, large drops of blood should slowly but spontaneously flow from the pricked site.

Source

Blood can be obtained from the **fingertips or earlobes** of adults and older children, and from the heel or plantar **surface of the big toe of infants.** The earlobe is not ideal for puncture as the flow of blood is slow and the concentration of cells and hemoglobin is higher in the earlobe.

Note: Blood obtained from the earlobe contains a higher concentration of hemoglobin and more cells than blood from the fingertips or venous blood. Hence, it is **not reliable for hemoglobin estimation and total leucocyte count**. However, blood from the earlobe is preferred for preparing blood films for differential count and to **study leucocyte abnormalities**, since larger cells are frequently trapped in the capillary bed of the earlobe due to the slower circulation in this area.

Requirements

1. Disposable sterile lancet (or 24G needle)
2. Alcohol
3. Dry gauze
4. Slides or pipettes

Various types of disposable lancets are used for skin puncture. Non-disposable lancets are not recommended because of the risk of transmission of infectious pathogens. 24G disposable needles can be used if lancets are not available. The **lancet is preferred** over a needle because the puncture (depth and size of the wound) is effectively performed and well controlled with lancets.

Procedure

▌Finger puncture

1. Assemble the necessary equipment (lancet device, alcohol, dry gauze, slides).
2. Make the subject sit comfortably.
3. Put on disposable rubber gloves.
4. Select the fingertip suitable for puncture.

Note: A fingertip free from calluses, infection, edema, and cyanosis is ideal for puncture.

5. Warm the puncture site by rubbing it.

Note: Warming the skin before puncturing improves circulation and ensures free flow of blood. This must always be done if the fingertip is cold.

6. Clean the skin of the tip of the finger using cotton or a piece of gauze touched with alcohol.

Note: This removes dirt and makes the area relatively sterile.

7. Allow the area to dry. The subject can shake his finger in the air to hasten drying.

Note: The finger should not be punctured **until the tip is completely dry** for the following reasons:
i. The formation of a spherical blood drop is essential for many procedures, especially for pipetting (sucking blood into the RBC, WBC or hemoglobin pipette). Blood does not form a drop on the fingertip if the skin is not dry; instead, it spreads sideways along with spirit.
ii. Sterilization with alcohol is effective only after it dries on the fingertip.
iii. Blood cells are hemolyzed when they come in contact with alcohol. Therefore, drying of the fingertip must be ensured for any investigation that requires the study of cells.

8. Hold the finger firmly and make a quick puncture about 3–5 mm deep with the lancet (Fig. 2.1).

Note: The puncture should be made at the middle of the tip, not too far down on the finger nor too close to the nail.

9. Wipe the first drop of blood using sterile dry gauze.

Note: The first drop is diluted with tissue fluid and discarded as it interferes with laboratory results. The succeeding drops are used for tests.

10. Allow the blood to flow slowly and freely. If it does not come out spontaneously, apply pressure gently so that a spherical drop is formed (Fig. 2.2).

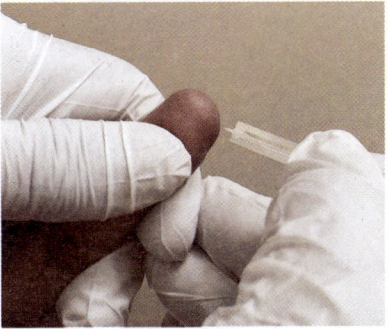 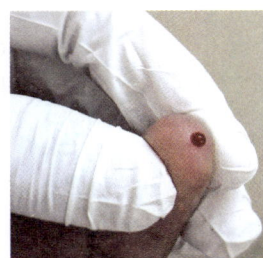

Fig. 2.1 Firmly holding the finger before making a finger prick using a lancet.

Fig. 2.2 Formation of a spherical drop of blood by the finger prick method. Gloves must be used while performing a finger prick on an unknown subject or patient.

Note: Blood should never be expressed by squeezing (milking) the finger as it causes the exudation of tissue fluid, which dilutes the blood.

11. Rapidly collect blood and use it immediately for laboratory studies before coagulation occurs.
12. Once the blood sample is collected, give the subject a sterile, dry piece of gauze or cotton to hold over the puncture site until the bleeding stops.
13. Remove gloves and wash hands.

Precautions

1. Sterile gloves should always be used while collecting blood from subjects or patients.
2. The fingertip should be warmed by rubbing it slightly to improve circulation.
3. Disposable lancets should be used.
4. The tip of the lancet should not touch anything until it punctures the skin of the subject.
5. The fingertip should not be squeezed because this dilutes the blood with tissue fluid.
6. The first drop of blood should be discarded as it is diluted with tissue fluid.
7. The middle three fingers are preferred for puncture because the venous bursa (palmar fascia) of the thumb and the little finger are continuous with that of the limb, whereas the **venous bursa of the middle three fingers are limited to the hand only**. Therefore, if infection occurs following puncture, it will be limited to the hands.

Earlobe puncture

1. Select and warm (by gentle rubbing) the puncture site.
2. Clean the earlobe with a cotton swab touched with spirit and gently hold it with one hand (Fig. 2.3).
3. Make a quick puncture (to a depth of about 2 mm) on the earlobe with the help of a sterile lancet.
4. Collect the blood that drips out spontaneously.
5. Apply pressure to stop bleeding.

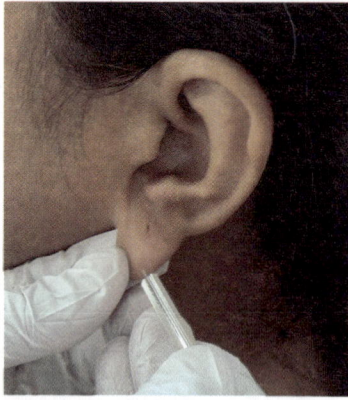

Fig. 2.3 Site and procedure of earlobe puncture.

Heel puncture

1. Select the puncture site (Fig. 2.4) and warm and clean it.

Note: Only perform the procedure once the heel is warm. If necessary, use warm water to raise the temperature of the heel.

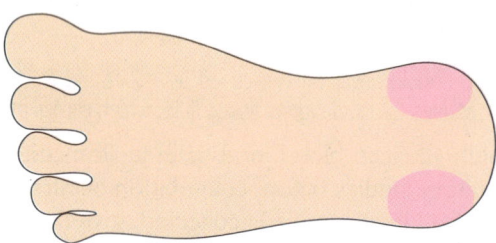

Fig. 2.4 Sites of heel puncture (shaded areas). The middle of the heel is spared.

2. Hold the heel firmly and puncture on the most medial or the most lateral portion of the plantar surface.

Note: The **central plantar area** and the **posterior curvature should not be punctured** in infants as this may cause injury to the underlying tarsal bones. The puncture should not be more than 2–4 mm deep.

3. Collect the blood that drips out.
4. Apply pressure to stop the bleeding.

Collection of Venous Blood

Source

Venous blood is typically collected by performing venipuncture of the vein of the forearm, wrist, or ankle. It is best withdrawn from an **antecubital (forearm) vein** because this vein is larger and fuller than those in the wrist, hand, and ankle. The veins of the wrist, hand, and ankle are used only if the forearm is not suitable for withdrawing blood. The **median cubital vein** is usually chosen for venipuncture because it *does not roll or slip* beneath the skin (Fig. 2.5).

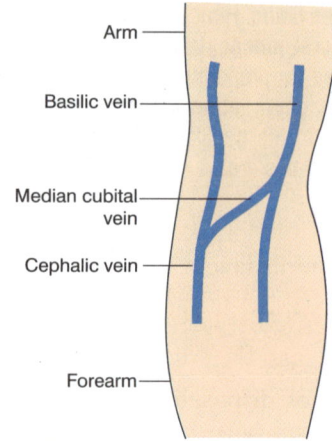

Fig. 2.5 The veins of the forearm: The median cubital vein is preferred for venipuncture.

Requirements

1. Disposable syringe and needle
2. Alcohol
3. Sterile gauze or cotton
4. Collection bottle containing anticoagulant
5. Disposable gloves
6. Tourniquet

Procedure

Venipuncture should be performed with proper care and skill. The veins should be made prominent by applying a tourniquet around the arm just above the elbow, just tight enough to stop blood flow. The subject should be instructed to clench their fist to increase the blood pressure in the area of the puncture.

1. Assemble all the materials required for blood collection—the disposable syringe and needle, alcohol, gauze or cotton, collection bottle, etc.
2. Determine the total amount of blood to be collected; for example, if a total hemogram is required, 2 ml of blood will be sufficient.
3. Keep the required anticoagulant (details described below) in the collection bottle.
4. Wash your hands and put on sterilized/disposable gloves.
5. Reassure the subject. Ask him to sit next to the table and place his arm on the table with the palm facing upwards.

Note: Never draw blood from a patient while they are standing.

6. Select the puncture site carefully after inspecting the arm. Using the index finger of your left hand, feel for the vein into which you will introduce the needle.
7. Apply a tourniquet above the subject's elbow and ask them to make a fist to make the vein prominent.
8. Clean the area with cotton touched with alcohol.

9. Remove the syringe and needle from the protective wrap and assemble them properly. See that the needle is fixed tightly with the syringe. Do not touch the needle.

Note: Ensure that the needle is not blocked and the syringe does not contain air.

10. Grasp the subject's elbow with your left hand and hold his arm fully extended. Anchor the vein with your thumb, drawing the skin tightly over the vein to prevent it from moving.

11. Hold the syringe in the right hand and position the needle to keep the bevel upward. Then, push the needle firmly and steadily into the center of the vein. First, enter the skin and then the vein at a 30–40° angle.

12. Push the needle along the line of the vein to a depth of 1–1.5 cm.

Note: As the needle enters the vein, a sudden loss of resistance is felt.

13. Look for the appearance of blood in the barrel. Pull back the piston slightly and allow the syringe to fill with the required amount of blood (Fig. 2.6).

14. Ask the subject to relax their hand and release the tourniquet.

Note: Always remove the tourniquet before taking the needle out of the vein to prevent the formation of a hematoma.

15. Withdraw the needle from the vein in one rapid movement.

16. Press down on the site with a sterile cotton swab and ask the subject to hold the swab in place for 3–5 minutes.

17. Remove the needle from the syringe and gently expel the blood into the container.

18. Immediately mix the blood gently but thoroughly with the anticoagulant to prevent clotting.

19. Promptly dispose of the syringe and needle set (if disposable) or rinse them with water.

20. Before the subject leaves the laboratory, ensure that the bleeding has stopped. Otherwise, ask him to continue to apply pressure until the bleeding stops.

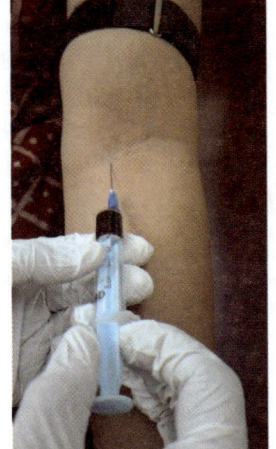

Fig. 2.6 Site and method of blood collection by venipuncture. Note that the application of the tourniquet makes the vein prominent.

Precautions

1. The collection bottle containing anticoagulant should be kept ready before collecting blood.
2. The subject should be seated comfortably and should be reassured.
3. Disposable gloves should always be used to prevent contamination.
4. A disposable syringe and needle should be used to draw the blood.
5. The puncture site should be cleaned with alcohol.
6. The vein should be made prominent before making a puncture.
7. The needle should be held at an angle of 30–40° and introduced into the vein steadily and firmly.
8. The tourniquet, if applied, should be removed before taking the needle out of the vein to prevent hematoma formation.
9. The patient should be instructed to press down on the puncture site with cotton wool for 3–5 minutes to prevent bleeding.
10. To prevent clotting, the blood from the syringe should be immediately transferred to the bottle containing the anticoagulant.

DISCUSSION

Causes of Misleading Results Related to Specimen Collection

It is essential to establish a standard procedure for the collection and handling of blood specimens, as the constituents of blood may get altered due to improper collection (Table 2.1).

Table 2.1 Factors that may alter the results due to improper collection procedure

A. Pre-collection	1. Physical activity like fast walking within 20 minutes of collection
	2. Smoking within 1 hour of collection
	3. Drugs within 8 hours / intake of a dietary supplement
	4. Food or water intake within 2 hours
	5. Urination within 30 minutes
	6. Stress
B. While collecting blood	1. Excessive negative pressure when drawing blood into the syringe
	2. Incorrect type of sample collection tube
	3. Hemoconcentration due to prolonged application of tourniquet
	4. Time of collection (morning/day/evening/night): diurnal variation
	5. Posture of subject (standing/sitting/lying)
	6. Capillary blood versus venous blood
C. Improper handling of specimen	1. Improper quantity (less or excess) of anticoagulants
	2. Inadequate mixing of blood with the anticoagulant
	3. Delay in dispatch to laboratory
	4. Inadequate specimen storage conditions
	5. Error in identification of subject
	6. Error in identification of specimen

Differences Between Capillary and Venous Blood

The composition of capillary and venous blood is not identical (Table 2.2). Though the blood obtained by skin puncture (capillary blood) is mainly capillary blood, it also contains some quantity of a mixture of blood from arterioles and venules and some interstitial and intracellular fluid. On the other hand, blood obtained by venipuncture is entirely venous blood. Arterial blood is usually not required for tests performed in the hematology laboratory for I MBBS Physiology students.

Anticoagulants

Anticoagulants prevent blood from clotting and are added to blood samples, particularly those collected via venipuncture, before sending them to laboratories for analysis. Several anticoagulants are available; some of those most commonly used in hematology are EDTA, trisodium citrate, double oxalate, sodium fluoride, and heparin. **EDTA is commonly used in hematology, while citrated blood is preferred for coagulation studies and blood banking.** The use of heparin and fluoride (oxalated) is more specific—heparin is used for blood gas and pH analysis, whereas sodium fluoride is used for plasma glucose testing.

Table 2.2   Differences between capillary and venous blood

		Capillary blood	Venous blood
1.	Collection method	Skin puncture of fingertip, earlobe, or heel	Venipuncture of superficial veins
2.	Type of specimen	Capillary blood mixed with a small quantity of blood from arterioles and venules	Venous blood
3.	Contamination with tissue fluid	May contain tissue fluid, especially if the finger is squeezed to collect blood	Does not contain tissue fluid
4.	Difference in counts	PCV, RBC and Hb concentrations of capillary blood are slightly less than that of venous blood. TLC and neutrophil counts are higher by 8%, and monocyte count by 12%, especially in children	Platelet count is higher in venous blood than in capillary blood, possibly due to the adhesion of platelets to the site of skin puncture
5.	Preferred	When blood is required for an individual count or when only a few tests are to be performed	When several hematologic tests have to be performed, requiring a larger volume of blood

EDTA (ethylenediamine tetra-acetic acid)

This is also known as **sequestrene or versene**. The sodium and potassium salts of EDTA are powerful anticoagulants.

Preparation

To prepare a 10% solution of dipotassium EDTA, dissolve 10 g of the salt in approximately 80 ml of water in a 100 ml volumetric flask, and then dilute to a final volume of 100 ml. Dipotassium EDTA is preferred over disodium EDTA due to its greater solubility.

Mechanism of action

Calcium is a crucial factor in the coagulation process. EDTA acts as an anticoagulant by chelating calcium ions in the blood, preventing clot formation.

Effective concentration

To achieve the chelating effect, a **concentration of 1.2 mg** of the anhydrous salt per ml of blood is required. **Excess of EDTA**, irrespective of its salts, affects both red cells and leucocytes, causing shrinkage and degenerative changes. If the concentration of the anticoagulant is high, it causes *distortion of cells*. EDTA in excess of 2 mg/ml of blood may result in a significant *decrease in packed cell volume* (PCV) by centrifugation and *increase in mean cell hemoglobin concentration* (MCHC). Platelets are also affected—they swell up and disintegrate, resulting in an *artificially high platelet count*, as the fragments are large enough to be counted as normal platelets. Therefore, care must be taken to ensure that the correct amount of EDTA is added and that blood is thoroughly mixed with the anticoagulant by repeated inversions of the container.

Uses

EDTA is suitable for all routine hematological investigations except coagulation studies.

Sodium Citrate

Trisodium citrate (32 g/l, $Na_3C_6H_5O_7 \cdot 2H_2O$) is the anticoagulant of choice for coagulation studies.

Preparation

A **0.106 M solution** of trisodium citrate is prepared in distilled water and then sterilized.

Mechanism of action

Sodium citrate prevents coagulation by inactivating calcium ions (chelating effect).

Effective concentration

Nine volumes of blood are added to one volume of sodium citrate (9:1) solution for anticoagulation studies. **If it is used in the estimation of ESR** (erythrocyte sedimentation rate), four volumes of venous blood are added to one volume of the sodium citrate (4:1) solution.

Uses

It is used for **coagulation studies** including prothrombin times and partial thromboplastin tests, in blood banks, and in the **estimation of ESR**, especially by the *Westergren method*.

Double oxalate

This is an anticoagulant containing ammonium oxalate and potassium oxalate (hence called double oxalate). Potassium oxalate alone causes shrinkage of red cells. Ammonium oxalate increases their volume and preserves their morphology, balancing the effect of potassium oxalate. For this reason, double oxalate is also called **balanced oxalate**.

Preparation

A solution containing 1.2% ammonium oxalate and 0.8% potassium oxalate is prepared. 0.25–0.5 ml of this solution is dispensed into penicillin bottles, evaporated in an oven at 60°C or incubator (37°C), and then stored for blood collection.

Mechanism of action

The oxalates in the double oxalate form an **insoluble complex with the calcium in the blood**, making it unavailable for clotting and thereby inhibiting coagulation.

Uses

Double oxalate is used for the **estimation of ESR and PCV** and investigations that require the volume of the cells to remain unaltered.

Sodium fluoride

Sodium fluoride is primarily used for **plasma glucose estimation**. Fluoride is an inhibitor of glycolytic enzymes and thus prevents the loss of glucose. However, it is not a strong anticoagulant and hence, is mixed with oxalate.

Oxalates

Oxalates of sodium, potassium, ammonium or lithium as dry additives act as anticoagulants. They form insoluble complexes with calcium and make it unavailable for clotting.

Heparin

Heparin is considered the **best natural anticoagulant** as it is already present in blood and does not introduce foreign substances into the sample.

Preparation

Heparin is available in **sodium, lithium, potassium, and ammonium salt** forms. A **stock solution** of suitable concentration is prepared, and the required amount is dispensed into penicillin bottles and dried at room temperature.

Mechanism of action

Heparin **prevents coagulation** for approximately 24 hours by *inhibiting the action of thrombin*, thus preventing the formation of fibrin from fibrinogen.

Concentration

Heparin is used at a concentration of 10–20 IU/ml of blood. In this concentration, it does not alter the size of red cells.

Uses

Heparin is used for *blood gas determination and pH assays*. It is the best anticoagulant for the **osmotic fragility test**. It is inferior to EDTA for general use and should not be used for counting leucocytes as it promotes their clumping. It is also not used for differential counts as it produces a blue background colour.

VIVA

1. *Name the methods of blood collection.* (Ans. Refer to page 4, text under the heading 'Methods of Collection'.)
2. *Name the sites of skin puncture for collecting capillary blood.* (Ans. Refer to page 4, under the heading 'Source'.)
3. *What are the important precautions for fingertip puncture?* (Ans. Refer to page 5, under the heading 'Precautions'.)
4. *Why are the middle three fingers preferred for fingertip puncture?* (Ans. Refer to page 6, under the heading 'Precautions'.)
5. *What are the advantages and disadvantages of earlobe puncture?* (Ans. Refer to page 5, read 'Note' under the heading 'Source'.)
6. *What are the indications for heel puncture?*
   (Ans. Heel puncture is primarily indicated for obtaining small blood samples from newborns and infants, usually for newborn screening tests or certain special investigations.)
7. *Which are the veins that are preferred for venipuncture?* (Ans. On page 6, refer to the text under the heading 'Source' below 'Collection of Venous Blood' and Fig. 2.5 on page 7.)
8. *What precautions should be followed while performing venipuncture?* (Ans. Refer to page 7, under the heading 'Precautions'.)
9. *List the factors that may alter the results of blood counts due to improper blood collection.* (Ans. Refer to Table 2.1 on page 8.)
10. *List the differences between capillary blood and venous blood.* (Ans. Refer to Table 2.2 on page 8.)
11. *Name the important anticoagulants. Explain the mechanisms of their action and their specific uses.* (Ans. Refer to pages 8–9.)

3 Estimation of Hemoglobin Concentration

Learning Objectives

After completing this practical, you will be able to (MUST KNOW):

1. Describe the clinical importance of the estimation of hemoglobin (Hb).
2. Estimate hemoglobin by Sahli's acid hematin method.
3. List the precautions and sources of error in the estimation of Hb.
4. List the advantages and disadvantages of Sahli's method.
5. Name the other methods used for the estimation of Hb.
6. List the normal values of Hb in males and females and in different age groups.
7. List the functions of Hb.
8. List the common conditions resulting in decreased and increased Hb concentration in the blood.
9. Define anemia.
10. List the common causes of anemia in developing countries.

You may also be able to (DESIRABLE TO KNOW):

1. Describe the synthesis and structure of Hb.
2. Classify Hb.
3. Describe different complexes and derivatives of Hb.
4. Explain the principle of other methods of Hb estimation.
5. Compare the merits and demerits of different methods.
6. Explain the variation of Hb concentration in different conditions.
7. Briefly describe the different types of anemia.

PY2.11: Estimate Hb, RBC, TLC, RBC indices, DLC, blood groups, and BT/CT.

INTRODUCTION

Hemoglobin (Hb) is a conjugated protein present in red blood cells. It carries O_2 from the lungs to the tissues and CO_2 from the tissues to the lungs. When the Hb molecule is fully saturated with oxygen, i.e., when four oxygen molecules combine with one hemoglobin molecule, it is called **oxyhemoglobin**. **One gram of hemoglobin carries 1.34 ml of oxygen**. Hemoglobin returning with carbon dioxide from the tissues is called **reduced hemoglobin**.

SYNTHESIS AND STRUCTURE OF HEMOGLOBIN

Hemoglobin is made up of two components: **heme and globin**. It is synthesized in the precursors of red cells during their development in the bone marrow. It appears in the early normoblast stage and attains maximum concentration in the late normoblast stage (for details, refer to Chapter 7).

Heme

Heme is a complex molecule, made up of a series of tetrapyrrole rings, terminating in protoporphyrin, with a central iron atom. After their normal lifespan (120 days), the red cells are destroyed by the reticuloendothelial cells, especially in the spleen, and the components of hemoglobin undergo metabolic degradation. The iron part of heme is recycled and used up again in hemoglobin synthesis. The only component of Hb that *cannot be recycled* is **protoporphyrin**, which forms **bilirubin**. Bilirubin is finally converted to various bile salts and pigments.

Globin

Globin is a protein substance that consists of four chains of amino acids (polypeptides). Each polypeptide chain is attached to a heme moiety to form a single hemoglobin molecule. After the degradation of hemoglobin, the globin component breaks down into its **amino acid constituents**, which are then recycled for hemoglobin synthesis.

TYPES OF HEMOGLOBIN

Hemoglobins can be broadly divided into normal and abnormal types.

1. **Normal Hb:** Adult Hb, fetal Hb, and embryonic Hb.
2. **Abnormal Hb:** HbS, HbC, HbD, HbE, and unstable hemoglobins

Normal Hemoglobins

Adult hemoglobins

▮ Hemoglobin A (HbA)

About 97 per cent of the hemoglobin of adult red cells is HbA. It consists of **two α and two β chains** with the structural formula $\alpha_2\beta_2$. HbA is detected in small amounts in the fetus as early as the eighth week of intrauterine life. During the first few months of postnatal life, HbA almost completely replaces HbF. The **adult pattern is fully established in six months**.

Hemoglobin A$_2$ (HbA$_2$)

This is the minor hemoglobin in the adult red cell. It has the structural formula $\alpha_2\delta_2$. HbA$_2$ is present in very small amounts at birth and reaches the **adult level of 3 per cent during the first year of life**. Its concentration increases in some types of anemia.

Fetal hemoglobins
Fetal hemoglobin (HbF)

HbF is the major hemoglobin in intrauterine life. It has the structural formula $\alpha_2\gamma_2$. HbF accounts for **70–90 per cent of hemoglobins at term**. It then falls rapidly to 25 per cent in one month, and **5 per cent in six months**. In some cases, the adult level of 1 per cent is not reached until puberty. HbF concentration in adults increases in some types of anemia, hemoglobinopathies, and sometimes, in leukemia.

Hemoglobin Bart's (Hb Bart's)

This is the minor hemoglobin present in fetal life. It consists of four gamma (γ) chains—γ_4. Hb Bart's concentration **increases during fetal life in thalassemia**.

Embryonic hemoglobins

These hemoglobins are confined to the very early stages (the embryonic stage) of development. There are **three embryonic hemoglobins**:

1. **Hb Gower 1** (consisting of two zeta and two epsilon chains—$\zeta_2\epsilon_2$)
2. **Hb Gower 2** (consisting of two alpha and two epsilon chains—$\alpha_2\epsilon_2$)
3. **Hb Portland** (consisting of two zeta and two gamma chains—$\zeta_2\gamma_2$)

Normal values

The following are the normal values of hemoglobin for adults:

1. **Males:** 14–18 (16 ± 2) g/dl of blood
2. **Females:** 12–16 (14 ± 2) g/dl of blood

In **newborns**, hemoglobin concentration is normally 14–20 g/dl. It decreases to 9–14 g/dl by about **two months** of age. By **ten years of age**, the normal hemoglobin concentration will be 12–14 g/dl. There may be a decrease in hemoglobin level after 60 years of age.

Abnormal Hemoglobins

There are four clinically significant abnormal hemoglobins: **HbS, HbC, HbD, and HbE**, each associated with different hereditary hemoglobinopathies. The most prevalent among them is **HbS**, which is found in **sickle cell anemia**. HbS has the structural formula $\alpha_2\beta_2$, but a single amino acid substitution occurs in the beta chain, where *valine replaces glutamic acid at the sixth position*.

Unstable hemoglobins are hemoglobin variants that undergo denaturation and precipitate in the red cells as **Heinz bodies**. Unstable hemoglobins are present in a type of **congenital non-spherocytic hemolytic anemia**.

HEMOGLOBIN COMPLEXES

Hb can combine with other substances besides oxygen, some normally and some abnormally. Some of the commonly encountered hemoglobin complexes are carbaminohemoglobin, carboxyhemoglobin, methemoglobin, sulfhemoglobin, and cyanmethemoglobin.

Carbaminohemoglobin

It is formed when **carbon dioxide (CO$_2$) combines with hemoglobin**. CO$_2$ combines with the amino groups in the polypeptide chains of globin, not with heme. The formation of this complex facilitates the transport of CO$_2$ from the tissues to the lungs.

Carboxyhemoglobin

When **carbon monoxide (CO) binds with hemoglobin**, it forms carboxyhemoglobin (HbCO). Hemoglobin has a significantly higher affinity for CO than for oxygen, allowing it to readily combine with CO even at low concentrations. Fortunately, this **process is reversible**—once CO is removed from the bloodstream, hemoglobin can resume binding with oxygen.

In healthy individuals, carboxyhemoglobin is present at very low levels. However, in smokers, its concentration ranges from 1 to 10 g/dL, impairing oxygen transport from the lungs to the tissues.

Methemoglobin

Methemoglobin is an abnormal Hb in which **iron is oxidised from its ferrous state to ferric state**. Consequently, it is incapable of carrying oxygen. Normally, methemoglobin is present in low concentrations but its formation increases in the presence of certain chemicals or drugs. The formation of methemoglobin is **also reversible**.

Sulfhemoglobin

This is an abnormal Hb complex formed by the **action of some drugs and chemicals such as sulphonamides**. The process is irreversible; once formed, sulfhemoglobin remains in the carrier RBC. It is incapable of transporting oxygen.

Cyanmethemoglobin (Hemiglobincyanide)

This is formed by the action of a chemical called **cyanide** (from potassium cyanide, KCN, etc.). The combination is reversible.

Hemiglobin is the hemoglobin in which the iron has been oxidised to the ferric state. *Hemiglobincyanide* is the methemoglobin bonded to cyanide ions.

> **Note:** To accurately measure the total Hb in the blood, it is essential to prepare a stable derivative that contains all the Hb forms (complexes) that are present in the blood. All forms of circulating hemoglobin are readily converted to hemoglobincyanide (cyanmethemoglobin), except for sulfhemoglobin, which is normally not present in blood. Therefore, the **cyanmethemoglobin method is the most accurate method** for the determination of hemoglobin.

Glycated Hemoglobin

When glucose attaches to Hb by a non-enzymatic process, it forms glycated Hb. In the fraction of HbA known as **HbA1c**, glucose is attached to terminal valine in the β chain. In normal individuals, glycosylated or glycated Hb (HbA1c) is present in low **concentrations—less than 5.7% of total Hb**. If the concentration of HbA1c is more than 6.5%, the person is said to be diabetic.

As per the **ADA (American Diabetic Association) criteria**:

1. HbA1c: 4–5.6%—**Normal**
2. HbA1c: 5.7–6.5%—**Prediabetes**
3. HbA1c: > 6.5%—**Diabetes**

> **Note:** Glycated Hb (HbA1c), indicates persistent hyperglycemia. When blood glucose is chronically **elevated for more than three months**, a higher amount of glycated Hb is formed. For this reason, the estimation of HbA1c is emphasized over fasting blood glucose for **assessing glycemic control in diabetic patients** on therapy.

HEMOGLOBIN DERIVATIVES

When red blood cells are destroyed in the tissue macrophage system, hemoglobin is degraded into heme and globin. Globin returns to the body's metabolic pool where its amino acids are subsequently reutilized. The porphyrin ring of heme is cleaved by the microsomal enzyme, heme oxidase, yielding **biliverdin**. This biliverdin is further reduced to form **bilirubin** by biliverdin reductase.

FUNCTIONS OF HEMOGLOBIN

Hemoglobin serves two important functions: the transport of gases and pH homeostasis. However, Hb also contributes to tissue blood flow.

1. **Transport of gasses**: Hb transports oxygen from the lungs to the tissues by forming oxyhemoglobin, and carbon dioxide from the tissues to the lungs by forming carbaminohemoglobin. When fully saturated, **1 g of Hb carries 1.34 ml of oxygen**.
2. **pH homeostasis**: Hemoglobin acts as an important buffer in maintaining blood pH. In fact, Hb is an important non-bicarbonate buffer system of the body and contributes to about 60% of the buffering capacity of blood.
3. **Regulation of blood flow:** To some extent, Hb contributes to the regulation of tissue blood flow. It has sufficient affinity for another gas in the blood, **nitric oxide (NO), which is a strong vasodilator**. In the tissue, as Hb picks up NO, vasoconstriction occurs due to the relative decrease in NO concentration, which in turn, decreases tissue blood flow. In the lungs, Hb picks up **super nitric oxide (SNO)** and by altering SNO level, controls pulmonary blood flow. However, the role of Hb in the regulation of systemic blood volume, peripheral resistance, and blood pressure is negligible.
4. **Stabilisation of tissue PO_2:** Hemoglobin helps maintain stable tissue PO_2 by ensuring an adequate supply of oxygen within the PO_2 range of 20–40 mmHg.

METHODS OF ESTIMATING HEMOGLOBIN

The different methods of estimating hemoglobin can be classified under the following categories:

1. Visual methods
    i. Sahli method
    ii. Dare method
    iii. Haden method
    iv. Wintrobe method
    v. Haldane method
    vi. Tallquist method
2. Gasometric method
3. Spectrophotometric method
    i. Oxyhemoglobin method
    ii. Cyanmethemoglobin method
4. Automated hemoglobinometry
5. Non-automated hemoglobinometry
6. Other methods
    i. Alkaline-hematin method
    ii. Specific gravity method
    iii. Comparator method

Visual Methods

Visual methods are more commonly used than photometric methods. However, the margin of error in these methods is higher than in other techniques. Due to this limitation, visual methods are generally not recommended for hemoglobin estimation in research. However, their ease of use and low cost make them widely practiced in clinical hematology laboratories and by students performing physiology practicals in medical colleges.

Sahli's Acid Hematin Method

Sahli's method is a visual technique for hemoglobin estimation, wherein hemoglobin in a blood sample is converted into acid hematin, producing a brown colour. Since **brown is easier for the human eye to match** than the red colour of hemoglobin, Sahli's method is one of the **most widely accepted** visual methods.

Principle

Hemoglobin is converted to acid hematin by the action of HCl. The acid hematin solution is further diluted until its colour exactly matches that of the permanent standard of the comparator block. The hemoglobin concentration is read directly from the calibration tube.

Requirements
◼ **Sahli's hemoglobinometer (Fig. 3.1)**
This contains a comparator, hemoglobin tube, hemoglobin pipette, and stirrer.

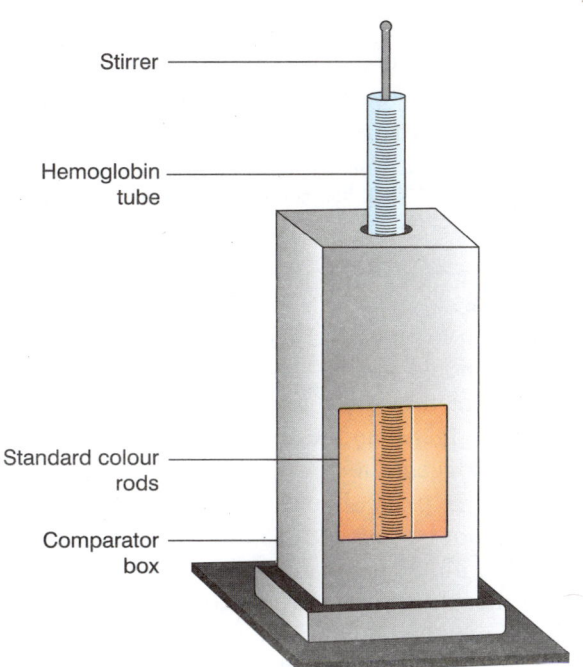

Fig. 3.1   Sahli's hemoglobinometer.

1. **Comparator:** It is a centrally located slot for the hemoglobin tube. Standard, non-fading, brown-tinted glass pieces are provided on either side for colour matching. A white, opaque glass at the back ensures uniform illumination.
2. **Hemoglobin tube:** Graduated on one side in grams per decilitre (g/dL) (ranging from 2 to 24) and on

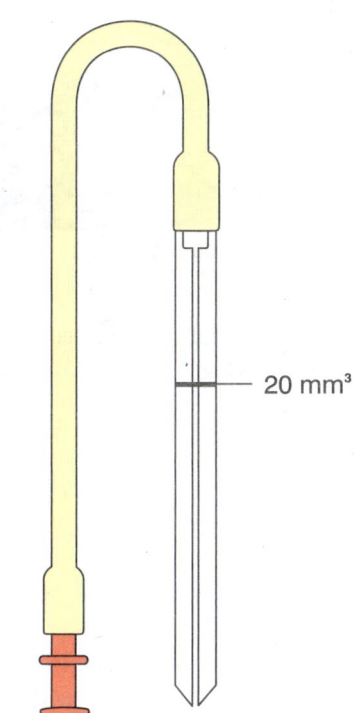

Fig. 3.2   The hemoglobin pipette.

the other side as a percentage (10% to 140%). Also known as the Sahli-Adams tube.
3. **Hemoglobin pipette** (Fig. 3.2)**:** The pipette bears only one mark indicating 20 mm³ (0.02 ml). It does not have a bulb.
4. **Stirrer:** It is a thin glass rod used for stirring the solution.

◼ **Other materials**
1. N/10 HCl
2. Distilled water
3. Dropper
4. Sterile materials to perform a finger prick

Procedure
1. Clean the hemoglobinometer tube and pipette and ensure that they are dry.
2. Fill the hemoglobinometer tube with N/10 HCl up to its lowest mark (10 per cent or 2 g%) with the help of a dropper.
3. Prick the finger observing all aseptic precautions and discard the first drop of blood.

Note: The prick should be deep enough to enable spontaneous flow of blood. Do not squeeze the finger to bring out the drop of blood.

4. Allow a large drop of blood to form on the fingertip, then dip the tip of the hemoglobinometer pipette into the drop and suck blood up to the 20 mm³ mark of the pipette (Fig. 3.3).

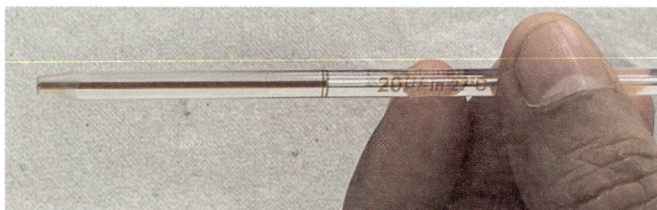

Fig. 3.3   Pipetting of blood exactly up to the 20 mm³ mark of the Hb pipette.

Note: When drawing blood into the pipette, take care to **prevent the entry of air bubbles** by keeping the tip immersed in the blood drop throughout the process. If an air bubble enters, discard the sample and obtain a new blood drop for re-pipetting. If blood is drawn above the 20 mm³ mark, adjust the level by gently tapping the pipette against a finger—avoid using absorbent materials like cotton wool, as they may alter the sample.

5. Wipe the tip of the pipette. Immediately transfer the 0.02 ml of blood from the pipette into the hemoglobinometer tube containing N/10 HCl by immersing the tip of the pipette in the acid solution and blowing out blood from the pipette. Rinse the pipette two to three times by drawing up and blowing out the acid solution. Withdraw the pipette from the tube.

Note: Make sure that no solution remains in the pipette.

6. Leave the solution in the tube in the hemoglobinometer for **about ten minutes** (for maximum conversion of hemoglobin to acid hematin, which occurs in the first ten minutes).

7. After 10 minutes, gradually dilute the solution with distilled water, mixing with the stirrer after each drop.

8. Continue dilution until the colour of the solution matches the standard in the comparator.

Note: After the addition of every drop of distilled water, the solution should be mixed, and the colour of the solution should be compared with the standard. While matching, the stirrer should be held above the level of the solution. However, **at no stage should the stirrer be taken out of the tube** (Fig. 3.4).

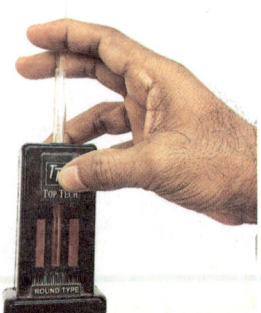

Fig. 3.4   Correct manner of holding the stirrer. Note that it is kept above the Hb solution in the pipette, but never taken entirely out of the pipette.

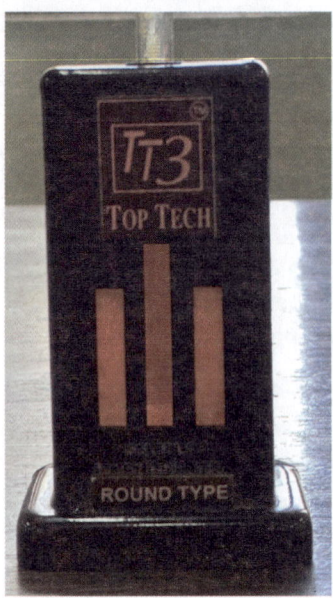

Fig. 3.5   Matching of the colour of Hb solution with that of the standard. The colour of the three bars should match exactly.

9. If the colour of the test solution is darker, continue dilution till it matches that of the standard (Fig. 3.5).

10. Note the reading when the colour of the solution exactly matches the colour of the standard, and express the hemoglobin concentration as g%.

Note: The reading of the lower meniscus of the solution should be noted as the result. One more drop of distilled water should be added, and the colour should be observed to check the result. The colour will be lighter than the standard if the previous reading was accurate.

Precautions

1. A large volume of N/10 HCl (above the 20 per cent mark) should not be taken in the tube. In cases of severe anemia, using too much HCl will produce a colour lighter than the standard, and there will be no way to concentrate it.

2. The finger prick should be done boldly. The finger should not be squeezed as this can cause tissue fluid to mix with the blood, leading to a falsely low result.

3. The first drop of blood should be discarded as it is mixed with tissue fluid.

4. Blood should be sucked exactly up to the 20 mm³ mark.

5. The tip of the pipette should be wiped before transferring blood from the pipette to the hemoglobinometer tube. Otherwise, the extra blood adhering to the tip of the pipette will give a false high reading.

6. Blood should be immediately transferred from the pipette into the tube containing HCl to prevent clotting in the pipette.

7. While transferring, the pipette should be rinsed several times to ensure that all the blood is delivered into the tube.

8. After transferring, the solution in the tube should be allowed to stand for a minimum of ten minutes for complete conversion of hemoglobin into acid hematin.

9. The colour of the acid hematin solution should be checked frequently (preferably after addition and mixing of every drop of distilled water) to prevent overdilution.

10. When the colour of the solution in the tube is compared with that of the standard, the **stirrer should be kept above the solution but should not be taken out of the tube**. If the stirrer is taken out of the tube, the solution sticking to the stirrer will be lost and will give a false low result. If the stirrer remains in the solution, the colour of the solution becomes lighter.

11. Comparison should always be done by holding the hemoglobinometer at eye level, at arm's length, and against good light (Fig. 3.6). The tube should be placed in the comparator in such a way that the graduation marks on it do not appear directly in front, as this could interfere with accurate colour matching.

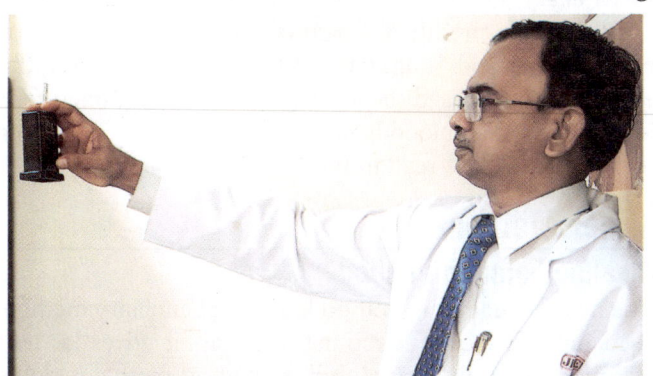

Fig. 3.6   Correct technique for observing and matching the colour of the Hb pipette with the standard. Note that the hemoglobinometer is held at eye level, at arm's length, and against a bright background.

Sources of error
■ Technical errors
1. Blood should be taken exactly up to the 20 mm³ mark and the tip of the pipette should be wiped off before introducing it into the HCl taken in the hemoglobinometer tube. Errors in this step may alter the concentration of blood in the tube.

2. It takes about ten minutes for Hb to be converted into acid hematin, with its characteristic brown colour. Reading the results too early results in errors in the reported concentration of Hb.

3. Errors also occur when the solution is not carefully diluted till the colour exactly matches that of the standard.

■ Errors inherent in the method
1. As it is a visual method, the matching of the colour may vary from observer to observer.

2. This test may not detect all types of hemoglobin in the blood.

3. The colour of the comparator standard may fade.

Observation and reporting
1. When the color of the solution exactly matches the color of the standard, note the reading and report Hb as gm%.

2. The hemoglobinometer tube provides readings in both percentage (%) and grams per decilitre (g/dL). Hemoglobin is usually **reported as grams per 100 ml of blood** (g/dL or g%). Reporting it as a percentage is discouraged, as different methods have varying reference standards. For example, 80 per cent of the normal in one method may be 98 per cent of the normal in another.

   The values for 100 per cent hemoglobin in five different visual testing methods are presented in Table 3.1.

Table 3.1   Hemoglobin percentages in different visual testing methods

Method	100% hemoglobin value (g/dL)
Sahli	16.3
Dare	16.0
Haden	15.6
Wintrobe	14.5
Haldane	13.8

If hemoglobin is reported as a percentage of the normal, the specific method used to estimate it should be stated.

Advantages
1. Sahli's method is easy to perform and convenient.
2. It is economical.
3. It is not very time-consuming (takes a maximum of fifteen minutes).

Disadvantages
1. Since this is a visual method, there is a high margin of error (about 5–10 per cent). This margin can be reduced by taking an average of three readings—first, when the colour is slightly darker than the standard; second, when the colour exactly matches the standard; and the third, when the colour is slightly lighter than the standard.

2. The colour of the standard may not always be reliable, especially if the apparatus used is old.

3. Sahli's acid hematin method does not estimate all the hemoglobins. It estimates only oxyhemoglobin and reduced hemoglobins, but not carboxyhemoglobin, methemoglobin, and sulfhemoglobin.

4. The acid hematin is not a true solution. Some degree of precipitation may be present at times, which may interfere with colour matching.

Other Visual Methods

Haldane method

In the Haldane method, red blood cells are hemolysed by mixing blood with a hypotonic solution such as distilled water. Carbon monoxide is then added to the solution, and its colour is compared to a standard reference.

Comparator method

This is a visual method similar to the acid hematin method, except that the diluent used is an alkali solution (ammonia solution 0.04 per cent).

After mixing the blood sample with dilute ammonia solution, the intensity of the *colour of the hemolysed solution of red blood cells is compared against a standard colour disc* in the comparator. However, this method shares the same limitations as Sahli's acid hematin method.

Tallquist method

This method involves the direct visual matching of the red colour of a drop of whole fresh blood on a filter paper with colour standards on a paper. Although it is one of the fastest methods, it is highly inaccurate and prone to significant errors.

Gasometric Method

The gasometric method, which utilises the Van Slyke apparatus, is considered the **most accurate method** for hemoglobin estimation. However, it is not routinely used in clinical laboratories due to its time-consuming nature and complexity. Instead, it serves as a reference method for standardising hemoglobin estimation techniques and is preferred for research purposes.

Spectrophotometric Methods

These methods are **rapid and yield accurate results**.

Oxyhemoglobin method

Ammonium hydroxide (0.04 ml/dl) is used to hemolyse the red cells and convert hemoglobin to oxyhemoglobin for measurement in the spectrophotometer. This conversion is complete and immediate, and the resulting colour is stable.

Cyanmethemoglobin method

This method employs **modified Drabkin's reagent**, which contains potassium ferricyanide, potassium cyanide, and sodium bicarbonate. Drabkin's reagent requires at least ten minutes for complete conversion of hemoglobin into cyanmethemoglobin. However, protein precipitation or incomplete hemolysis can cause turbidity. A modified version of Drabkin's reagent substitutes potassium phosphate for sodium bicarbonate, reducing the conversion time to three minutes, minimising turbidity, and enhancing red blood cell lysis.

Automated Hemoglobinometry

Automated hematology analysers are commonly used for hemoglobin estimation in modern laboratories. These devices utilise electronic techniques for precise measurement. **Automated pipettors and dilutors** are often incorporated into these instruments to ensure accuracy. The principles applied in automated hemoglobinometry are similar to those used in manual methods.

Non-automated Hemoglobinometry

Disposable, self-filling, self-measuring dilution micropipettes, such as the **Unopette,** are commercially available for the determination of hemoglobin. These systems are easy to use and are available with a series of different diluting fluids for different purposes.

The Unopette system for hemoglobin determination consists of a self-filling, self-measuring pipette attached to a plastic holder. The pipette is automatically filled with blood by capillary action. A plastic container called a reservoir is filled with modified Drabkin's reagent. The pipette containing blood is inserted into the reagent reservoir, emptied and rinsed according to the manufacturer's instructions. The blood is mixed well with the reagent and is then ready to be read in the spectrophotometer.

Other Methods

Alkaline hematin method

The alkaline hematin method is a useful ancillary method, used under special circumstances as it gives a **true estimate of total hemoglobin**, including methemoglobin and sulfhemoglobin. A true solution is obtained, and plasma proteins and lipids have little effect on the colour. The principle is to **convert hemoglobin into alkaline hematin**, which is present in the true solution. There are two variations of this method: the standard method and the acid-alkaline method.

Specific gravity method

This method is based on the principle that when a drop of whole blood is dropped into a solution of **copper sulphate of a given specific gravity**, the drop will maintain its density for approximately 15 seconds. The density of a blood drop is directly proportional to the amount of hemoglobin it contains. If the drop is denser than the copper sulphate solution, it will sink to the bottom instead of floating on the surface.

The specific gravity method is **not a quantitative test**. However, it is quick and easy and a reasonably acceptable technique ***to screen blood donors*** for possible anemia. It is also used to detect hematocrit.

DISCUSSION

Physiological Significance

Hemoglobin, a crucial component of red blood cells, constitutes more than 90% of their dry weight. Its red pigment gives erythrocytes their characteristic colour. The primary function of hemoglobin is oxygen transport from the lungs to tissues. A deficiency in hemoglobin leads to **hypoxia**, impairing tissue oxygenation.

When hemoglobin is released into the plasma, *as seen in hemolysis*, it is filtered through the renal tubules and appears in the urine (**hemoglobinuria**). Hemoglobin casts can obstruct renal tubules, causing *acute tubular necrosis* (acute renal failure). Hemoglobin in the blood (**hemoglobinemia**) exerts an osmotic effect and *increases blood viscosity*, affecting cardiac output and altering the dynamics of blood flow.

Clinical Significance

Hemoglobin estimation is one of the most frequently ordered laboratory tests in clinical practice. It is performed routinely in outpatient clinics as well as hospital settings, often as a bedside test. **Preoperative hemoglobin evaluation** is mandatory before any surgical intervention. Hemoglobin estimation is primarily used **to detect anemia**, as it is more convenient and less time-consuming than total RBC counts. Anemia is diagnosed when hemoglobin levels fall below the normal range for a person's age and sex. It is essential to interpret hemoglobin values within the appropriate reference range for each individual. **Glycated Hb** (HbA1c) is estimated to assess the glycation status of a diabetic patient.

Conditions That Alter Hemoglobin Concentration

Conditions that decrease Hb concentration

▮ Physiological

1. Hemoglobin is **reduced in pregnancy** due to hemodilution.
2. **Children** have lower values than adults.
3. **Women have lower values** than men because the total RBC count is lower in women. This is because of the inhibition of erythropoiesis by estrogen in females and the cyclical loss of blood in the reproductive age group. In males, testosterone stimulates erythropoiesis.

▮ Pathological

1. Hemoglobin levels are decreased in **different types of anemia**.
2. **A relative decrease in Hb concentration occurs in different pathological conditions** that produce hemodilution. For example, hemoglobin concentration is lowered due to excess ADH secretion as seen in pituitary tumours.

Conditions that increase Hb concentration

▮ Physiological

1. Hb concentration increases **at high altitudes** (due to hypoxia).
2. **Newborns and infants** have higher Hb concentrations than adults.
3. **Excessive sweating** increases Hb concentration (due to hemoconcentration).

▮ Pathological

1. Hb is higher in **conditions that produce hemoconcentration** (due to loss of body fluid); for example, severe diarrhea, vomiting.
2. Hemoglobin concentration also increases in **conditions that produce hypoxia**, for example, congenital heart disease and emphysema.
3. Hb concentration increases in **polycythemia vera**.

Types of Anemia

Anemia is defined as a decrease in hemoglobin concentration or RBC count below the normal range for an individual's age and sex. It is classified based on morphology (red blood cell indices) or etiology (underlying cause).

Morphological types

▮ Hypochromic microcytic anemia

Values of MCV, MCH, and MCHC are below normal. This manifests as **microcytosis and hypochromia** of red cells in the blood film. This occurs due to a defect in red cell formation in which hemoglobin synthesis is impaired to a greater extent than the synthesis of other cellular components.

The most common causes of this condition are **iron deficiency anemia**—in which there is inadequate iron for the formation of the heme component of hemoglobin and **thalassemia**—in which the formation of the globin component of hemoglobin is defective.

▮ Normochromic normocytic anemia

In this type of anemia, the MCV, MCH, and MCHC are within the normal range and the size of the RBCs and hemoglobin concentration are normal in the blood film. It usually occurs in the following cases:

1. Due to substantial blood loss (**blood loss anemia**)
2. Due to hemolysis (**hemolytic anemia**)
3. When red cell production is impaired by bone marrow failure, chronic kidney failure, chronic inflammation, or infection (**aplastic anemia**)

Macrocytic anemia

In this type of anemia, the MCV is above the upper limit of the normal, which corresponds to macrocytosis of red cells in the blood film. The **MCH is also higher** than the normal. However, the MCHC is normal or sometimes, lower. The red cells are usually normochromic. A classic example of this type of anemia is **megaloblastic anemia**, which occurs due to the *deficiency of vitamin B12 or folic acid*.

Etiological types

1. Blood loss
2. Impaired red cell production
   - Inadequate supply of nutrients (deficiency of iron, vitamins, and proteins)
   - Aplastic anemia
   - Anemia associated with chronic diseases
   - Anemia associated with renal failure
   - Anemia due to inherited diseases (e.g., thalassemia)
3. Excessive red cell destruction (hemolysis)

OSPE

Dilute blood (from the given sample) for the estimation of hemoglobin concentration.

Steps

1. Select a clean and dry hemoglobin tube.
2. Fill up N/10 HCl up to the 10 per cent mark.
3. Select a hemoglobin pipette and ensure that it is dry.
4. Dip the tip of the hemoglobinometer pipette into the sample and suck blood up to the 20 mm³ mark of the pipette.
5. Thoroughly mix blood in the sample by shaking.
6. Wipe the tip of the pipette.
7. Blow the blood into the acid solution in the hemoglobin tube. Wash out the blood from the pipette by repeatedly drawing in and blowing out of the diluting fluid (two to three times).
8. Note the time (the mixture is kept for ten minutes for the conversion of Hb to acid hematin).

VIVA

1. *What is the normal value of hemoglobin in an adult?* (Ans. Refer to page 11, under the heading 'Normal Values'.)
2. *Why is the hemoglobin content of blood lower in women?* (Ans. Refer to page 17, under the heading 'Conditions that decrease Hb Conc. – Physiological'.)
3. *What is the principle of hemoglobin estimation in Sahli's acid hematin method?* (Ans. Refer to page 13, under the heading 'Principle'.)
4. *What difference would it make if N/10 HCl is taken above the 20 per cent mark?*
   (Ans. If more HCl is taken, the colour of the undiluted solution may be lighter than the standard, especially if there is severe anemia.)
5. *Can N/10 HCl be used for dilution?*
   (Ans. Yes, because it will not change the colour of the solution. However, tap water should not be used as it causes turbidity and interferes with the colour of the solution.)
6. *Why is the result preferably expressed in g/dl rather than in per cent?* (Ans. Refer to page 15, under the heading 'Reporting'.)
7. *What are the precautions to be observed during hemoglobin estimation?* (Ans. Refer to page 15, under the heading 'Precautions'.)
8. *Why should the stirrer be kept above the solution but not taken out of the tube while matching the colour?* (Ans. Refer to page 15, point no. 10, under the heading 'Precautions'.)
9. *Why should the tip of the pipette be wiped before transferring blood from the pipette into the N/10 HCl in the tube?* (Ans. Refer to page 14, point no. 5, under the heading 'Precautions'.)
10. *Why should absorbent material not be used for adjusting the level to the 20 mm³ mark if excess blood is sucked into the pipette?* (Ans. Refer to page 14, the 'Note' below point no. 4 under the heading 'Procedure'.)
11. *Why should ten minutes be allowed before diluting the solution of blood and HCl?* (Ans. Refer to page 14, point no. 6, under the heading 'Procedure'.)
12. *What are the advantages and disadvantages of Sahli's acid hematin method? What are the possible errors in this method?* (Ans. Refer to page 15, under the heading 'Sources of Error, Advantages, Disadvantages'.)
13. *What are the other methods of hemoglobin estimation?* (Ans. Refer to page 16, under the heading 'Other Methods'.)
14. *Which is the quickest method of hemoglobin estimation?*
    (Ans. The quickest method is Tallquist's method as it only compares the colour of the sample blood with that of the standard. However, it is not an accurate method.)
15. *Which method is most accurate for hemoglobin estimation and why?*
    (Ans. The most accurate method is the gasometric method using Van Slyke apparatus. However, it is time-consuming and complicated and hence, is not routinely used in laboratories. Of the routinely used tests, the most accurate method is the cyanmethemoglobin method because it detects all forms of hemoglobin, including sulfhemoglobin and methemoglobin.)

16. *What are the functions of hemoglobin?* (Ans. Refer to page 12, under the heading 'Functions of Hb'.)
17. *What is the oxygen-carrying capacity of hemoglobin?* (Ans. Refer to page 12, point no. 1, under the heading 'Functions of Hb'.)
18. *What are the types of hemoglobins?* (Ans. Refer to pages 10–11, under the heading 'Types of Hb'.)
19. *What is the structure of normal adult hemoglobin (HbA)?* (Ans. Refer to pages 10–11, under the heading 'Adult Hemoglobins'.)
20. *At what stage in erythropoiesis does hemoglobin appear in the red cells?*
    (Ans. Hemoglobin appears in the early normoblast stage of erythropoiesis; then, its concentration increases and attains its maximum in the late normoblast stage.)
21. *What is the fate of hemoglobin in the body?* (Ans. Refer to page 12, under the heading 'Hb Derivatives'.)
22. *What is anemia? What are the types of anemia?* (Ans. Refer to page 17, under the heading 'Types of Anemia'.)
23. *What is the most common cause of anemia in developing countries like India, and why?*
    (Ans. Iron deficiency anemia is the most common cause of anemia. It is highly prevalent due to socioeconomic factors, poor nutrition, and cultural habits.)
24. *Give a physiological cause for anemia. What is the physiological basis of anemia in this condition?* (Ans. Refer to page 17, under the heading 'conditions that decrease Hb conc'.)
25. *What is megaloblastic anemia and how is it produced?* (Ans. Refer to page 18, under the heading 'Macrocytic Anemia'.)
26. *What is pernicious anemia?*
    (Ans. When megaloblastic anemia occurs due to vitamin B12 deficiency caused by decreased intrinsic factor secretion from the parietal cells of the stomach.)
27. *What is aplastic anemia?* (Ans. Refer to page 18, under the heading 'Normochromic normocytic anemia'.)
28. *What is the normal value of HbA1c and what is the clinical importance of HbA1c estimation?* (Ans. Refer to page 12, under the heading 'Hb Complexes'.)

4 | Determination of Hematocrit

Learning Objectives

After completing this practical, you will be able to (MUST KNOW):
1. Explain the importance of the determination of hematocrit in clinical medicine.
2. Name the methods of determining hematocrit.
3. Identify the Wintrobe tube.
4. Fill the Wintrobe tube properly with the blood provided.
5. Determine PCV by the Wintrobe method.
6. List the possible sources of error in this method.
7. List the normal values of PCV in men and women.
8. Name the common conditions in which PCV is altered.

You may also be able to (DESIRABLE TO KNOW):
1. Describe the microhematocrit method for the determination of PCV.
2. State the principle and advantages of determination of hematocrit by automated methods.
3. List the physiological bases of alteration.

PY2.12: Describe the tests for ESR, osmotic fragility, and hematocrit. Note the findings and interpret the test results.

INTRODUCTION

Hematocrit, which literally translates into 'blood separation', is a measure of the percentage of the volume of packed red cells. Also known as **packed cell volume (PCV)**, hematocrit is a reliable index of the red cell population in the blood. The manually estimated PCV is considered more accurate than the manually performed red cell count due to the lower margin of error in its determination. It provides valuable information about the red cells. Therefore, it should always be correlated with the number of red cells and their hemoglobin content.

Hematocrit is used for the **detection and classification of various types of anemias** along with other parameters (hemoglobin and red cell count) of red cell indices.

Normal Values of Hematocrit

1. **Adult male:** 46% (40–50%)
2. **Adult female:** 42% (37–47%)

METHODS OF DETERMINING HEMATOCRIT

Two manual methods are used for determining hematocrit: the **macrohematocrit method and the microhematocrit method**. The microhematocrit method is preferred due to its efficiency and because it requires less time, labour, and blood. The macrohematocrit method is known as the Wintrobe method. Hematocrit is also measured by automated techniques, which have virtually replaced the manual methods in advanced laboratories.

Macrohematocrit Method (Wintrobe Method)

Since this method requires a large volume of blood, only venous blood is used.

Principle

In a Wintrobe tube, anticoagulated blood is filled up to the graduation mark and centrifuged for the prescribed length of time. The volume of packed cells is read directly from the graduation mark on the Wintrobe tube.

Requirements

1. **Wintrobe tube:** This is a 110 mm-long, narrow, thick-walled test tube with a 3 mm internal bore. The tube bears graduations marking 0 to 10 cm (100 mm) on either side, in ascending and descending orders (Fig. 4.1). Thus, at the top of the tube, 0 and 10 cm coincide. The scale with 0–10 from top to bottom is used to measure erythrocyte sedimentation rate (ESR), whereas the side with markings from 0–10 from bottom to top is used for hematocrit determination. The tube holds approximately 1 ml of blood.
2. **Centrifuge machine:** The centrifuge should be capable of producing a force of 2300 G. Insufficient force results in falsely high hematocrit readings, while excessive force may cause falsely low values. The centrifuge should be standardised for speed and time by taking a reference blood sample and determining the time and speed necessary to obtain the reference value.
3. **Pasteur pipette:** It is a 22 cm-long glass tube with a long, thin nozzle measuring about 13 cm in length. It is used to transfer blood from the container to fill the Wintrobe

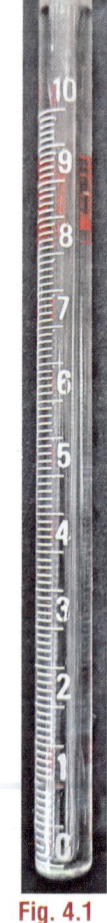

Fig. 4.1
Wintrobe tube.

tube. If a Pasteur pipette is not available, a **syringe with a Pasteur needle** (needle with a nozzle >13 cm) can be used.

4. **Blood sample:** A sample of venous blood to which ***EDTA or double oxalate anticoagulant*** has been added is used for the study.

Procedure

1. Thoroughly mix the blood specimen by repeated inversion. Collect blood in the Pasteur pipette or Pasteur needle carefully, ensuring that there is no entry of air bubbles into the pipette or needle (Fig. 4.2).

2. Fill the Wintrobe tube with blood with the help of the Pasteur pipette up to the 10 cm mark (which represents 100 per cent) (Fig. 4.3). If the level of blood in the tube crosses the 10 cm mark, use a dropper to remove the extra blood. Do not use a cotton swab, blotting paper, or any other absorbent material for this purpose as these may introduce errors. Alternatively, deduct the excess volume of blood (recorded on top of the tube) from the final result.

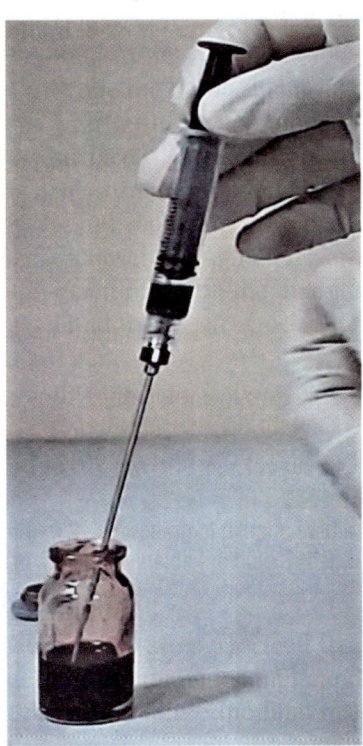
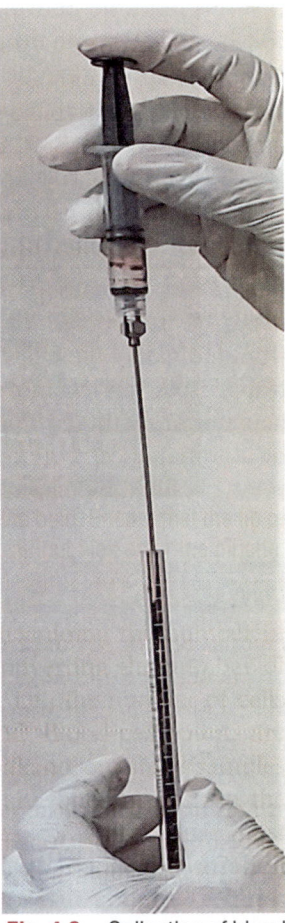

Fig. 4.2 Collection of blood for estimation of hematocrit by the Wintrobe method: A syringe with a long nozzle needle (>13 cm length) is used. The tip of the needle should enter the blood column in the vial so that air bubbles do not enter the syringe. The donning of gloves is a must when a hospital sample is being used.

Fig. 4.3 Collection of blood in the Wintrobe tube exactly up to the 10 cm mark.

Note: Filling the Wintrobe tube requires special care since air bubbles may be trapped and cause damage to the red blood cells. To avoid this, place the tip of the pipette at the bottom of the Wintrobe tube and fill from the bottom, gradually withdrawing the pipette as the blood goes in. Try to **keep the tip of the pipette under the rising column of blood** to avoid foaming.

3. Place the Wintrobe tube in a centrifuge cup and balance it with a second Wintrobe tube containing water in the opposite cup.

4. Start the centrifuge at a low speed, and then gradually increase to the required speed. Centrifuge for 30 minutes at 3000 rpm.

5. After 30 minutes, turn off the centrifuge and allow it to stop naturally—do not use the brake.

6. Remove the Wintrobe tube and read the PCV directly from the graduation marks, where each numbered graduation mark represents 10%.

Precautions

1. The hematocrit should ideally be measured within six hours of blood collection.

2. Thorough mixing of the blood sample should be ensured before measurement.

3. Hemolyzed specimens should be avoided, as they may yield false low results.

4. An appropriate anticoagulant in the correct concentration should be used to prevent distortion of red cell size and shape.

5. If the blood exceeds the 10 cm mark, the excess should be removed with a dropper rather than with absorbent materials.

6. If air bubbles enter the tube during filling, all the blood should be removed from the tube and it should then be refilled.

7. Adequate centrifugation time should be allowed to ensure proper red cell packing.

8. The buffy coat (white cell layer) should not be included in the final reading.

Observations and reporting

After centrifugation, the hematocrit value is recorded as the percentage of packed red cells. For example, if the red cell column reaches just above the 4 cm mark, the hematocrit is recorded as 41%.

Note: The buffy coat (refer to Fig. 1.1, Chapter 1) is the thin grey-white layer of white cells at the top of the red cell column. Do not include this while reading the height of the red cell column.

True hematocrit: Red cells are not fully packed even after centrifugation, as about 2% of plasma remains trapped between them. This effect is more pronounced in conditions like spherocytosis and sickle cell anemia. To obtain the true hematocrit, the observed value is multiplied by 0.98.

Additionally, venous blood hematocrit is approximately 3% higher than arterial blood hematocrit (details given in the answer to question 11 at the end of the chapter).

Advantages

1. ESR (by the Wintrobe method) can be determined simultaneously, using the same sample. To do this, the Wintrobe tube filled with blood is kept vertically in the Wintrobe rack for one hour (see Chapter 14). After the ESR reading has been noted, the tube is centrifuged to determine the hematocrit.
2. It is not an expensive method.

Microhematocrit Method

This method requires only a small volume of blood, making it ideal for cases in which only small specimens can be collected (for example, pediatric patients and burn patients). It can be performed using free-flowing capillary blood from a finger puncture or EDTA-anticoagulated venous blood. Since centrifugation occurs at high speed, results are obtained quickly.

Principle

Anticoagulated blood is centrifuged in a sealed capillary tube, and the volume of packed red cells and percentage of whole blood (level of plasma) are determined by a special hematocrit reader.

Requirements

1. **Capillary hematocrit tubes:** These tubes are approximately 75 mm in length, and have an internal diameter of approximately 1 mm. For anticoagulated venous blood, simple capillary tubes can be used. For blood collected by skin puncture, heparinized tubes should be used.
2. **Microhematocrit centrifuge:** This is a special centrifuge that runs at high speeds (approx. 12,000 rpm) and is capable of producing a force of 12,000 G.
3. **Hematocrit reader:** There are several hematocrit readers available. The simplest one is the card reader, which can be made by hand.
4. **Modelling clay:** This is used to seal the end of the hematocrit tubes.
5. **Sterile skin puncture equipment:** Includes disposable lancets, alcohol, and sterile needles.

Procedure

1. Perform a sterile skin puncture and allow blood to enter the capillary tube by capillary action.

> **Note:** Use a plain tube for anticoagulated venous blood or a heparinized tube for skin puncture. The blood should flow freely in this case. Fill three-quarters of the tube.

2. Seal the dry end of the tube using plastic sealing clay or heat-sealing.
3. Place two sealed tubes in opposite radial grooves of the centrifuge to balance the load.
4. Turn the centrifuge on for five minutes at 12,000 rpm.
5. After the centrifuge stops, remove the tubes and measure PCV using the microhematocrit reader.

Precautions

1. The blood sample must be collected properly.
2. Anticoagulated blood should be used within six hours of collection.
3. The blood should not be clotted or hemolyzed.
4. Centrifugation must be sufficient to yield proper red cell packing.

Advantages

1. This procedure requires very little blood and hence, can easily be performed for pediatric patients and patients suffering from hemoconcentration or blood loss, as in the case of burns.
2. It is not time-consuming.
3. It can be used in mass surveys because a large number of specimens can be handled simultaneously.
4. Capillary tubes are easy to fill.
5. The tubes are cheap, the method is cost-effective, and replicates are easily obtainable.

Automated Method

Automated hematocrit measurements can be obtained using electronic cell counters. This result is computed from individual red cell volumes and is not affected by the trapped plasma left in the red cell column of the manual hematocrit methods. Thus, the hematocrit value obtained by automated cell counters is accurate and lower than the value obtained by manual methods.

DISCUSSION

Hematocrit, or packed cell volume (PCV), is the percentage of packed red blood cells obtained after centrifugation. When blood is centrifuged in a tube, the centrifugal force causes the red cells to accumulate at the bottom of the tube as they are heavier than plasma. However, if the cells are deformed (as in hereditary spherocytosis or sickle cell disease), more plasma remains between the packed cells, giving a false high result.

Physiological and Clinical Significance

1. Hematocrit is a **reasonable index of the red cell population or Hb content** of blood (Fig. 4.4).

Therefore, it is used to detect conditions in which the red cell count increases (polycythemia) or decreases (anemia). Hematocrit measurement is more useful and reliable than the red cell count performed manually because it has a lower margin of error.

2. The value of hematocrit is used in **determination of blood indices,** especially MCV (mean corpuscular volume) and MCHC (mean corpuscular hemoglobin concentration). Blood indices help in the diagnosis and classification of various types of anemia.

3. Hematocrit is an important factor that determines the **viscosity of blood. Increase in hematocrit** increases blood viscosity, as observed in polycythemia. This increases peripheral resistance, which in turn decreases cardiac output as the afterload on the heart increases. Conversely, **decrease in hematocrit**, as seen in anemia, decreases the peripheral resistance that increases cardiac output. This also makes circulation hyperdynamic.

Conditions That Alter Hematocrit

Conditions that decrease hematocrit
Physiological
1. Pregnancy (due to hemodilution)
2. Excess water intake
3. Gender (lower in women as the red cell count is less in them)

Pathological
1. Various types of anemia
2. Conditions in which there is hemodilution and expansion of plasma volume; for example, hyperaldosteronism

Conditions that increase hematocrit
Physiological
1. High altitude (due to hypoxia)
2. Newborns and infants
3. Excessive sweating (due to hemoconcentration)

Pathological
1. Decreased oxygen supply to the tissues (hypoxia), for example, congenital heart disease and emphysema
2. Polycythemia
3. Conditions in which there is hemoconcentration, for example, severe vomiting and diarrhea (due to dehydration)

OSPE
Load a Wintrobe tube with the blood supplied for the estimation of hematocrit.
Steps:
1. Select an appropriate Wintrobe tube.
2. Clean and dry the tube thoroughly.
3. Mix blood thoroughly by swirling or repeatedly inverting the tube.
4. Draw blood into the Pasteur pipette.
5. Fill the Wintrobe tube slowly by placing the tip of the pipette at the bottom inner wall of the tube. Fill the tube from the bottom upwards, withdrawing the pipette gradually as the blood level rises. Keep the pipette tip under the surface of the rising blood column to prevent foaming.
6. Fill exactly up to the 0 mark. If excess blood is added, use a dropper to remove it—never use absorbent materials like cotton or gauze, as they can introduce errors.
7. Place the filled Wintrobe tube in the centrifuge cups for processing.

VIVA

1. *What is hematocrit? What is the significance of hematocrit?* (Ans. Refer to pages 22–23, under the headings 'Discussion' and 'Physiological and Clinical Significance'.)
2. *What are the different methods of estimating hematocrit?* (Ans. Refer to page 20, under the heading 'Methods'.)
3. *What are the sources of error in the microhematocrit method? What precautions should be taken?* (Ans. Refer to page 21, under the heading 'Precautions'.)
4. *What is the ideal anticoagulant to be used for hematocrit determination and why?* (Ans. Refer to page 21, under the sub-heading 'Blood Sample'.)
5. *Why is an anticoagulant used in a recommended concentration for the estimation of hematocrit?*
   (Ans. The use of a high concentration of anticoagulant gives a false low result, because excess EDTA may cause hemolysis.)
6. *Why should the hematocrit ideally be determined within six hours of collecting blood?*
   (Ans. If the blood is kept beyond six hours, red cell metabolism alters their size and shape, and hemolysis may begin. If testing cannot be done within six hours, the sample should be stored in a refrigerator.)
7. *What are the sources of error in the Wintrobe hematocrit method?*
   (Ans. i. Improper mixing of blood, ii. improper anticoagulant and improper concentration of anticoagulant, iii. inadequate centrifugation, and iv. reading of hematocrit with buffy coat.)

8. *What is the normal value of hematocrit in adults?* (Ans. Refer to page 20, under the subheading 'Normal Values'.)
9. *Why is the hematocrit value lower in women?* (Ans. Refer to page 23, under the heading 'Conditions that decrease hematocrit – Physiological', point No. 3'.)
10. *What are the physiological and pathological conditions that alter hematocrit value?* (Ans. Refer to page 23, under the heading 'Conditions that Alter Hematocrit'.)
11. *Why is the hematocrit value of venous blood slightly higher than that of arterial blood?*
     (Ans. Venous blood has a hematocrit value approximately 3% higher than arterial blood due to two main reasons:
   i.   At the tissue level, CO_2 is added to blood, creating an osmotically active particle, either bicarbonate or chloride (due to chloride shift). This increases intracellular osmolarity, causing red cells to take up water and swell, which increases hematocrit.
   ii. A small volume of fluid from arterial blood returns to circulation via the lymphatic system rather than through veins, slightly concentrating the venous blood.)

5 | Study of the Compound Microscope

Learning Objectives

After completing this practical, you will be able to (MUST KNOW):

1. Identify different parts of the compound microscope.
2. List the uses of different parts of the microscope.
3. Make microscopic adjustments to view the object under low-power, high-power, and oil-immersion objectives.
4. List the precautions to be taken while using the microscope.
5. Handle the microscope carefully.

You may also be able to (DESIRABLE TO KNOW):

1. Describe the principle of microscopy.
2. Explain the physical principles of construction of the compound microscope.
3. Provide the solutions for common problems encountered in microscopy.
4. Explain the basic working principles of other types of microscopes.

INTRODUCTION

A microscope magnifies the image of an object. The modern compound microscope (**light microscope**) is one of the most frequently used equipment in medical laboratories for students. The microscope is commonly used in the physiology laboratory to study the morphology of blood cells and for making different cell counts.

Improper use of a microscope leads to loss of clarity of the image, which results in loss of definition. Therefore, it must be kept in excellent condition, optically and mechanically, with routine care. To achieve this, users must understand the optical principles of microscopy, the basic construction of the microscope, and how to properly maintain the instrument. Additionally, it is essential to read the manufacturer's manual and operating instructions before operating the microscope.

Physical Terms

The compound microscope consists of two magnifying lenses: **the objective and the eyepiece**. It is used to magnify an object to a point where it can be seen with the human eye. The physical terms fundamental to microscopy are the **resolution**, the **working distance**, and the **numerical aperture**.

1. **Resolution:** The limit of useful magnification of a microscope is set by its **resolving power**, that is, its **ability to reveal closely adjacent structural details as separate and distinct**. Resolution, therefore, describes how small individual objects can lie close to each other and still be recognisable.

Generally, the human eye can separate (or resolve) dots that are 0.25 mm apart; **the light microscope can separate dots that are 0.25 mm apart, and the electron microscope can separate dots that are 0.5 nm apart.**

> **Note:** 1 nanometre (nm) = 0.001 micrometre (μm)
> = **0.000 001** mm

Resolving power is expressed quantitatively as the microscope's **limit of resolution (LR)**, that is, the **minimum distance between two visible bodies at which they are seen as separate and not in contact with one another.** The LR is determined according to the following formula:

$$LR = \frac{0.61 \times W}{NA}$$

Where W is the wavelength of the light rays and NA is the numerical aperture of the objective in use.

For example, if green light (wavelength 0.55 μm) and an oil-immersion objective (NA 1.3) are used, the LR will be 0.25 μm (0.61 × 0.55 / 1.3 = 0.25 μm).

2. **Working distance:** This is the **distance between the objective and the objective slide.** The working distance decreases with increasing magnification. It is 0.15–1.5 mm in the case of the oil-immersion objective, 0.5–4 mm in the case of a high-power objective, and 5–15 mm for a low-power objective.

3. **Numerical aperture (NA):** The numerical aperture of a lens is the **ratio of the diameter of the lens to its focal length**. Every lens has a constant numerical aperture, and this value is dependent on the radius of the lens and its focal length (the distance from the object being viewed to the lens or the objective).

The NA of a lens is an **index of its resolving power**. As the NA increases, the resolution (or distance from each other at which objects can be distinguished) decreases. Thus, the greater the NA, the greater the resolving power of the lens. The NA for low-power, high-power, and oil-immersion objectives are 0.30, 0.65, and 1.30 respectively.

NA also serves as an **index of the light-gathering capacity** of a lens, that is, the amount of light entering the objective. The NA can be decreased by decreasing the amount of light that passes through a lens. Therefore, the illumination must also be increased in the same order when the objectives are changed from low-power to high-power.

PARTS OF A COMPOUND MICROSCOPE

There are two common types of compound microscopes: **monocular and binocular**. The main difference between them is the number of eyepieces—monocular microscopes have one eyepiece (ocular), while binocular microscopes have two. The structure of the compound microscope can be discussed under four broad systems:
1. The support system (the framework)
2. The illumination system
3. The magnification system
4. The adjustment system

The Support System

The support system is the framework of the microscope that holds its components. The framework consists of several units (Fig. 5.1).
1. **Base:** The base supports the microscope and is horseshoe-shaped to provide maximum stability.
2. **Pillars:** Two upright pillars project upwards from the base, and the handle of the microscope is hinged to the pillars.
3. **Handle (arm):** The curved arm supports the magnifying and adjusting systems. It is also the handle by which the microscope can be carried without damaging the delicate parts. The microscope can be tilted at the hinged joint of the arm as desired.
4. **Body tube:** The body tube is the part through which the light passes to the eyepiece. The length of the tube is usually 160 mm. This is the tube that actually conducts the image.
5. **Stage:** The fixed stage is the horizontal platform on which the object being observed is placed. The centre of the stage has an aperture through which the converging cone of light passes. Most microscopes have a mechanical stage which makes it much easier to manipulate the objects being observed. It is calibrated and fitted on the fixed stage. There is a spring-mounted clip to hold the slide or the counting

chamber in position, and two screws for moving these transversely or forwards and backwards.
6. **Nosepiece:** The **fixed nosepiece** is attached to the lower end of the body tube. Beneath it is the **revolving nosepiece**, which carries multiple objective lenses of varying magnification.

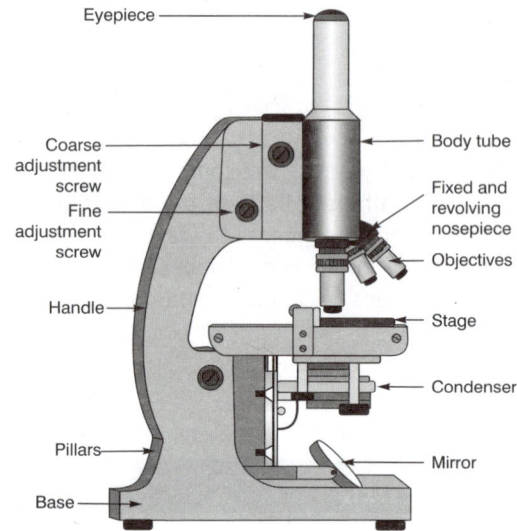

Fig. 5.1   Parts of a compound microscope.

The Illumination System

A microscope cannot function optimally without proper illumination. The illumination system provides uniform and soft-bright illumination of the entire field viewed under the microscope. The illumination system is, therefore, an important part of the compound light microscope.

There are six types of illumination systems based on which microscopes work:
1. **Bright-field or light microscope:** This uses white light, either external sunlight or an internal tungsten filament lamp, as the source of illumination. When viewed under the microscope, objects look dark or coloured in contrast to a bright background.
2. **Dark-field microscope:** Employs a special dark-field condenser that lights up the object against a dark background, like stars in the night sky.
3. **Fluorescent microscope:** Uses a special ultraviolet lamp as the source of illumination. The objects are dyed with a flourescent dye, which makes them glow when exposed to UV radiation.
4. **Polarizing microscope:** Uses polarized light to detect structures in materials that rotate light.
5. **Phase-contrast microscope:** Enhances contrast in transparent, unstained specimens by converting phase shifts in light into changes in brightness.
6. **Interference-contrast microscope:** Produces high-contrast, pseudo-3D images of unstained specimens by using differences in optical path length.

The illumination system of a compound microscope consists of a light source, a condenser, and an iris diaphragm.

Light source

The illumination system of a microscope begins with a source of light, which may be either internal or external.

1. **Internal source:** Most modern compound microscopes have a built-in light source with an electric lamp, which provides control of illumination. The lamp housing contains a frosted tungsten lamp, which is placed directly under the stage.
2. **External source:** In the students' compound microscope, there is no in-built light source. These microscopes use an external source of light. This can be from an electric lamp housed in a lamp box with a window, or from the sun. The rays of light are reflected by a mirror towards the object. The mirror is located at the base of the microscope. It has two surfaces, **plane and concave**. The plane mirror is used for the oil-immersion objective, whereas the concave mirror is used for the low- and high-power objectives.

Condenser

The condenser focuses light rays reflected from the mirror onto the object under examination and also helps in resolving the image. It is mounted below the stage with a rack and pinion mechanism for adjusting its focus. Microscopes generally use a substage **Abbe-type condenser**. This is composed of two lenses uncorrected for spherical and chromatic aberration. Therefore, for better microscopic examination, a **good quality achromatic condenser** should be used.

The condenser can be raised and lowered beneath the stage by turning the adjustment screw. It should be correctly aligned to focus light properly on the specimen since it has a fixed **numerical aperture (NA)**. The NA of the condenser should be equal to or slightly less than that of the objective lens in use. By adjusting the height of the condenser, its NA can be altered. Therefore, its position must be adjusted for each objective to ensure optimal light focus and resolution.

When a low-power objective is used, the condenser is positioned at the lowest level; with a high-power objective, it is raised optimally; and with an oil-immersion objective, it is raised fully. Most modern microscopes do not need condenser adjustment because the condenser is fixed at the highest position, and illumination is controlled primarily by opening or closing the **iris diaphragm**.

Iris diaphragm

The iris diaphragm regulates the amount of light that passes through the material under observation. It is located at the bottom of the condenser. It has a **central aperture** that can be opened for more light or closed for less light as required by means of a lever provided with a shutter.

The size of the aperture regulates the amount of light that passes to the field under observation. Regulation of the light by such means affects the numerical aperture of the condenser. By reducing the field size with the help of the iris diaphragm, the numerical aperture of the condenser is decreased.

Thus, **proper illumination procedure** includes a combination of **light intensity regulation, light source position, condenser position, and field size regulation**.

The Magnification System

The magnification system plays an extremely important role in microscopy because it magnifies the image of the object under view. The compound microscope consists of two magnifying lenses: **the eyepiece and the objective**. The total magnification provided by a compound microscope is the product of the magnification contributed by the objective and that provided by the eyepiece. The eyepiece forms a virtual magnified image of the real magnified image formed by the objective.

Eyepiece

The eyepiece or the **ocular** is a lens that magnifies the image formed by the objective. It fits into the top of the body tube. Most microscopes are provided with two eyepieces, 5× and 10×, with magnifying powers of 5 and 10 respectively. However, 2×, 8×, and 20× eyepieces are also available. Microscopes fitted with a single eyepiece are called **monocular microscopes** (Fig. 5.2), while those with two eyepieces are known as **binocular microscopes** (Fig. 5.3). **The magnification produced by the eyepiece multiplied by the magnification produced by the objective gives the total magnification of the object being viewed.**

Objectives

Objectives are the most important part of the magnification system. Usually, three objectives are screwed onto the revolving nosepiece in a compound microscope. The nosepiece is a pivot that enables a quick change of objectives.

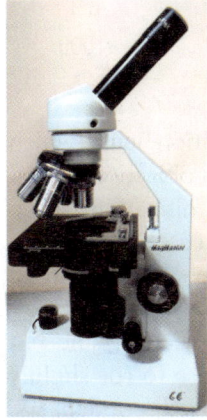

Fig. 5.2 The monocular microscope.

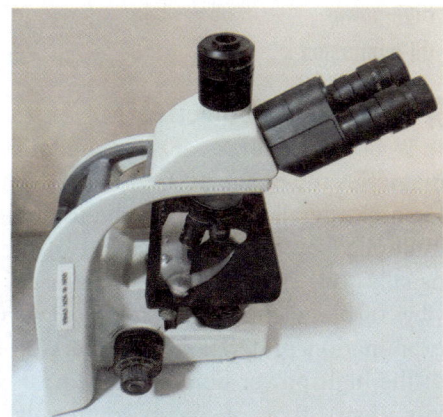

Fig. 5.3 The binocular research microscope.

The **three objectives** are (a) 10×: low-power objective, (b) 40× or 45×: high-power objective, and (c) 90× or 100×: oil-immersion objective (Fig. 5.4).

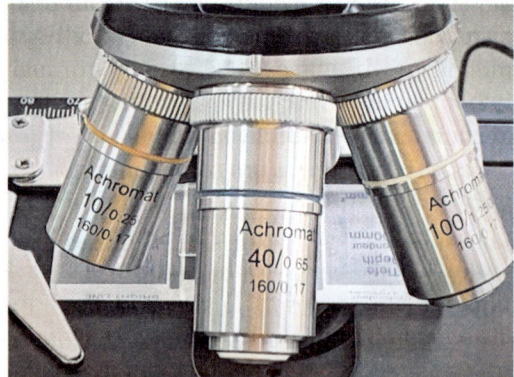

Fig. 5.4   Objectives of a microscope: Low-power objective (10×), high-power objective (40×), and oil-immersion objective (100×).

■ Low-power objective

The low-power objective, usually 10×, enlarges the image tenfold and is typically used for initial focusing and general observation. Some microscopes also have very low-power objectives (3× or 4×), known as **scanning objectives**, for an overall view of tissue sections.

The NA of the low-power objective is always less than that of the condenser in most microscopes. Therefore, to achieve focus, the **numerical apertures should be more closely matched by reducing the light on the specimen**. This can be achieved by lowering the condenser and closing the iris diaphragm (iris slightly opened). The NA of objectives is related to the magnification capacity of the microscope (Table 5.1).

Table 5.1   Relation of NA of objectives to magnification.

Objective	NA	Magnification		
		Objective	Eyepiece	Total
Low-power	0.30	10	10	100
High-power	0.65	45	10	450
Oil-immersion	1.30	100	10	1000

■ High-power objective

It is usually a 40× or 45× magnification lens, which magnifies the image 40 or 45 times. This objective is used for more detailed study, as the total magnification (when multiplied by the magnification of the 10× eyepiece) is usually 400 or 450 times. It is used to obtain a broad view of blood films or histological sections prior to their examination under the oil-immersion objective. The NA of the high-power objective is almost close to (or slightly less than) that of most commonly used condensers. **Therefore, the condenser should be slightly raised, and the iris partially opened to achieve maximum focus.**

■ Oil-immersion objective

The **oil-immersion objective** is typically a 90× or 100× lens, which magnifies the specimen 90 or 100 times. When in use, this objective nearly touches the slide (Fig. 5.5). It requires a specific type of oil known as **immersion oil**, which is applied between the slide and the objective lens. The most commonly used immersion oil is **cedarwood oil**. The use of oil increases the NA and thereby enhances the resolving power of the microscope.

Oil is used to increase the numerical aperture and thereby, the resolving power of the objective. Light travels through air at a greater speed than through glass; when it passes through immersion oil, light travels at the same speed as through glass. Thus, oil is used to decrease the speed at which light travels to increase the effective numerical aperture of the objective. It also decreases the diffraction of light rays.

Since the numerical aperture of the oil-immersion objective is always greater than that of the condenser, the **condenser should be placed at the highest position**, and the iris **diaphragm should be fully open** (Table 5.2). The oil-immersion lens gives a total magnification of **1000 times or 900 times with a 10× eyepiece**. Therefore, it is generally used for detailed morphological examination of blood films or histological slides.

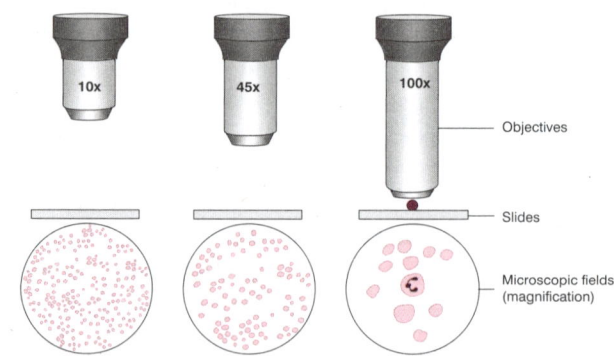

Fig. 5.5   Distance (working distance) between the objective lenses and the object in the three types of objectives. Note the magnification obtained under the three objectives.

Table 5.2   Adjustments in the microscope for using different objectives.

Objective	Mirror	Condenser position	State of iris diaphragm
Low-power	Concave	Lowest	Partially closed
High-power	Concave	Slightly raised	Partially opened
Oil-immersion	Plane	Fully raised	Fully opened

The Adjusting System

The adjusting system consists of two adjustment systems: the **coarse adjustment system** and the **fine adjustment** system. The coarse adjustment system is used to obtain an approximate focus, whereas the fine adjustment system is used to obtain fine focus of the object after coarse adjustment.

Coarse adjustment system

Two **coarse adjustment screws** are used for making coarse adjustments. These screw are mounted on the top of the handle by a double-sided micrometre mechanism, one on each side. If one screw is rotated, its member on the opposite side also rotates at the same time. Therefore, there is no need to operate the adjustment screws from both sides simultaneously. If the left hand is used for handling the adjustment screw, the right hand can be used for manipulating the body tube or the mechanical stage. The body tube or stage can be raised or lowered quickly with the coarse adjustment screw.

Fine adjustment system

Two **fine adjustment screws** are used for making fine adjustments. Usually, these screws are mounted on the handle below the coarse adjustment screws by double-sided micrometre mechanisms, one on each side. These screws are operated for fine adjustment and exact focusing of the object.

METHOD OF OPERATING A COMPOUND MICROSCOPE

Principle

In the compound microscope, a focused beam of light scans the specimen or object placed on a glass slide on the stage of the microscope. Parts of the specimen that are optically dense, have a high refractive index, or are coloured with a stain cast a potential image like a shadow, which is magnified in different stages as it passes up the microscope to the eye.

Requirements

1. Microscope
2. Light source
3. Blood film

Procedure

The microscope should be handled carefully. Before using the microscope, examine it thoroughly. The student should follow the steps given below while using a compound microscope.

1. Place the microscope on the working table in the **upright position** and **adjust the height and position of your chair** so that you are comfortable and prepared for prolonged viewing. The eyepieces of the microscope should level with and be close to your eyes while you are sitting upright (Fig. 5.6). Place your forearms on the table so that you can easily handle the

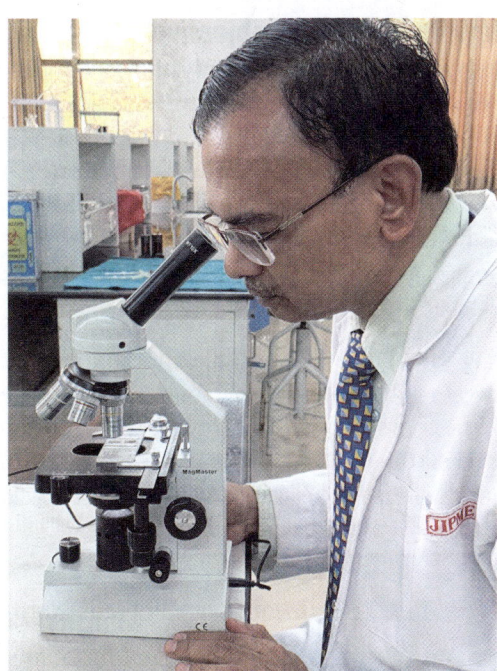

Fig. 5.6 Working with the microscope. Note that the eye position should be at the level of the eyepiece in the upright sitting position; an examiner using spectacles should wear them while viewing through the eyepiece. (*Courtesy:* Physiology Department, Hematology Laboratory, JIPMER, Puducherry, India.)

adjustment screws. You need not remove your glasses if you use them constantly.

Note: Observers who wear glasses should take care to prevent their spectacles from touching and scratching the lenses of the eyepieces.

2. Check that the eyepieces and objective lenses are clean and free of dust or oil. Use a **fresh lens tissue** for cleaning.

Note: Only benzol or xylol should be used to remove hardened oil.

3. Provide adequate illumination. If you have to use an external lamp, place it about 20 cm away from the microscope, switch on the lamp, and allow the light to fall on the mirror. If you have to use natural light, place the microscope near a window for maximum illumination.

4. Select and adjust the mirror for optimal illumination according to the objective to be used. Direct the path of light to pass through the hole of the stage with maximum intensity while setting the mirror (look from the side to check illumination).

5. Place the slide with the object on the stage such that it is held by the stage clips and pressed down at both ends so as to be in close contact with the surface of the stage.

6. After preliminary screening under the low-power objective, proceed to examine the film under the high-power objective.

Viewing with low-power objective

1. Bring the low-power objective (10×) into position by revolving the nosepiece (the objective must click into place).
2. Adjust the illumination to improve contrast. Use the concave mirror, bring the condenser to the lowest position, and slightly open the iris.

Note: For the low-power objective, the illumination is cut down to the minimum by reducing the aperture size.

3. Using the stage control dials, bring the object of interest to the centre of the stage.
4. Use the coarse adjustment screw to focus the specimen on the slide.

Note: Never use the fine adjustment screw until the specimen has been made visible and brought nearly into focus with the coarse adjustment screw.

5. Use the fine adjustment only to obtain and maintain exact focus. Place one hand on the focusing knob (coarse or fine, one at a time) and the other on the screw to move the stage.
6. Bring the object of interest to the centre of the stage.

Examining the film with the high-power objective

1. Bring the high-power objective (40× or 45×) into position by rotating the nosepiece; make sure that the objective clicks into place.
2. Use the concave mirror, raise the condenser slightly, and check that the iris diaphragm is partially open so that the illumination is properly centred. Increase the illumination as needed.
3. Repeat the process of focusing as described earlier by using the coarse adjustment and fine adjustment screws in sequence.

Note: Since the high-power objective typically does not come into contact with the slide (carefully check the distance between the slide and the objective at its lowest point), the use of the coarse and fine adjustment knobs may not be so critical and they can be switched freely.

Using the oil-immersion objective

1. Swing the high-power objective away from the stage and place a tiny drop of immersion oil on the slide, directly in the path of light.
2. Switch the mirror to its plane side.
3. Raise the condenser as much as possible (so that it is just below the stage) and open the iris fully to obtain maximum illumination.
4. Turn the nosepiece and set the oil-immersion objective in position; make sure that the objective has clicked into place.
5. Use the fine adjustment knob to get the object in focus. If this fails, look from the side, keep the eye level with the slide, and lower the objective carefully with the coarse adjustment knob until the oil-immersion objective

touches the oil. Lower the objective further and stop when the oil-immersion objective touches the slide (caution: avoid pressing hard on the preparation). First, focus the object with the coarse adjustment knob while increasing the gap between the slide and the objective. Finally, focus the object with the help of the fine adjustment knob.

Precautions

1. The microscope should be placed on a **stable and even surface**.
2. The **height of the observer's chair** should be raised to a position that allows for comfortable handling of the microscope.
3. Objectives and eyepieces should be **free from dust and oil**. Xylol or benzol should be used to remove hardened oil. Lenses should never be touched with the fingers.
4. If **natural light** is used, the microscope should be kept near the window; if a **lamp** is used, it should be kept about 20 cm from the microscope to prevent heating of the microscope.
5. The mirror, the position of the condenser, and the aperture of the iris should be checked in order to get proper illumination.
6. **When the objective lens is changed, it should click into position**. Otherwise, it may not stay securely aligned.
7. **The coarse adjustment screw should never be used while looking through the microscope lens**. Coarse adjustments should be made while viewing the microscope from the side with the naked eye.
8. Examination of the specimen under **low and high power should always precede** examination under the **oil-immersion objective**.
9. The **stage of the microscope should always be brought down** before bringing the oil-immersion objective into position. Otherwise, it may damage the preparation.
10. The **distance between the slide and the objective should always be checked** while using the coarse adjustment screw, especially for high-power and oil-immersion objectives.
11. The stage should always be kept clean and free of specimen material, stain, oil, and water.
12. The microscope should be **kept covered** when not in use.

Observations

Briefly mention your findings of the cell components of the blood smear as observed under low- and high-power and oil-immersion objectives. Also list the difficulties you faced during the procedure.

DISCUSSION
Common Difficulties in Microscopy

This section deals with the common difficulties faced by beginners and some tips to work around them.

Inability to achieve focus or obtain a clear image

1. The failure to achieve focus may be due to the slide not being brought close enough to the objective to remain within its focal distance. Alternatively, there may be no visible material on the small area of the slide within the field of the objective. First, move the slide so that the material to be focused on is brought into the field of vision. This will ensure that there is visible material to focus on. Then, with the eyes level with the stage, use the coarse adjustment to raise the slide until it again comes as close as possible to the objective without touching it. Finally, with your eyes on the eyepieces, use the coarse adjustment to move the objective away from the slide until the specimen is seen in focus.

2. Check that no dirt or dried oil has adhered to the objective lens. If it has, clean the lens thoroughly.

3. Check that the slide carrying the object has not been placed upside down on the stage. If it has, reverse it.

4. Check that the immersion oil has not become sticky. If so, wipe off the old oil and replace it.

5. Check whether the specimen is covered with a layer of dried oil or dirt (left on it by a previous viewer). If it is, clean it with a lens paper moistened with benzol or xylol.

6. Check whether the coverslip placed on the specimen is too thick or whether the mountant is so thick that the objective cannot reach close enough to the specimen to bring it within its focal length.

7. If none of the above steps improves the performance of the microscope, you should consider the possibility that the objective may be faulty. Exchange the objective with one from a good microscope, and if a sharp image is obtained, discard the faulty one.

Dark shadow in the field/poor image definition

1. Often caused by a dirty eyepiece. If the shadow moves when the eyepiece is rotated, remove and clean the eyepiece.

2. Air bubbles in the immersion oil can also cause shadows. Remove the oil and apply a fresh drop.

Poor illumination

1. Check whether the condenser is appropriately positioned, that is, racked fully upwards. Sometimes, it slips downwards in its mounting ring. It should be pushed up so that it can be racked up to within 1 mm below the specimen slide for the oil-immersion objective.

2. Check whether the iris is kept fully open while using an oil-immersion objective.

3. Check that the illumination is properly centered. Ensure that the concave surface of the mirror faces the light while using the low- and high-power objectives and the plane surface faces the light while using the oil-immersion objective, and that it is in the correct position to reflect light centrally into the condenser.

Unclear image under the oil-immersion objective

1. It suggests a problem with the slide or with the objective. First, check the slide to see whether it contains dirt. If so, clean it with benzol.

2. Check the objective, and if required, clean it properly.

3. Check for air bubbles in the specimen by holding the slide against the light.

Object not coming into focus despite fine adjustment

This happens when the fine adjustment screw reaches the end of the thread before the object is brought to focus. To correct this, turn back the fine adjustment screw in the reverse direction for several turns and then focus the object carefully with the coarse adjustment knob to find the focus. Finally, sharpen the focus by turning the fine adjustment knob.

Note: It is a good practice to keep the fine adjustment screw in the middle position. To check the position, turn the fine adjustment screw to either extreme end, then turn it back, counting each turn until the screw reaches the midpoint.

Oval field of view

Check if the objective is placed in the correct position. Note that whenever the objective is changed, it must click into position.

Routine Care and Maintenance of the Microscope

A microscope, if properly maintained, can be used for many years. Fungal growth and scratches (caused by dust particles) on the lens damage microscopes in a short time. The following points must be noted carefully for routine use of the microscope:

1. When transporting the microscope, carry it by holding the arm with one hand and supporting the base with the other.

2. When not in use, cover the microscope with a plastic dust cover. At the end of the day, blow off dust using an air syringe and store it in a warm, dry place. Avoid storing the microscope in its wooden box.

3. Remove oil from the oil-immersion objective immediately after use by wiping it with a clean lens paper.

4. Clean the eyepiece frequently because it is vulnerable to dirt since it is placed at the top of the microscope and usually comes in contact with the observer's eye. An air syringe can be used for this purpose.

5. Do not remove the eyepiece from the microscope for a long time; otherwise, dust will enter the body tube and get deposited on the rear lens of the objectives.

6. While working with the oil-immersion objective, do not pull out the specimen-slide from the stage without lowering the stage or swinging out the objective; the slide may scratch the objective. Also remember that you should not push the oil-immersion objective on the slide; it may damage both the slide and the objective.

7. While handling the fine and coarse adjustments to achieve focus, if the screws offer unusual resistance, do not use force to overcome it, as it may damage the screw and the pinion mechanism. It is better to contact the mechanic.

8. Before storing the microscope after work, clean the lenses.

Cleaning lenses

1. Never touch the lenses with your fingers.
2. Lenses are cleaned with special care to avoid dust scratches.
3. If the lens is taken out for cleaning (eyepiece or objective), keep it on a clean surface. Pull the eyepiece out from the tube while the objective is unscrewed from the nosepiece.
4. First, blow off the dust particles from the surface of the lens with the help of an air syringe or a rubber bulb or a paintbrush. Then, gently rub it with a clean lens paper.
5. While cleaning the lens, breathe on it through the mouth but do not clean it by spitting or blowing on it.
6. The oil-immersion objective requires proper cleaning. Use clean tissue paper for removing oil by repeated gentle rubbing on the surface. Move the cloth across and not circularly.

Note: Do not use organic solvents like ethanol and xylene frequently because the solvent may dissolve the cement holding the lens in the socket.

Other Types of Microscopes

Some microscopes are not routinely used in laboratories. They are designed for specific purposes and have some advantages over compound microscopes. They are based on different illumination systems—the character of light delivered to the specimen in different systems varies.

Dark-field microscope

A special condenser is used in this microscope, which allows light waves to pass across the specimen rather than through it. As a result, the field in view looks dark, as light does not pass from the condenser to the objective. When an object is placed on the stage, light that hits the object is deflected through the objective, creating an image that is viewed through the eyepiece. Thus, the object under study appears light against a dark background. This microscope is usually used in the microbiology laboratory to study spirochetes in exudates from **leptospiral or syphilitic infections**.

Fluorescence microscope

Certain compounds, when irradiated by light of short wavelengths (like ultraviolet light), absorb the radiation and re-emit light energy of a longer wavelength, i.e., visible light. This phenomenon is called **fluorescence**.

In a fluorescence microscope, the material in the specimen that fluoresces becomes visible. The fluorescence microscope is a dark-field microscope, which has been modified by incorporating two special filters. The condenser is preceded by an **exciter filter** that allows only light with shorter wavelengths to pass through the specimen. If the specimen contains an object that fluoresces, it absorbs the short wavelength light and emits light of a longer wavelength. The **barrier filter** placed in the microscope tube or eyepiece, filters only the wavelength of emitted light for the particular fluorescent system. The fluorescence microscope is usually used in **immunology laboratories to study fluorescent antibodies**.

Polarizing microscope

A polarizing microscope differs from an ordinary microscope in that it has two polarizing devices, a **polarizer and an analyzer**. The polarizer (the filter) absorbs light waves radiating in all directions and allows light waves from a particular direction to pass through the filter. The polarizer is usually placed between the light source and the specimen and the analyzer is placed between the objective and the eyepiece. The polarizer and the analyzer are rotated until the two are at right angles to each other. This causes the disappearance of light because light waves are cancelled when they are at right angles to each other. However, some objects have the property of **birefringence**, that is, the ability to rotate (polarize) light. These objects bend light and can be seen in this microscope, appearing bright against a dark background.

Phase-contrast microscope

An important property of light is its phase. If two light waves are completely in phase, they show interference; the resultant amplitude is greater, and brighter light is seen. When an object is seen without staining, the indirect waves passing through the object are retarded.

The principle of the phase-contrast microscope lies in further retardation of these indirect waves. This is achieved by inserting a phase plate within the objective lens. Since some diffracted light passes through the grooves of the plate, a halo appears around the object. The advantage of this microscope is that the cells or the organisms can be observed in wet preparations (without prior dehydration or staining).

As the name of the system indicates, the structures observed show added contrast compared to the bright-field microscope. The retardation of the speed of light makes the system sensitive to differences in refractive indices. Objects with different refractive indices show added differences in the intensity and shade of light passing through them. Therefore, one can observe unstained wet preparations with good resolution and detail. This microscope is used in hematology for counting platelets by using a direct method.

Interference-contrast microscope

This microscope yields a three-dimensional image of the object. A special beam-splitting prism is added to the condenser. The two split beams are then polarized; one passes through the specimen, altering the amplitude of the light wave, and the other (which serves as a reference) does not pass through the specimen. The two dissimilar light beams then pass separately through the objective and are recombined by a second prism. This recombination of light waves provides the three-dimensional image. It is very useful for wet preparations such as urinary sediments, showing finer details without the need for special staining.

Electron microscope

The electron microscope uses a beam of electrons instead of light rays. The magnified image is visible on a fluorescent screen and can be recorded on a photographic film. The magnification obtained is very high. It casts an image on the photographic plate at a magnification of about 5000 to 20,000× to be the same x as used in the next sentence. The negative is then enlarged to about 10 times, thus enabling a total magnification of about 120,000× or more. In this microscope, electromagnetic fields are used in place of lenses. This is usually used for the study of finer details of organisms, cells, or tissues.

OSPE

I.   Make microscopic adjustments for focusing a film under a low-power objective.

Steps
1.   Switch the mirror to its concave side.
2.   Slightly open the iris diaphragm.
3.   Bring the low-power objective into position.
4.   Use the fine adjustment screw for final focusing.
5.   Bring the condenser to its lowest position.
6.   Place the slide on the stage of the microscope.
7.   Make coarse adjustments to focus the image.

II.   Make microscopic adjustments for focusing a film under a high-power objective.

Steps
1.   Use the concave side of the mirror.
2.   Partially open the iris diaphragm.
3.   Bring the high-power objective into position.
4.   Use the fine adjustment screw for final focusing.
5.   Slightly raise the condenser.
6.   Place the slide on the stage of the microscope.
7.   Make coarse adjustments to focus the image.

Note: To achieve better focus under a high-power objective, it is better to first focus the film under a low-power objective.

III. Make microscopic adjustments for focusing a film under an oil-immersion objective.

Steps
1.   Switch the mirror to its plane side.
2.   Open the iris diaphragm fully.
3.   Place a drop of oil at the centre of the smear.
4.   Move the slide on the stage of the microscope to bring the centre of the slide under view so that the objective touches the oil.
5.   Make coarse adjustments to focus the image.
6.   Bring the condenser to its highest position.
7.   Bring the oil-immersion objective into position, so that the objective touches the oil.
8.   Use the fine adjustment screw for final focusing.

Note: To get the focus easily under an oil-immersion objective, it is better to examine the films first in low- and high-power objectives.

VIVA

1.   *Who invented the compound and simple microscopes?*

(**Ans.** The table below presents the names of the inventors and the year of the different types of microscopes.)

Year	Inventor	Microscope type	Magnification
1590–1595	Hans and Zacharias Janssen	Compound (bi-convex eyepiece/plano-convex objective)	3X to 9X
1609	Galileo Galilei	Compound (bi-concave eyepiece/bi-convex objective)	Up to 30X
Late 1600s	Robert Hooke/Christopher Cock	Compound (bi-convex eyepiece and objective with removable field lens)	Up to 50X
1676	Antonie van Leeuwenhoek	Simple microscope (single bi-convex lens)	70X to 275X

2. *What is the principle of microscopy?* (Ans. Refer to page 29, under the heading 'Method of Use...', Subheading 'Principle'.)

3. *What does the term 'resolution' mean?* (Ans. Refer to page 25, under the subheading 'Resolution'.)

4. *What is the use of the terms numerical aperture (NA) and working distance in microscopy?* (Ans. Refer to page 25, under the subheading 'Working Distance, NA'.)

5. *How are different adjustments made in the microscope while using different types of objectives?* (Ans. Refer to page 28, Table 5.2)

6. *What are the functions of the condenser and iris diaphragm?* (Ans. Refer to page 27, under the heading 'Condenser, Iris Diaphragm'.)

7. *How is the NA of objectives related to magnification?* (Ans. Refer to page 28, Table 5.1)

8. *Why is a special grade of oil (immersion oil) used in the oil-immersion objective?*
    (Ans. Immersion oil [cedarwood oil or liquid paraffin] is used to increase the NA and thereby, the resolving power of the objective. Light travels through air at a greater speed than through glass. Thus, to increase the effective NA of the objective, oil is used to slow down the speed at which light travels [the speed of light is measured in terms of the refractive index], increasing the gathering power of the lens and decreasing the diffraction of light rays. The refractive indices of air, glass, and immersion oil are 1.00, 1.515, and 1.515 respectively.)

9. *Why should the eyepiece, objective, and condenser lenses never be cleaned with paper tissue, gauze, or ordinary cloth?*
    (Ans. Optical lenses are softer than regular glass and can be scratched by abrasive materials like tissue, gauze, or cloth. For this reason, only lens paper should be used for cleaning. Before wiping, the surface of the lens should be checked to ensure that it is free of dust or particles that could scratch the glass; any dust that is present should be blown off gently with an air syringe.)

10. *Why should the oil be removed from the oil-immersion objective immediately after use?*
    (Ans. Oil is removed from the oil-immersion objective by wiping it with a clean lens paper immediately after use. If the oil is not removed, it may dry on the lens surface or seep inside, potentially damaging the objective.)

11. *What microscopic adjustments are made when the field of view is not clear?* (Ans. Refer to page 31, under the heading 'Common Difficulties in Microscopy, Inability to obtain clear image'.)

12. *What is the cause of dark shadows in the field of view, and how can this be prevented?* (Ans. Refer to page 31, under the heading 'Common Difficulties in Microscopy, Dark shadows'.)

13. *What microscopic adjustments are made if the image is not clear in the oil-immersion objective?* (Ans. Refer to page 31, under the heading 'Common Difficulties in Microscopy, Presence of unclear image....')

14. *What is the cause of an oval field of view and how do you correct it?* (Ans. Refer to page 31, under the heading 'Common Difficulties in Microscopy, point no. 6, Field of view'.)

15. *In microscopy, what does the term 'parfocal' mean?*
    (Ans. Parfocal means that once an image is focused under one objective, switching to another objective keeps the image nearly in focus. After focusing under low power, you can shift to high power or oil-immersion with minimal adjustment—usually, a full turn of the fine adjustment screw (about 1 micron) brings it into sharp focus.)

6 | Hemocytometry

Learning Objectives

After completing this practical, you will be able to (MUST KNOW):

1. Identify RBC and WBC pipettes.
2. Focus on the RBC and WBC squares of the Neubauer chamber using low-power and high-power objectives of the microscope.
3. Dilute blood appropriately using RBC and WBC pipettes.
4. List the precautions to take while diluting blood.
5. Charge the Neubauer chamber correctly.
6. List the precautions for charging the chamber.
7. Calculate the area and volume of RBC and WBC squares.

You may also be able to (DESIRABLE TO KNOW):

1. Explain possible sources of error during blood dilution in pipettes and their impact on results.

INTRODUCTION

The formed elements of blood are counted by hemocytometry. The apparatus used is called the **hemocytometer**, which consists of diluting pipettes and counting chambers. The procedures used for the enumeration of blood cells include the manual method of hemocytometry and the use of electronic counting devices. The cells counted in routine practice are red cells, white cells, and platelets.

Manual techniques lend themselves to the enumeration of all small separate bodies such as spermatozoa, eosinophils, and cells in the cerebrospinal fluid. In the manual method, the hemocytometer is used for counting, whereas in electronic methods, **automated electronic counting** devices are used. The electronic counting device bypasses the element of human error and is also statistically more accurate because it can count many more cells.

Units for Reporting

Since the enumerated constituents are reported in units per litre of blood, the number of cells actually counted must be converted to the number present per litre of blood. An alternative and more commonly used unit is **cells per cubic millimetre (mm³)** or **microlitre (µL)**, since 1 µl is essentially equal to 1 mm³. Though the report is usually expressed per cubic millimetre of blood, the reporting unit of choice is cells per litre of blood.

$1 \text{ mm}^3 = 1 \text{ µl} = 10^{-6} \text{ l}$

Therefore, $1 \text{ µl} \times 10^6 = 1 \text{ litre}$

METHODS

Hemocytometry involves two main steps: (i) **pipetting** – diluting blood in the pipette and (ii) **charging** – charging the Neubauer chamber with the diluted blood sample.

Pipetting

Principle

A measured unit of blood is diluted quantitatively with diluents using special measuring devices (pipettes).

Requirements

Pipettes

To ensure proper dilution of the sample to be used for counting blood cells, blood must be precisely measured and diluted with specially calibrated pipettes. Two types of pipettes are used for blood cell counts: RBC pipettes and WBC pipettes (Fig. 6.1). In hematology, a third type—the **hemoglobin pipette**—is used only for hemoglobin estimation, not for cell counting.

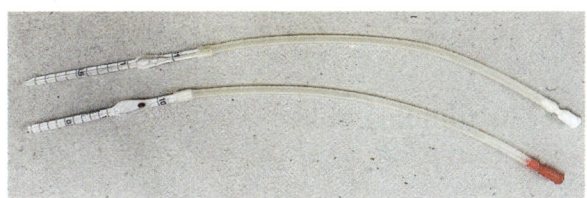

Fig. 6.1 RBC pipette and WBC pipette. Note that the RBC pipette has a red bead in the bulb and a red mouthpiece, and the WBC pipette has a white bead in the bulb and a white mouthpiece.

RBC pipette: This is used for counting red cells. It has a stem, bulb, rubber tube, and mouthpiece. The stem has two markings, 0.5 and 1. The **stem** widens into a **bulb** with a **red bead** in it (Fig. 6.2), which helps in identifying the pipette and mixing the fluid with blood in the bulb of the pipette. The capacity of the bulb is 100 parts (from the 1 to 101 mark). The bulb narrows above ('101' is marked just above the bulb); to this end, a rubber tube that ends in a mouthpiece is attached (Fig. 6.3). The mouthpiece is red in colour. As the lumen diameter in the stem of the RBC pipette is smaller than that of the WBC pipette, the RBC pipette is sometimes called a **slow-speed pipette.**

WBC pipette: This is used for counting white blood cells. It is similar to the RBC pipette except that the *capacity of the bulb is less* (10 parts) and the bulb contains a **white bead**. The mark above the bulb is '11' (Fig. 6.4). The **mouthpiece is white** in colour. In the WBC pipette, the lumen diameter of the stem is more than that of RBC pipettes (Table 6.1). Hence, the WBC pipette is sometimes called a **fast-speed pipette.**

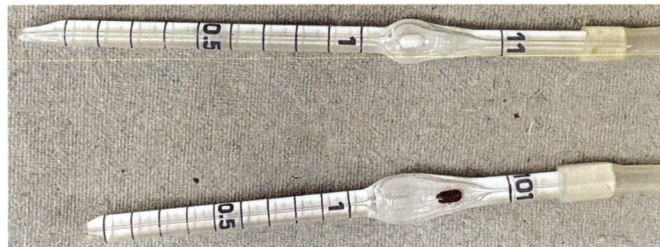

Fig. 6.2 The stem part of RBC pipette and WBC pipette. Note that the RBC pipette has a red bead in the bulb and a 101 mark after the upper part of the bulb, and the WBC pipette has a white bead in the bulb and a 11 mark after the upper part of the bulb.

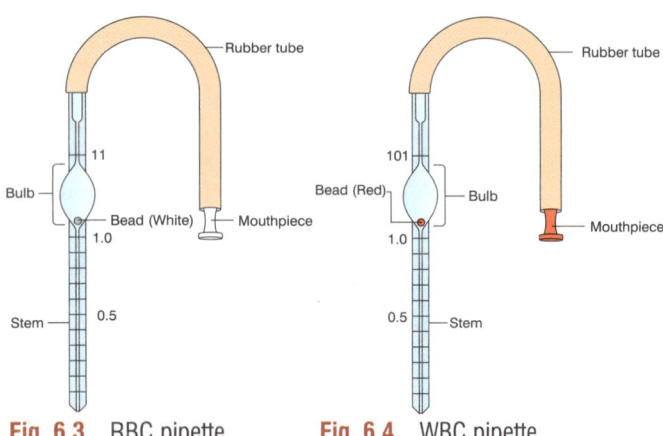

Fig. 6.3 RBC pipette.   **Fig. 6.4** WBC pipette.

Diluents (diluting fluids)

Different diluents are used depending on the cell type being counted. Each diluent is described in the chapters dealing with the respective cell count procedures.

Table 6.1 Differences between RBC and WBC pipettes.

	RBC pipette	WBC pipette
Calibrations	0.5 to 1.0 in the stem, 101 above the bulb	0.5 to 1.0 in the stem, 11 above the bulb
Bulb	Larger—capacity of 100 parts, contains red bead	Smaller—capacity of 10 parts, contains white bead
Mouthpiece	Red	White
Stem lumen diameter	Less	More
Dilution	0.5 in 100, or 1 in 200	0.5 in 10, or 1 in 20
Speed of flow of fluid	As the pipette is narrow and the diameter of the stem diameter is small, it takes time for a drop to form at the tip of the pipette at the time of charging (slow-speed pipette)	As the pipette is wider and the diameter of the stem diameter is larger, it takes less time for a drop to form at the tip at the time of charging (fast/high-speed pipette)

Procedure

1. Clean the pipette and ensure that it is dry.
2. Collect the diluting fluid in a watch glass from a stock bottle.
3. Prick the fingertip (as described in Chapter 2) after taking all aseptic precautions to obtain a free flow of blood.
4. Discard (wipe off) the first drop of blood.
5. Let a large drop of blood accumulate on the fingertip (Fig. 6.5).
6. Hold the pipette tilted at an angle of about 60° (Fig. 6.6) or horizontally (Fig. 6.7) and dip its tip into the drop of blood. Allow blood to enter into the pipette by capillary action or suck gently on the mouthpiece to draw blood up to the required mark (0.5) on the stem of the pipette. If more than the required amount of blood is drawn into the pipette, **tap it gently against a fingernail or palm or touch the tip with non-absorbent material keeping the pipette horizontal** to bring the blood to the desired 0.5 mark (Fig. 6.8).

Note: Do not blow out the extra blood or use absorbent materials like cotton wool to absorb excess blood.

7. Wipe off the tip of the pipette to remove the extra blood sticking to it.
8. Maintain the blood level at the 0.5 mark and place the tip of the pipette in the diluting fluid well below the surface of the liquid.

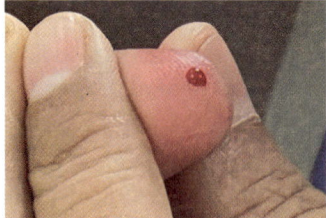

Fig. 6.5 Forming a drop of blood by pricking the tip of the finger.

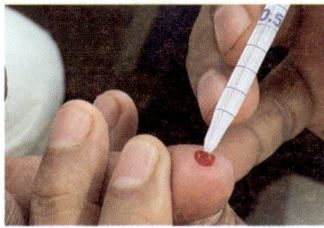

Fig. 6.6 Dipping the pipette into the blood drop from one side at an angle of about 60°.

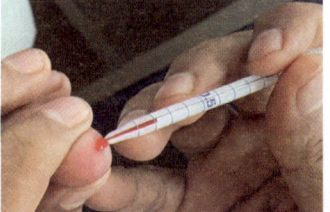

Fig. 6.7 Process of pipetting: when the pipette is held horizontally, blood usually enters into it by capillary action. If this does not happen automatically, blood may be gently sucked into the pipette.

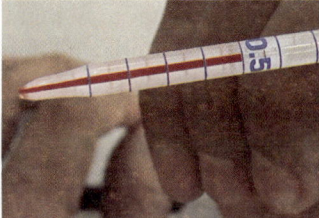

Fig. 6.8 Pipetting of blood exactly up to the 0.5 mark.

Note: Do not directly draw the diluting fluid from the stock bottle as it may contaminate the solution with the cells.

9. Using constant suction, draw the diluting fluid into the pipette (Fig. 6.9). Draw the mixture exactly to the top mark ('101' or '11') above the bulb. While the bulb is being filled, you may tap the pipette with a finger to knock the bead down below the surface of the solution in the bulb to prevent the formation of bubbles.

10. Maintain the level of the mixture exactly at the mark by closing the pipette tip with the index finger. Holding the pipette in the horizontal position is also important.

11. Mix the contents of the bulb thoroughly for 2–3 minutes by rotating the pipette with its tip pressing against the palm of the left hand (the rubber tube may be removed to facilitate mixing).

Note: The contents of the pipette may also be mixed by holding and rotating it between the palms. However, this involves some risk of leakage, especially if the pipette is not held horizontally.

12. Place the pipette on a horizontal surface. The pipette is now ready for charging.

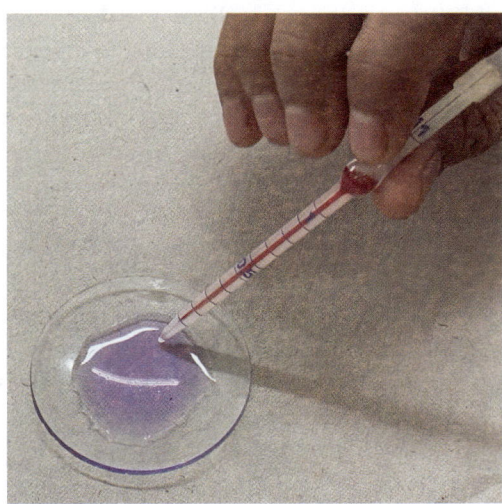

Fig. 6.9   Pipetting of diluting fluid into the bulb. Ensure that the tip of the pipette is inside the fluid; otherwise, air bubbles enter the pipette.

Precautions

Cell counts are performed by determining the number of cells in the diluted sample and converting the number of cells counted into the final result, i.e., the number of cells in 1 litre or in 1 ml of whole blood. Blood cell counts are performed on minute quantities taken from small samples of an individual's blood. Errors are inherent even in the best methods. Therefore, the steps in the procedure must be followed as carefully as possible to reduce the variation of the final result from the actual or true count.

1. Pipettes should be **clean, dry and without chipped or broken tips**.

2. The **puncture should be deep** enough for **free flow** of blood. The first drop should be discarded because it contains tissue fluid.

3. A **large drop of blood** should form on the fingertip to provide adequate blood to fill up to the 0.5 mark of the pipette at a time.

4. The tip of the **pipette should dip into the blood drop**, otherwise, while sucking blood into the pipette, air bubbles also enter along with blood.

5. Blood should be taken **exactly up to the 0.5 mark**. If blood is present above the mark, **absorbent material, such as gauze or cotton, should not be used** to adjust the blood level because these materials absorb the water content of the blood and cause blood to concentrate.

6. The **tip of the pipette should be wiped off**. Otherwise, the extra blood attached to the tip enters the pipette along with diluent when the diluting fluid is sucked in.

7. Blood in the pipette should be **diluted immediately**, otherwise it will clot.

8. Contaminated diluting fluids should not be used. **Blood should not be allowed to get into the diluent because this will affect subsequent cell counts with the same diluent**. Therefore, the diluent should not be drawn into the pipette directly from the bottle. Rather, the fluid should be taken in a watch glass from where it should be drawn into the pipette.

9. The tip of the pipette should **dip inside the diluting fluid** throughout the process of filling the bulb, otherwise air bubbles enter the pipette.

10. The upper dilution mark on the pipette **should not be exceeded by more than 1 mm**, and the mixture should not be corrected back to the top mark if overdiluted because this would cause the cells from the bulb to be forced to enter into the lower stem of the pipette.

11. If blood is to be used from a blood sample, the **preserved blood sample should not be hemolysed nor should it contain a fibrin clot**. It should be **mixed** (preferably by gentle shaking) before use.

Charging the Counting Chamber
Principle

A mixture of blood and diluting fluid is introduced onto the central platform of the counting chamber, beneath a coverslip.

Requirements

1. Counting chamber
2. Pipette containing the mixture
3. Coverslip

▉ Counting chamber

The counting chamber in common use is the **improved Neubauer chamber**. This chamber consists of a thick glass slide divided into two central platforms by an H-shaped groove (Fig. 6.10). The central platform is slightly lower than the sides, ensuring that when a coverslip is placed, it covers the central platform and rests on the side platforms.

The depth, i.e., the distance between the undersurface of the coverslip and the central platform is 1/10 mm (Fig. 6.11). When the chamber is charged with diluted blood, a thin film of fluid of known volume is spread on the central platform, and this is used for performing the cell counts.

The counting grid: On the central platforms are engraved ruled squares used for various cell counts. The ruled area on each central platform is called a **counting grid**.

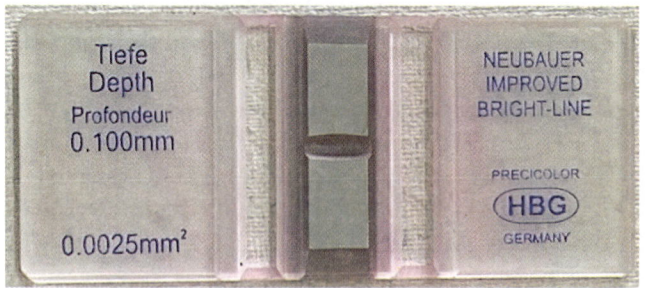

Fig. 6.10   Improved Neubauer chamber (Bright-line).

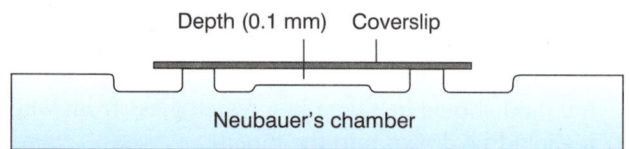

Fig. 6.11   Side view of Neubauer chamber showing the space between the undersurface of the coverslip and the surface of the platform (0.1 mm deep).

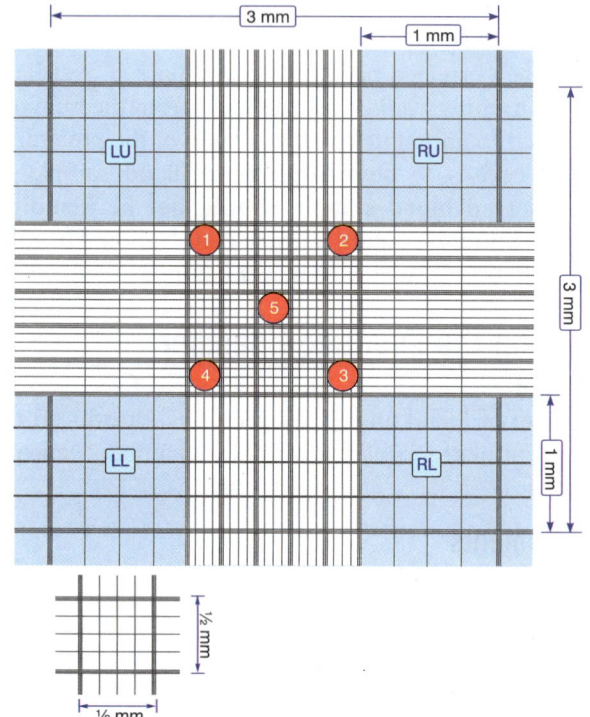

Fig. 6.12   Improved Neubauer's chamber (LU: left upper; RU: right upper; LL: left lower; RL: right lower WBC squares; 1, 2, 3, 4, and 5: RBC squares).

The ruled area is a square measuring 3 mm × 3 mm (Fig. 6.12). This area is divided into nine large squares, each having an area of 1 mm² (1 mm × 1 mm). The **four large corner squares are used for WBC count,** while the **large 1 mm square in the centre is used for RBC count**.

Each WBC square is further subdivided into 16 smaller squares, each measuring 1/16 mm². The 1 mm² central RBC square is divided into 25 medium-sized squares by means of triple lines (the Old Neubauer chamber has 16 medium-sized central squares). Each medium-sized square measures 1/5 mm in length and has an area of 1/5 × 1/5 = 1/25 mm². The medium-sized squares of the four corners and the central medium-sized square are used for the RBC count. The area of the five medium-sized squares is 1/25 × 5 = 1/5 mm². Since the depth of the chamber is 1/10 mm, the volume of the five medium-sized squares is 1/5 × 1/10 = 1/50 mm³ (Fig. 6.12).

Each medium-sized square is further divided into 16 small squares, that is, 25 × 16 = 400 small squares. The side of the smallest RBC square measures 1/20 mm. Therefore, the area of the smallest RBC square is 1/20 × 1/20 = 1/400 mm². Since the depth under the coverslip is 1/10 mm, the volume of the smallest RBC square is 1/400 × 1/10 = 1/4000 mm³. The red cells are counted in 80 small squares (5 medium-sized squares); the volume of 80 small-sized RBC squares is 1/4000 × 80 = 1/50 mm³.

Other counting chambers: These include the **Thoma chamber and Old Neubauer chambers**. Neither of these is currently used.

1. In the **Thoma chamber**, the central platform is depressed and circular. The grid is only 1 mm², consisting of 25 groups of 16 smaller squares each. The corner 1 mm squares are absent.

2. The **Old Neubauer chamber** has nine 1 mm squares. The four larger corner squares consisting of 16 squares each are meant for WBC counting, and the central 1 mm² area has 16 groups of 16 squares each, meant for RBC counting. In the improved Neubauer chamber, 25 groups of 16 smaller squares are available for RBC counting. However, in both the chambers, medium squares are separated by triple lines.

Procedure

1. Clean the Neubauer chamber and the coverslip.
2. Place the coverslip on the central platform of the chamber (Fig. 6.13).
3. Mix the contents of the pipette bulb thoroughly to ensure that the cells are well distributed/suspended in the fluid-cell mixture.

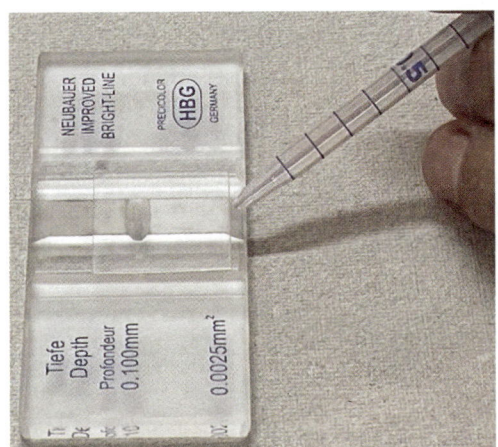

Fig. 6.13   Proper placement of the coverslip on the Neubauer chamber's central platform.

> **Note:** Cells in the bulb settle down in the lower part of the bulb in a short time. Therefore, mixing the contents of the pipette is an essential step to ensure proper cell-fluid mixing before charging.

4. Discard the first two drops of fluid from the pipette as it contains only the diluting fluid.
5. Place the tip of the pipette on the surface of the chamber touching the edge of the coverslip at an angle of 45°. Allow the diluted blood to flow under the coverslip by capillary action (Fig. 6.14A, B, C). Remove the pipette quickly from the edge of the coverslip as soon as the counting platform is filled with diluted blood. Take care to avoid the entry of air bubbles and fluid overflow into the gutters.

> **Note:** The mixture should completely cover the platform but should not enter the gutters (Fig. 6.15). If air bubbles enter the platform or fluid enters the gutters, discard the specimen and recharge.

6. Allow the cells to settle for 2–3 minutes before placing the charged chamber on the stage of the microscope for counting. Count the cells (red cells, white cells, platelets) as described in the relevant chapters.

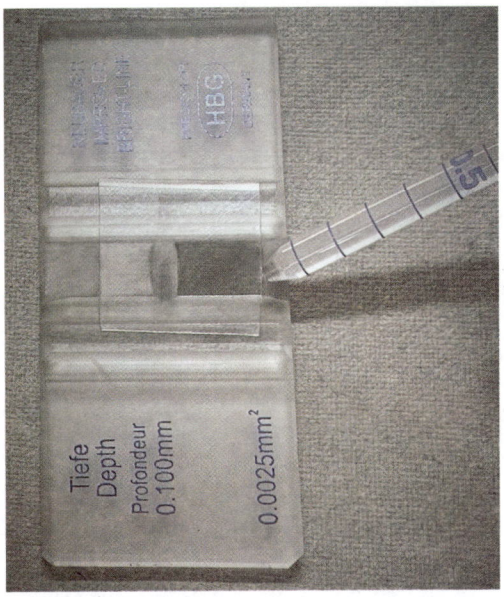

Fig. 6.15   Properly charged chamber—fluid remains on the platform without entering the gutters.

Precautions

1. The chamber and the coverslip should be properly cleaned.
2. The contents of the bulb must be thoroughly mixed before charging.
3. The first two drops of fluid must be discarded from the pipette before charging as the stem of the pipette contains only diluting fluid.
4. Air bubbles should not enter the platform of the chamber while charging.
5. The chamber should not be overcharged (fluid overflows into the gutters) or undercharged (fluid does not spread on the entire central platform). If the chamber is overcharged, the cells may enter the gutter and settle there, which gives false low results. If the chamber is undercharged, the cells may not be found in the peripheral squares (Fig. 6.16 A, B, and C).

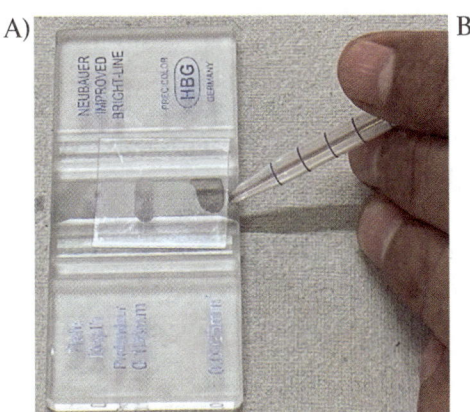 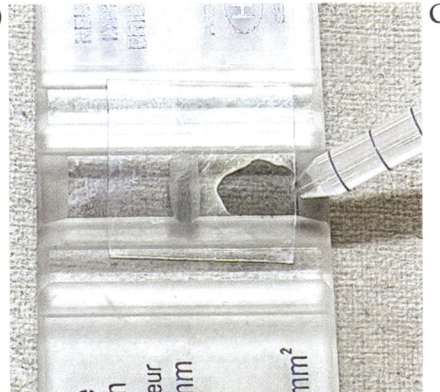 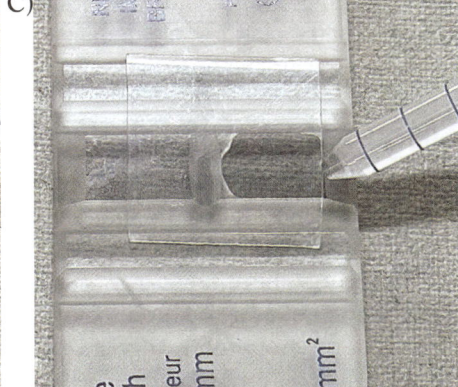

Fig. 6.14A, B, C   Charging (in progress) of the Neubauer chamber. The tip of the pipette is kept at the edge of the coverslip at a 45° angle, and the fluid from the pipette is released under control beneath the coverslip.

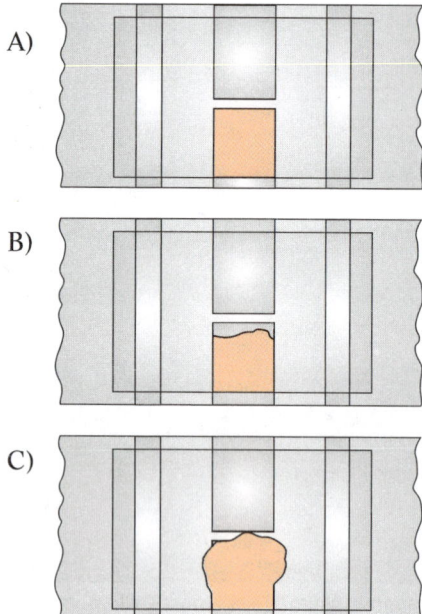

Fig. 6.16 Charging of Neubauer chamber (only the central part of the chamber is shown): (A) Normal (ideal) charging; (B) undercharging; (C) overcharging.

DISCUSSION

Students should practice pipetting and charging repeatedly. However, before learning this, they should learn to focus the RBC and WBC squares of the chamber under the low-power and high-power objectives of the microscope. While focusing the chamber, especially under the high-power objective, care should be taken not to break the chamber. In fact, the chamber should have been focused under the low-power microscope before charging, so that focusing becomes easy after charging.

Beginners would find it difficult to directly bring to focus a charged chamber. Therefore, they should first bring to focus the uncharged chamber to locate the desired squares and then take out the chamber from the stage of the microscope for charging without disturbing the setting of the microscope. After charging the chamber, they can place the charged chamber on the platform of the microscope and easily bring it into focus using the fine adjustment screws.

Sources of Error in Cell Counting

Errors in cell count could be due to: i) **pipetting error** (blood pipetted above or below the 0.5 marks), ii) **dilution error** (incorrect amount of diluent pipetted), iii) **charging/chamber error** (improper charging of the chamber), and iv) **counting/field error** (double counting or not following the L-pattern). Manual counting has an inherent **error of 5–7%**, particularly in the hands of students. Therefore, in practice, automated counters are preferred.

Automated Cell Counters

These advanced instruments provide accurate and efficient cell counting for high-volume lab use. These counters work on the principle of **electrical impedance** (**Coulter principle**), wherein cells suspended in a conductive fluid pass through a small aperture. Each cell causes a change in electrical resistance, allowing for precise counting.

Advantages
1. High-performance and fast
2. Accurate and precise
3. Removes subjectivity and variability
4. Time-saving with features like autosave, built-in calculators, and rapid capture

OSPE

I. Dilute the given sample of blood for RBC count.

Steps
1. Select an appropriate pipette and clean and dry it.
2. Take diluting fluid in a watch glass.
3. Shake the blood sample to mix it properly.
4. Place the tip of the pipette inside the blood sample or blood drop and suck blood exactly up to the 0.5 mark. If blood is sucked above the mark, adjust the level by tapping the tip of the pipette against a fingernail or by touching the tip of the pipette with non-absorbent material.
5. Wipe the tip of the pipette.
6. Maintaining the blood level at the 0.5 mark, place the tip of the pipette in the diluting fluid and suck fluid exactly up to the 101 mark. Take care to prevent the entry of air bubbles into the pipette.
7. Mix the contents of the bulb of the pipette by rotating the pipette with its tip pressed against the fingers.
8. Place the pipette on a horizontal surface.

II. Dilute the given sample of blood for WBC count.
1. Same as OSPE I except that the student uses the WBC pipette and WBC diluting fluid.

III. Charge the Neubauer chamber with the diluted blood from the supplied pipette.

Steps
1. Clean the Neubauer chamber and the coverslip.
2. Place the coverslip on the central platform of the chamber.
3. Mix the contents of the bulb thoroughly.
4. Discard the first two drops of fluid from the pipette.
5. Place the tip of the pipette on the surface of the chamber touching the edge of the coverslip at an

angle of 45° and allow the diluted blood to flow under the coverslip by capillary action.

6. Remove the pipette quickly from the edge of the coverslip as soon as the counting platform is filled with diluted blood. Take care to prevent overcharging or undercharging the chamber.

7. Place the charged chamber on a flat surface.

VIVA

1. *What are the uses of the hemocytometer in hematology?* (Ans. Refer to page 35, under the heading 'Introduction'.)

2. *How do you identify the RBC and WBC diluting pipettes?* (Ans. Refer to page 36, and Fig. 6.3 and 6.4.)

3. *What are the steps for diluting blood for various cell counts?* (Ans. Refer to page 36, under the heading 'Procedure'.)

4. *What are the precautions taken for pipetting?* (Ans. Refer to page 37, under the heading 'Precautions'.)

5. *How do you bring down the level of blood in the pipette if it exceeds the 0.5 mark?* (Ans. Refer to page 36, under the heading 'Procedure', point no. 6.)

6. *Why is the diluting fluid not sucked directly from the stock bottle?* (Ans. Refer to page 36, under the heading 'Procedure'; the note under point no. 8.)

7. *How do you prevent the entry of air bubbles into the pipette while diluting the blood?* (Ans. Refer to page 37, under the heading 'Procedure', point no. 9.)

8. *How do you calculate the area and volume of RBC and WBC squares?* (Ans. Refer to page 38, under the heading 'Counting Grid'.)

9. *What are the steps for charging the Neubauer chamber?* (Ans. Refer to page 38–39, under the heading 'Procedure'.)

10. *What are the precautions taken for charging the chamber with diluted blood?* (Ans. Refer to page 39, under the heading 'Precaution'.)

11. *Why are the contents of the bulb mixed thoroughly before charging?* (Ans. Refer to page 38, under the heading 'Procedure', point no. 3.)

12. *What are the functions of the bead in the bulb of the pipette?* (Ans. Refer to page 35, under the subheading 'RBC Pipette; see the description of 'bead'.)

13. *Why are the first two drops of fluid discarded from the pipette before charging?* (Ans. Refer to page 37, under the heading 'Precautions', point no. 3.)

14. *What do the terms overcharging and undercharging mean and what is their significance?* (Ans. Refer to page 39, under the heading 'Precautions', point no. 5 and Fig. 6.16.)

15. *For practising charging, why should a student preferably start with the RBC pipette and then move on to the WBC pipette?* (Ans. The RBC pipette has a narrower stem and releases drops slowly [slow-speed pipette], giving a beginner more time to release fluid from the pipette into the chamber. The WBC pipette, with a wider stem, releases drops more quickly and may cause spillage in unskilled hands [fast-speed pipette].)

16. *What are the differences between RBC and WBC pipettes?* (Ans. Refer to page 36, and Table 6.1.)

17. *Explain the principle and advantages of automated cell counters.* (Ans. Refer to page 40, under the heading 'Automated Cell Counters'.)

18. *Can pipettes be used for counting purposes other than their respective cell counts?* (Ans. The RBC pipette can be used for platelet and WBC counts [very high in leukemia] and the WBC pipette can be used for counting spermatozoa in semen.)

7 | Total RBC Count

Learning Objectives

After completing this practical, you will be able to (MUST KNOW):

1. Explain the significance of performing an RBC count in practical physiology.
2. Identify the RBC diluting pipette.
3. Accurately draw blood up to the 0.5 mark of the pipette.
4. Properly dilute the blood using the appropriate diluting fluid.
5. Load (charge) the Neubauer counting chamber.
6. Perform a manual RBC count.
7. Calculate the total RBC count and express the result in cells/mm³ of blood.
8. Enumerate the precautions necessary for conducting an accurate RBC count.
9. Describe the composition and function of each constituent of the RBC diluting fluid.
10. Outline the steps and regulatory mechanisms involved in red cell production.
11. List the physiological functions of red blood cells.
12. State the normal RBC count values in adults.
13. Define polycythemia and anemia.
14. Identify common causes of alterations in RBC count.

You may also be able to (DESIRABLE TO KNOW):

1. Name other RBC diluting fluids, their composition, and advantages.
2. Explain the principles of automated RBC counting methods.
3. Classify different types of polycythemia and anemia.
4. Discuss the physiological basis for variations in RBC count under different conditions.
5. Describe the stages and regulatory mechanisms of erythropoiesis.
6. Explain the causes and underlying mechanisms of polycythemia and anemia.

PY2.11: Estimate Hb, RBC, TLC, RBC indices, DLC, blood groups, and BT/CT.

INTRODUCTION

The human red blood cell (erythrocyte) is normally a circular, non-nucleated, biconcave disc that contains hemoglobin. The surface area of the red cell is much greater than that of a sphere of the same size. Thus the **exchange of oxygen and carbon dioxide is maximal** with the **biconcave configuration**. This shape also helps it *to withstand osmotic lysis* and to *easily pass through narrow capillaries*.

Red Cell Dimensions

Shape: Biconcave disc
Size: 7.5 (7 to 8) μm in diameter
Thickness: 2.0 μm
Surface area: 140 μm²

Formation of Red Blood Cells

The development of red cells is known as **erythropoiesis**. In postnatal life, this process occurs primarily in the bone marrow. During fetal life, erythropoiesis occurs in the spleen, liver, thymus, and bone marrow. In children, cells are produced in the marrow cavities of all the bones. By the age of 20, the marrow in the cavities of the long bones, except for the upper humerus and femur, becomes inactive. The **active cellular marrow** is called the **red marrow**; the **inactive marrow** that is infiltrated with fat is called the **yellow marrow**.

The stages of erythropoiesis are presented in Fig. 7.1.

As the cell matures in the bone marrow, its diameter decreases and the nucleus becomes denser and smaller and finally disappears from the cell. Meanwhile, the hemoglobin concentration increases, and the cytoplasm progressively changes from blue to orange on a stained blood film. The entire sequence of maturation from the early precursor to a circulating red cell takes **3–5 days**.

Erythropoiesis is subject to **feedback control**. It is inhibited by a rise in the circulating red cells and is stimulated by a decreased red cell count. This alteration is mediated by a number of factors that influence the secretion of **erythropoietin**, a hormone secreted by the kidney. **Interleukins (IL1, IL3, IL6) and GM-CSF** also affect the development of red cells.

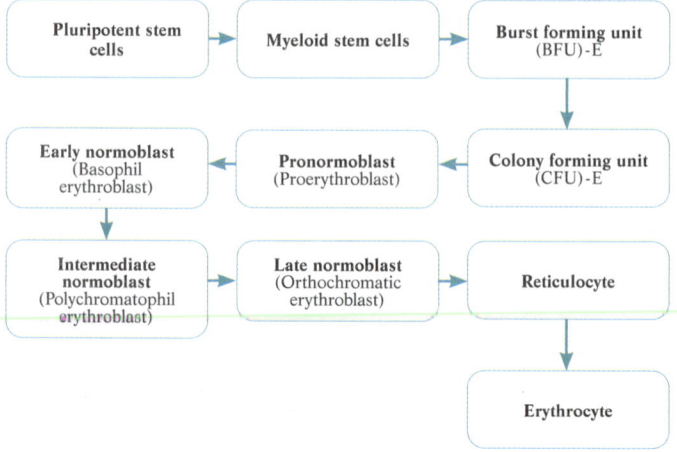

Fig. 7.1 The stages of erythropoiesis.

Functions of RBCs

The chief function of RBCs is to **carry oxygen from the lungs to the tissues of the body and carbon dioxide from the tissues to the lungs**. Red cells contribute to **blood viscosity** and thereby, to the peripheral resistance of blood. The viscosity of blood is low in anemia and high in polycythemia.

Lifespan and Fate of RBCs

The average lifespan of red cells is about **120 days**. The bone marrow releases new red cells into circulation every day. The dead red cells are broken down by the reticuloendothelial system. The globin part of Hb is broken down into amino acids, which are returned to the protein storage pool of the body. They are also essential for the retention and reuse or storage, to be recycled for hemoglobin synthesis.

Normal RBC Count

1. **Males**: 5.2 million/mm³ of blood (range: 4.5–6.0 million/mm³)
2. **Females**: 4.7 million/mm³ of blood (range: 4.0–5.5 million/mm³)

The RBC count is highest in newborns (6–8 million per mm³ of blood). The count rapidly decreases thereafter and is lowest at about two to four months of life (3–4 million per mm³). The count slowly increases from one year of life to reach 5 million per mm³ at about ten years.

METHODS OF COUNTING RBCs

Red cells are counted by two methods: **manual (non-automated)** and **automated.** Manual cell counting is less accurate but is still widely used in developing countries since automated counting is expensive.

Manual Method
Principle
The blood specimen is diluted (usually 200 times) with the diluting fluid, which does not remove white cells but allows red cells to be counted in a known volume of fluid. Finally, the number of cells in undiluted blood is calculated and reported as the number of red cells per mm³ of whole blood.

Requirements
▌Apparatus
1. Microscope
2. Hemocytometer (RBC diluting pipette and counting chamber)
3. Equipment for sterile finger prick
4. Watch glass
5. Coverslip

▌RBC diluting fluid
The red cell diluting fluid is isotonic and, therefore, prevents hemolysis. Of the different diluting fluids used for red cell count, the **most frequently used is Hayem's fluid**.

1. Hayem's fluid
- **Sodium chloride**: 0.5 g—maintains osmolarity
- **Sodium sulphate**: 2.5 g—prevents aggregation of RBCs
- **Mercuric chloride**: 0.25 g—acts as a preservative (it is antifungal and antibacterial)
- **Distilled water**: 100 ml—acts as a solvent
  Dissolve thoroughly in a beaker with a stirrer.

2. Dacie's fluid
This is an alternative to Hayem's fluid.
- Trisodium citrate: 3.13 g
- Commercial formaldehyde (37% formalin): 1.0 ml (**Caution:** Formaldehyde is corrosive and should be handled with care.)
- Distilled water: 100 ml
  Dissolve thoroughly with a stirrer, in a beaker.
  Dacie's fluid is preferred in some laboratories because of the following advantages:
- Simple preparation
- Long shelf-life without sterilisation
- Red cells retain their morphology and do not agglutinate
- Since cells are well-preserved, counts may be performed several hours after the blood has been diluted

3. Isotonic saline
If the above two diluting fluids are not available, isotonic saline may be used. Counting should be done immediately after dilution because isotonic saline does not contain any agent to prevent the aggregation of red cells.

Procedure
1. Assemble all the required equipment and ensure that the pipettes, coverslip, and Neubauer chamber are thoroughly clean and dry.
2. Pour an adequate amount of RBC diluting fluid into a watch glass.
3. Prick the finger under aseptic conditions (as described in Chapter 3) to make a medium-sized blood drop (Fig. 7.4) and suck blood into the pipette (see Chapter 6, Fig. 6.6–6.8) and dilute it following the step-by-step procedure of pipetting described in Chapter 6.
4. Hold the pipette horizontally and close both ends. Then, gently mix the contents of the bulb. For mixing, shake the pipette at right angles to its long axis for a few seconds. The red bead in the pipette should move from one side to the other during the mixing.

5. After mixing, keep the pipette in a horizontal position to prevent any loss of its contents until the cell count is performed.
6. Discard the first two drops of fluid from the pipette.
7. Charge the Neubauer chamber as described in Chapter 6 (refer to Fig. 6.13–6.15) and allow two minutes for the cells to settle.
8. Place the charged chamber on the stage of the microscope and adjust the microscope for observation under low power.
9. Focus the central square of the Neubauer chamber under the low-power objective, and check for uniform distribution of cells. If the cells are not uniformly distributed (Fig. 7.2), clean the Neubauer chamber and recharge it.
10. Focus the RBC squares under the high-power objective. Count the cells in five medium RBC squares in sequence as described in Fig. 7.3A (four corner squares and the central medium-sized RBC squares) i.e., 16 × 5 = 80 small RBC squares.

> **Note:** Care should be taken not to count the same cells again. To avoid this, the **rules of counting** should be followed: the red cells present in the square and on its left and lower lines are counted, and those on its right and upper lines are ignored. This is called '**L pattern' counting** (Fig. 7.3B). However, the 'inverted L pattern' can also be followed: counting cells present on the left and upper lines of the square and avoiding those present on the right and lower lines.
> Only one pattern should be followed for the entire count (not a combination of the two). Ideally, the same method should be practised by all the students in a class to maintain uniformity and avoid confusion.

11. Draw the RBC squares in your notebook and enter the observation. Calculate the final result.

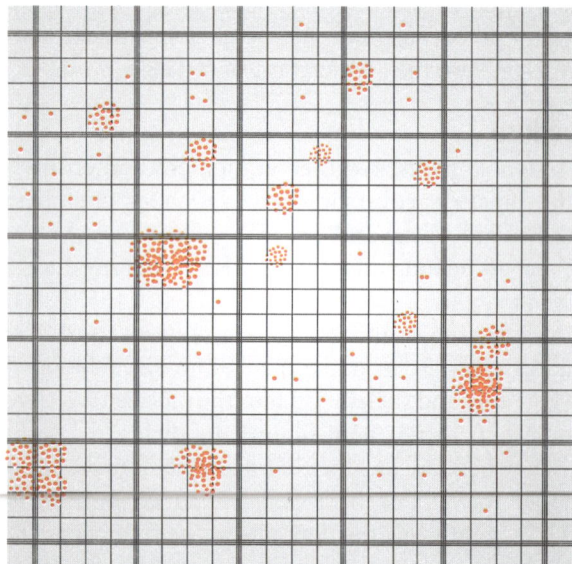

Fig. 7.2 Non-uniform distribution of red cells (as seen under low power). Note that cells are clumped in a few places and sparse in other places.

Dilution obtained

The volume in the bulb is 100 (101 − 1 = 100). The stem of the pipette (from the tip of the pipette to mark 1) contains diluting fluid that does not participate in dilution. Dilution (mixing of blood with diluting fluid) occurs only in the bulb. Thus, 100 volumes of diluted blood (in the bulb) contain 0.5 volumes of blood and 99.5 volumes of diluting fluid, resulting in a dilution of 0.5 in 100. Therefore, the dilution obtained is 1 in 200 or 200 times.

Calculation

Area of 5 medium squares = $(1/25) \times 5 = 1/5$ mm²

Volume of 5 medium squares = $(1/5) \times (1/10)$
$$= 1/50 \text{ mm}^3$$
$$(\text{depth is } 1/10 \text{ mm})$$

Dilution factor = 1:200

Let us say the cells in $1/50$ mm³ volume of diluted blood is n. Therefore, cells in 1 mm³ volume of diluted blood $= n \times 50$

Therefore, cells in 1 mm³ volume of undiluted blood $= n \times 50 \times 200 = n \times 10,000$

Where n is the total number of cells counted in 5 medium-sized RBC squares.

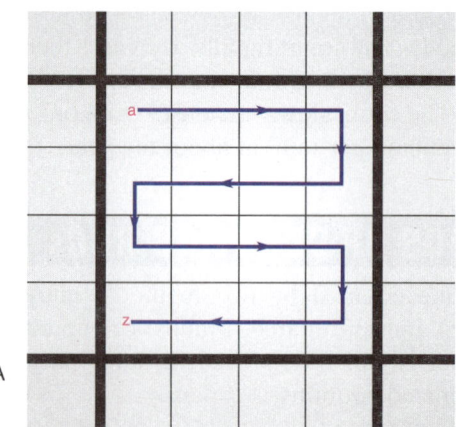

A

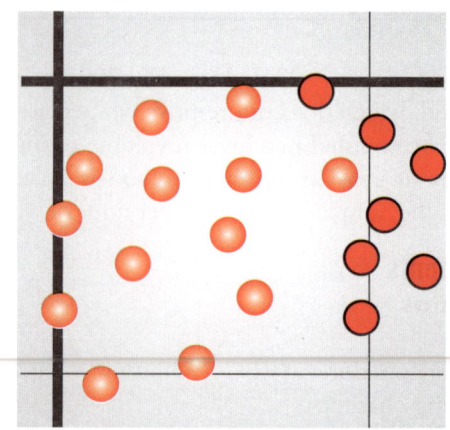

B

Fig. 7.3 Pattern of counting red cells in a medium RBC square: **(A)** direction of counting as indicated by arrows and **(B)** cells to be counted as shown in a small square.

Precautions

1. The pipette, coverslip, and Neubauer chamber should be thoroughly clean and dry.
2. The puncture should be deep enough to allow spontaneous flow of blood (refer to Fig. 6.5, Chapter 6). The finger should not be squeezed, as doing so expresses tissue fluid.
3. If blood is taken from a sample, it should be mixed properly prior to pipetting.
4. The first drop of blood should be wiped off as it is mixed with tissue fluid.
5. The tip of the pipette should gently touch the blood drop (Fig. 7.4), and blood should be drawn exactly up to the 0.5 mark (Fig. 7.5). The blood column (from the tip of the pipette to the 0.5 mark) should not be fragmented, nor should it contain air bubbles. If blood is drawn above the mark, the pipette is gently tapped against the fingertip or nail bed to bring the blood to the required level.
6. Absorbent material should never be used for this purpose as it absorbs water from blood and makes it more concentrated.
7. The tip of the pipette should always be wiped clean before diluting the blood. This should always be done; otherwise, the extra blood sticking to the tip of the pipette will be sucked into the bulb along with the diluting fluid, resulting in a falsely high result.
8. Blood in the pipette should be diluted quickly but steadily (Fig. 7.6) to avoid the formation of blood clots in the pipette.
9. The RBC diluting fluid should be sucked exactly up to the 101 mark. If the fluid is drawn much above the mark (more than 1 mm), it should not be adjusted back to the mark as it forces cells in the bulb to enter into the stem of the pipette. This affects the dilution and cell concentration in the bulb. It is better to discard the contents of the pipette, clean it, and restart the procedure.

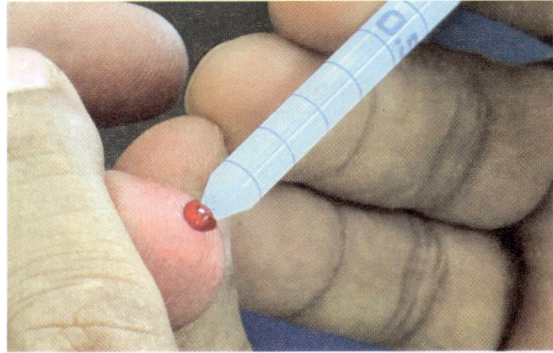

Fig. 7.4 Obtaining a medium-sized blood drop for RBC count by finger pricking. The tip of the pipette should gently touch the drop from the side.

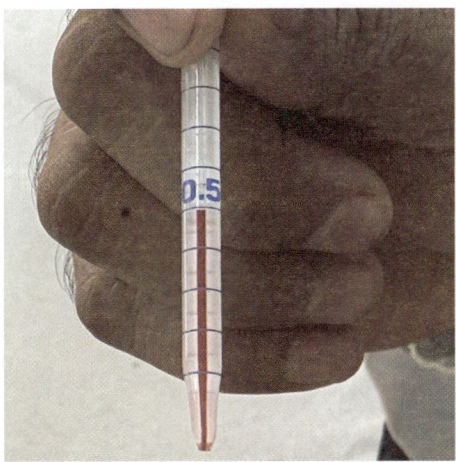

Fig. 7.5 Pipetting of blood exactly up to the 0.5 mark in the stem of the RBC pipette.

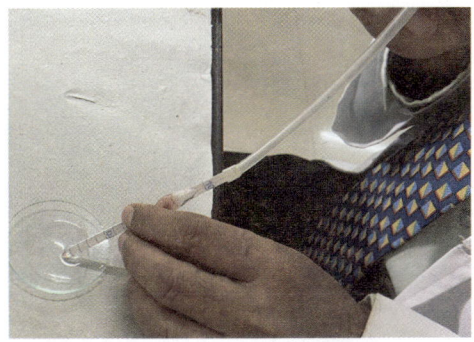

Fig. 7.6 Dilute the blood in the pipette quickly but steadily to avoid clotting in the pipette.

10. Before charging the chamber, the contents of the bulb are gently mixed.
11. The first two drops of fluid are discarded as the fluid in the stem does not contain cells.
12. The chamber should neither be overcharged nor undercharged. If it is overcharged, the contents should be discarded, the chamber cleaned and then recharged.
13. If the distribution of cells is not uniform, the contents should be discarded and the chamber recharged.
14. The same cells should not be counted twice. This can be ensured by following the rules of counting.

Observation and results

1. Draw the five medium-sized RBC squares in your notebook as shown below and enter the number of cells counted in each medium square containing 16 small squares (refer to Fig. 6.12, Chapter 6, for the orientation of the RBC squares).
2. Total the number of cells counted. This is expressed as n.
3. Calculate the final result using the formula: $n \times 10,000 =$ _____ .
4. Report your results as follows: "The total RBC count of the given blood sample is _____/mm³ of blood."

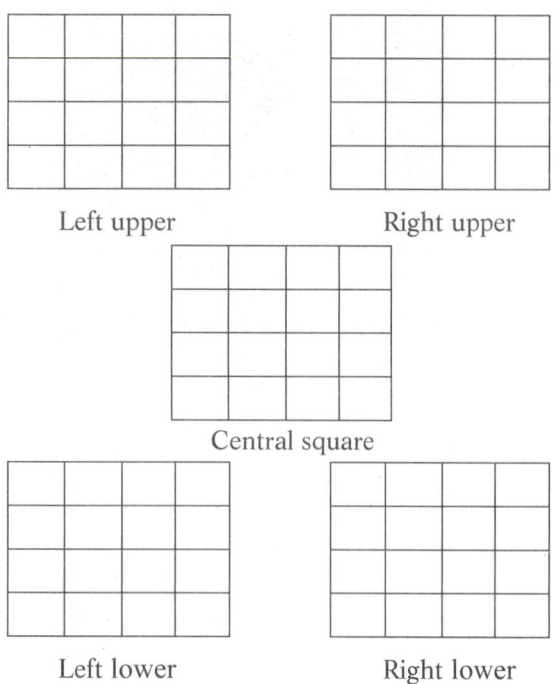

Left upper   Right upper

Central square

Left lower   Right lower

Sources of error

The margin of error in manual total RBC counting is 15–30%. This can be reduced by counting more cells. Errors are categorised as **inherent and technical**.

Errors inherent in the method

1. **Error of visual red cell count:** Errors decrease with with an increase in the total number of cells counted. Both sides of the Neubauer chamber can be charged, and counting can be performed on both chambers. The average of the two counts can be taken for the final calculation. This decreases the error.
2. **Error due to distribution of cells** Distribution can never be perfectly uniform even with near-perfect mixing and charging. This gives rise to errors.

Technical errors

1. **Dilution error:** Inaccurate volume measurement of blood or diluent.
2. **Pipette error:** Use of defective pipettes (e.g., with incorrect markings or improper bulb size).
3. **Chamber error**: Defective Neubauer chambers (e.g., inaccurate grid or depth).
4. **Charging error**: Improper charging (overcharging or undercharging) of the Neubauer chamber.
5. **Counting error**: Improper counting (missing some cells while counting or counting some cells twice).
6. **Calculation error:** Errors in calculation.

Automated Methods

There are two automated methods: **(i) impedance counting and (ii) light scattering technology**. As these methods are not usually practised in laboratories in Indian medical colleges, only their basic principles are described here.

Impedance counting

First described by Wallace Coulter in 1956, this method is based on the principle that red blood cells are poor conductors of electricity, whereas certain electrolytic diluents conduct electricity well.

Blood is highly diluted in a buffered electrolyte solution. An external vacuum initiates the movement of a mercury siphon, which causes a large volume of the sample to flow through an aperture tube of specific dimensions. By means of a constant source of electricity, a direct current is maintained between two electrodes, one in the sample beaker or the chamber surrounding the aperture tube, and the other inside the aperture tube. When a blood cell passes through the aperture, it displaces some of the conducting fluid and increases the electrical resistance. This produces a corresponding change in potential between the electrodes, which lasts as long as the red cells pass through the aperture. **The height of the pulses produced indicates the volume of the cells passing through.** The pulses are displayed on an oscillograph screen.

Light scattering technology

Red cells are counted by means of electro-optical detectors. A diluted cell suspension flows through an aperture so that the cells pass by a light source in a single file, scattering light. This scattered light is detected by a **photomultiplier or photodiode**, which converts it into **electrical impulses that are then accumulated and counted**. The amount of light scattered is proportional to the surface area and, therefore, the volume of the cells, so that the height of the electrical pulses can be used to estimate the cell volume.

DISCUSSION

Clinical Significance

The total RBC count is performed to assess the red cell mass in blood. Changes in erythrocyte number are frequently detected in clinical practice by ordering the estimation of hemoglobin rather than total RBC count because the estimation of hemoglobin is **easy and relatively inexpensive**. Moreover, the total RBC count by the **manual method is likely to be erroneous** (>20 per cent). The total RBC count is still performed in some conditions to detect the red cell population, especially if the count is expected to be very high, as in **polycythemia**.

Conditions That Alter Total RBC Count

Conditions that decrease RBC count

Physiological

1. Pregnancy (due to hemodilution).
2. Lower counts in children than in adults.
3. Women have lower RBC counts than men. The count is higher in men because male sex hormones stimulate erythropoiesis. It is lower in women because **estrogen inhibits erythropoiesis**, and there is cyclical loss of blood during the reproductive years.

Pathological

1. Different types of anemia.
2. Relative decrease in RBC count occurs in different pathological conditions that produce hemodilution, e.g., excess ADH secretion as occurs in posterior pituitary tumours.

Conditions that increase RBC count

Physiological

1. High altitude (due to hypoxia).
2. Newborns have high RBC counts.
3. Excessive sweating (due to hemoconcentration).

Pathological

1. Conditions that produce hemoconcentration (due to loss of body fluid), for example, severe diarrhea, and vomiting.
2. Conditions that produce chronic hypoxia, for example, congenital heart disease and emphysema.
3. Polycythemia vera.

Polycythemia

The term polycythemia, strictly speaking, implies elevated levels of all the cellular elements of blood, though it is usually used to describe an increase in the red cell count alone. Polycythemia may result from an increase in the total number of red cells in the body (**true polycythemia**) or from a reduction in the plasma volume relative to the volume of the red cells (**relative polycythemia**). True polycythemia may be due to a primary disorder of the hemopoietic tissue which produces an excess of red cells (**polycythemia vera**) or may be secondary to excessive stimulation of erythropoiesis by erythropoietin (**secondary polycythemia**).

Causes of polycythemia

I. True polycythemia
    1. Polycythemia vera
    2. Secondary polycythemia
        a. Secondary to tissue hypoxia
           i. High altitude
           ii. Congenital heart disease
           iii. Chronic pulmonary disease
        b. Secondary to inappropriately increased erythropoietin production
           i. Kidney tumours
           ii. Liver tumours
           iii. Pheochromocytoma
           iv. Virilizing ovarian tumour
II. Relative polycythemia
    1. Dehydration
    2. Redistribution of body fluids

Anemia

A decrease in RBC number or hemoglobin content below normal levels is known as anemia (refer to Chapter 3 for details).

OSPE

I. Dilute blood (from the given sample) for total RBC count.

Steps

1. Select the appropriate RBC pipette and ensure that it is clean and dry.
2. Mix blood thoroughly.
3. Pipette blood exactly up to the 0.5 mark.
4. If blood is drawn above the mark, remove the extra blood by tapping the pipette with a fingernail (not with absorbent material).
5. Wipe the tip of the pipette.
6. Suck diluting fluid up to the 101 mark. While drawing the fluid, avoid the entry of air bubbles.
7. Gently mix the contents of the bulb and place the pipette horizontally on the table.

II. Charge the Neubauer chamber for total RBC count.

Steps

1. Clean the coverslip and Neubauer chamber.
2. Place the coverslip on the platform of the Neubauer chamber.
3. Mix the contents of the bulb of the RBC pipette.
4. Discard the first two drops of the fluid from the pipette.
5. Touch the tip of the pipette at the edge of the coverslip.
6. Slowly release fluid from the pipette (fluid moves by capillary action) in such a way that the fluid spreads just beneath the coverslip and does not spill into the gutters or contain air bubbles.

VIVA

1. *Explain the composition and function of each component of Hayem's fluid. What other fluid can be used as a RBC diluting fluid?* (Ans. Refer to page 43, under the subheading 'Hayem's Fluid'.)
2. *What are the advantages of using Dacie's diluting fluid?* (Ans. Refer to page 43 under the subheading 'Dacie's Fluid'.)
3. *What are the precautions to be taken while performing an RBC count?* (Ans. Refer to page 45, under the heading 'Precautions'.)
4. *What are the functions of the red bead in the bulb of the pipette?*
    (Ans. The red bead has two functions—it helps in mixing the contents of the bulb and helps in the identification of the RBC pipette.)
5. *What is the significance of the different markings present on the RBC pipette?*
    (Ans. There are three markings on the RBC pipette: 0.5, 1, and 101. The 0.5 mark is the mark up to which blood is sucked. The 101 mark is the mark up to which the diluting fluid is sucked to obtain a dilution of 1 in 200. In cases of polycythemia, dilution may have to be increased, and in case of anemia, dilution may have to be decreased. The 1 mark is used for pipetting blood in conditions of severe anemia where more blood is taken for dilution. In such conditions, blood is sucked up to the 1 mark and then diluted up to the 101 mark to achieve a dilution of 1 in 100.)
6. *When is the RBC pipette used for white cell counting? What are the other uses of the RBC pipette?*
    (Ans. An RBC pipette is used for counting WBCs in cases of leukemia, wherein leucocytes are counted not in thousands but in lakhs or millions per mm^3 of blood. In leukemia, blood is sucked up to mark 1 in the RBC pipette and then diluted to the 101 mark, producing a dilution of 1 in 100. The RBC pipette is also used for sperm counts and platelet counts.)
7. *Why are the first two drops of the solution from the pipette discarded before charging the Neubauer chamber?* (Ans. Refer to page 45, under the heading 'Precautions, see point no. 11'.)
8. *Why is the dilution obtained 1 in 200, not 1 in 202?* (Ans. Refer to page 44 under the heading 'Dilution Obtained'.)
9. *What are the sources of error in RBC count?* (Ans. Refer to page 45, under the heading 'Sources of Error'.)
10. *What happens to WBCs in the RBC count?*
    (Ans. WBCs are not lysed by the diluting fluid, so they remain visible during the count. However, they don't affect the RBC count because they are very few in number compared to RBCs [about 1 WBC per 700 RBCs]. Since fewer than 700 RBCs are usually counted, WBCs are rarely present in the counting area.)
11. *How do you remove a blood clot from the pipette?*
    (Ans. First, the clot is dissolved and removed using a strong acid or H_2O_2. Then, the pipette is cleaned with distilled water. The pipette can be rinsed with alcohol or ether for rapid drying.)
12. *Explain the function of the coverslip for charging and counting.*
    (Ans. The coverslip, due to its flat and smooth surface, facilitates the uniform spread of diluted blood in the chamber beneath. By surface tension, it holds the diluted blood on the platform and prevents its spillage into the gutter, unless overcharged.)
13. *Should both sides of the chamber be charged? Why?* (Ans. Preferably yes. If cell distribution is uneven or counting on one side fails, the other side can be used. Counting on both sides also improves accuracy. Simultaneously charging both sides ensures balance and uniform depth.)
14. *How do you differentiate red cells from debris or dust particles?*
    (Ans. Debris is irregular in shape and size. Dust particles may be attached to eye piece, objective or present in the diluent. If attached to eye piece, they rotate with the rotation of eye piece. They are irregular in shape and size. Red cells are round and uniformly shaped, with a central halo-like appearance due to the thinness of that area. RBC counting is done using high-power objective to distinguish between red cells and debris/dust particles.)
15. *Why should the rules of counting be followed?*
    (Ans. The rules of counting are followed to avoid counting the same cell twice. Either the 'L' [count the red cells present in the square and those present on its left and lower lines and ignore those on its right and upper lines] or 'inverted L' pattern [count cells on the left and upper lines and ignore those on the right and lower lines of the square] should be used consistently, not a combination of the two.)
16. *What are the values of normal red cell count in adults and why is there a difference between the sexes?* (Ans. Refer to page 46, under the heading 'Conditions that decrease RBC Count - Physiological, see point no 3'.)
17. *What are the functions of red cells?* (Ans. Refer to page 43, under the heading 'Functions of Red Cells'.)
18. *Explain proper charging, overcharging, and undercharging.* (Ans. Refer to Chapter 6, page 39, under the heading 'Precautions, point no. 5'.)
19. *Why should a chipped coverslip never be used?*
    (Ans. A chipped or broken coverslip doesn't cover the chamber evenly, leading to improper distribution of cells.)

20. *Why are both sides of the Neubauer chamber charged?*

(Ans. **i.** Ensures uniform coverslip placement; **ii.** reduces counting errors; **iii.** allows result comparison between sides; **iv.** opposite side can be used for TLC with WBC fluid.)

21. *Why is it difficult to see the grid lines and cells at the same focus?*

(Ans. Grid lines and cells lie at different levels in the 0.1 mm space, requiring fine focus adjustment to view both clearly.)

22. *Can red cells be counted under low power?*

(Ans. Yes, by experienced observers. But students should use high power.)

23. *What are the sites of red cell formation before and after birth?*

(Ans. **Before birth:**

- Mesoblastic stage: In yolk sac mesoderm [intravascular].
- Hepatic stage: From 3rd month, the liver and spleen are the main sites.
- Myeloid stage: From the 5th month, the bone marrow becomes the primary site.

After birth:

- Initially in all bone marrows.
- By age 20, active in flat bones and ends of long bones.
- Under increased demand, the liver and spleen may resume production [extramedullary hematopoiesis].)

24. *What are the stages of erythropoiesis?* (Ans. Refer to page 42, under the heading 'Formations – see the Flowchart'.)

25. *What are the factors that regulate erythropoiesis?*

(Ans. The factors involved in regulation of erythropoiesis can be classified as follows:

- Environmental
- Hypoxia
- Hormonal: Erythropoietin, androgens, ACTH, thyroid hormones, TSH, growth hormone, estrogen [all these hormones stimulate erythropoiesis except estrogen, which inhibits it]
- Hemolysates [products of hemolysis]
- Products of red cell destruction stimulate erythropoiesis
- Vitamins: Vitamin B12, folic acid, ascorbic acid
- Metals: Iron, cobalt, copper, iodine
- Proteins: Albumin)

26. *What are the conditions that alter RBC count?* (Ans. Refer to page 47, under the heading 'Conditions that alter RBC count'.)

27. *What is anemia and what are the types?* (Ans. Refer to chapter 3, page 17, under the heading 'Types of Anemia'.)

28. *What is the most common cause of anemia in developing countries?*

(Ans. Nutritional anemia, especially iron deficiency anemia, due to poor socioeconomic status.)

29. *What is polycythemia and what are its causes?* (Ans. Refer to page 47, under the heading 'Polycythemia'.)

30. *What is the fate of red cells?* (Ans. Refer to page 43, under the heading 'Lifespan and fate'.)

31. *What is stem cell therapy and stem cell harvesting?*

(Ans. Stem cell therapy involves transplanting stem cells [usually from bone marrow] to treat conditions like leukemia. Harvesting involves collecting stem cells from umbilical cords or embryos for use in diseases like Parkinson's, Alzheimer's, diabetes, etc.)

8 | Determination of Red Blood Cell Indices

Learning Objectives

After completing this practical, you will be able to (MUST KNOW):
1. Explain the importance of calculating red cell indices in clinical hematology.
2. Calculate different red cell indices.
3. State the normal values of MCV, MCH, and MCHC.
4. Name the common conditions in which these indices are altered.

You may also be able to (DESIRABLE TO KNOW):
1. Correlate the change in red cell indices in different clinical conditions.
2. Explain the physiological basis of these changes.

PY2.11: Estimate Hb, RBC, TLC, RBC indices, DLC, blood, groups, and BT/CT.

INTRODUCTION

From the estimated hemoglobin content, packed cell volume (PCV), and red cell count, other values can be derived that reflect red cell volume, hemoglobin content, and hemoglobin concentration in red cells. These values are commonly referred to as **red blood cell indices**: mean corpuscular volume (MCV), mean corpuscular hemoglobin (MCH), and mean corpuscular hemoglobin concentration (MCHC).

The MCV defines the volume or size of the average RBC; the MCH defines the weight of hemoglobin in the average RBC; and the MCHC defines the hemoglobin concentration or colour of the average RBC.

Another quantitative measurement of red cells, the mean corpuscular diameter (MCD), is made directly. A derived measurement determined electronically is the red cell distribution width (RDW). This is a measurement of red cell variability.

Physiological and Clinical Significance

The determination of these indices is of considerable clinical importance and is widely used in the **classification of anemia**. When the red cell indices are calculated from manually determined values for hemoglobin, hematocrit, and red cell counting, the major disadvantage results from the errors associated with manual counts. When electronic counting devices are used, the error is significantly reduced. Indices calculated directly by electronic methods have been found to be more accurate. In recent years, electronic counting of indices is routinely practiced in advanced laboratories.

It is important to verify all indices against observations of stained films. When the red cell indices are used in conjunction with an examination of the stained blood film, a clear picture of red cell morphology is obtained. Since red cells are very small and the amount of hemoglobin in a single cell is minute, the units used for red cell indices are **picograms (pg)** and **femtolitres (fl)**.

METHODS OF DETERMINING RBC INDICES

Red cell indices are determined by two methods: 1) **indirectly** by calculating the indices from PCV, hemoglobin, and red cell count and 2) **directly** by automated counting.

Procedure

The procedures for hemoglobin estimation, RBC count, and PCV determination are followed as described in Chapters 3, 7, and 4 respectively. The results obtained are used for calculating red cell indices as described in this section.

Mean corpuscular volume (MCV)

MCV is the average volume of a red cell expressed in femtolitre or cubic micrometre ($1\ fl = 10^{-15}\ l = 1\ \mu m^3$).

$$MCV(fl) = \frac{Hematocrit(per\ cent) \times 10}{RBC\ count\ in\ millions\ /\ mm^3}$$

Where factor 10 is introduced to convert the hematocrit reading (in per cent) from the volume of packed red cells per 100 ml to volume per litre.

For example, if the hematocrit reading is 45 per cent, and the red cell count is 5 million/mm³ of blood, then the MCV will be 90 fl.

$$MCV = (45 \times 10) \div 5 = 90\ fl$$

Normal value: The normal value of MCV for adults is **78–96 fl**.

Derivation of the formula

$45\% = 45/100 = 45 \times 10/1000 = 45 \times 10 \times 10^{-3}$

$5 \text{ million/mm}^3 = 5 \times 10^6/10^{-6}\text{l} = 5 \times 10^{12}\text{l}$

(since 1 million = 10^6, 1 mm^3 = 10^{-6}l)

Therefore, MCV = $(45 \times 10 \times 10^{-3}) \div (5 \times 10^{12}/\text{l})$

$$= \frac{45 \times 10}{5} \times 10^{-3} \times 10^{-12}\text{l}$$

$$= \frac{45 \times 10}{5} 10^{-15}\text{l} = 90 \text{ fl}$$

Significance

The manual estimation of red cells is not very reliable, nor is the determination of MCV. Automated electronic counting devices measure the electrical impedance caused by each red cell as it passes through the counting devices. The extent of impedance provides an accurate indication of the volume of each cell. Such machines not only indicate the profile of the distribution of the volume of red cells but also provide a highly reproducible value for the MCV, making them more reliable than manual methods.

Mean corpuscular hemoglobin (MCH)

The MCH is the average weight of the hemoglobin content in a red cell expressed in picograms (1 pg = 10^{-12} g).

$$\text{MCH(pg)} = \frac{\text{Hb (g/dl)} \times 10}{\text{RBC count in millions/mm}^3}$$

For example, if the hemoglobin content is 14 g/dl and the RBC count is 5 million/mm^3:

MCH = $(14 \times 10) \div 5 = 28$ pg

Normal value: The normal range for MCH is **27–33 pg**. It may be as high as 50 pg in macrocytic anemia or as low as 20 pg or less in hypochromic microcytic anemia.

Derivation of the formula

14 g/dl = 14 g/100 ml = 14×10 g/1000 ml

$= 14 \times 10$ g/l

5 million/mm^3 = 5×10^{12}/l

(since 1 million = 10^6, 1 mm^3 = 10^{-6} l)

MCH = $\dfrac{14 \times 10}{5 \times 10^{12}/\text{l}}$ g/l = $\dfrac{14 \times 10\text{ g/l}}{5} \times 10^{-12}\text{l}$

$= \dfrac{14 \times 10}{5} 10^{-12}$ g = 28×10^{-12} g = 28 pg

Mean corpuscular hemoglobin concentration (MCHC)

The MCHC is an expression of the average hemoglobin concentration per unit volume of packed red cells. It is expressed as g/dl or per cent.

$$\text{MCHC(per cent)} = \frac{\text{Hb (g/100 ml)}}{\text{PCV/100 ml}} \times 100$$

For example, if the hemoglobin content is 15 g/dl and hematocrit is 45 per cent:

MCHC = $15/45 \times 100 = 33.3$ per cent.

Normal value: The normal range of MCHC is **30–37 g/dl** (or per cent).

Significance

An MCHC above 40 per cent indicates errors in the instrument or in the calculation of the manual measurements used, since an MCHC value of 37 per cent is near the upper limit for hemoglobin solubility. This limits the physiologic upper limit of the MCHC. MCHC is a more reliable index than other indices because its calculation does not involve the RBC count. Therefore, the error associated with RBC counting is excluded in MCHC.

In **hypochromic anemias**, the hemoglobin concentration is reduced, and values as low as 20–25 per cent are not uncommon.

Colour index (CI)

This is the ratio of hemoglobin per cent and RBC per cent.

$$\text{CI} = \frac{\text{Hb per cent}}{\text{RBC per cent}}$$

$$= \frac{\text{Estimated Hb/100 per cent of Hb}}{\text{Calculated RBC count/100 per cent of RBC}}$$

(100 per cent of Hb = 14.8 g/100 ml; 100 per cent of RBC = 5 million/mm^3)

For example, if estimated Hb = 12 g/100 ml and calculated RBC count is 4 million/mm^3,

$$\text{CI} = \frac{12/14.8}{4/5} = \frac{12}{14.8} \times \frac{5}{4} = 1.01$$

Normal value: The normal range of CI is between **0.85 and 1.10. CI less than 0.85 indicates hypochromic anemia.**

Red cell distribution width (RDW)

RDW is a quantitative measure of **anisocytosis**.

RDW per cent = (Standard deviation + mean cell volume) × 100

Normal value: The **normal value** is 11.5 to 14.5%.

DISCUSSION

MCV

The MCV indicates whether RBCs are **microcytic, normocytic, or macrocytic**. If the MCV is less than 80 fl, the red cells are microcytic. If it is greater than 96 fl, the red cells will be macrocytic. If it is within the normal range, the red cells are normocytic. The chief source of error in the determination of MCV is the considerable error in the manual red cell count.

Microcytosis

When the MCV is subnormal (below 80 fl), the condition is called microcytosis.

■ Causes

Microcytosis occurs due to decreased synthesis of hemoglobin due to:

1. Iron deficiency (as in iron deficiency anemia [IDA]
2. Globin deficiency (as in thalassemia)

Microcytosis frequently occurs in **anemia due to hypoproteinemia and iron deficiency**.

Macrocytosis

When MCV is elevated (above 96 fl), the condition is called macrocytosis.

■ Causes

1. Megaloblastosis of the bone marrow due to the deficiency of vitamin B12 and folate deficiency
2. Liver disease, alcoholism, etc.

MCH

MCH indicates the **mean amount of hemoglobin per red cell**. Subnormal MCH levels are seen in microcytosis, but MCH is significantly low when microcytosis is associated with hypochromia (decreased concentration of hemoglobin in red cells). This is seen in iron deficiency and thalassemia minor.

MCHC

MCHC reflects a parameter entirely different from MCH. It indicates the **average hemoglobin concentration per unit volume of packed red cells**.

1. **Decreased MCHC:** Subnormal MCHC indicates an abnormality in which interference with hemoglobin formation is more than that of other constituents of red cells. This is commonly seen in *iron deficiency or thalassemia*.
2. **Increased MCHC:** Reflects dehydration of the red cells, which is commonly seen in *spherocytosis*.

Colour Index (CI)

CI is the ratio of hemoglobin percentage to red blood cell (RBC) percentage; CI decreases if Hb per cent is low and increases if Hb per cent is high. CI indicates the Hb content of RBC. It is not a good index of hemoglobin content because when the Hb per cent and the RBC per cent change proportionately, the CI may not change as it is calculated as the ratio of both these parameters. CI is **low in iron deficiency anemia** and **high in macrocytic anemia**.

Red Cell Distribution Width (RDW)

RDW is a quantitative measure of anisocytosis.

Significance: RDW is used in differentiating anemia due to iron deficiency anemia (IDA) and thalassemia. It is *increased in IDA* (along with low MCV) and in *megaloblastic anemia* (with high MCV). In the presence of the *thalassemia trait*, RDW is *normal with low MCV*.

VIVA

1. *What are the different red cell indices?* (Ans. Refer to page 50, under the heading 'Introduction'.)
2. *What is the practical utility of red cell indices in clinical hematology?* (Ans. Refer to page 50, under the heading 'Introduction' and subheading 'Physiological and Clinical Significance'.)
3. *Define MCV, MCH, and MCHC.* (Ans. Refer to pages 50 and 51, under the headings 'MCV', 'MCH', and 'MCHC'.)
4. *How are MCV, MCH, and MCHC calculated?* (Ans. Refer to pages 50 and 51, under the headings 'MCV', 'MCH', and 'MCHC'.)
5. *What is the significance of calculating MCV?* (Ans. Refer to page 51, under the heading 'MCV' and subheading 'Significance'.)
6. *Explain macrocytosis and microcytosis and the causes of these conditions.* (Ans. Refer to page 51 and 52, under the heading 'MCV' and subheadings 'Macrocytosis' and 'Microcytosis'.)
7. *What does MCH indicate? What is the significance of calculating it?* (Ans. Refer to page 51, under the heading 'MCH' and page 52, under the heading 'Discussion' and subheading 'MCH'.)
8. *What does MCHC represent? What is the significance of calculating it?* (Ans. Refer to Page 51, under the heading 'MCHC'.)
9. *Why is MCHC more reliable than other indices?* (Ans. Refer to page 51, under the heading 'MCHC' and the subheading 'Significance'.)
10. *Why does MCHC have a physiological upper limit?*
    (Ans. Because red cells cannot contain hemoglobin beyond a certain limit [metabolic limit], anemia can never be hyperchromic.)
11. *Why is the colour index not a good indicator of hemoglobin content of the red cells?* (Ans. Refer to page 52, under the heading 'Color Index'.)
12. *Classify anemia based on blood indices.*
    (Ans. Described in Chapter 3, page 17).
13. *What is red cell distribution width (RDW) and its significance?* (Ans. Refer to pages 51 and 52, under the heading 'Red Cell Distribution Width'.)

9 | Total Leucocyte Count

Learning Objectives

After completing this practical, you will be able to (MUST KNOW):

1. Explain the importance of performing total leucocyte count (TLC) in practical physiology.
2. Describe the structure and functions of leucocytes.
3. Perform TLC using the manual method (based on the principle of hemocytometry).
4. List the precautions and sources of error in TLC.
5. State the composition and function of each constituent of Turk's fluid.
6. State the normal range of TLC.
7. Define leukocytosis, leukocytopenia, and leukemia.
8. List the common causes of leukocytosis and leukocytopenia.
9. Name the different types of leukemia.

You may also be able to (DESIRABLE TO KNOW):

1. Describe the steps of leukopoiesis.
2. Explain the fate of leucocytes.
3. State the principle of the automated method for TLC.
4. Discuss the variations in leucocyte count under different conditions.
5. Briefly describe the types of leukemia.

PY2.11: Estimate Hb, RBC, TLC, RBC indices, DLC, blood groups, and BT/CT.

INTRODUCTION

Leucocytes (white blood cells) are nucleated cells that are involved in the defence mechanisms of the body. White cells use the bloodstream primarily as a means of transport to reach their sites of function in the body tissues. Leucocytes are classified as granulocytes and agranulocytes. Neutrophils, eosinophils, and basophils are **granulocytes**, and lymphocytes and monocytes are **agranulocytes**.

FORMATION OF LEUCOCYTES

The development of leucocytes is called **leukopoiesis**. *In the embryo*, white blood cells develop in the mesoderm and migrate secondarily into the blood vessels. *After birth*, granulocytes develop exclusively in the bone marrow. Lymphocytes and monocytes also develop from stem cells in the bone marrow. *In adults*, lymphocytes are primarily produced in lymphoid tissues (such as lymph nodes and the spleen) and secondarily in the bone marrow. Leucocytes develop from **two types of stem cells**:

1. *Myeloid stem cells*—form granulocytes and monocytes
2. *Lymphoid stem cells*—form lymphocytes (Fig. 9.1)

The number of circulating leucocytes is very precisely controlled. The substances that regulate the development of leucocytes are grossly called ***leucopoietins*** or **leucocyte-promoting factors**. These substances are various types of *interleukins* (produced by monocytes, macrophages, and endothelial cells), *colony-stimulating* factors (produced by monocytes and T lymphocytes), *prostaglandins* (produced by monocytes), other *cytokines, and lactoferrin*.

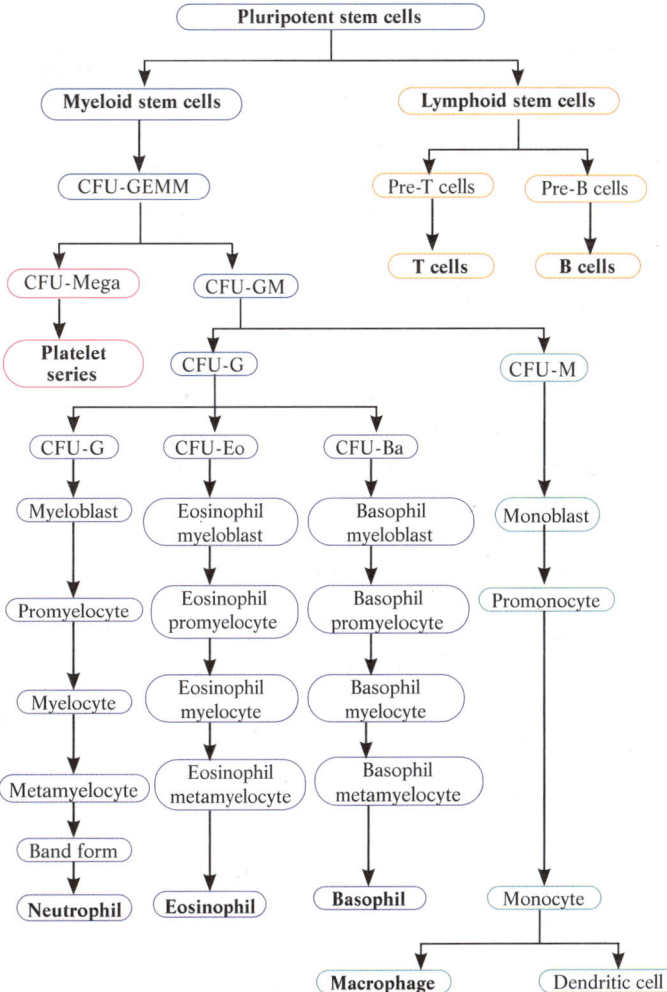

Fig. 9.1 Sequence of development of granulocytes.

FUNCTIONS OF LEUCOCYTES

Granulocytes act as **phagocytic scavengers**. They engulf and destroy invading microorganisms and clear the body of unwanted particulate materials such as dead and injured tissue cells.

1. **Neutrophils** are said to be the ***first line of defence against acute bacterial invasion***. They kill organisms by phagocytosis.
2. **Eosinophils** are the body's *defence against allergies*.
3. **Monocytes** are also phagocytes and are thought to be the ***second line of defence against microbial invasion***. They enter tissues, form tissue macrophages (mononuclear phagocyte system), and then phagocytose microorganisms in tissues.
4. **Lymphocytes** and **plasma cells** act as immunocytes and ***maintain the body's immunity***. Plasma cells are not normally found in blood, but they are formed from B lymphocytes under specific immunologic stimulation.
   - ***Plasma cells produce antibodies*** that destroy or inactivate antigens.

LIFE HISTORY OF LEUCOCYTES

The lifespan of granulocytes is about four to eight days. Lymphocytes survive for about 80 to 100 days. Monocytes, after performing their activities in the circulation for a few hours, enter different tissues, where they transform themselves into tissue macrophages and stay in the tissues for a long time (a few months or years).

Phases

The life cycle of leucocytes has **three phases**—marrow phase, circulation phase, and tissue phase.

1. **Marrow phase**: This is the phase of development of leucocytes. In this phase, there are two pools: the **mitosis pool** (development of myeloblasts into myelocytes) and the **maturation pool** (development of metamyelocytes to matured cells).
2. **Circulation phase**: Many leucocytes, especially neutrophils, stick to the endothelial margin of blood vessels (***margination pool***), while the remaining circulate in the blood (***active circulation pool***). Neutrophils have a half-life of about six hours in the circulation.
3. **Tissue phase**: After activities in circulation, leucocytes enter the tissues (tissue pool). Monocytes in the tissue form the ***mononuclear phagocyte system*** (previously known as the *reticuloendothelial system*).

NORMAL COUNT

- **Adults:** 4,000–11,000/mm³ of blood
- **Newborns:** 10,000–25,000/mm³ of blood

- **Infants:** 6,000–18,000/mm³ of blood
- **Children:** 5,000–15,000/mm³ of blood
  These values do not differ between the sexes.

METHODS OF COUNTING

White blood cells are counted by two methods: non-automated (manual) and automated. The manual cell count is less accurate, but is still used widely in developing countries, especially in the laboratories of medical colleges.

Manual Method

Principle

Blood is diluted with an acid solution that removes red cells by hemolysis and accentuates the nuclei of white cells. The counting of the white cells then becomes easy. Counting is done using a microscope under the low-power objective. With knowledge of the volume of fluid examined and the dilution of the blood obtained, the number of white cells per mm³ of undiluted whole blood is calculated.

Requirements
Apparatus

1. Microscope
2. Hemocytometer (WBC diluting pipette and counting chamber)
3. Equipment for sterile finger prick
4. Watch glass
5. Coverslip

WBC diluting fluid

It is also known as **Türk's fluid** (Fig. 9.2).

1. *1% glacial acetic acid solution*—causes destruction of red cells (hemolysis).
2. *Gentian violet stain or aqueous methylene blue* (0.3 per cent w/v)—stains the nuclei of leucocytes.
3. *Distilled water*—acts as a solvent.

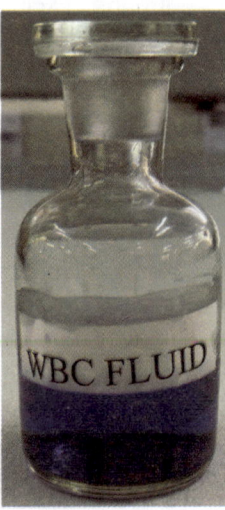

Fig. 9.2   WBC diluting fluid (Türk's fluid).

Procedure

1. Clean and dry the pipette, watch glass, coverslip and Neubauer chamber thoroughly.
2. Take enough WBC diluting fluid in a watch glass.
3. Prick the finger under aseptic conditions and wipe off the first drop of blood. Allow a good-sized blood drop to form on the fingertip spontaneously (do not squeeze).
4. Touch the blood drop with the tip of the pipette (refer to Fig. 6.6, Chapter 6) and suck blood *exactly up to the 0.5 mark* (Fig. 9.3A). If blood is drawn above the 0.5 mark, bring the blood column to the 0.5 mark by tapping the tip of the pipette on the palm or finger, or by using non-absorbent material. Do not use gauze or cotton for this adjustment, because the liquid portion of the sample inside the stem will be drawn into the absorbent material, leaving a higher concentration of cells inside the stem.
5. *Wipe the tip of the pipette* and maintain the blood level at the 0.5 mark by holding the pipette horizontally.
6. Dip the tip of the pipette into the diluting fluid (in the watch glass) *well below the surface of the liquid* (Fig. 9.3B).
7. Suck WBC diluting fluid *exactly up to the 11 mark*. While the bulb is being filled, you may tap the pipette with a finger to knock the bead down, below the surface of the solution in the bulb. This will prevent the formation of bubbles.
8. While removing the pipette from the diluent, maintain the level of the mixture at the 11 mark by closing the pipette tip with the index finger.
9. Hold the pipette horizontally and close both its ends. Then, *gently mix the contents* of the bulb. For mixing, shake the pipette at right angles to its long axis for a few seconds. The glass bead in the pipette should move from one side to the other.

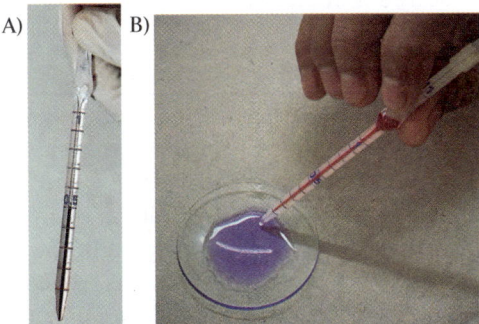

Fig. 9.3 **(A)** Pipetting of blood up to the 0.5 mark and **(B)** process of pipetting WBC diluting fluid into the bulb of the pipette. While drawing the fluid, maintain steady suction and keep the tip submerged to avoid air bubbles.

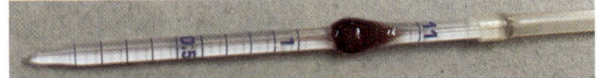

Fig. 9.4 Horizontal placement of the WBC pipette containing the fluid mixture after completion of pipetting. Note that the upper level of the fluid mixture is at the 11 mark.

10. After mixing, *place the pipette in a horizontal position* (Fig. 9.4) to prevent any loss of its contents until the cell count is completed.
11. *Discard the first two drops* of fluid from the pipette, as the fluid in the stem does not contain cells.
12. Charge the Neubauer chamber as described in Chapter 6 and allow two minutes for the cells to settle.
13. Place the charged chamber on the stage of the microscope and adjust it for observation under low power.
14. Focus the Neubauer chamber under the low-power objective and check for uniform distribution of cells in the WBC squares. If the cells are not uniformly distributed, clean the chamber and recharge it.
15. Count the total number of WBCs in the four corner squares under the low-power objective (see Fig. 6.12, Chapter 6, for the orientation of WBC squares). To avoid counting the same cells again, follow the '*rules of counting*'. Using the 'L pattern' counting, count the white cells present in the square and those on its left and lower lines. Ignore those on its right and upper lines. 'Γ (inverted L) pattern' counting may also be followed, i.e., count the cells on the left and upper lines of the square in addition to cells inside the square. Do not follow the 'L pattern' for a few squares and the 'Γ pattern' for other squares. Follow one pattern for the entire counting. Preferably, the same method should be practiced by all the students of a class.

Note: WBCs appear similar to clumped red cell debris or stained particles. They are identified as clear, nucleated, and refractile bodies.

16. Draw the WBC squares in your notebook and enter the observation. Calculate the final result.

Dilution obtained

The volume of the bulb is 10 (11 − 1 = 10). The stem of the pipette (from the tip of the pipette to mark 1) contains diluting fluid that does not contribute to the dilution. Dilution (mixing of blood with diluting fluid) occurs only in the bulb. Thus, 10 volumes of diluted blood (in the bulb) contain 0.5 volumes of blood and 9.5 volumes of diluting fluid, giving a dilution of 0.5 in 10. Therefore, the dilution obtained is 1 in 20 or 20 times.

Calculation

Area of 4 WBC squares = 4 × 1 = 4 mm²
Volume of 4 WBC squares = 4 × 1/10 = 4/10 mm³
Dilution factor = 1:20
Cells in 4/10 mm³ volume of diluted blood = n
Therefore, cells in 1 mm³ volume of diluted blood = n × (10/4)
Therefore, cells in 1 mm³ volume of undiluted blood = n × (10/4) × 20 = **n × 50**

Precautions

(Same as those taken for RBC count; see Chapter 7 for details.)

1. The pipette, coverslip, and Neubauer chamber should be thoroughly cleaned and dried.
2. The prick should be at least 3 mm deep. It should not be squeezed to express blood.
3. The first drop of blood should be wiped off.
4. Blood should be drawn *exactly up to the 0.5 mark*.
5. The *tip of the pipette should be wiped*.
6. The WBC diluting fluid should be drawn *exactly up to the 11 mark*.
7. Air bubbles should not enter while pipetting the fluid.
8. Before charging the chamber, the contents of the bulb of the pipette should be *gently mixed*.
9. The *first two drops of fluid should be discarded*.
10. The chamber should not be overcharged or undercharged.
11. *Air bubbles should not be allowed to enter* the chamber.
12. Once the counting chamber is filled (charged), the counting should be completed as early as possible before the fluid begins to dry.
13. If the distribution of cells is not uniform, discard and recharge.
14. Avoid counting the same cells twice.

Observation and results

1. Draw the four WBC squares in your notebook and record the number of cells counted in each (each WBC square has 16 small squares; refer to Fig. 6.12, Chapter 6 for orientation of WBC squares).
2. Total the number of cells counted, which is expresssed as *n*.
3. Calculate the final result using the formula:
   n × 50 = _____
4. Report the result as: "TLC of the given blood sample is _____/mm³ of blood."

Sources of error

Fortunately, errors in the leucocyte count are not as critical as errors in the red cell counts. Even an error of 20 per cent does not affect the result much. The possible sources of error may be errors inherent to the method or technical errors.

▋ Errors inherent to the method

1. **Error in visual counting:** One potential error is mistaking dirt or clumped red cell debris for leucocytes. This can be avoided by making a second count on the opposite side of the Neubauer chamber.
2. **Error due to distribution of cells:** Distribution can never be perfectly uniform, even with thorough mixing and charging. If there is clumping of leucocytes, recharge the chamber.

▋ Technical errors

1. **Dilution error:** Improper volume measurement of blood and diluent
2. **Pipetting error:** Use of defective pipettes
3. **Charging error:** Improper charging of the chamber
4. **Counting error:** Improper counting
5. **Calculation error:** Wrong calculation

Additional information

In case of a very high leucocyte count, as seen in leukemia, dilution may have to be increased to 100 times or more. The RBC pipette can be used for this purpose.

Blood is sucked up to the '1' mark of the RBC pipette and then diluted 100 times. The calculation is made according to the dilution.

Automated Method

Automated WBC counting is performed by either impedance counting or light-scattering technology. The principle is the same as described in Chapter 7.

DISCUSSION

Physiological Significance

Total leucocyte count is used to assess the subject's ability to mount a defence against microbial invasion.

Leucocytes are the **mobile defenders of the body**. They can pass through the vascular endothelium and enter tissues by *diapedesis*. Once in the tissues, the white cells migrate to the site of injury in response to chemical substances released by microorganisms or injured or infected cells. This process of migration is called *chemotaxis*, and the substances that promote migration are called *chemoattractants*.

Once they reach the site of invasion, white cells engulf and digest the foreign substances by *phagocytosis*. All granulocytes, especially neutrophils, and monocytes kill organisms by phagocytosis. Lymphocytes are the principal cells of the body's immune system.

Clinical Significance

Total leucocyte count is a part of the routine hematologic investigations used to assess the *nature and severity of an infection*, the extent of spread of the disease, and the body's defence capability. In some diseases, alteration in leucocyte count alone may be diagnostic, but frequently, the leucocyte count is ordered with other investigations, especially with the differential leucocyte count, to aid in diagnosis. When the total leucocyte count increases above the normal, the condition is called **leucocytosis**, and when the count decreases below normal, it is called **leucocytopenia**.

Conditions That Alter Total Leucocyte Count

Leucocytosis

▋ Physiological

1. **Newborns and infants:** The WBC count is as high as 15,000–20,000/mm³.

2. **Physical exercise**: During exercise, circulation becomes more dynamic, causing **disruption of margination of leucocytes** along the vascular endothelium. As a result, leucocytes shift from the margination pool into the circulating pool (general circulation). This is known as **shift leucocytosis**. It is not due to increased cell formation.

3. **After food intake:** The body's metabolism increases, which results in an increase in the body's temperature. Because of this, circulation improves. This causes the disruption of the margination of leucocytes and results in leukocytosis.

4. **Exposure to the sun and increased environmental temperature** result in leucocytosis.

5. **Pregnancy:** Leucocytosis occurs despite hemodilution. The exact cause is unknown but may be due to increased physiological stress associated with pregnancy and the inflammatory response for supporting the growing fetus.

6. **Parturition:** Leucocytosis occurs due to the combined effects of tissue injury, hemorrhage, and severe exertion.

7. Pain, nausea and vomiting

8. Menstruation

9. Emotion and anxiety

▌ Pathological

1. **Acute bacterial infections:** Infection with pyogenic bacteria (localised or generalised) is the commonest cause; examples are boils, abscesses, and pneumonia. However, there are a few bacterial infections in which the leucocyte count decreases. One of the typical examples of leukocytopenia in acute bacterial infection is typhoid fever.

2. **Chronic bacterial infections**, e.g., tuberculosis

3. Tissue injury: Infarction, burns, or surgery

4. Hemorrhage

5. Neoplasia

6. *Stress states and hyperactivity*: Convulsions and severe colic

7. *Inflammatory disorders*: Includes certain collagen diseases and rheumatic fever

8. *Metabolic disorders*, e.g., diabetic ketoacidosis

9. Corticosteroid therapy

10. *Viral infections*, e.g., infectious mononucleosis

Leucocytopenia
▌ Physiological

Physiological decrease in leucocyte count is very rare. Exposure to severe cold may sometimes lower the total WBC count.

▌ Pathological

1. **Infections:** Typhoid fever, paratyphoid fever, and early phases of viral infections such as infectious hepatitis.

2. **Overwhelming sepsis:** In severe sepsis, the consumption of neutrophils exceeds their production.

3. **Replacement of hemopoietic tissue in the bone marrow by neoplastic infiltrative cells:** As seen in acute leukemia, lymphoma, multiple myeloma, and myelofibrosis.

4. **Aplastic anemia:** Hypoplasia of the bone marrow decreases all the cell counts.

5. **Cytotoxic therapy:** Treatment of malignant diseases by cytotoxic drugs causes a decrease in the WBC counts.

6. **Drugs** (especially in sensitive individuals): Chloramphenicol, sulpha drugs, and aspirin.

7. Hypersplenism

8. Starvation and malnutrition

9. Radiation
   Leukocytopenia usually occurs due to neutropenia.

Leukemia
Leukemia is a cancerous disease of the blood-forming tissues, involving the uncontrolled proliferation of one or more types of hematopoietic cells, which progressively displace the normal cellular elements.

▌ Definition
Leukemia is a malignant neoplasia of hemopoietic cells characterised by abnormal proliferation of leucocytes and their precursors. It results in the appearance of abnormal and immature cells with very high leukocytosis in the peripheral blood and the infiltration of tissues by leukemic cells. Total leucocyte count is typically very high, except in the **subleukemic or aleukemic form of leukemia**.

▌ Classification
Leukemia is broadly classified into two main categories: **myeloid** (myelocytic) and **lymphocytic** leukemia. These two types are further classified into acute and chronic forms on the basis of the clinical course and the number of blast cells present.

Acute lymphoblastic leukemia (ALL)
ALL is primarily a **disease of children and young adults**. It constitutes *80 per cent of childhood acute leukemias*. The most common mode of presentation is with symptoms of anemia or hemorrhage, infective lesions of the mouth and pharynx, fever, prostration, headache, and malaise. There is *generalised lymphadenopathy, splenomegaly, and hepatomegaly*. The typical **blood picture** consists of anemia, thrombocytopenia, and moderate or marked increase in leucocytes, the majority of which are blast cells (**lymphoblasts**; 60–80 per cent).

Acute myeloblastic leukemia (AML)
AML primarily affects adults between the **ages of 15 and 40 years**. It constitutes only 20 per cent of childhood leukemias. The presentation is similar to

ALL, but lymphadenopathy and hepatosplenomegaly are uncommon. The **blood picture** consists of anemia, thrombocytopenia, and moderate-to-high leukocytosis. More than 60 per cent of leucocytes in the peripheral blood are blast (*myeloblast*) cells.

Chronic myeloid leukemia (CML)

CML is primarily a disease of adults of 30–60 years with peak incidence in the **fourth and fifth decades of life**. Onset is usually slow with non-specific features like anemia, weight loss, weakness, and easy fatigability. *Splenomegaly is the outstanding physical sign*. Hepatomegaly may be present, but lymph node enlargement is rare. *Markedly elevated total leucocyte count*, usually more than one lakh cells per mm³ of blood, is seen. Neutrophils and metamyelocytes constitute most of the circulating cells. *Blast cells are rarely present except in blastic crises*.

Chronic lymphocytic leukemia (CLL)

CLL is the *most indolent of all leukemias*. It typically occurs in persons over **50 years of age**. Men are affected twice as frequently as women. Patients present with non-specific symptoms. *Lymphadenopathy* is the outstanding physical sign. Hepatosplenomegaly may be present. Mild to severe increase in leucocyte count is seen. *More than 90 per cent of leucocytes are lymphocytes*.

Leukemoid and Leukoerythoblastic Reactions, and Leukostasis

Leukemoid reaction

This is a condition in which the *leucocyte count is very high*, and may be more than 50,000 per mm³ of blood. This occurs rarely, in severe infections, especially in children and may occur in acute hemolysis, acute hemorrhage, and malignant diseases such as carcinoma of the breast, lungs, and kidney. A few immature cells may be seen in the peripheral blood. *This is not leukemia, but the blood picture resembles chronic leukemia*. Therefore, it is called **leukemoid reaction**. It is differentiated from leukemia by demonstrating **high leucocyte alkaline phosphatase (LAP)** in blood, which is depressed in CML.

Leukoerythoblastic reaction

This is similar to the leukemoid reaction, but includes **nucleated red blood cells (erythroblasts)** in the blood smear. This indicates the involvement of the *erythrocytic series*. It may occur in cases of severe hypoxia, severe anemia, and malignancies infiltrating the bone marrow.

Leukostasis

When the leucocyte count is above 100,000 per mm³ of blood, thrombi consisting chiefly of leucocytes may get lodged in the brain, lung, and heart. This is called leukostasis.

The risk of leukostasis is highest when blood is transfused before reducing TLC in extreme leukocytosis.

OSPE

I.   Dilute the blood (from the given sample) for a total leucocyte count.

Steps

1. Select an appropriate WBC pipette and ensure that it is dry and clean.
2. Take adequate diluting fluid in the watch glass.
3. Mix blood thoroughly by gently shaking the sample.
4. Suck blood exactly up to the 0.5 mark. If blood is drawn above the mark, remove the extra blood by tapping it with a fingertip (not by touching with absorbent material).
5. Wipe the tip of the pipette.
6. Suck the diluting fluid up to the 11 mark. While drawing the fluid, avoid the entry of air bubbles.
7. Gently mix the contents of the bulb and place the pipette horizontally on the table.

II. Charge the Neubauer chamber for total WBC count.

Steps

1. Clean the coverslip and Neubauer chamber.
2. Place the coverslip on the platform of the Neubauer chamber.
3. Mix the contents of the bulb of the WBC pipette.
4. Discard two drops of the fluid from the pipette.
5. Touch the tip of the pipette with the edge of the coverslip.
6. Slowly release fluid from the pipette (fluid moves by capillary action) in such a way that the fluid spreads just beneath the coverslip and does not spill into the gutters and does not contain air bubbles.

VIVA

1. *Which diluting fluid is used for determining total leucocyte count and what is its composition? What is the function of each component?* (Ans. Refer to page 54, under the subheading 'WBC Diluting Fluid'.)

2. *Why is the term 'glacial' used for acetic acid in Turk's fluid? What is its significance?*
    (Ans. The term *glacial* refers to pure acetic acid. Only glacial [pure] acetic acid produces the characteristic shine [halo-like refractility] around WBCs due to nuclear swelling. This refractility helps differentiate leucocytes from dust particles.)

3. *Why are two drops of fluid discarded from the pipette before charging the Neubauer's chamber?* (Ans. Refer to page 55, under the heading 'Procedure', point no. 11.)

4. *Why is the dilution obtained 1 in 20 and not 1 in 22?* (Ans. Refer to page 55, under the heading 'Dilution Obtained'.)

5. *In which condition is the RBC pipette used for white cell counting?* (Ans. Refer to page 56, under the heading 'Additional Information'.)

6. *Why are the red cells not seen while counting WBCs?*
    (Ans. Red cells are hemolyzed by acetic acid, hence not seen. Sometimes, remnants of red cells are faintly visible, and they are called ghost cells.)

7. *Can any other acid or agent be used for hemolyzing the red cells.*
    (Ans. No, other agents will not be useful. A weaker acid will take more time to lyze red cells, and a stronger acid will lyze the WBCs in addition to destroying red cells.)

8. *What are the precautions for performing total leucocyte count?* (Ans. Refer to pages 55-56, text under the heading 'Precautions'.)

9. *What are the possible sources of error in total leucocyte count?* (Ans. Refer to page 56, text under the heading 'Sources of Error'.)

10. *How will you differentiate WBC pipette from RBC pipette?* (Ans. Refer to Chapter 6, Table 6.1.)

11. *What are the other uses of WBC pipette?*
    (Ans. WBC pipette can be used for counting RBC in case of severe anemia. It can be used for counting sperm and bacteria.)

12. *What are the functions of the white bead present in the WBC pipette?*
    (Ans. i. Facilitates mixing of blood with diluent in the bulb, ii. identification of WBC pipette, and iii. indicates whether the pipette is dry or wet. In a dry pipette, the bead rolls freely and in a wet pipette, it sticks to the wall of the bulb.)

13. *What are the functions of leucocytes?* (Ans. Refer to page 54, under the heading 'Functions of Leucocytes'.)

14. *What is the physiological significance of performing a total leucocyte count?* (Ans. Refer to page 56, under the heading 'Discussion – Physiological Significance'.)

15. *What are the causes of physiological leucocytosis?* (Ans. Refer to page 56, under the heading 'Leucocytosis - Physiological'.)

16. *What is TLC in adults, newborns, infants and children?* (Ans. Refer to page 54, under the heading 'Normal Count'.)

17. *What is absolute leucocyte count?*
    (Ans. Absolute leucocyte count is done for individual leucocytes, for which differential leucocyte count (DLC) is done along with TLC. Then the specific cell counted in DLC/100 is multiplied by the TLC, to obtain absolute count of that leucocyte. For example, if TLC is 7000, and neutrophil is 55% in DLC, absolute count of neutrophil = 55/100 x 7000.)

18. *What is the mechanism of leucocytosis in physical exercise?* (Ans. Refer to page 57, under the heading 'Leucocytosis – Physiological, point no. 2'.)

19. *What are the pathological causes of leucocytosis?* (Ans. Refer to page 57, text under the heading 'Leucocytosis - Pathological'.)

20. *What are the pathological causes of leukocytopenia?* (Ans. Refer to page 57, text under the heading 'Leukocytopenia - Pathological'.)

21. *What is leukemia? What are the types of leukemia?* (Ans. Refer to page 57, text under the heading 'Leukemia – Definition, Classification'.)

22. *What are the most frequently occurring leukemias in children and in adults?*
    (Ans. ALL in children and CML in adults.)

23. *What is the principle of bone marrow transplantation (BMT)? What are the indications?*
    (Ans. BMT is the intravenous transfusion of red bone marrow from a healthy donor to the recipient. Usually, the marrow is taken from the ileac crest. However, the donor's marrow should match with the recipient's. The stem cells of the donor settle in the recipient's marrow, proliferate and produce cells of different cell lines. This is usually indicated in some form of leukemia, malignancies, severe hemolytic anemia, genetic disorders, and severe combined immunodeficiency diseases.)

24. *What is leukemoid reaction? How does it differ from leukemia?* (Ans. Refer to page 58, under the heading 'Leukemoid Reaction'.)

25. *What is leukoerythroblastic reaction?* (Ans. Refer to page 65, text under the heading 'Leukoerythroblastic Reaction'.)

26. *How are leucocytes produced (give broad steps of leucopoiesis)?* (Ans. Refer to page 53, under the heading 'Formation of Leucocytes', and see Fig. 9.1.)

27. *How is leukopoiesis regulated? What are the leukopoietic growth factors (leukopoietins)?* (Ans. Refer to page 53, under the heading 'Formation of Leucocytes'.)

28. *What is the lifespan of leucocytes?* (Ans. Refer to page 54, under the heading 'Life History of Leucocytes'.)

29. *What is the fate (different phases in the life history) of various leucocytes?* (Ans. Refer to page 54, under the heading 'Life History of Leucocytes – Phases'.)

30. *What is mononuclear phagocyte system? What are its components?*

    (Ans: Monocytes that enter tissues become macrophages, collectively known as the **mononuclear phagocyte system** (MPS). They destroy microbes via phagocytosis. The cells of MPS in different tissues are as follows:)

A. In blood	B. In tissues
– Monocytes	– Kupffer cells in liver
C. In bone marrow	– Osteoclasts in bone marrow
– Monoblasts, Promonocytes	– Alveolar macrophages in lungs
	– Histiocytes in connective tissue
	– Microglia in brain
	– Red pulp macrophages in spleen
	– Macrophages in lymph nodes and thymus
	– Mesangial cells in kidney
	– Dendritic cells/histiocytes in skin

10 | Preparation and Examination of Blood Smears

Learning Objectives

After completing this practical, you will be able to (MUST KNOW):
1. List the uses of a peripheral blood smear.
2. Select the appropriate spreader for preparing blood smears.
3. Prepare an ideal smear using the wedge method.
4. Fix and stain the smear appropriately.
5. Enumerate the characteristics of a good-quality smear.
6. Name the constituents of Leishman stain and describe their functions.
7. Identify possible sources of error in smear preparation and the precautions to be taken to avoid these.
8. Recognise red blood cells, platelets, and different types of leucocytes on a stained smear.
9. Describe the identifying features of each type of blood cell.
10. Distinguish between neutrophils and eosinophils and between large lymphocytes and monocytes.

You may also be able to (DESIRABLE TO KNOW):
1. Explain the common sources and implications of errors in smear preparation.
2. Name the alternative stains used for staining blood smears.
3. Explain the principle and advantages of other smear preparation methods.
4. List the causes of defective staining and the measures to prevent them.

INTRODUCTION

Microscopic examination of peripheral blood smear is a routine hematologic investigation. It involves *preparing, staining, and examining* a thin film of blood on a glass slide. The blood film is often called **peripheral blood smear**. The cellular components of blood are noted while examining a blood smear under a microscope.

A unique feature of a blood smear is that it can be *retained and preserved as an original record* in the laboratory to recheck for errors or evaluate the progress in the clinical status of the patient or to assess the response of the patient to treatment. Thus, it can be reused after days, months, or years. No other routine hematologic test can be reassessed. Therefore, a peripheral smear is a **permanent record**.

Uses of Blood Smears

1. A peripheral smear made for **differential count of leucocytes** provides information not only about them but also about the other cellular elements of blood.
2. It is used to study the *morphology of red cells and platelets*.
3. It is used to detect the presence of *various parasites* like malarial parasites and microfilaria.
4. Peripheral blood smear is also used to verify *hemoglobin status, hematocrit, and the red cell count* of the subject.

Because the blood film has many uses, a smear must be carefully prepared and studied.

METHODS OF PREPARING A SMEAR

A blood smear is prepared in **two stages**:
1. Making a blood smear
2. Fixing and staining the blood smear

Making a Blood Smear

There are **three primary techniques**:
1. Glass slide (wedge) method
2. Cover glass method
3. Centrifugal method

The wedge (glass slide method) method is most commonly used in routine practice.

Wedge or glass slide method

This method is so named for the shape of the smear, which resembles a wedge.

Principle

A drop of blood is spread into a thin film using a spreader slide, forming a wedge-shaped smear.

Requirements

1. Glass slides
2. **Spreader**, which is a specially designed glass slide with a *smooth edge*, the breadth of which is slightly

less than that of usual glass slides (if a spreader is not available, a glass slide with a smooth edge can be used)

3. Equipment for sterile finger puncture

▮ Procedure

1. Select four clean and grease-free glass slides and *select one to use as a spreader*.
2. Clean the tip of the middle finger with alcohol, allow it to air dry, and then prick the fingertip with a sterile lancet.
3. Discard the first drop of blood.
4. Place a drop of blood centrally at one end (say the right end) of a slide, about 1 cm from the edge of the slide, in such a way that only the top of the blood drop touches the slide. Ensure that the skin of the finger does not touch the slide.

Note: If the finger touches the slide, moisture or oil from the skin of the finger may spoil the smear.

5. Place the specimen slide on the flat surface of a table, and hold it in position at the left end (the end opposite the blood drop) with the middle or index finger and thumb of the left hand.
6. Place the smooth, clean edge of the spreader slide on the specimen slide just in front of the drop of blood (Fig. 10.1A). There should be an approximate angle of *30–45° between the two slides*.
7. Using the right hand, draw the spreader back until it touches the drop of blood. Let the blood run along the edge of the spreader (Fig. 10.1B). The *spreader can be slightly shaken sideways* to facilitate the **smooth spread of blood** along the edge of the spreader.
8. When the blood has spread evenly across the edge of the spreader slide, *push the spreader to the other end of the slide* with a **smooth, quick, and controlled movement.**

Note: All the blood in the drop should be used up before you reach the other end of the slide.

9. **Keep the angle of the spreader constant throughout the process.** As the spreader moves, a thin film of blood will be deposited behind it. The blood film should cover half to three-fourths of the slide when properly prepared (Fig. 10.1C). It should also be noted that **no blood is left at the end of the smear** (the blood should be used completely in making the smear), otherwise, the distribution of cells becomes unequal (**for explanation**, see precaution 8).
10. Turn the spreader slide over (this gives another clean edge) and prepare a second blood film using the same procedure.

Note: At least two films should be made from a single blood specimen. A third smear can also be prepared.

11. **Dry the blood smears quickly** by waving them in the air. If the moisture is too high, as occurs in the rainy season, dry the films by waving them rapidly about 5 cm above the flame of a spirit lamp. Never put the slide directly over the flame as excess heat may damage it. Adequate drying is essential to preserve the quality of the film. Hence, before staining the slide, make sure that the **film is completely dry**, otherwise, the stain washes off when the slide is washed after staining.

Note: If the smears are not dried quickly, the blood cells will shrink and appear distorted.

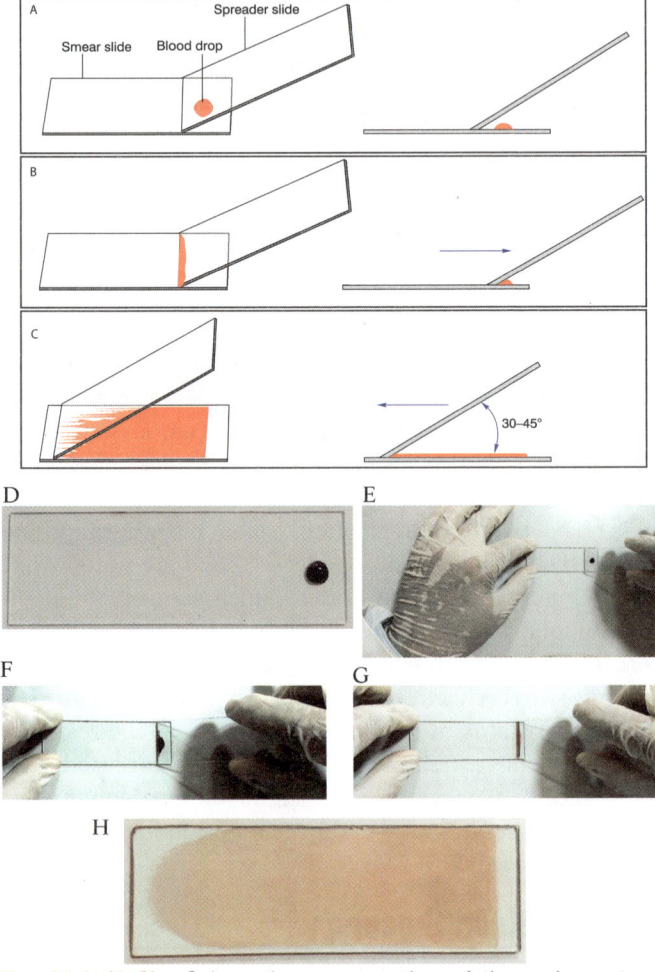

Fig. 10.1 (A-C) Schematic representation of the various steps in the preparation of blood smear (arrows indicate the direction of movement of the spreader slide). **(D-H)** The five photographs demonstrate the five major steps in making a blood smear.

▮ Precautions

1. The glass slides must be scrupulously cleaned. Dirty slides prevent the making of an even smear.
2. The first drop of blood should be discarded as it contains tissue fluid and is rich in neutrophils.

3. The drop of blood should not be obtained by squeezing. The puncture should be deep enough to form a blood drop spontaneously.

4. A *medium-sized blood drop* should be used. If the drop is small, the size of the smear decreases, and if it is too large, some blood will be left at the tail end of the smear.

5. The *smear should be made immediately* after placing the drop of blood on the slide. Delaying will result in an uneven distribution of white cells on the film. Rouleaux formation by the red cells and clumping of platelets occurs if the blood is not spread immediately. The blood may also clot.

6. The spreader slide must be *moved steadily and confidently* with a single, quick and smooth movement. Loss of contact between the spreader slide and smear slide yields poor smears. Pressing too much on the spreader slide results in the accumulation of white cells and platelets at the end of the smear. Pushing the spreader slide with an uneven movement results in thicker and thinner areas in the body of the smear (Fig. 10.2C). The smear *should not be made very fast or slow*. The smear becomes thick if made very fast or thin if made slow. With practice, the student will learn the optimum speed.

7. Before the smear is made (before the spreader slide is moved), it should be ensured that the *blood has spread uniformly along the edge of the spreader*; otherwise, a thick, narrow smear results (Fig. 10.2B).

8. The *entire amount of blood* taken on the slide should be used in making the film. The film should gradually fade away at the feather edge, and no blood should be left at the tail end of the smear (Fig. 10.2A). A *defined border* at the end of the smear indicates that most of the *white cells have piled up at the end*. When this occurs, the heavier neutrophils accumulate at the end to a greater extent than the other white cells, resulting in

an uneven distribution of white cells in the body of the smear. Platelets also tend to accumulate at the end of the smear if some blood is left (not used in the smear), decreasing the number in the body of the smear.

9. The **angle** between the spreader slide and the smear slide should be *about 45°*. The angle of holding the spreader slide determines the thickness of the film. *Increasing the angle yields a thicker smear, whereas decreasing it produces a thin smear*.

10. The smear should be **completely dry**. A wet smear will not stick to the slide while staining. Cells become distorted if the smear takes a long time to dry.

Cover glass method
Principle
A drop of blood is spread between two cover glasses as they are pulled in opposite directions.

Disadvantages
1. It is more time-consuming than the wedge method.
2. It is difficult to learn and perform correctly.
3. Requires more careful handling of the preparation than the wedge method.

Centrifugal blood smear method
With the use of a cytocentrifuge, a monolayer of cells can be prepared. These centrifuges facilitate rapid spreading of the cells across a slide.

Principle
A drop of blood is spun outward from a central point, resulting in an evenly dispersed monolayer of cells. The blood spreads across the slide by virtue of the high torque and low inertia of motion.

Advantages
1. Only a small volume of blood is used.
2. Cellular destruction and artefacts that occur in the glass slide method are eliminated.
3. Cells are evenly distributed and less distorted.
4. A smear of single-layer thickness is easily obtained.

Fixing and Staining a Smear
Principle
The staining method for blood films fixes dead cells, whereas supravital staining is used for living cells. Fixation is the process by which blood cells are made to adhere to the slide, and staining is the process by which the cells (cytoplasm and nuclei) are stained. Blood cells are fixed by methanol. It is advisable to stain the smear soon after making it. If it cannot be stained within a few hours, the smear should be fixed by immersing it in absolute methyl alcohol (methanol) for 2–3 seconds, and then air-drying it.

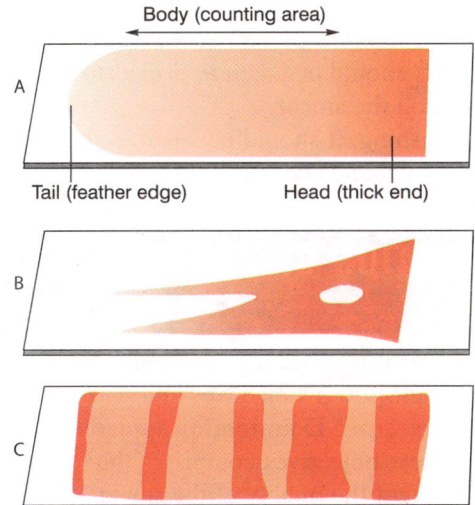

Fig. 10.2 (A) Ideal smear; (B and C) sub-ideal smears.

Requirements

■ Apparatus

1. **Staining rack**: This consists of two glass rods placed in parallel, about 5 cm apart, on a tray. The glass rods hold the slides, and the tray holds the stain and water poured on the slides.
2. Distilled water
3. Pasteur pipette
4. Blood smears

■ Leishman stain

This is a mixture of methylene blue and eosin in acetone-free methyl alcohol.

1. **Methylene blue** stains the acidic part of the (basic dye) cell, that is, the nuclei (DNA) and cytoplasm (RNA) of WBCs and granules of basophils.
2. **Eosin (acidic dye)** stains the basic part of the cell— eosinophilic granules and Hb of red cells.
3. **Methyl alcohol** fixes the smear to the slide. It is **acetone-free** because *acetone causes lysis of the cell* (breaks the cell membrane).

■ Alternative stains

Other stains that can be used in place of the Leishman stain are the following:

1. **Wright stain**: This is a *modified Romanowsky stain* that is quite similar to the Leishman stain, producing the same colour reaction with the cellular components of blood.
2. **May–Grunwald and Giemsa stain**: The slide is first stained with May–Grunwald stain for 5 minutes, then with Giemsa stain for 10 minutes. Staining of the cells is similar to Leishman staining.
3. **Field stain**: Originally used for thick films for malarial parasites in field studies. Staining is rapid and convenient and is used for rapid screening of blood smears.

Procedure

1. Place the slides on the staining rack with the blood smear (dull side of the slide) facing up. If a staining rack is not available, place two glass rods over a tray to hold the slide.
2. Pour 8–12 drops of Leishman stain on the slide, *just enough to cover the smear*.
3. Note the time and leave it for 1½ to 2 minutes.

Note: During this period, the alcohol in the stain fixes the cells (**fixation time**).

4. With the help of a dropper, add double the amount of distilled water over the smear, taking care that the *water does not spill*.
5. Mix the stain and water evenly by blowing gently or by blowing air through a Pasteur pipette.

Note: A **metallic shiny layer (greenish scum)** should form on the top of this mixture.

6. Note the time and leave it for 7–10 minutes.

Note: This is the time when staining occurs (**staining time**). Staining time may have to be adjusted according to the intensity of the stain. Reduce the time if it is overstained, and increase the time if it is poorly stained.

7. Pour off the stain and wash the slide gently and thoroughly under tap water.

Note: Make sure that the stream of water does not fall directly on the smear. While discarding the stain, ensure that there is **no greenish scum sticking to the surface** of the smear.

8. Shake off all water adhering to the slide and place the slide in an upright position in a drying rack.

Note: Keep the smeared surface of the slide face down. This prevents dust from settling on the smear.

Precautions

1. The smear *should dry completely* before staining. Unless completely dry, the smear will not stick to the slide and is removed while washing.
2. An adequate quantity (8–10 drops) of stain should be poured on the smear and the stain should cover the entire smear. *Do not pour excess stain* (it should just cover the smear).
3. *Adequate fixing time* should be allowed (check the recommended time of fixation for the given sample of stain).
4. The distilled water should just cover the slide. Care should be taken to *prevent spill-over of the mixture* of water and stain.
5. It is important that the *staining rack be kept on a level surface* so that the stain is uniform throughout the film and the mixture does not spill over.
6. Water and stain should be *mixed by gentle blowing*. This should be done immediately after pouring the distilled water.
7. The exact timing for staining should be followed (check the recommended time).
8. When the mixture of stained water is poured off the slide, care should be taken *to prevent the deposition of scum* on the smear.
9. While washing, it should be ensured that *the smear is not directly under the stream of water*.

EXAMINATION OF A STAINED BLOOD SMEAR

After the smear is prepared, it is examined under the low-power and high-power objectives and then under the oil-immersion objective. **Examination under the low-power and high-power objectives** comprises the following:

1. Evaluation of the quality of the smear
2. Rough estimation of the red cell and leucocyte numbers

3. Distribution of the cells in the smear
4. A scan of the film
   Examination under the oil-immersion objective comprises the following:
1. Examination of the erythrocytes for alterations and variations in morphology
2. Evaluation of platelet numbers and morphology
3. Differential count of leucocytes

Steps of Examination

The examination of a smear takes place in three steps: general scanning, selection of the site for examination, and identification and count of cells.

General scanning

First, examine the stained blood smear under *low-power objective* for screening. This allows you to scan the entire slide of blood smear quickly. Note the background colour and distribution of white cells. In an ideal stained smear, **three zones** can be identified (Fig. 10.2A):
1. The thick area or the 'head' of the smear
2. The 'body' of the smear
3. The thin end or 'tail' of the smear

Towards the tail end, the red cells lie singly, and neutrophils and monocytes predominate. **In the body**, the red cells overlap to a certain extent, and the lymphocytes predominate. *Towards the head end*, the red cells considerably overlap, and eosinophils predominate. This non-uniform distribution of various types of leucocytes is inherent to the smear prepared by the glass slide method. Therefore, the smear should be **examined in a zigzag fashion** (refer to Fig. 11.1) across the length of the smear but not along its breadth to get an accurate differential count. If the scanning indicates the very irregular distribution of leucocytes (neutrophils and monocytes are fully concentrated in the tail), the smear will yield an inaccurate differential count. In this case, make a new smear. The scanning of the entire slide also helps to *detect the presence of large abnormal cells* like megakaryoblasts and parasites like microfilariae.

Selection of site for examination

If the **smear is an ideal one** (*one-cell thickness, red cells not overlapping and not wide apart*), it should be examined throughout its length, excluding the extreme, thin portion of the tail and the very thick portion of the head.

If the **smear is not an ideal one** (which often happens in practice), select the portion of the blood smear where the red cells just touch each other or slightly overlap but are not piled on top of one another. This area is usually found **near the feather edge** (between the body and tail) of the film.

Place **a drop of immersion oil on the slide** directly on the smear (not on a coverslip). Now switch to the oil-immersion objective. Ensure that the objective makes contact with the oil. Look through the microscope and increase the light by opening the iris as needed.

Identification of Cells

Various types of blood cells are identified on the basis of the following characteristics that become apparent after staining with the Leishman stain. Even if the smear is not properly stained, the shape and size of the cells provide sufficient clues for their identification (Fig. 10.3).

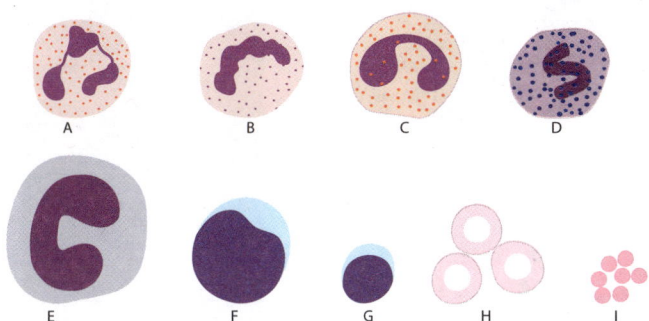

Fig. 10.3 Cells observed in a normal peripheral smear: (A) segmented neutrophil; (B) band neutrophil; (C) eosinophil; (D) basophil; (E) monocyte; (F) large lymphocyte; (G) small lymphocyte; (H) red cells; (I) platelets.

■ I. Red blood cells

Appearance: Red cells appear as round bodies containing no nucleus, granules, or discrete materials.

Staining: They stain orange-red. The red colour is darker at the edges of the cell than in the centre (giving the appearance of a central halo). This variation is caused by the biconcave shape of the cells which contain less hemoglobin in their (thinner) centres.

Size: The diameter of the cells is about 7.2 μm.

■ II. Platelets

Appearance: Under high-power, they look like dirt and stain deposits. Under oil-immersion, they look like pin heads. They contain no nuclei. On fine adjustment, platelets look refractile; this is a characteristic feature that distinguishes them from deposited stained particles.

Staining: They stain mauve-pink.

Distribution: Usually, they are present in groups or aggregates (many platelets lying close to each other). However, the presence of a single (isolated) platelet is not unusual.

Size: They are the smallest cells in the peripheral smear. The diameter of platelets is 2–4 μm.

■ III. Leucocytes

i. Neutrophils *(Fig. 10.4)*

Size: Neutrophils are about 10–14 μm.

Nucleus: They are multilobed (2–6 lobes), and the lobes are connected by thin strands. In the **band form**, the nucleus is sausage-shaped (also called **stab form**).

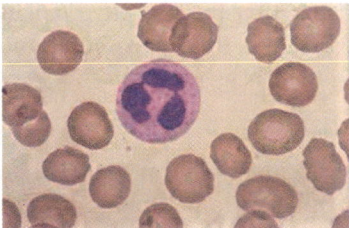
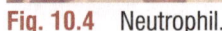

Fig. 10.4   Neutrophil.

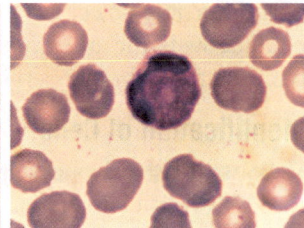

Fig. 10.5   Eosinophil.

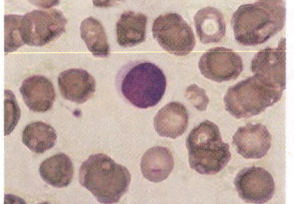

Fig. 10.8   Small lymphocyte.

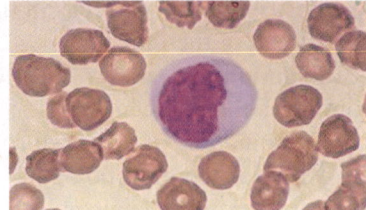

Fig. 10.9   Monocyte.

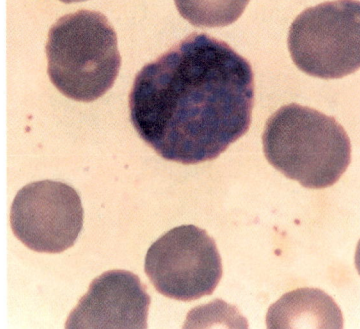

Fig. 10.6   Basophil.

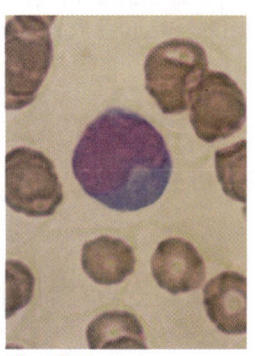

Fig. 10.7   Large lymphocyte.

Cytoplasm: Looks pale pink and contains fine pink granules.

ii. Eosinophils *(Fig. 10.5)*

Size: About 10–14 µm.
Nucleus: Usually bilobed; lobes are connected by a thick strand, giving the appearance of spectacles (spectacle-shaped nucleus).
Cytoplasm: Stains faintly pink with coarse brick-red or red-orange granules. The cytoplasm is usually not visible as it is obscured by granules.

iii. Basophils *(Fig. 10.6)*

Size: About 10–14 µm.
Nucleus: Usually bilobed or trilobed. However, lobes are usually not distinctly visible because the cell is studded with granules.
Cytoplasm: Contains numerous coarse granules that are blue-black. They fill the cells and obscure the nucleus.

iv. Large lymphocytes *(Fig. 10.7)*

Size: 10–14 µm.
Nucleus: Occupies 80–90 per cent of the cell. It is eccentrically placed, and oval or round with or without a dent. It is homogeneous (compact) and violet in colour.
Cytoplasm: Clear blue cytoplasm; usually contains no granules.

v. Small lymphocytes *(Fig. 10.8)*

Size: 6–9 µm (same as or slightly larger than red cells).
Nucleus: Occupies almost the whole cell. It is homogeneous (compact) and deep violet in colour.
Cytoplasm: May not be present; sometimes, there may be a thin rim of clear blue cytoplasm present at the periphery. There are no granules.

vi. Monocytes *(Fig. 10.9)*

Size: 12–24 µm; the largest leucocytes.
Nucleus: Occupies 50 per cent of the cell and is centrally or slightly eccentrically placed. It is usually kidney-shaped or horseshoe-shaped, but may be round, oval, dumb-bell shaped, or irregular. It is non-homogeneous (spongy) in appearance and pinkish-violet in colour
Cytoplasm: Has a ground-glass (hazy, turbid) appearance and grey-blue in colour. It usually contains no granules; sometimes (15–30 per cent of monocytes), fine granules may be present.

Observation and Results

1. Note your observation on the quality of your smear (good or bad). Mention the criteria of an ideal smear (details in the 'Discussion' section).
2. Make a note of the structure and function of each leucocyte.
3. Report any abnormal cell or parasite observed during the general screening of the smear or its detailed examination.
4. Note your observations of the identification the WBCs in a tabular form with details of the structure and functions of the cells observed (as presented in Table 10.1).

The differences in structure and function of leucocytes are summarised in Table 10.1.

DISCUSSION

A bad smear results from a lack of sincerity and interest in making the smear. If all the steps for preparing and staining the smear are properly followed, the smear will definitely be a good one. Even a good smear will be spoiled if not stained properly.

Staining Defects

The following staining defects are frequently observed.

1. **Presence of more precipitated stained particles:** This occurs due to either *improper washing or the use of an old stain* that has not been properly filtered. Improper washing means inadequate washing of metallic scum. It can be corrected by using a freshly prepared or adequately filtered stain and ensuring proper washing. The smear should be washed for about one minute.

Table 10.1   Structure and functions of various leucocytes in the differential leucocyte count (DLC).

Leucocytes	% in DLC	Structure	Functions
Neutrophils	50–70%	10–14 μm diameter; nucleus is multilobed; lobes connected by thin strands of chromatin; cytoplasm has fine, pink granules	Phagocytosis of organisms (first line of defence against bacterial infection)
Eosinophils	1–4%	10–14 μm diameter; nucleus is bilobed; coarse brick-red granules in cytoplasm	Combat the effects of histamine in allergic reactions, kill parasitic worms
Basophils	0–1%	10–14 μm diameter; nucleus is bilobed and irregular in shape; large cytoplasmic granules are deep blue-purple	Release heparin, histamine, and serotonin in allergic reactions that promote overall inflammatory response
Lymphocytes	20–40%	Small lymphocytes are 6–9 μm in diameter; large lymphocytes are 10–14 μm in diameter; nucleus is round or slightly indented; cytoplasm forms a clear rim around the nucleus; nuclear–cytoplasmic ratio is 80:20	Mediate immune responses
Monocytes	2–8%	12–25 μm diameter; nucleus is oval or kidney-shaped or horseshoe-shaped; cytoplasm turbid in appearance; nuclear–cytoplasmic ratio is 50:50	Phagocytosis (second line of defence); more phagocytic after transforming into tissue macrophages

2. **Excessively red appearance**: This occurs due to *understaining, overwashing, or the use of a highly acidic stain or water* (for staining). It can be rectified by increasing the fixing and staining time and properly washing the smear. *Buffered* (pH 6.8) or distilled water should be used for staining.

3. **Excessively blue appearance**: This results from *overfixing, overstaining, inadequate washing*, or the use of a **highly alkaline stain or water** (for staining). It can be rectified by decreasing the fixing and staining time, properly washing the smear, and using a proper stain and water.

4. **Faded appearance of the cells**: This results from **overwashing, understaining, or underfixing** or from an *improperly made stain*.

Morphological Differences Between Leucocytes

Usually, students confuse neutrophils with eosinophils and large lymphocytes with monocytes. The important differentiating features of these cells are presented in Table 10.2.

Criteria of an Ideal Smear

1. A good blood smear should cover one-half to three-quarters of the length of the slide.

2. It should be thickest at the origin and gradually thin out rather than having alternate thick and thin areas. The thin end of the smear should have a good feather

Table 10.2   Differences between neutrophils and eosinophils; and large lymphocytes and monocytes.

Features	Neutrophils	Eosinophils
Size	Double the size of red cells	Double the size of red cells
Nucleus	Multilobed (2–6 lobes); lobes connected by thin strands	Usually bilobed; lobes connected by a thick strand (has a spectacle-like appearance)
Cytoplasm	Contains fine pink granules	Contain coarse brick-red granules
	Large lymphocyte	**Monocyte**
Size	About double the size of red cells	Triple the size of red cells or larger
Nucleus	Oval or round, usually with a dent Compact (homogeneous) Eccentric Occupies 80–90 per cent of the cell	Kidney or horse-shoe shaped nucleus, but may be round, oval or dumb-bell-shaped Spongy (non-homogeneous) Centrally placed Occupies 50 per cent of the cell
Cytoplasm	Clear, sky blue, contains no granules	Hazy, ground-glass in appearance, sometimes (15–20% monocytes); may contain fine granules
Nuclear–cytoplasmic ratio	80:20	50:50

edge, i.e., the film should fade away without a defined border at the end. It should be tongue-shaped.

3. There should be no streaks or gaps in the smear.
4. It should be one-cell thick (of red cells), i.e., the red cells should not overlap, nor should they be too far from each other. If a film is thick, the cells pile up. The **thickness of the film** is determined by:
   i. **Size of the drop of blood used**—a thick film results when the drop of blood is large, and a thin film from a small drop of blood.
   ii. **The speed of the stroke used to move the spreader slide**—a thick film results from fast spreader movement, and a thin film from slow movement.
   iii. **The angle at which the spreader slide is moved**—a thick film results when the angle is greater than 45°, and a thin film results when the angle is less than 30°.
5. It appears salmon pink to the naked eye if stained properly.

6. It should not contain precipitated stained particles.
7. When examined microscopically, the background or space between the cells should be clear, the red cells should appear light red-orange, the platelets should look pink, and the nucleus, cytoplasm, and granules should be stained with the right colour.

Preparation of Thick and Thin Smears

Thick smears are chiefly prepared for the *detection of microfilariae* in the peripheral blood. A drop of blood is placed at the centre of the slide and spread with the corner of another slide. The film is allowed to dry for 30 minutes at 37°C and then stained. The entire film is scanned using a low-power objective.

A **thin smear** is prepared for the *identification of species of the parasite*, for which a drop of blood is spread thinly across a slide, allowing a single layer of the cell to be examined.

OSPE

I.   Prepare a smear from the given sample of blood.
Steps
1. Clean four slides.
2. Select a spreader.
3. Mix the blood thoroughly.
4. Place a drop of blood at one end of a slide.
5. Hold the opposite end of the slide between the middle or index finger and the thumb of the left hand.
6. Place the spreader in front of the drop of blood at an angle of 30–45° and then draw the spreader back until it touches the drop of blood. Wait for the blood to spread along the edge of the spreader or slightly shake the spreader to facilitate spreading.
7. Push the spreader with a steady, smooth, and quick movement to the other end of the slide to make an ideal smear (examiner to look for thickness and size of the smear).
8. Immediately dry the smear by waving the slide in the air.

II.   Stain the supplied smear for DLC.
Steps
1. Select an ideal smear.
2. Place the slide horizontally across the two glass rods on the staining tray.
3. Select the Leishman stain.
4. Add 8–12 drops of the stain to the smear (the stain should be adequate to cover the smear) and note the time.
5. After 1½ minutes, add distilled water, and double the amount of stain on the smear, taking care not to spill the mixture.

6. Mix the stain with water by blowing gently or with the help of a Pasteur pipette. Take care to prevent spill-over of the mixture.

III.   Focus a neutrophil in the given smear under the oil-immersion objective.
Steps
1. Select an ideal smear.
2. Place the slide on the stage of the microscope and scan the smear under the low-power objective by making necessary microscopic adjustments (concave mirror, condenser at lowest position and iris partially closed) and select the proper site for further examination under the oil-immersion objective.
3. Place a drop of oil on the chosen site and change to the oil-immersion objective.
4. Make other microscopic adjustments (change to plane mirror, raise the condenser to maximum height, and open the iris fully) for examination under the oil-immersion objective.
5. Focus on the neutrophil and make fine adjustments to get a clear picture of the cell.

IV.   Focus an eosinophil in the given smear under the oil-immersion objective.
1. Steps are the same as for OSPE III, except that the student focuses on the eosinophil.

V.   Focus a large lymphocyte in the given smear under the oil-immersion objective.
1. The steps are the same as for OSPE III, except that the student focuses on the large lymphocyte.

VI.   Focus a monocyte in the given smear under the oil-immersion objective.
1. The seps are the same as for OSPE III, except that the student focuses on the monocyte.

VIVA

1. *What are the methods of preparing a blood smear?* (Ans. Refer to page 61, under the heading 'Methods of Preparation of a Smear'.)
2. *Why is the glass slide method called the wedge method?* (Ans. Refer to page 61, under the heading 'Wedge...Method'.)
3. *What are the advantages of making a smear by the centrifugal method?* (Ans. Refer to page 63, under the heading 'Centrifugal...Method', read Advantages.)
4. *How is a spreader selected for making a smear?* (Ans. Refer to page 61, under the heading 'Requirements', point no. 2.)
5. *Why should the angle between the spreader and the specimen slide be between 30° and 45°?* (Ans. Refer to page 63, under the heading 'Precautions', point no. 9.)
6. *Why should the smear be dried quickly after preparing it?* (Ans. Refer to page 62, under the heading 'Procedure', see 'Note' below point no. 11.)
7. *What is the method of drying the blood smear?* (Ans. Refer to page 62, under the heading 'Procedure', point no. 11.)
8. *What are the precautions to be taken while preparing a blood smear?* (Ans. Refer to page 62, text under the heading 'Precautions'.)
9. *Why is the smear immediately made after placing the drop of blood on the slide?* (Ans. Refer to page 62, under the heading 'Precautions', point no. 5'.)
10. *Why is the smear made by a steady and smooth movement of the spreader?* (Ans. Refer to page 62, under the heading 'Precautions', point no. 6'.)
11. *Why should the initial drop of blood be fully used in making a smear?* (Ans. Refer to page 62, text under the heading 'Precautions, point no. 8'.)
12. *Name the factors that determine the thickness of a smear.* (Ans. Refer to page 67, text under the heading 'Criteria of an Ideal Smear', point no. 4.)
13. *Why is the fixing done immediately after making a smear?*
(Ans. Fixing is done immediately to preserve the morphology of blood cells by adhering them to the slide before they begin to degrade. Leishman stain contains methanol, which acts as a fixative and fixes dead cells to the slide [unlike supravital staining, which fixes living cells]. Delayed fixing can lead to distortion and poor staining quality. Therefore, staining the smear promptly ensures proper fixation and accurate examination.)
14. *What is the method of fixing a smear if staining is to be delayed?*
(Ans. If the smear cannot be stained within a few hours, it should at least be fixed by immersion in absolute methyl alcohol [methanol] for 2–3 seconds and then air-dried.)
15. *Which is the stain usually used in staining the blood smear? What are its constituents and the functions of each constituent?*
(Ans. Refer to page 70, under the heading 'Requirements', read about the Leishman stain.)
16. *Why is the alcohol present in the Leishman stain acetone-free?*
(Ans. It is acetone-free because acetone breaks the cell membrane and causes lysis of the cells.)
17. *Why is distilled water added to the stain after fixation?*
(Ans. In the first two minutes, methanol in the stain causes the fixation of cells. Since stains only work in their ionized form, distilled water is added to them after fixation ionize the stain [ionization of methylene blue and eosin].)
18. *Why is water not used as a solvent for the Leishman stain?*
(Ans. Staining of cells is done only after they are fixed, by adding distilled water. Water opposes fixation of cells. If water is present in the stain, the cells will stain but will not fix to the smear. Therefore, stain is water-free. Water also enhances rouleaux formation of red cells, but this rarely happens after the smear is made.)
19. *What is buffered water and why is it preferred to distilled water for staining? Can tap water be used for the purpose?*
(Ans. Buffered water is a phosphate buffer. As ionization of stain particles occurs maximally at pH 6.8, the pH of buffer water is 6.8. Tap water is not used as it contains impurities.)
20. *Name the other stains that can also be used for staining the smear.* (Ans. Refer to page 64, under the heading 'Requirements', read 'Alternate Stains'.)
21. *In which special circumstances is the Field stain used?* (Ans. Refer to page 64, under the heading 'Requirements', read Other Stains....subheading 'Field stain')
22. *What are the precautions for staining a smear?* (Ans. Refer to page 64, text under the heading 'Precautions'.)
23. *Why is the stain diluted with distilled water after 1½ to 2 minutes and not earlier?* (Ans. Refer to page 64, under the heading 'Requirements', read point no. 3 and the 'Note' below it – Fixation Time.)
24. *What is the significance of the appearance of scum on the staining fluid after addition of distilled water?* (Ans. It indicates that the staining has been done properly. If the greenish scum does not float on the diluted stained surface, this indicates that the scum is deposited on the surface of the smear. In that case, the cells look hazy when examined under a microscope.)

25. *Why is the smear examined under low-power objective before being examined under an oil-immersion objective?* (Ans. Refer to page 65, under the heading 'Steps of Examination', read 'General Scanning'.)

26. *What is the purpose of general scanning of the smear prior to DLC?* (Ans. Refer to page 65, under the heading 'General Scanning'.)

27. *Which is the most ideal area of the smear for DLC and why?* (Ans. Refer to page 72, under the heading 'Steps of Examination', read 'General Scanning'.)

28. *What are the uses of a blood smear?*
(Ans. A blood smear is used for: i. DLC and detection of abnormalities of leucocytes if present, for example, immature and abnormal leucocytes as seen in different leukemias; ii. study of red cell morphology [size, shape, hemoglobin content]; iii. rough estimation of red cells and PCV; iv. the determination of indirect platelet count and morphology of platelets; v. detection of the presence of parasites, for example, malarial parasite, microfilariae and so on; vi. to differentiate the sexes by identifying the presence of Barr body in the nucleus of neutrophils [it needs special staining].)

29. *How do you identify red blood cells and platelets in a smear?* (Ans. Refer to page 65, under the heading 'Red Blood Cells' and 'Platelets'.)

30. *How will you differentiate neutrophils from eosinophils?* (Ans. Refer to page 67, Table 10.2.)

31. *How will you differentiate large lymphocytes from monocytes?* (Ans. Refer to page 67, Table 10.2.)

32. *What are the criteria of an ideal smear?* (Ans. Refer to page 67, under the heading 'Criteria of an Ideal Smear'.)

33. *What are the causes of deposition of precipitated stains in the smear and how do you prevent it?* (Ans. Refer to page 66, under the heading 'Staining Defects', point no. 1.)

34. *What are the causes of excessive red or blue appearance of the smear and how do you prevent it?* (Ans. Refer to page 67, 'Staining Defects', points no. 2 and 3.)

35. *What are the causes of the faded appearance of the cells in the smear and how do you prevent it?* (Ans. Refer to page 67, 'Staining Defects', point no. 4.)

36. *What is punctate basophilia (basophilic stippling) and what does it indicate?*
(Ans. Punctate basophilia or basophilic stippling is the presence of numerous basophilic granules in red cells. It indicates disturbed rather than increased erythropoiesis. It occurs in thalassemia, megaloblastic anemia, infections, liver disease, poisoning by lead and heavy metals, unstable hemoglobins and pyrimidine 5'-nucleotidase deficiency.)

37. *What are Dhol bodies, and what do they indicate?*
(Ans. **Dhol bodies** are small, round or oval, pale blue-grey bodies usually found in the periphery of neutrophils. They consist of ribosomes and endoplasmic reticulum. Their presence indicates bacterial infections. But they are also seen in tissue damage, inflammation and pregnancy.)

38. *What other information can be obtained from a blood smear?*
(Ans. i. Diagnosis of malaria by demonstrating malaria parasites in smear; ii. diagnosis of filaria by demonstrating filaria parasites or larva in smear; iii. diagnosis of leukemia, by demonstrating abnormal leucocytes, blast cells; iv. sex determination by demonstrating Barr bodies [sex chromatin appearing like drum sticks] attached to nucleus of neutrophil; v. red cell morphological abnormalities in the diagnosis of anemia; vi. platelet population in smear.)

11 | Differential Leucocyte Count

Learning Objectives

After completing this practical, you will be able to (MUST KNOW):

1. Describe the importance of performing DLC in practical physiology.
2. Select a good spreader slide.
3. Prepare a good smear for making DLC.
4. Identify leucocytes.
5. Perform a differential count within the stipulated time.

6. Describe the structure of various leucocytes.
7. List the common causes of alterations in leucocyte counts.

You may also be able to (DESIRABLE TO KNOW):

1. Explain the functions of different leucocytes.
2. State the physiological basis of alterations in cell counts in different clinical conditions.

PY2.11: Estimate Hb, RBC, TLC, RBC indices, DLC, blood groups, and BT/CT.

INTRODUCTION

The types and numbers of each type of leucocyte counted are traditionally reported as percentages. The determination of the **percentage distribution of leucocytes in peripheral blood** is known as *differential leucocyte count (DLC)*.

Leucocytes are divided into granulocytes and agranulocytes. Neutrophils, eosinophils, and basophils are **granulocytes**, and lymphocytes and monocytes are **agranulocytes**. The size of leucocytes and the characteristics of the nucleus and the cytoplasm of the cells are considered for the identification of leucocytes. The **features of the nucleus** include its shape and size compared to the rest of the cell and the pattern of chromatins in the nucleus. The **features of the cytoplasm** include the presence or absence of granules, the nature of granules and their staining characteristics and colour, and the relative amount of cytoplasm.

STRUCTURE AND FUNCTIONS OF LEUCOCYTES

Neutrophils

Neutrophils are the commonest leucocytes. They constitute 50–70% of the total leucocytes. Typically, there are **two types**: segmented and band neutrophils.

Segmented neutrophils: The structure of neutrophils is described in Chapter 10 (see Fig. 10.4, Chapter 10). About two-thirds of the granules are specific neutrophilic granules, while the remaining one-third are azurophilic granules.

Neutrophils are *actively phagocytic*. Their granules have many *hydrolytic enzymes* and appear to be lysosomal in character. **Phagocytosis** occurs through a series of events, which include **opsonization, chemotaxis, ingestion, and degranulation**. During phagocytosis, a *number of chemicals* are released, such as hydrogen peroxide, and hypochlorite and hydroxyl radicals, all of which are *strongly bactericidal*. Neutrophils form the **first line of defence** against acute bacterial infections.

Band neutrophils: Band neutrophils are younger neutrophils that account for 2–5 per cent of the total neutrophils. The nucleus may be rod or band-shaped, with slight indentations, but without definite lobes (see Fig. 10.3B, Chapter 10) The **number of granules is more** in band neutrophils than in segmented neutrophils. They are **more actively phagocytic**.

Eosinophils

Eosinophils constitute 1–4% of total leucocytes. Their structure is discussed in Chapter 10 (Fig. 10.5). Eosinophilic granules are coarse and highly refractile, a feature that is often valuable in distinguishing them from neutrophil granules.

Functions: Eosinophils are involved in *defending the body from allergic reactions*. Eosinophil granules contain a number of chemicals like MBP (major basic proteins), protein X, ECF-A (eosinophil chemotactic factor of anaphylaxis), and lysozymes that neutralize allergens and are also larvicidal and parasiticidal.

Basophils

Basophils constitute 0.5% of the total leucocytes. The structure of basophils is described in Chapter 10 (see Fig. 10.6). The cytoplasm is often studded with coarse, deeply stained blue-black granules.

Functions: Basophils mediate *allergic reactions*. Basophil granules contain heparin, histamine, and a slow-reacting substance (SRS). The cells are phagocytic. They contribute to the prevention of minute intravascular clot formation.

Monocytes

Monocytes are the largest leucocytes, measuring 12–25 μm in diameter (for detailed structure, see Fig. 10.9). They constitute 2–8% of the total leucocytes. Their nucleus is large and occupies 50% of the cell, the *nuclear-cytoplasmic ratio* being 50:50. *Nuclear chromatins* are sharply segregated and distributed in a linear arrangement of delicate strands, which gives the nucleus a *stringy appearance*. The **cytoplasm has a ground-glass appearance,** and sometimes, contains extremely fine pink granules.

Functions: Monocytes are *actively phagocytic*. They are the *second line of defence* of the body, protecting it against bacteria, viruses, fungi, and parasites. They also participate in immunity. They act as *antigen-presenting cells* and secrete a *number of cytokines* that mediate various immunologic responses. They remain in circulation for a few hours and then migrate into the tissues, and transform into *tissue macrophages*.

Lymphocytes

Lymphocytes constitute 20–40% of leucocytes in adults. *Structurally, lymphocytes are of two types:* small and large (structures described in Chapter 10, Figs. 10.7 and 10.8, respectively). The majority (80%) of circulating lymphocytes are small. In **small lymphocytes**, the intracellular space is largely occupied by the nucleus, with a thin rim of peripheral cytoplasm. In **large lymphocytes**, the nucleus occupies around 80% of the cell (*nuclear–cytoplasmic ratio* is 80:20). The nucleus contains homogeneous chromatin with some clumping at the nuclear periphery. This gives the nucleus of lymphocytes a **compact appearance** in contrast to the spongy appearance of the nucleus of monocytes. The cytoplasm is clear and navy blue in colour, and usually does not contain granules.

Functions: Lymphocytes mediate the immunologic responses of the body. Functionally, lymphocytes are divided into **two categories**: T lymphocytes and B lymphocytes. *The majority (80%) of the circulating lymphocytes are T lymphocytes.* **T lymphocytes** mediate **cellular immunity**, which is concerned with viral and fungal infections, parasitic infestation, cancer cells, transplant rejection and the rejection of tumour cells. **B lymphocytes** mediate **humoral immunity** by producing antibodies concerned with protecting the body against bacterial and other infections. B cells, on specific immunologic stimulation, transform into **plasma cells** that synthesise antibodies. Therefore, plasma cells are not normally found in the blood.

NORMAL COUNTS

For a differential leucocyte count, a minimum of 100 cells should be counted. Ideally, 200 or more cells should be counted to find out a more accurate percentage of each type of leucocyte. The percentage distribution of cells in a normal leucocyte count in adults is as follows:

1. **Neutrophil:** 50–70 per cent
2. **Eosinophil:** 1–4 per cent
3. **Basophil:** 0–1 per cent
4. **Lymphocyte:** 20–40 per cent
5. **Monocyte:** 2–8 per cent

Infants and children have fewer neutrophils (40–60 per cent) and more lymphocytes (25–55 per cent).

METHOD OF COUNTING LEUCOCYTES

Principle

A blood film stained with Leishman stain is examined under an oil-immersion objective, and the different types of white blood cells are identified. The percentage distribution of these cells is then determined.

Requirements

1. Glass slides
2. Leishman stain
3. Microscope
4. Distilled water
5. Pasteur pipette

Procedure

1. **Prepare a blood smear** and stain it with Leishman stain as described in Chapter 10.
2. First, examine the smear under a low-power objective for **general scanning,** assessing the quality of the smear, and studying the pattern of distribution of the cells.
3. Place a drop of cedarwood oil at the *feather edge* of the smear. Bring the oil-immersion objective into position and make the lower end of the objective touch the drop of oil. Using the fine adjustment screw, adjust the objective and focus the cells.
4. For **counting cells,** start from one end of the smear and move the slide in a **zigzag manner** (Fig. 11.1). Count individual white cells that you come across and enter your observation in a table (as described below) in your rough notebook. Continue counting until 100 cells are counted.
5. Calculate the percentage of each leucocyte and report your observation.

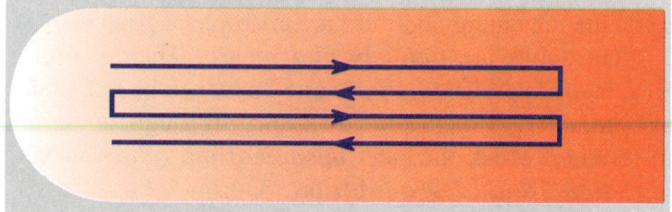

Fig. 11.1 Zigzag method used for differential leucocyte count. The arrows in the blood smear indicate the direction of counting.

Neutrophils	ⵍ⊦I	ⵍ⊦I	ⵍ⊦⊦	ⵍ⊦⊦	ⵍ⊦⊦	Iⵍ⊦	Iⵍ⊦	Iⵍ⊦	Iⵍ⊦	Iⵍ⊦	ⵍ⊦⊦	=	55 cells
Eosinophils	ⵍ⊦I	ⵍ⊦I	ⵍ⊦⊦									=	15 cells
Basophils												=	nil
Lymphocyte	ⵍ⊦I	ⵍ⊦I	ⵍ⊦⊦	ⵍ⊦⊦	ⵍ⊦⊦							=	25 cells
Monocytes	ⵍ⊦I											=	5 cells
											Total	=	**100 cells**

Neutrophils	55 per cent
Eosinophils	15 per cent
Basophils	0 per cent
Lymphocytes	25 per cent
Monocytes	5 per cent

Observation and Results

Different leucocytes are placed in groups of 5, five lines indicating five cells (four vertical lines and one oblique line placed over the four lines indicates the fifth cell). In this way, 100 cells are counted. An example of such counting is shown below.

Alternatively, a **table of 100 small squares** can be drawn and each cell counted can be entered in the small squares of the table, till 100 cells are filled. On the right side of the table, against each row, the number of different leucocytes present in that row can be entered in separate columns and finally, the percentage can be taken as shown below.

N	N	N	L	L	N	N	N	E	M
N	L	L	N	L	E	E	N	N	N
N	N	N	L	E	N	E	M	N	N
N	L	L	E	N	N	N	L	N	N
N	N	N	L	L	L	N	E	N	E
N	N	N	L	L	N	N	N	N	M
N	L	L	N	E	E	N	L	E	N
N	N	N	L	L	N	E	M	N	N
N	L	L	E	E	N	M	L	N	N
N	N	N	L	L	L	N	E	N	N

Inference: In the example above, there is moderate eosinophilia of 15 per cent. Other leucocyte values are within the normal range.

Precautions

All the precautions described in the previous chapter are applicable to this practical. In addition, the following precautions should be observed:

1. The quality of the smear should be assessed before starting the count. The smear should be discarded if it is not good, and a fresh smear should be prepared.
2. Cells should be counted across the length of the smear, except the extreme ends (head and tail).
3. Counting should be done in a zigzag pattern to prevent the double counting of a cell.
4. A minimum of 100 cells should be counted.
5. The slide should be preserved for future rechecking of the result.

DISCUSSION

Differential count is a frequently ordered investigation in clinical medicine. Usually, it is performed along with other hematologic tests like total leucocyte count to assess the ability of the subject to defend his body from microbial invasion and to assist in diagnosing the diseases.

Clinical Significance

Differential count is vital for the diagnosis of a number of diseases involving leucocytes or red cells. Its primary use is to identify changes in the distribution of white cells, which

N	E	B	L	M
6	1	0	2	1
5	2	0	3	0
6	2	0	1	1
6	1	0	3	0
5	2	0	3	0
7	0	0	2	1
4	3	0	3	0
6	1	0	2	1
4	2	0	3	1
6	1	0	3	0
55	**15**	**0**	**25**	**5**

may be related to a particular disease like a specific infection (e.g., typhoid) or a malignant condition (e.g., leukemia). An *increase in specific white cells* (neutrophilia, eosinophilia, lymphocytosis, and monocytosis) or *decrease in cells* (neutropenia, eosinopenia, lymphocytopenia, and monocytopenia) are based on the differential count.

Other uses: Studying a blood smear also reveals the following: i) *morphological abnormalities* of blood cells, ii) the **presence of abnormal cells**, iii) the presence of *blood parasites*, iv) the *approximate estimation of other cells* (RBCs and platelets), v) the *hemoglobin status and type of anemia* and checking the reports on blood indices, vi) female sex can be determined by demonstrating the **Barr** body (chromatin of the sex chromosome) attached to a lobe of the nucleus of the neutrophil, appearing like a drumstick.

Conditions That Alter Different Cell Counts

I. Neutrophilia
Physiological
1. Exercise
2. Pregnancy
3. Parturition
4. Food intake
5. Emotional stress
6. Exposure to cold

Pathological
1. **Acute pyogenic infections**, e.g., tonsillitis and pneumonia
2. **Non-infective inflammations**, e.g., rheumatic fever
3. **Non-inflammatory conditions**, e.g., myocardial infarction and pulmonary embolism
4. **Acute hemorrhage**
5. **Muscle trauma**, e.g., following surgery
6. **Leukemia**, e.g., chronic myeloid leukemia
7. Toxic conditions, e.g., uremia and hepatic coma
8. Corticosteroid therapy

II. Neutropenia
Physiological
Physiological neutropenia is very rare. Sometimes, it occurs after chronic exposure to severe cold.

Pathological
1. Starvation and debility
2. **Typhoid** and paratyphoid fever
3. **Aplastic anemia** (bone marrow failure)
4. Parasitic infections like malaria and kala azar
5. **Viral infections** like measles, influenza, and viral hepatitis
6. Hypersplenism
7. **Drug-induced** neutropenia, e.g., chemotherapeutic drugs

III. Eosinophilia
1. **Allergic conditions**
   - Bronchial asthma
   - Urticaria
   - Food allergy
   - Hay fever
2. **Parasitic infestations**
   - Hookworm
   - Filariasis
   - Hydatid disease
3. **Skin diseases**
   - Psoriasis
   - Pemphigus

4. **Collagen diseases**
   - Periarteritis nodosa
5. Hodgkin's disease
6. **Addison's disease**
7. Certain leukemias

IV. Eosinopenia
1. ACTH therapy
2. Cushing's disease
3. Acute pyogenic infections
4. Aplastic anemia

V. Basophilia
1. Chronic myeloid leukemia
2. Polycythemia

VI. Basophilopenia
It is a rare condition seen in severe septicemia or aplastic anemia.

VII. Lymphocytosis
1. **Chronic infections**
   - Tuberculosis
   - Pertussis (whooping cough)
   - Syphilis
   - Brucellosis
2. **Infectious mononucleosis**
3. **Lymphocytic leukemia**
4. **Lymphomas**
5. Viral infections

VIII. Lymphocytopenia
1. Immunosuppressive therapy
2. ACTH therapy
3. Hodgkin's disease
4. Bone marrow failure

IX. Monocytosis
1. Protozoan diseases
   - Malaria
   - Kala azar
2. Hodgkin's disease
3. Monocytic or myelomonocytic leukemia
4. ACTH therapy

X. Monocytopenia
1. Bone marrow failure
2. Aplastic anemia
3. Septicemia

OSPE

The OSPEs discussed in the previous chapter are also applicable to this chapter.

VIVA

All the questions **listed in the previous chapter** are also applicable to this chapter. The following are some additional questions:

1. *What are the functions of neutrophils, eosinophils, and basophils?* (Ans. Refer to page 71, under the heading 'Structure and Functions of Leucocytes' and the subheadings 'Functions' under Neutrophils, Eosinophils, and Basophils.)

2. *What are the functions of lymphocytes and monocytes?* (Ans. Refer to pages 71 and 72, under the heading 'Structure and Functions of Leucocytes', read the subheading 'Functions' under Lymphocytes and Monocytes.)

3. *What is the normal percentage distribution of different leucocytes in peripheral blood?* (Ans. Refer to page 72, under the heading 'Normal Counts'.)

4. *What is the clinical significance of performing DLC?* (Ans. Refer to page 71, under the heading 'Discussion', read 'Clinical Significance'.)

5. *List the conditions in which leucocytes increase and decrease.* (Ans. Refer to page 74 under the heading 'Conditions That Alter Different Cell Count'.)

6. *Apart from identifying alterations in specific cell counts, what are the other uses of DLC?* (Ans. Refer to page 73, under the heading 'Discussion' read 'Other Uses' in 'Clinical Significance'.)

7. *Can a subject's sex be determined by examining their blood smear?* (Ans. Refer to page 73, under the heading 'Clinical Significance', read 'Other Uses'.)

8. *What is the peroxidase reaction? What type of leucocytes produce this reaction?*
    (Ans. The peroxidase reaction [peroxidase stain] occurs when a dry blood film is treated with a solution of benzidine and sodium nitroprusside dissolved in ethyl alcohol and then hydrogen peroxide. After thoroughly washing with water, the film is counter-stained with Leishman stain in the usual manner. The peroxidase reaction detects the presence of oxidizing enzymes in the cytoplasm of the myeloid series of WBCs. Oxidase granules are seen in myelocytes and myeloblasts. The lymphoid series of cells is peroxidase-negative. This peroxidase reaction helps in distinguishing immature cells of the myeloid series from lymphoid series in cases of leukemia.)

9. *How is the absolute count of each type of leucocyte calculated using the value of TLC and DLC?*
    (Ans. Absolute count of a cell is equal to the number of that cell counted in DLC divided by $100 \times$ TLC. For example, if TLC = $7000/mm^3$ of blood, DLC is as follows:)
    Neutrophils: 55 per cent   Lymphocytes: 25 per cent

    Eosinophils: 15 per cent   Monocytes: 5 per cent   Basophils: 0 per cent

    Absolute counts of the various leucocytes are as follows:

    Neutrophils = $(55/100) \times 7000 = 3850/mm^3$ of blood

    Eosinophils = $(15/100) \times 7000 = 1050/mm^3$ of blood

    Lymphocytes = $(25/100) \times 7000 = 1750/mm^3$ of blood

    Monocytes = $(5/100) \times 7000 = 350/mm^3$ of blood

12 | Arneth (Cooke-Arneth) Count

Learning Objectives

After completing this practical, you will be able to (MUST KNOW):

1. Identify neutrophils at various stages of development.
2. State the percentage distribution of neutrophils at various stages.
3. Perform the Arneth count.
4. List the precautions taken while performing the Arneth count.

5. List the functions of neutrophils.
6. Explain the meaning and causes of 'shift to right' and 'shift to left'.

You may also be able to (DESIRABLE TO KNOW):

1. Explain the clinical significance of the Arneth count.
2. Explain the mechanisms of 'shift to right' and 'shift to left' that occur in various conditions.

INTRODUCTION

Arneth count (also called Cooke–Arneth count) is a method of **determining the percentage distribution of different types of neutrophils** on the basis of the number of their nuclear lobes. Joseph Arneth, a German physiologist, classified neutrophils into **five types** (stages), according to the number of lobes in their nuclei (Fig. 12.1):

1. **N1 (Stage 1):** The nucleus is unilobed. This stage is called the **band neutrophil** because the nucleus is rod- or band-shaped. There may be slight indentations, but distinct lobes (clearly separated lobes by thin strands) are not found. In some neutrophils, the nucleus may be U-shaped (called **stab neutrophils** or **Schaff cells**).
2. **N2 (Stage 2):** The nucleus is bilobed (two lobes separated by a thin strand).
3. **N3 (Stage 3):** The nucleus is trilobed (three lobes separated by thin strands).
4. **N4 (Stage 4):** The nucleus is tetralobed (four lobes separated by thin strands).
5. **N5 (Stage 5):** The nucleus is pentalobed (five lobes separated by thin strands).

Rarely, **N6** (six lobes) and **N7** (seven lobes) stages may be encountered.

This staging of neutrophils is based on the **degree of maturity**. The younger neutrophils contain fewer nuclear lobes than the older ones.

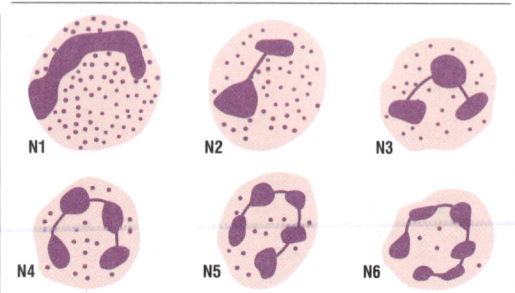

Fig. 12.1 Stages of neutrophils. Note that with maturation, the number of nuclear lobes increases, but the number of granules and the size of the cell decrease.

Sometimes it is difficult to stage neutrophils, especially when the lobes of the nucleus are folded. In such situations, **two other features** may be considered: (1) **the number of granules** and (2) **the cell size**. The *younger cells contain more granules than older cells.* As they participate in physiologic activities, cells lose their granules (degranulation) and therefore, the older cells contain fewer granules. Hence, neutrophils of stage 6 or 7 contain very few or no granules. *The size of the cell also decreases as age advances.* In older cells (N5, N6, and N7), the nucleus may also exhibit features of degeneration in the form of fragmentation (of lobes) and pyknosis.

Normal Counts

N1: 2–10 per cent
N2: 20–30 per cent
N3: 40–50 per cent
N4: 10–15 per cent
N5: 2–5 per cent

METHOD OF PERFORMING THE ARNETH COUNT

Principle

Neutrophils are grouped into different stages based on the number of nuclear lobes they possess. The percentage distribution of different stages of neutrophils is determined by examining a stained smear under an oil-immersion objective.

Requirements

This is the same as that used for differential leucocyte count (Chapter 11).

Procedure

1. Prepare a blood smear and stain it with Leishman stain as described under DLC.

2. Examine the smear under a low-power objective to assess the distribution of cells.

3. Count neutrophils under an oil-immersion objective as N1, N2, N3, N4, and N5 for neutrophils of stages 1, 2, 3, 4, and 5, respectively.

Note: While counting the cells, start from one end of the smear and proceed in a zigzag manner as described under DLC.

4. Count at **least 100 neutrophils** and enter your observation in a tabular format (in 100 small squares).

Observation and Results

1. Count 100 neutrophils and enter your observations as N1–N5 in a **tabular format** in 100 small squares (as shown below).

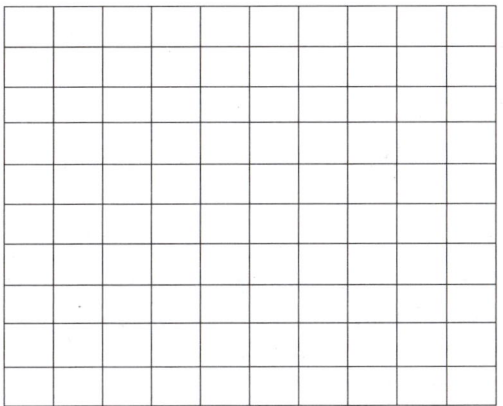

2. Count the % of each N1 to N5, similar to that of DLC as described in Chapter 11.

3. Express your values as the percentage of neutrophils counted:
    N1: Cells with single-lobed nucleus_____%
    N2: Cells with bilobed nucleus_____%
    N3: Cells with trilobed nucleus_____%
    N4: Cells with tetralobed nucleus_____%
    N5: Cells with pentalobed nucleus_____%

4. Note the **percentage distribution** of various stages of neutrophils and **plot them on a graph** (Fig. 12.2). The curve that is obtained by plotting this graph is called the **Arneth curve**.

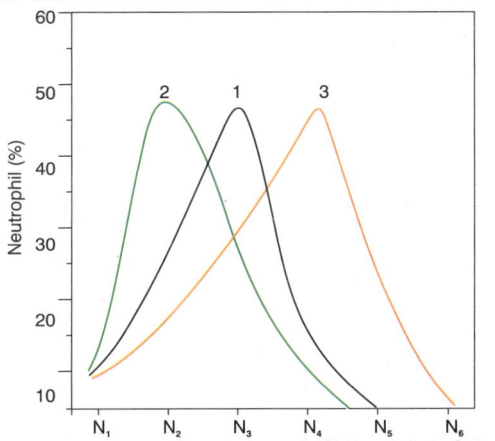

Fig. 12.2 Arneth curve (1: Normal count; 2: Shift to left; 3: Shift to right).

Precautions

1. The smear should be one-cell thick.
2. Staining should be proper.
3. The **lobes of the neutrophils** should be counted accurately.
4. If there is confusion in staging a neutrophil, the **number of granules and the size of the cell** should be considered.
5. At least 100 neutrophils should be counted.

DISCUSSION

Neutrophils are **actively phagocytic cells** in the blood. They are the **body's first line of defence** against acute bacterial infections. They are actively mobile; therefore, they migrate immediately to the site of infection and kill the organisms. In acute infections, the neutrophil count increases in proportion to the degree of assault.

Physiological Significance

Arneth count is not usually ordered in clinical practice. In some clinical conditions, it is used to determine the number of younger or older neutrophils in circulation. When there are more younger cells, the change is called **shift to left**; and when there are more older cells, the change is called **shift to right**. In shift to left, the total cells counted in N1 and N2 are more than 50 per cent, and in shift to right, the total cells counted in N4 and N5 is more than 20 per cent. Since Arneth count reveals the production of neutrophils, it **indirectly reflects the activity of the bone marrow**.

Shift to left (regenerative shift)

This indicates that the **bone marrow is hyperactive**; therefore, the circulating neutrophils are largely N1 and N2. This shift occurs due to the active response of the bone marrow to different stimuli to form and release more neutrophils into the circulation. The band forms increase in number, which may sometimes be accompanied by the presence of immature neutrophils.

- If **immature neutrophils** are present along with the younger neutrophils, the condition is called a **leukoblastotic reaction**.

- **Toxic changes** may manifest in neutrophils in the form of **basophilic stippling**, deep blue staining of the neutrophil granules like that of basophil granules (basophilic stippling is seen in red cells in lead poisoning).

Because the shift to left occurs due to increased production of cells, this is also called the **regenerative shift**.

Shift to right (degenerative shift)

This indicates the presence of older cells in the circulation. It occurs due to **decreased production of cells** by the bone marrow (*inadequate hematopoiesis*) as occurs in **aplastic anemia**.

- Sometimes, neutrophils of stage 6 or 7 may also appear in the blood.
- Neutrophils may undergo **toxic changes** in the form of the presence of *basophilic granules* (dark blue granules that resemble basophilic granules), vacuolisation of cytoplasm, **hypersegmentation** (more than five lobes) of the nucleus, and degeneration and pyknosis of the nucleus.

Since shift to right occurs due to hypofunction of the bone marrow, this is also called the **degenerative shift**.

Conditions That Affect Arneth Count

Shift to left

1. Acute pyogenic infections
2. Tuberculosis (In tuberculosis, lymphocytosis occurs. However, in Arneth count, a shift to left is observed. This may be due to increased destruction of older neutrophils)
3. Hemorrhage
4. Irradiation (exposure to radiation)—low-dose irradiation stimulates the bone marrow and increases the production of cells; however, exposure of the bone marrow to a high dose of irradiation causes a shift to right because the bone marrow is suppressed

Shift to right

1. Megaloblastic anemia
2. Aplastic anemia
3. Septicemia
4. Uremia

OSPE

Focus a neutrophil of stage 3 in the supplied slide under an oil-immersion objective.

Steps

1. Select an ideal smear.
2. Place the slide on the stage of the microscope and scan the smear under a low-power objective by making the necessary microscopic adjustments (concave mirror, condenser at the lowest position, and iris partially closed).
3. Select the appropriate site in the smear for further examination under an oil-immersion objective.
4. Place a drop of oil on the chosen site and change to the oil-immersion objective.
5. Make other microscopic adjustments (change to plane mirror, raise the condenser, and open the iris fully) to examine the slide under the oil-immersion objective.
6. Place in focus a neutrophil of stage 3 and make fine adjustments to get a clear picture of the cell.

VIVA

All the questions provided at the **end of Chapters 10 and 11** also apply to this chapter.

1. *What are the functions of neutrophils?* (Ans. Refer to page 77, read the first para under 'Discussion'.)
2. *What is the half-life of neutrophils in circulation? How long do they survive in tissues?*
   (Ans. Neutrophils have a half-life of about six hours in circulation. After migrating to tissues, they survive there for a few days and do not return to circulation.)
3. *What precautions should be taken while performing the Arneth count?* (Ans. Refer to page 77, read the list of 'Precautions'.)
4. *What is the normal percentage distribution of neutrophils in different stages?* (Ans. See page 76, under the heading 'Normal Count'.)
5. *What is the relationship between the number of nuclear lobes and the age of neutrophils?*
   (Ans. As neutrophils grow older, the number of nuclear lobes increases. Younger neutrophils have fewer nuclear lobes than older neutrophils.)
6. *Apart from nuclear lobes, what are the other features that help in staging neutrophils?* (Ans. Refer to page 76, under the heading 'Introduction'.)
7. *What is the Physiological significance of the Arneth count?* (Ans. Refer to page 77, under the heading 'Physiological Significance'.)
8. *What is basophilic stippling of neutrophils? What does it signify?* (Ans. Refer to page 77, under the heading 'Shift to Left'.)
9. *In what conditions is a 'shift to left' observed?* (Ans. Refer to page 77, under the heading 'Conditions that Affect...' and subheading 'Shift to left'.)
10. *In what conditions is a 'shift to right' observed?* (Ans. Refer to page 78, under the heading 'Conditions that Affect...' and subheading 'Shift to right'.)

13 | Absolute Eosinophil Count

Learning Objectives

After completing this practical, you will be able to (MUST KNOW):

1. Describe the importance of performing absolute eosinophil count (AEC) in practical physiology.
2. Describe the structure and functions of eosinophils.
3. State the normal value of AEC.
4. Count eosinophils using the principle of hemocytometry.
5. List the precautions taken while performing AEC.
6. Explain the composition and function of each constituent of the Pilot solution.

7. List the common causes of eosinophilia and eosinopenia.

You may also be able to (DESIRABLE TO KNOW):

1. Explain the principle of indirect absolute eosinophil count.
2. Describe other diluting fluids used for eosinophil count.
3. Name the chemicals present in the granules of eosinophils and list their functions.
4. State the physiological basis of alterations in the eosinophil count in different conditions.

INTRODUCTION

The absolute number of eosinophils in circulation is estimated by performing **indirect and direct absolute counts**. The **indirect method** of absolute eosinophil count (AEC) is done by calculating the number of eosinophils as a percentage of the total leucocytes present in the circulation. For this, two tests need to be performed: a **differential count and a total leucocyte count**. The sources of error are greater in the indirect count as it multiplies the margin of error of the two methods.

The **direct method** of absolute eosinophil count is done by using the principle of hemocytometry. The direct count is more accurate.

STRUCTURE, DEVELOPMENT, AND LIFE CYCLE OF EOSINOPHILS

Eosinophils have the same size as neutrophils (10–14 μm) and usually have a bilobed nucleus and large, coarse granules that stain deep red or brick-red (Fig. 13.1). In the absolute count, other leucocytes and red cells are destroyed, making it easy to distinguish eosinophils. Development of eosinophils occurs along the same lines as that of other granulocytes (see Fig. 9.1, Chapter 9). Production of eosinophils is regulated by **GM-CSF** and **interleukins IL3 and IL5**.

Once released into the bloodstream, the **half-life of eosinophils** in circulation if **4.5 to 8 hours**. Then, they move into tissues, where they survive for 8–12 days. Like neutrophils, eosinophils are mobile cells whose movement is directed by chemotactic factors derived from a variety of sources including mast cells and lymphocytes.

FUNCTIONS

1. Eosinophils are present in large numbers in **parasitic infestations**, in which they appear to serve an important defence function. Eosinophil granules contain a number of chemicals, some of which directly kill the larvae of parasites (*larvicidal*) and adult parasites (*parasiticidal*).

Granular contents: The granules of eosinophils contain the following chemicals.

- **Major basic protein (MBP):** The MBP makes up 50 per cent of the mass of the granules. It is a potent tissue toxin that kills larvae and adult parasites.
- **Eosinophilic cationic protein (ECP):** The ECP is a bactericidal and larvicidal agent.
- **Eosinophil peroxidase:** This enzyme participates in inflammatory activities.
- **Aryl sulphatase B:** This enzyme inactivates leukotrienes that are involved in hypersensitivity reactions. It also inactivates the slow-releasing substance A.

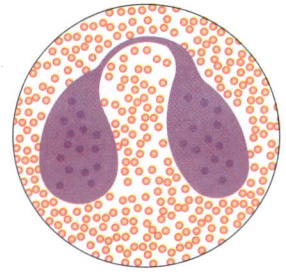

Fig. 13.1 Structure of an eosinophil. Note the presence of brick-red, coarse granules.

- *Lysophospholipase:* This is a membrane-bound enzyme that causes hydrolysis of intracellular lipoproteins.
- *Histaminase:* It causes the degradation of histamine.

2. The eosinophil count increases in patients suffering from **allergic diseases** in which exposure to abnormal exogenous or endogenous antigens leads to an immunologic reaction. In these allergic conditions, eosinophils dampen the host's response by limiting the antigen-induced release of mediators of inflammation.

3. Eosinophils are also **phagocytic**, and destroy organisms through oxidative mechanisms similar but not identical to those of neutrophils. Eosinophils can phagocytose bacteria, fungi, and inert particles, but are less efficient than neutrophils.

Normal Count

The normal range is **40 to 440 per ml of blood**. There is no variation with sex and age.

METHODS OF COUNTING EOSINOPHILS

Absolute count of eosinophils is done by two methods: (1) directly, by using the principle of hemocytometry and (2) indirectly, by studying the smear and total leucocyte count.

1. Direct Method

Principle

Blood is diluted 10 times in a WBC pipette with a special diluting fluid, which removes red cells and stains the eosinophils. The diluted blood specimen is then charged in a counting chamber, and the cells are counted under a high-power objective. The population of eosinophils is then calculated for undiluted blood.

Requirements

Equipment

1. Microscope
2. **Hemocytometer (WBC pipette and counting chamber)**: Three counting chambers are commonly used.
   i.   Fuchs–Rosenthal counting chamber
   ii. Neubauer counting chamber
   iii. Speir counting chamber

The **Fuchs–Rosenthal counting chamber** is preferred because it is specially designed for the eosinophil count. It has a depth of 0.2 mm to accommodate more diluting fluid.

The **Speir chamber** is very similar to the Fuchs–Rosenthal counting chamber. However, as these chambers are not usually available, the Neubauer chamber is commonly used in our laboratories.

3. Materials for sterile finger puncture
4. Watch glass
5. Filter paper
6. Petri dish

Reagents (diluting fluids)

There are **three diluting fluids** available for eosinophil count: *Pilot solution, Randolph solution, and Dunger solution*.

Pilot solution

This is the most frequently used diluting fluid.
Composition
1. *Phloxine B* (1% solution in water): 10 ml—stains eosinophil granules.
2. *Propylene glycol*: 50 ml—lyses the red cells.
3. *Sodium carbonate solution* (10% solution in water): 1 ml—lyses all white cells except (with water) eosinophils.
4. *Heparin*: 100 units—prevents coagulation. Heparin is usually not added to the solution as red cells are lysed by propylene glycol. However, to prevent clumping of red cell fragments, heparin should be added to the solution.
5. *Distilled water*: 40 ml.

Randolph solution

This is very similar to the Pilot solution except that methylene blue is added to help in differentiating other leucocytes (blue) from eosinophils (orange-red).

Dunger solution

Composition
1. *Aqueous eosin (1%)*: Stains eosinophils
2. *Acetone: Fixes white cells*
3. *Distilled water: Lyses red cells*

This solution does not remove other white cells, which appear as grey bodies.

Specimen

Capillary blood or EDTA-anticoagulated venous blood is used.

Procedure

1. Clean the watch glass, coverslip, WBC pipette, and Neubauer's chamber thoroughly and ensure that they are dry.
2. Pour adequate Pilot fluid into a watch glass.

3. Prick the fingertip under aseptic conditions.
4. Suck blood exactly up to the 0.5 mark, and clean the tip of the pipette.
5. Suck Pilot fluid up to the 11 mark.
6. Shake the pipette for at least 2 minutes to mix the blood thoroughly with the diluting fluid.
7. **Keep the pipette in horizontal position for 15 minutes under the cover of a petri dish lined with moist filter paper**.
8. After 15 minutes, take out the pipette, mix the solution by gently shaking the pipette, and discard 2–3 drops of the solution from the pipette.
9. Charge the Neubauer chamber (as described in Chapter 6).
10. Count eosinophils in **four WBC squares** under the high-power objective of the microscope.
11. Enter your observations in a rough notebook in similarly drawn squares (as shown below).

Calculation

The dilution of the blood is 1 in 20. Therefore, the number of eosinophils counted per mm^3 of blood will be **$n \times 50$** (for details, see Chapter 9), where **n** represents the total number of cells counted.

Observation and results

1. Draw four WBC squares, each having 16 small squares, as drawn below.
2. Enter the number of WBCs as observed in the WBC squares of the Neubauer chamber into the drawn representative squares.
3. Total the numbers of cells in the four WBC squares (this is **n**).

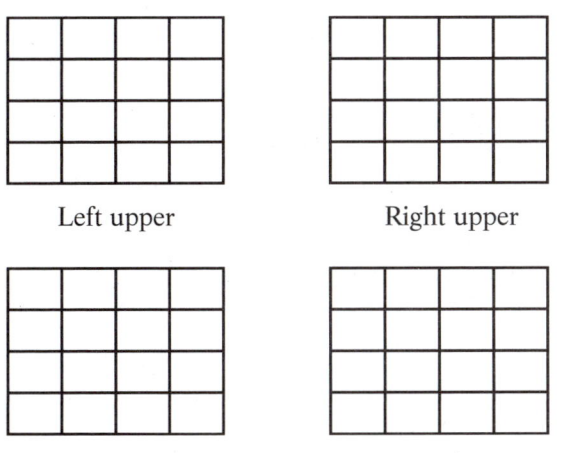

Left upper   Right upper

Left lower   Right lower

4. Calculate the total number with the formula **$n \times 50$** = ___ cells /mm^3 of blood.
5. Report your result as: 'AEC of the given sample of blood is ___ cells /mm^3 of blood.'

Precautions and sources of error

All the precautions observed while pipetting and charging the chamber (as described in Chapter 6) should be followed for this experiment too. In addition, the following **extra precautions** should also be observed.

1. Counting with capillary blood gives a higher result (about 10–20 per cent more) than with venous blood.
2. Counting should be done **within 30 minutes of charging** the chamber because eosinophils slowly disintegrate in the diluting fluid.
3. To mix the contents of the pipette, the pipette should be shaken gently to avoid undue rupture of the eosinophil membranes.
4. After diluting the blood, the pipette should be kept **under the cover of a petri dish lined with moist filter paper** for *15 minutes* (staining time) to prevent evaporation.
5. The indirect counting method should be performed simultaneously to check the result of direct counting.

2. Indirect Method

In the indirect method, the value of the total leucocyte count is required in addition to the value of the eosinophil percentage obtained from the differential count.

$$AEC = \frac{Differential\ count \times Total\ leucocyte\ count}{100}$$

For example, if the eosinophil in DLC is 4% and the TLC is 7000/mm^3 of blood, then:

$$AEC = (4/100) \times 7000 = 280/mm^3\ of\ blood.$$

Note: If the results of the direct and indirect methods differ significantly, the absolute count of eosinophils by the direct method should be repeated.

DISCUSSION

Clinical Significance

The number of eosinophils in blood is altered significantly in different **allergic diseases and parasitic infestations**. The eosinophil count is also taken as an index of **ACTH activity** in the blood. If ACTH is injected intramuscularly in a subject with normal adrenocortical function, it results in the *reduction of the total number of circulating eosinophils*. This effect has been used as a **test of adrenocortical function** and is called the **Thorn test**. It is not a specific test, and its value is limited.

The increase in eosinophil count is called **eosinophilia** and the decrease in count is called **eosinopenia**.

Conditions That Alter Eosinophil Count

Eosinophilia

1. Allergic diseases
   - Bronchial asthma
   - Hay fever
   - Food allergy

2. Parasitic infestations
   - Hookworm
   - Roundworm
   - Tapeworm
   - Filarial worm
3. Skin diseases
   - Eczema
   - Pemphigus
   - Dermatitis herpetiformis
4. Tropical pulmonary eosinophilia and Loeffler's syndrome

5. Malignant neoplasia
   - Eosinophilic leukemia
   - Lymphoproliferative disorders, e.g., Hodgkin's disease
   - Secondary carcinomas
6. Addison's disease

Eosinopenia
1. Cushing syndrome
2. Aplastic anemia
3. ACTH therapy

VIVA

Apart from the questions given below, all the **questions pertaining to hemocytometry, pipetting, and charging of Neubauer chamber** can be asked in this practical.

1. *What are the methods to obtain an absolute eosinophil count?* (Ans. Refer to page 80, under the heading 'Methods of Counting'.)
2. *Other than Neubauer chamber, what other counting chambers are used for absolute eosinophil count? What are their advantages?* (Ans. Refer to page 80, under the heading 'Requirements' and subhead 'Equipment', point no. 2.)
3. *What are the different diluting fluids used for absolute eosinophil count?* (Ans. Refer to page 80, under 'Requirements' and the subheading 'Reagents'.)
4. *What is the composition of the Pilot solution? What are the functions of each constituent?* (Ans. Refer to page 80, under 'Requirements' and the subheading 'Reagents'...Pilot Solution.)
5. *After diluting the blood, why is the pipette kept under the cover of a petri dish lined with moistened filter paper?* (Ans. Refer to page 80, under the heading 'Precautions', point no. 4.)
6. *Why should the counting be performed within half an hour of diluting the blood?* (Ans. Refer to page 81, under the heading 'Precautions', point no. 2.)
7. *Why should the pipette be shaken gently to mix blood with the diluting fluid?* (Ans. Refer to page 81, under the heading 'Precautions', point no. 3.)
8. *What are the precautions and sources of error while performing an absolute eosinophil count?* (Ans. Refer to page 81, under the heading 'Precautions and Sources of Error'.)
9. *How are eosinophils counted by the indirect method?* (Ans. Refer to page 81, under the heading 'Indirect Method'.)
10. *Why is the direct count preferred over the indirect count for obtaining the absolute value of eosinophils?* (Ans. Refer to page 79, under the heading 'Introduction'.)
11. *What is the structure of an eosinophil? What chemicals are present in the eosinophil granules?* (Ans. Refer to pages 79 and 80, under the heading 'Structure....' and 'Function'...Granular contents.)
12. *What is the half-life and fate of eosinophils?* (Ans. Refer to page 79, under the heading 'Life cycle'.)
13. *What are the functions of eosinophils?* (Ans. Refer to page 79, under the heading 'Functions'.)
14. *What is the normal eosinophil count?* (Ans. Refer to page 80, under the heading 'Normal Count'.)
15. *What is the clinical significance of this investigation?* (Ans. Refer to page 81, under the heading 'Clinical Significance'.)
16. *Name the conditions that alter the eosinophil count.* (Ans. Refer to pages 81 and 82, under the heading 'Conditions that alter eosinophil count'.)
17. *What is the **Thorn test**? What is its significance?* (Ans. Refer to page 81, under the heading 'Clinical Significance'.)

14 | Determination of Erythrocyte Sedimentation Rate

Learning Objectives

After completing this practical, you will be able to (MUST KNOW):
1. Explain the importance of determining ESR in practical physiology.
2. Explain what ESR is and how it differs from PCV.
3. List the factors that affect ESR.
4. List the methods of determining ESR.
5. Identify the Westergren pipette and Wintrobe tube.
6. Load ESR tubes with blood.
7. List the precautions and sources of error in the determination of ESR.

8. State the normal value of ESR in males and females with each method.
9. Name the common conditions in which there are alterations of ESR.

You may also be able to (DESIRABLE TO KNOW):
1. Explain the role of fibrinogen and other factors in determining ESR.
2. Explain the physiological basis of variation in ESR in different physiological and pathological conditions.

PY2.12: Describe the test for ESR, osmotic fragility, and hematocrit. Note the findings and interpret the test results.

INTRODUCTION

Erythrocyte sedimentation rate (ESR) is a commonly ordered hematological investigation. Though it is not a specific diagnostic investigation, it has enormous clinical utility and significance in health and diseases.

Definition: *The rate at which red cells sediment when anticoagulated blood is allowed to stand vertically in a narrow tube for one hour is known as erythrocyte sedimentation rate (ESR).* Students should not confuse ESR with PCV (hematocrit). In the case of hematocrit, the packing of red cells is accomplished by centrifugation, while in ESR, the column of red cells settles by gravity.

Principle

Red cells, being heavier (specific gravity 1.095) than colloid plasma (specific gravity 1.032), sediment gradually in the tube containing anti-coagulated blood. However, sedimentation of red cells occurs primarily due to **rouleau** (singular **rouleaux**) **formation**. Rouleaux is the piling up of red cells like a stack of coins. When red cells form rouleau, together they become heavier as they sit on one another. Sedimentation is faster when the size and number of rouleau are large. Therefore, any factor that facilitates rouleaux formation increases ESR, and any factor that inhibits it decreases ESR.

Stages of sedimentation

The sedimentation or settling of red cells occurs in three stages:

1. **First stage:** Red cells pile up and form rouleaux. This happens in about 10 minutes.
2. **Second stage:** Rouleau, being heavier, start settling to the bottom, and the process lasts for about 30 to 45 minutes.
3. **Third stage:** Packing of red cells/rouleau at the bottom of the red column. This stage lasts for about 10 minutes.

Factors Affecting ESR

ESR chiefly depends on **four factors:** (1) the size of the rouleau, (2) plasma factors, (3) the shape and number of red cells, and (4) technical and mechanical factors.

Size of the rouleau

ESR primarily depends on the *size or mass of the sedimenting particles*, that is, the **rouleaux**. The *larger the particle, the faster it falls.* The size of the falling particles depends on the formation of red cell aggregates, that is, rouleaux formation.

Plasma factors

1. **Plasma proteins:** The size of the rouleaux depends on the presence of certain factors in the plasma, especially the **fibrinogen and globulin** content. Normally, red cells tend to repel each other because they are negatively charged due to the negative electrostatic charges imparted by sialic acid moieties on the cell membrane. This repulsion force is known as **zeta potential**. Fibrinogen *neutralises the charges on the red cells* and makes them sticky. Therefore, when the fibrinogen concentration increases in the plasma, the *repelling force on the red cells is removed*; this facilitates rouleaux formation. In some pathological conditions,

in addition to fibrinogen, other plasma factors called **acute-phase reactants** increase in the blood. These phase reactants also neutralize the charges on the red cell surface and facilitate rouleaux formation. A rise in **C-reactive protein** in the plasma in acute rheumatic fever is an example of such acute phase reactants.

2. **Viscosity**: When the medium in which red cells settle becomes thick (**more viscous**), the rate of *sedimentation decreases*; conversely, when the medium becomes thin (**less viscous**), the rate of *sedimentation increases*. Thus, in the conditions in which the viscosity of blood increases, the ESR decreases, and in conditions in which viscosity decreases, ESR increases. The **viscosity of blood increases in polycythemia and decreases in anemia**. Therefore, *ESR is low in polycythemia and high in anemia.*

Shape and number of red cells

Red cells are biconcave discs, which favours rouleaux formation. A **change in the shape of red cells opposes** rouleaux formation. Therefore, in **sickle cell disease and hereditary spherocytosis, the ESR is low** in spite of anemia. Polycythemia lowers ESR, and anemia raises ESR.

Technical and mechanical factors

Some technical and mechanical factors also affect ESR:
1. **Temperature**: The rate of sedimentation *increases with temperature*. Increase in temperature increases ESR *by decreasing the viscosity of blood.*
2. **Position of the pipette**: ESR pipettes are kept vertical in the rack. Slanting of the tubes in the rack facilitates ESR.

NORMAL VALUES

Wintrobe method
1. Males: 0–9 mm/h
2. Females: 0–20 mm/h

Westergren method
1. Males: 3–5 mm/h
2. Females: 5–12 mm/h

Age-adjusted ESR: In elderly individuals, the upper limit of normal ESR can be calculated, in which ESR is adjusted for age by the age-adjusted formula.

For men, it is age in years divided by 2, e.g., for a 70-year-old man, ESR = 70/2 = 35 mm/hr

For women, it is (age in years + 10) divided by 2, e.g., for a 70-year-old woman, ESR = (70+10)/2 = 40 mm/hr

METHODS OF DETERMINING ESR

Traditionally, there are **two methods** of determining ESR: **the Westergren method and the Wintrobe method**. The Westergren method is more sensitive and provides more accurate values than the Wintrobe method because it uses longer and narrower tubes for ESR measurement.

Westergren Method

Principle

Anticoagulated blood is taken in a pipette and left undisturbed in a vertical position. The level of the column of blood is noted at the beginning (0 h) and after 1 and 2 hours. The distance the column moves as expressed by mm of clear plasma is noted as the ESR (mm/h).

Requirements
▌Apparatus
1. **Westergren pipette**: This is an open-ended tube. It is 300 mm in length with an internal bore of 2.55 mm. It is graduated from 0–200 mm along the lower two-thirds of its length. The graduated volume of the pipette is 1.0 ml. The pipettes are held vertically in the Westergren rack after filling them with blood. The rack is provided with rubber pads at the lower end and metal clips at the upper end (Fig. 14.1).
2. **Westergren rack**: This is a special rack designed to hold Westergren pipettes in a vertical position. It is constructed in such a way that the rubber stoppers attached to springs close the open ends of the tubes when they are placed in the rack (Fig. 14.1).

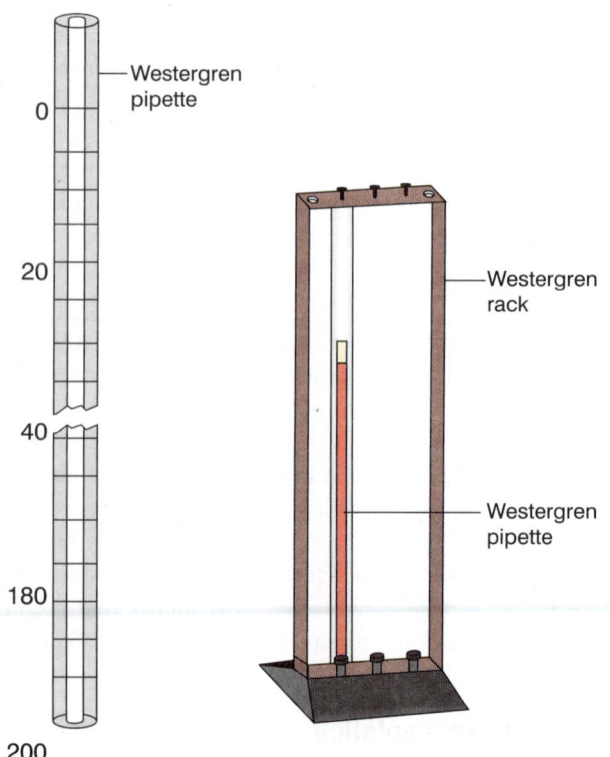

Fig. 14.1 Westergren pipette and rack.

▉ Blood sample

Anticoagulated blood is collected for the study. *Sodium citrate solution (3.8%)* is the preferred anticoagulant. The ratio of blood to the anticoagulant is **4:1**, i.e., 4 parts blood (say 2.0 ml) mixed with 1 part anticoagulant (0.5 ml). EDTA can also be used as the anticoagulant.

Procedure

1. Mix the blood thoroughly by inversion or swirling.
2. Fill the citrated blood into the Westergren pipette **up to the 0 mark**, making sure that *there is no air bubble* in the blood column. The Westergren pipette can either be filled by applying suction by sucking through the mouth (not usually recommended) or by means of a rubber bulb, if available.
3. **Immediately close the upper end** of the Westergren tube to prevent the blood from running down.

> **Note:** The upper level of the blood column should coincide with the 0 mark of the pipette. If a difference exists, it should be noted and adjusted accordingly with the final result.

4. Place the Westergren tube in the rubber pad of the Westergren rack and **fix it vertically** with the metal clips provided on the rack (Fig. 14.2).

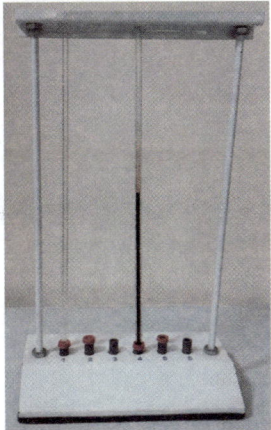

Fig. 14.2 Westergren pipette kept in the rack vertically after filling. This filled pipette has been kept for one hour. An empty pipette is kept to the left of the filled one.

5. Note the time and allow the tube to stand undisturbed for 1 hour.
6. Record your observations (note the level to which the red cell column has fallen) after 1 hour.

> **Note:** Ideally, observations should also be recorded at the end of the second hour.

Observation and results

1. At the end of one hour, record your observation by noting the level to which the red cell column has fallen in the pipette, which is determined by reading the mm of clear plasma above the red cells.
2. *Report your result as:* "The ESR of the given sample of blood is ___mm at the end of the 1st hour (Westergren method)", and state whether the ESR reported is normal, low, or high.

Remember that ESR in males is 3–5 mm/h and in females is 5–12 mm/h by the Westergren method.

Corrected ESR: ESR is corrected when *hematocrit is low* (below 35%). The corrected Westergren ESR value is obtained by **Fabry's formula**:

$$\text{Corrected ESR} = \frac{\text{Measured ESR} \times 15}{(55 - \text{Hematocrit})}$$

1. The Westergren can overestimate ESR in samples with low hematocrit. Fabry's formula helps to correct this bias.
2. When the ESR is near the upper limit, the correction factor that is usually allowed for low hematocrit (anemia) is applied to obtain the corrected ESR.

Precautions

1. The **concentration of the anticoagulant** should be appropriate.
2. Blood should be properly mixed before pipetting.
3. The pipette should be clean and dry.
4. Blood should be filled **exactly up to the 0 mark** and **should not contain air bubbles**. If the upper level of the blood is above the 0 mark (say 2 mm), care must be taken to add the additional distance travelled by the blood column (2 mm) in the final report. This means that if the reading is 12 mm after 1 hour, it should be reported as 14 mm/1st h.
5. The tube should be **kept vertically** in the rack.
6. Readings should be taken at the end of the first and second hours.

▉ Sources of error

1. The **concentration of the anticoagulant affects ESR value**. A false low value is reported in case of higher concentration of anticoagulant.
2. **Be accurate about timing.** Do not take a reading after 30 minutes and report it as a one-hour reading by multiplying by two. The rate of sedimentation is slow in the beginning and fast after about 45 minutes. A one-hour reading gives the final picture. Therefore, the reading should be taken only after one hour.
3. **Temperature** directly affects ESR. High temperatures lead to false high values; conversely, low temperatures give false low values. Therefore, the **specimen must be brought to room temperature before setting up the test**.
4. **Tilting of the tube** increases the ESR.

Advantage

It is more sensitive because the tube is sufficiently long. Especially when the ESR is high, like >80 mm, a longer tube only can accommodate a sufficient height of the blood column for the adequate sedimentation to happen across a greater length of the tube and ESR to be expressed fully. The Westergren tube, being longer, has this advantage.

Disadvantages

1. Some argue that the anticoagulant (citrate solution) used in Westergren method dilutes the red cells, which by itself, tends to raise ESR. However, fibrinogen, globulin, and other phase reactants are also simultaneously diluted, which tends to lower ESR. Therefore, the use of citrate solution is not a big disadvantage.
2. The Westergren method may overestimate ESR in samples with low hematocrit (below 35%). In such cases, Fabry's formula should be applied to correct the ESR and minimise this bias.

Wintrobe Method

This method is not usually followed for the determination of ESR in clinical practice. It is used in some laboratories because it simultaneously yields two values from the same sample, i.e., ESR and hematocrit. The ESR reading is taken in the first hour. Then, the tube is centrifuged for the hematocrit value. The Wintrobe tube is made in such a way that both readings are available on two different graduations marked on the tube. However, the ESR result by this method is not as accurate as that of the Westergren method.

Principle

The principle is the same as that of the Westergren method.

Requirements
▮ Apparatus

1. **Wintrobe tube:** This is a thick-walled cylindrical tube measuring 11 cm in length with an internal bore of 3 mm diameter. The tube is graduated in mm in both directions from 0 to 10 cm. The marking 0–10 from above downwards is used for reading ESR. The marking 0–10 from below upwards is used for reading hematocrit (Fig. 14.3A and B).
2. **Wintrobe rack:** This is a wooden rack with holes at the top for holding Wintrobe tubes (Fig. 14.4).
3. **Pasteur pipette:** This is a pipette with a long neck (Fig. 14.5) used for filling Wintrobe tubes. A syringe with a long needle will also serve the purpose of filling

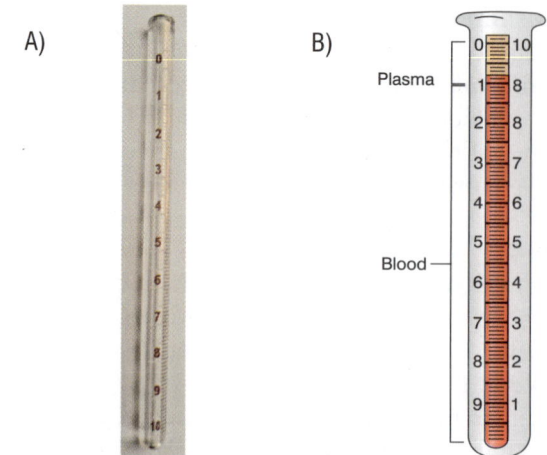

Fig. 14.3   (A) Wintrobe tube and (B) schematic diagram of Wintrobe tube filled with blood.

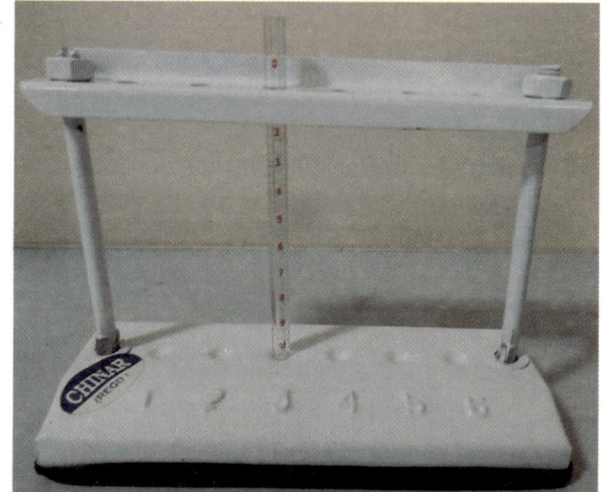

Fig. 14.4   Wintrobe tube kept in the Wintrobe rack.

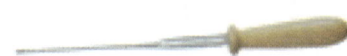

Fig. 14.5   Pasture pipette

▮ Blood sample

Fresh EDTA-anticoagulated blood is used for this method. Note that blood is not diluted in this method. Double oxalate is also used as an anticoagulant in this method.

Procedure

1. Mix the blood thoroughly by repeated inversion or swirling for at least two minutes.
2. With a long-necked Pasteur pipette or a special syringe, *fill the Wintrobe tube up to the 0 mark.* For this, the tip of the pipette should be introduced right down to the bottom of the Wintrobe tube, and the blood should be slowly forced out of the pipette into the tube from below upwards (Fig. 14.6).

3. While filling, draw out the pipette tip from the tube to prevent air bubble formation.
4. Place the Wintrobe tube in an **absolutely vertical position** in the rack (Fig. 14.7).
5. Note the time.
6. Note the reading of the erythrocyte column at the end of one hour and report the ESR as mm/1st hr.

Observation and results

1. At the end of one hour, record your observation by noting the level to which the red cell column has fallen in the pipette, which is determined by reading the mm of clear plasma above the red cells.
2. *Report your result as:* "The ESR of the given sample of blood is ....mm at the end of 1st hour (Wintrobe method)", and state whether the ESR reported is normal, low, or high.

   Remember that ESR in males is 0–9 mm/h and in females is 0–20 mm/h by the Wintrobe method.

Precautions

1. The Wintrobe tube should be absolutely clean and dry.
2. Hemolyzed blood should not be used.
3. Blood should be **mixed properly** before pipetting.
4. Blood should be filled **exactly up to the 0 mark**. If blood is drawn above the mark, absorbent material should not be used to adjust the level. Instead, a dropper should be used for this purpose.
5. The blood column **should not contain air bubbles** or blood clots.
6. The tube should be **kept vertically** in the rack.
7. The reading should be taken after an hour.
8. While filling the pipette, **the tip of the pipette should be kept below the level of blood**.

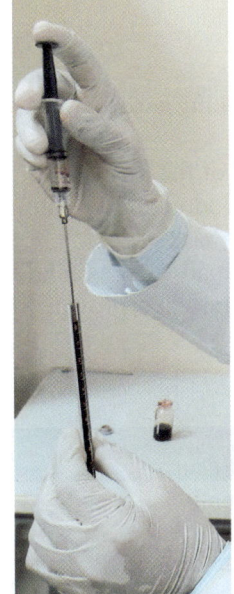

Fig. 14.6 Loading blood in the Wintrobe tube. Note that the tip of the long needle has to be kept below the rising column of blood in the pipette to prevent the entry of air bubbles.

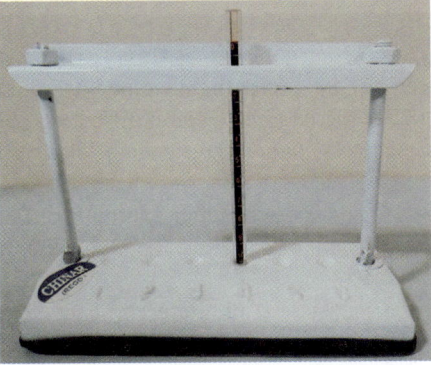

Fig. 14.7 The Wintrobe tube kept vertically in the rack immediately after filling the pipette. Note that the blood is filled exactly up to the zero mark.

Sources of error

1. **The timing should be accurate.** A reading taken after 30 minutes should not be reported as a one-hour reading by multiplying it by two. The rate of sedimentation is slow in the beginning and fast after about 45 minutes. A one-hour reading gives the final picture. Therefore, the reading should be taken only after one hour.
2. **Temperature** directly affects ESR. High temperatures lead to false high values. Therefore, the specimen must be brought to room temperature before setting up the test.
3. **Tilting** of the tube increases the ESR rate.

Advantage

In the same sample of oxalated blood in the Wintrobe tube, first ESR can be estimated and then PCV can be determined by centrifuging it. Hence, in cases of anemia, the appropriate correction factor can be applied.

Disadvantage

It is less sensitive since the tube is not long. Especially when the ESR is high, like >50 mm, a longer tube is needed to accommodate a sufficient height of the blood column for the adequate sedimentation to happen across a greater length of the tube and ESR to be expressed fully. The Wintrobe tube, being shorter, has this disadvantage.

DISCUSSION

Clinical Significance

ESR is generally the index of inflammation in the body. It increases in **inflammatory conditions**, be it infective or non- infective. A *rise in plasma fibrinogen* as occurs in acute infections (pneumonia), a *rise in plasma globulin* as seen in chronic infections (like tuberculosis), and a **rise in phase reactants** as seen in non-infective inflammations (like rheumatoid arthritis)—all result in increased ESR. Conversely, it decreases with a decline in inflammatory activity. ESR also increases in **malignant diseases** like carcinoma and leukemia.

Conditions That Alter ESR

Increased ESR
Physiological

1. **Age**—ESR is low in newborns and infants because of physiological polycythemia (0–2 mm/hr at birth, Westergren); it increases after the age of 50 years
2. **Gender**—ESR is higher in females than in males, which could be due to hormonal fluctuations during the menstrual cycle which influence the fibrinogen level; it can also be due to the lower Hb level in females
3. **Pregnancy**—ESR is higher due to increased fibrinogen and globulin

4. **After a meal**—ESR is higher after eating; therefore, a fasting blood sample for ESR measurement is collected early in the morning on an empty stomach
5. **Body temperature**—increase in body temperature decreases viscosity and increases ESR

▌Pathological

1. Acute infection (e.g., pneumonia)
2. Chronic infection (e.g., tuberculosis)
3. Acute non-infective inflammation (e.g., gout)
4. Collagen vascular (connective tissue) diseases (e.g., rheumatoid arthritis and systemic lupus erythematosus)
5. Malignant disease (e.g., carcinoma of the breast and leukemia)
6. Anemia
7. Trauma—large-scale tissue injury

Decreased ESR
▌Physiological

1. High altitude—ESR tend to decrease at high altitude due to increased hematocrit (hypoxia-induced polycythemia)

▌Pathological

1. Polycythemia—increased red cell mass increases viscosity and reduces ESR; examples are congenital heart disease, COPD, congestive heart failure, etc.
2. Afibrinogenemia
3. Sickle cell anemia
4. Hereditary spherocytosis

Zeta Sedimentation Ratio (ZSR)

Blood in special capillary tubes is spun in the vertical position for four 45-second cycles in a centrifugal device called the **Zetafuge**. This leads to rapid compaction of red cells, allowing rouleaux to form and sediment in just three minutes. The capillary tube is then read like a microhematocrit. The value obtained is referred to as **zetacrit**. The *true hematocrit is then divided by the zetacrit* to calculate the zeta sedimentation ratio, which is expressed as a percentage, which is known as ZSR. The **normal ZSR value 40–50%** for both males and females.

The interpretation is easier as ZSR is not affected by anemia. It is an equally sensitive test as the recording of ESR. The advantages of ZSR are that it requires only 100 microlitres of blood and its measurement is considerably faster. As zetafuge is not commonly available now, recording ZSR becomes difficult, though it is a satisfactory alternative to ESR.

OSPE

I. Load the Wintrobe tube with the supplied blood for determining ESR.
Steps
1. Select and clean the tube.
2. Mix the blood.
3. With the help of a Pasteur pipette, fill the Wintrobe tube (starting from the bottom) with blood up to the 0 mark, taking care to avoid air bubble formation.
4. Place the Wintrobe tube vertically in the stand.
5. Note the time.

II. Load the Westergren pipette with the supplied blood for determining ESR.
Steps
1. Mix the blood.
2. Pipette blood up to the 0 mark, taking care to avoid air bubble formation.
3. Immediately close the upper end of the pipette.
4. Observe the upper end of the blood column. Note the difference, if any, from the 0 mark.
5. Place the pipette on the rubber pad of the stand and fix it vertically with the metal clips provided on the rack.
6. Note the time.

VIVA

1. *What is ESR? How does it differ from hematocrit?* (**Ans.** Refer to page 83, under the heading 'Introduction'.)
2. *What are the factors that affect ESR?* (**Ans.** Refer to page 83, under the heading 'Factors Affecting ESR'.)
3. *What is the role of plasma fibrinogen in ESR?* (**Ans.** Refer to page 83, under the heading 'Plasma Factors'...1. Plasma Proteins.)
4. *What are the methods of determining ESR?* (**Ans.** Refer to page 84, under the heading 'Methods of Determination'.)
5. *Why should the anticoagulant concentration be appropriate for ESR estimation?* (**Ans.** Refer to page 85, under the heading 'Requirements', see the subheading 'Blood sample'.)
6. *What are the precautions and sources of error in the Wintrobe method?* (**Ans.** Refer to page 87, under the heading 'Precautions' and subheading 'Sources of error'.)
7. *What are the precautions and sources of error in the Westergren method?* (**Ans.** Refer to page 85, under the heading 'Precautions' and subheading 'Sources of error'.)
8. *Why is the Westergren method more accurate than the Wintrobe method?* (**Ans.** Refer to page 84, read the 1st para under 'Methods of Determination'.)

9.   *What is the clinical significance of determining ESR?* (Ans. Refer to page 87, under the heading 'Clinical Significance'.)

10. *Why is the blood collected on an empty stomach for determining ESR?*
     (Ans. A fasting blood sample is collected while the subject is on an empty stomach for determining ESR. This is because food, especially proteins and some fatty foods, can result in an increase in ESR.)

11. *What are the physiological conditions in which ESR is increased?* (Ans. Refer to page 87, under the heading 'Conditions That Alter ESR', and subheading 'Increased ESR'.)

12. *What are the diseases in which ESR increases and decreases?* (Ans. Refer to page 88, text under the heading 'Conditions That Alter ESR'.)

13. *What is ZSR and what is its importance?* (Ans. Refer to page 88, under the heading 'ZSR'.)

14. *Can the oxalate mixture be used for the Westergren method and citrate for the Wintrobe method?*
     (Ans. No, this cannot be done. Anticoagulants have been standardized for specific methods. Sodium citrate cannot be used for the Wintrobe method because it would dilute the blood too much for the height of the tube, resulting in a falsely high value.)

15. *What are the advantages and disadvantages of the Westergren method?* (Ans. Refer to page 86, under the headings 'Advantage' and 'Disadvantages'.)

16. *What are the advantages and disadvantages of the Wintrobe method?* (Ans. Refer to page 87, under the headings 'Advantage' and 'Disadvantages'.)

17. *What is corrected ESR? In what conditions is ESR corrected?* (Ans. Refer to page 85, under the subheading 'Corrected ESR'.)

18. *What is Fabry's formula for ESR correction?* (Ans. Refer to page 85, under the subheading 'Corrected ESR'.)

19. *What is age-adjusted ESR and how is it determined for males and females?* (Ans. Refer to page 84, under the heading 'Normal Values' and the subheading 'Age-adjusted ESR'.)

20. *What is zeta potential? What is its significance?*
     (Ans. RBCs repel each other as they are negatively charged due to the negative electrostatic charges imparted by sialic acid moieties on the cell membrane. This repulsion force is known as zeta potential. Fibrinogen and other phase reactants neutralize this zeta potential and make red cells sticky; this facilitates rouleau formation, which facilitates the sedimentation rate [increase ESR]).

15 | Determination of Blood Group

Learning Objectives

After completing this practical, you will be able to (MUST KNOW):

1. Describe the clinical significance of blood group determination.
2. Name the blood groups of the ABO and Rh systems.
3. State the physiological significance of the ABO and Rh systems.
4. State Landsteiner's law.
5. State the principle of blood group determination.
6. Determine blood groups by using anti-A and anti-B antisera.
7. List the precautions taken while determining the blood group.
8. List the common indications of blood transfusion.
9. List the common hazards of transfusion.
10. Name the diseases transmitted by blood transfusion.
11. Explain universal donor and universal recipient.
12. Explain the importance of cross-matching.

You may also be able to (DESIRABLE TO KNOW):

1. Name and explain the importance of other blood group systems.
2. State the physiological basis of the development of blood groups.
3. Explain the physiological basis of major and minor cross-matching.
4. List and explain all the effects of mismatched transfusion.
5. Explain how blood is stored in blood banks.
6. Explain the physiological changes in red cells during storage and after transfusion.
7. List the cause, features, treatment, and prevention of erythroblastosis fetalis.
8. Name the diseases associated with different blood groups.

PY2.11: Estimate Hb, RBC, TLC, RBC indices, DLC, blood groups, and BT/CT.

INTRODUCTION

There are more than 300 blood group antigens. These are grouped into about 45 blood group systems. Many of these antigens are not significant immunologically and many of them have cold antibodies that do not react at body temperature. The antigens that are involved in blood groups are called **agglutinogens**, and the antibodies that are produced against these antigens are called **agglutinins**. Clinically, the important blood group systems are: (1) the **ABO system** and (2) the **Rh system**. The **MN system** is important from the medicolegal point of view.

The ABO System

The ABO blood group system is the most important of all blood group systems because of the presence, from birth, of natural A and B antibodies in individuals who lack the corresponding antigen on their red cells. In addition, transfusion of incompatible ABO blood immediately leads to serious consequences.

Agglutinogens: In this system, there are *two antigens, antigen A and antigen B*. Based on the presence or absence of these antigens on the red cells, blood groups are classified as follows:

1. **Group A:** Antigen A is present
2. **Group B:** Antigen B is present
3. **Group AB:** Both antigens A and B are present
4. **Group O:** Neither antigen A nor B is present

The A antigen is of two types, **A and A1**. Therefore, Group A is further divided into two subgroups:

1. Group A1: Containing both A and A1 antigens
2. Group A2: Containing only the A antigen

Thus, the AB blood group is subdivided into the **A1B and A2B blood groups**.

A and B agglutinogens are complex oligosaccharides that differ in their terminal sugars. On the RBC membrane, they are glycolipids, and in tissues and body fluids, they are soluble glycoproteins.

Agglutinins: The antibodies in the ABO system are of two types: **anti-A (α) and anti-B (β)**. These antibodies are naturally occurring and are *present in the blood of individuals **in whom the respective antigens are absent***. Thus, Group A (having A agglutinogen on the red cell membrane) individuals will have anti-B and Group B (having B agglutinogen on the red cell membrane) individuals will have anti-A agglutinins in their plasma. The AB group will have no antibody, and Group O will possess both antibodies (Table 15.1).

Physiological basis: The H antigen

H antigen is a fucose-containing antigen that is **found in all individuals.** Usually, the H antigen has **no antigenic activity.** In the case of **antigen A**, a transferase places N-acetylgalactosamine as the terminal sugar on antigen H. In **antigen B,** the terminal sugar is galactose.

In Group AB, both the transferases are present. **Group O individuals** have neither of the enzymes, and so, antigen H persists. As H antigen has no antigenic activity, it is identified as the capital letter O. Since, H antigen is not antigenic, there are *no corresponding antibodies.*

Therefore, an individual with blood group O having no antigens of the ABO system has no antigenic activity at all, and hence, is identified as 'O'. It appears that group O persons produce a protein that has no transferase activity, which results from a single base deletion in the corresponding gene.

Table 15.1 Antigens (Ag) and antibodies (Ab) in the ABO system and their reactions with anti-sera.

Blood group	Antigen on RBC membrane	Antibody in serum	Reaction with anti-serum A	Reaction with anti-serum B
A	A	Anti-B	–	+
B	B	Anti-A	+	–
AB	A, B	No antibodies	+	+
O	No antigen	Anti-A, Anti-B	–	–

Distribution of the ABO blood groups

In the Indian population, the distribution of the ABO blood group is approximately as follows:

A: 22.88%

B: 32.6%

AB: 7.74%

O: 37.12%

Among the A blood groups, the distribution of **A1 group is 75%, and that of A2 is 25%.**

Landsteiner's law

In 1091, Karl Landsteiner devised a law that states that **if an agglutinogen is present on the red cell membrane, the corresponding agglutinin must be absent in the plasma**; if the agglutinogen is absent in the red cells, the corresponding agglutinin must be present in the plasma. The second half of the definition may not be applicable to all blood group systems. For example, *in Rh-negative individuals,* the absence of the Rh agglutinogen in the red cells is not accompanied by the presence of anti-Rh agglutinin in the serum.

The RH (Rhesus) System

This system was first discovered in Rhesus monkeys; hence it is called the Rh system. In this system, there are *six antigens*, but *no naturally occurring antibodies*. The antigens are C, D, E, c, d and e. Of these six antigens, immunologically, **D is the most significant**. Therefore, the Rh system has two blood groups:

1. **Rh-positive:** D antigen present
2. **Rh-negative:** D antigen absent

The Rh (D) is present only on red cells and not in body fluids and tissues. The antibody in this system is called the **anti-D antibody** and is produced only when an Rh-negative individual receives Rh-positive blood. Anti-D antibodies develop slowly in the first encounter and then rapidly in subsequent encounters. The differences between ABO antibodies and Rh antibodies are presented in Table 15.2.

In the Indian population, approximately 94.13% are Rh-positive and 5.87% are Rh-negative.

Table 15.2 Differences between antibodies of the ABO and Rh systems.

Antibodies of ABO system	Antibodies of Rh system
The anti-A anti-B antibodies are of the larger **IgM type** They cannot cross the placenta	Rh antibodies are of the **IgG type** They easily cross placenta
These antibodies react best with antigens at low temperatures of 5–20°C Hence called *cold antibodies*	These antibodies react best with antigens at body temperature Hence called *warm antibodies*
ABO incompatibility between mother and fetus does not occur	Rh incompatibility between mother and fetus occurs

Other Blood Group Systems

1. **MN system:** This system comprises three blood groups: M, N, and MN. It is often used in *paternity testing*, It can only determine who is not the father of a baby but cannot confirm who is. For example, if the baby's blood group is M and the presumed father's is N, then it can definitely be said that N is not the father of M. However, it can never be specifically said who the father of the baby is. The determination of other blood groups assists in establishing paternity. MN groups are also useful for **anthropological and genetic studies**.

2. **Lewis system:** The *two antigens* of the Lewis system are **Lea and Leb**. These are not really red cell antigens because they are produced in plasma and then absorbed into red cells. These antibodies are of the IgM type. They do not cross the placental barrier and, therefore, do not cause hemolytic disease of the newborn.

3. **Ii system:** There are *two antigens* in the Ii system, **I and i**. This system differs from other classifications in several ways:
   i. At birth, the I antigen is poorly developed, but fetal and neonatal red cells are rich in i antigens.
   ii. There occurs a gradual changeover from i to I in the first two years of life.
   iii. In conditions like hemoglobinopathies, red cells show increased i antigen without any decrease in the I antigen.

4. **Duffy system:** There are *two blood group antigens* in this system, **Fya and Fyb,** and three blood types: **Fya, Fyb, and Fyab**. A close relationship has been

established between the **Duffy blood group and malaria:**

i. The Fyab blood group is resistant to *Plasmodium vivax*

ii. Fya and Fyb groups are susceptible to vivax malaria

This is because the Fya and Fyb antigens, if present separately on the red cell membrane, increase the entry of the malarial parasite into the red cells.

5. **Kell system:** In this system, there is only one antigen called the **K antigen**. People with K-positive blood group (containing K antigen on the red cell membrane) are *susceptible to chronic granulomatous diseases*.

METHODS OF DETERMINING BLOOD GROUP

Principle

Red cells contain different types of agglutinogens while plasma contains agglutinins. The subject's red cells are allowed to react with commercially made agglutinins. The presence or absence of the clumping of red cells with different agglutinins determines the blood groups.

Requirements

1. **Anti-A serum** (containing anti-A agglutinin), **anti-B serum** (containing anti-B agglutinin), and **anti-D serum** (Fig. 15.1): Anti-A is a blue liquid in a bottle with a blue cap; anti-B is a yellow liquid in a bottle with a yellow cap, and anti-D is straw-coloured in a bottle with a black cap.

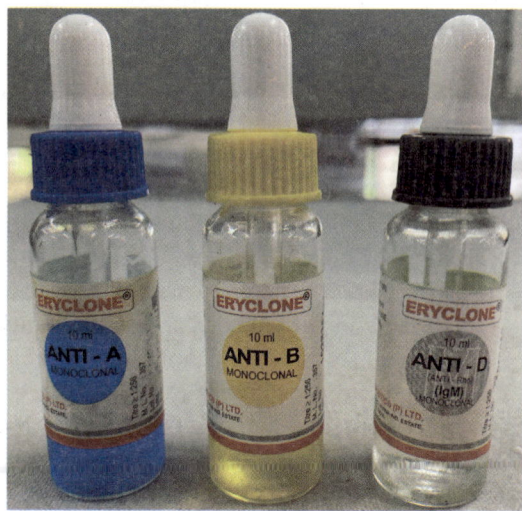

Fig. 15.1 Three antisera bottles. Anti-A is blue in colour, and the cap of the bottle is blue. Anti-B is yellow, and its bottle cap is yellow. Anti-D is straw-coloured, and the cap of the bottle is black.

2. Test tubes
3. Slides
4. 0.9 per cent saline
5. Microscope
6. Equipment for sterile finger prick
7. Capillary pipette
8. Glass-marking pencil
9. Glass rods

Procedure

1. Take 2 ml of 0.9 per cent saline solution in a test tube.
2. Make a sterile finger prick and collect a large drop of blood into the test tube containing the saline solution.
3. Mix the solution to obtain a **red cell suspension**.
4. On one of the slides, place a drop of anti-A serum on its left half and **label it 'anti-A'** with the help of the glass-marking pencil (Fig. 15.2). On the left half of another slide, place a drop of anti-B serum and **label it 'anti-B'**. On the left half of one more slide, place a drop of anti-D serum and **label it as 'anti-D'**.
5. Place a drop of saline on the right half of each slide and **mark it as control (C)**.
6. To each of these drops, **add a drop of red cell suspension** using a capillary pipette.
7. **Mix the red cell suspension** with the sera *using separate glass rods* or by gently shaking the slides. Wait for 5–10 minutes.
8. Observe the serum-cell mixtures **for agglutination (clumping)**. Compare them with the cells in the saline controls (Fig. 15.3).
9. Confirm your findings under the low-power objective.

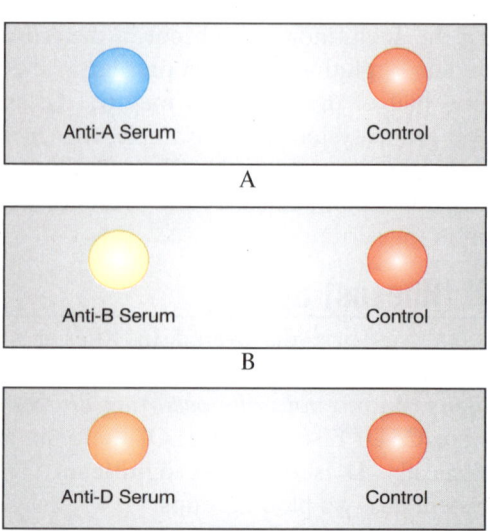

Fig. 15.2 Placement of antisera and control fluid (red cell suspension in normal saline) on testing slides: (A) anti-A serum and control; (B) anti-B serum and control; and (C) anti-C serum and control.

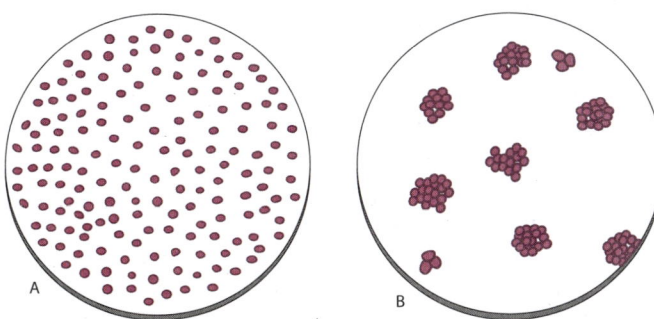

Fig. 15.3 Confirmation of blood grouping under low-power microscope: (A) no agglutination (cells are uniformly distributed) and (B) agglutination present.

Note: The serum–cell mixture should be examined before it dries up to differentiate clumping (actual agglutination) from rouleaux formation of red cells.

10. Record the presence or absence of agglutination on each slide and interpret the result as shown in Fig. 15.4.

Note: A **false positive** result should be excluded by comparing the test with the control (both should show clumping of cells). **False negative** results may occur because of decreased immunocompetence of antisera because of improperly stored antisera.

Fig. 15.4 Determination of blood group. Agglutination is marked by clumping of red cells and non-agglutination by the absence of clumping (uniform distribution of RBC).

Observation and Results

1. Observe the presence or absence of agglutination on each slide.
2. Microscopically confirm the clumping of red cells under a low-power objective.
3. Compare the test with the cells of the saline control.
4. Report the results according to the findings. For example, if the ABO blood group is A and Rh blood group is positive, it should be reported as: "The blood group of the individual is A+".

5. For practice of the concept of blood grouping, prepare a tubular format showing how the red cell suspension added to anti-sera A and B yields agglutination or no agglutination and accordingly determine the blood group. (Table 15.3).

Table 15.3 Presence or absence of agglutination as a determinant of blood group.

Anti-A serum	Anti-B serum	Agglutinogens (on RBC)	Blood group
+	–	A	A
–	+	B	B
+	+	AB	AB
–	–	Nil	O

+: agglutination; – : no agglutination

Precautions

1. The slides must be labelled correctly.
2. While mixing the red cell suspension with antisera, care must be taken **not to mix anti-A and anti-B sera with the same glass rod**.
3. If there is no clumping on either of the slides, 15 minutes should be allowed to pass before reporting the result.
4. The observations should finally be checked under a microscope.
5. A *control should always be used* to **exclude false positive results**.
6. Blood should always be diluted for the blood grouping test. The use of undiluted blood may yield false positive results (rouleaux formation may be confused with clumping). Dilution of blood decreases rouleaux formation.
7. The cell–sera suspension should be examined for clumping before the preparation dries up.

DISCUSSION

To be able to donate or receive blood, an individual should know his or her blood group. This may be required in many medical emergencies. Therefore, usually the blood group is always noted on the identity card of a person. The blood group is always determined prior to any surgical intervention.

Physiological and Clinical Significance
Uses of blood grouping

1. To ensure **compatible blood transfusion**
2. To *eliminate hemolytic disease of the newborn* due to **Rh incompatibility** (details below)
3. To solve **paternity disputes**: The ABO, Rh, and MN systems are used to settle paternity disputes. It

is possible to prove that the person could not have been the father, but not that he is the father. *DNA fingerprinting* is done to confirm and settle such disputes. Antigen A and B are dominant, whereas O is recessive.

4. To detect **susceptibility to diseases**: *Blood groups prone to different diseases:*
   Group A: Carcinoma of stomach
   Group O: Duodenal ulcer
   Fya & Fyb: Vivax malaria
   Group K: Chronic granulomatous diseases
   Rh-negative group: Autoimmune hemolytic anemia
   Group Li: Hemoglobinopathies

5. **Genetic studies:** Molecular typing of blood group genes is a powerful tool, preventing alloantibody formation, with potential advantages for identifying rare blood types and finding better antigen matches for chronically transfused patients. This has led to the development of various DNA tests to predict blood group antigens. Blood type is not affected by disease, drugs, climate, or occupations. Hence, blood typing and the genetic analysis of blood types are used by scientists in different genetic studies to understand the pathophysiology of many genetic diseases.

6. **Selection of donor for tissue/organ transplantation:** In organ transplantation, three tests are carried out for donor-recipient compatibility: blood typing, tissue typing, and cross-matching.

7. **Medicolegal uses:** A blood stain on a victim's body or clothing can be used to identify suspects in cases of murder, sexual assault, or other medicolegal investigations.

8. **Personality trait:** Blood group is linked to the personality and behaviour of an individual (for more information, see PMC article: PMID: 14250420).

Blood Transfusion

Indications: Blood transfusion is required in many diseases and medical emergencies.

1. **Acute blood loss:** This usually occurs in trauma, major surgeries, and hemorrhagic shock. **Whole blood** is generally preferred.

2. **Anemia:** Blood may need to be transfused in cases of severe anemia or anemia due to various causes of decreased production or increased hemolysis, and anemia in specific conditions such as CKD, CHF, etc. In such cases, packed red cells are usually preferred.

3. **Bleeding disorders:** These include thrombocytopenia, platelet function defects, and bleeding conditions such as hemophilia, Von Willebrand disease, and bleeding associated with other diseases such as GI bleeding, bleeding from the genitourinary tracts, respiratory tract, etc.

4. **Bone marrow failure:** Seen in leukemia, aplastic anemia, or bone marrow infiltration by neoplastic cells. In bone marrow failure, fresh blood and specific blood components are required. Red cells are administered along with granulocytes to fight infections.

5. **Preparation for surgeries:** For some major surgeries, transfusion is administered beforehand to increase the patient's Hb level before surgery.

6. **Specific clotting factor deficiencies:** Fresh frozen plasma is preferred in such cases. In hemophilia, cryoprecipitate (rich in factor VIII and fibrinogen) is administered.

Procedure: Blood grouping and cross-matching are always done before blood transfusion to ensure a safe and compatible transfusion. A satisfactory compatibility procedure should include:

1. ABO and Rh typing
2. Cross-matching
3. Antibody screening of the patient (to detect the presence of clinically significant antibodies)

Cross-matching: There are two types of cross-matching:

1. **Major cross-matching:** The *cells of the donor* are directly matched against the *plasma of the recipient*. It is important to ensure that antibodies present in the recipient's plasma do not harm the donor's red cells.

2. **Minor cross-matching:** The donor's plasma is checked against the red cells of the recipient. It is called minor cross-matching because it is not very important since a small volume of the donor's plasma is diluted in a large volume of the recipient's plasma. Therefore, the titre of antibodies present in the donor's plasma falls to such a low level after transfusion that they are quite unlikely to damage the recipient's red cells.

Universal donor and recipient

1. **Universal donor:** Persons with **blood group O-negative** are considered to be universal donors because their red cells contain no antigens. Therefore, their blood can be given safely to anyone.

2. **Universal recipient:** Persons with **blood group AB-positive** are considered to be universal recipients because their plasma contains no antibodies. Therefore, they can receive blood from anyone.

Storage of Blood for Transfusion

Procedure: Blood is stored in the blood bank **at 4°C**. *Disodium hydrogen citrate* is used instead of trisodium citrate as anticoagulant because this favours the fall of pH, which is required for the survival of red cells. Stored blood should ideally be used within two weeks of storage. Blood should not be used if it is stored for more than four weeks because gross hemolysis occurs after this period.

Changes in RBCs during storage: Red cells undergo rapid changes during storage in simple citrate solution, even at 4°C. During cold storage, the changes that occur are chiefly due to the reduction of the metabolism of cells.

1. **Increase in sodium and decrease in potassium concentration** in the red cells. This occurs due to decreased active transport of ions across the cell membrane due to decreased Na^+–K^+ pump activity. This results in a net increase in the total base and water content of the cell.

2. **Cells swell up and become more spherocytic**, resulting in spontaneous hemolysis.

3. The **ATP content in the cell decreases,** and inorganic phosphate concentration increases. This is due to an imbalance between the phosphorylation and dephosphorylation processes in the cells.

Changes in stored blood after transfusion: Within 24 hours of transfusion, the cell metabolism greatly increases; consequently, sodium is extruded from the cells and potassium is drawn back into the cells. The volume, shape, and fragility of the red cells revert to normal within 24–48 hours. Red cells show 80 per cent survival 24 hours after transfusion, if the transfusion is given within 14 days of storage of the blood. But the survival rate greatly decreases if the blood is stored for more than two weeks. Therefore, it is ideal to use blood within 14 days of storage.

Hazards of Blood Transfusion

I. **Due to mismatched transfusion:** When an incompatible blood group is transfused, it leads to the agglutination of the donor's red cells and the **hemolysis**. The severity of the reaction depends on the degree of hemolysis. Possible complications include:

1. Shivering and fever
2. Hemoglobinemia and hemoglobinuria
3. Jaundice
4. Acute renal failure, which occurs due to:
   i. Hemoglobin casts blocking the renal tubules and damaging the tubes
   ii. Release of toxic substances from lysed red cells, causing renal vasoconstriction
   iii. Circulatory shock
5. Hyperkalemia (due to the release of potassium ions from red cells), which causes cardiac problems

II. **Due to faulty transfusion technique:**

1. *Thrombophlebitis*: This is a common complication in those receiving repeated transfusions.
2. *Air embolism*: Air enters the venous circulation, gets lodged at the outlet of the right ventricle and blocks the flow of blood to the lungs. Death may occur in severe cases. The use of plastic bags has reduced this complication.

III. **Due to massive transfusion:** This occurs when more than 10 units of blood are transfused within 24 hours or when the total blood volume is exchanged within 24 hours. Cardiac arrhythmias or cardiac arrest may occur due to high potassium levels in stored blood.

IV. **Febrile reaction:** The patient feels cold and may develop rigor due to raised body temperature. This occurs chiefly due to the presence of pyrogens in the transfusion apparatus.

V. **Allergic reactions:** This is less frequent and is characterised by itching, erythema, nausea, vomiting and, in severe cases, anaphylactic reactions.

VI. **Transmission of diseases:** There is a risk of transmitting infections such as hepatitis, malaria, AIDS, and syphilis through blood transfusion.

Rh Incompatibility

If an Rh-negative individual receives Rh-positive blood, there will be no immediate reaction because Rh-negative individuals do not normally have anti-Rh antibodies. However, the donor's red cells induce an immune response in the recipient to syntheise anti-Rh antibodies. These *take about 2–4 months to reach a significant titre,* by which time, the donor's red cells die a natural death. Thus, anti-Rh antibody cannot harm the recipient's red cells, because the recipient's red cells contain no Rh antigens. However, if the same person **receives a subsequent Rh-positive transfusion,** anti-Rh antibodies are synthesised immediately in large amounts by the recipient's memory cells, causing a *mismatch reaction*.

Erythroblastosis fetalis

Etiopathogenesis: Erythroblastosis fetalis is a hemolytic disease of the newborn that occurs due to Rh incompatibility when an **Rh-negative mother carries an Rh-positive fetus.** Usually, no reaction occurs in the first pregnancy. However, if the mother has received transfusion of Rh-positive blood in the past, the reaction may occur in the first pregnancy. A small amount of blood leaking into maternal circulation at the time of delivery induces the formation of anti-Rh agglutinins in the mother. In subsequent pregnancies, the mother's agglutinin crosses the placenta to the fetus and causes hemolysis in the fetus.

Clinical features: *Severe hemolysis* may result in the death of the fetus in utero or if the fetus is born alive, he may have the following features:

1. Anemia
2. Jaundice
3. Edema (**hydrops fetalis**)
4. **Kernicterus:** This is a neurologic syndrome that occurs due to the *deposition of bile pigments in the basal ganglia*. Bile pigments cannot cross the blood–brain barrier (BBB) in adults but can do so

in fetuses and infants because the BBB is not fully developed.

5. Presence of **erythroblasts** (nucleated red cells) in the blood

Treatment: The best treatment is to carry out an **exchange transfusion** soon after birth.

Prevention: The disease is prevented by **administering a single dose of anti-Rh antibodies** in the form of Rh immunoglobulin during the postpartum period following the first delivery. The disease can also be prevented through **passive immunisation** of the mother with a small dose of Rh immunoglobulins during pregnancy.

VIVA

1. *What is the physiological basis of blood group determination?* (Ans. Refer to page 90, under the heading 'ABO System', and the subheading 'Physiological basis. . .'.)

2. *What are the precautions taken for the determination of ABO blood groups?* (Ans. Refer to page 93, under the heading 'Precautions'.)

3. *How is the clumping (agglutination) of red cells confirmed?*
(Ans. Agglutination is confirmed under the low-power objective of a microscope.)

4. *Explain agglutination, its mechanism, and its effects.*
(Ans. Agglutination is the clumping of red cells that leads to hemolysis. It occurs in three stages:
i. **Sensitisation:** Antibodies get attached to the surface of antigens. A single ABO antibody (IgM type) has 10 binding sites and can thus cross-link 10 red cells. An Rh antibody has two binding sites and can link to two red cells.
ii. **Clumping:** Immediately after sensitisation, red cells form clumps; this is followed by hemolysis.
iii. **Hemolysis:** The Ag–Ab complex also activates the complement system, which releases proteolytic enzymes [lytic complex] that promote hemolysis.)

5. *What is the mode of inheritance of blood groups?*
(Ans. Blood groups are genetically determined. In general, the presence of a blood group antigen is a codominant characteristic. Therefore, the antigen is present in the phenotype regardless of the genotype [whether homozygous or heterozygous]. However, the homozygous or heterozygous state determines the type of contribution an individual can make to their progeny. Thus, a child's blood group may be different from that of both his parents.)

6. *What is Landsteiner's law ? What are the exceptions to this law?* (Ans. Refer to page 91, under the heading 'Landsteiner Law'.)

7. *What is meant by the terms 'universal donor' and a 'universal recipient'?* (Ans. Refer to page 94, under 'Universal Donor and Recipient'.)

8. *What is cross-matching of blood ? What is its clinical significance?* (Ans. Refer to page 94, under 'Blood Transfusion', read 'Cross-matching'.)

9. *Why is minor cross-matching usually not done for blood transfusion?* (Ans. Refer to page 94, see 'Blood Transfusion', read Cross-Matching.)

10. *What is Rh incompatibility and how does it differ from ABO incompatibility?*
(Ans. Rh incompatibility occurs when an Rh-negative person receives Rh-positive blood. In the first transfusion, there's usually no immediate reaction, but the body starts producing anti-Rh antibodies. If the person receives Rh-positive blood again, these antibodies cause a quick and serious reaction. In contrast, ABO incompatibility causes an immediate reaction during the first transfusion because anti-A or anti-B antibodies are already present in the plasma.)

11. *What is erythroblastosis fetalis ? How can it be prevented?* (Ans. Refer to page 94, under the heading 'Erythroblastosis Fetalis'.)

12. *How is blood stored in the blood bank?*
(Ans. Blood is collected from the donor in a labelled plastic bag or glass bottle. Disodium hydrogen citrate is used as an anticoagulant because it favours the survival of red cells by decreasing the pH of the blood. Blood banks store blood at 4°C.)

13. *What are the physiological changes that occur in the red cells during storage?* (Ans. Refer to page 93, under the heading 'Storage of blood for transfusion', and subheading 'Changes in RBCs during storage'.)

14. *What is the cause of hemolysis of stored blood?* (Ans. Refer to page 93, under 'Storage of blood for transfusion', points 1 and 2 under subheading 'Changes in RBCs during storage'.)

15. *What are cold and warm antibodies for blood group antigens? What are the differences between them?*
(Ans. 'Cold' and 'warm' antibodies refer to the types of antibodies involved in different blood group systems and the temperatures at which they react best. The differences between them are presented in Table 5.2 on page 90.)

16. *What is the importance of using a control on each side of the three test slides?*
(Ans. The control sample for blood group testing in each case is only a suspension of red cells in normal saline. It is used as a control to avoid 'false positive' and 'false negative' results.)

17. *What are false positive and false negative results?*
(Ans. These are errors in blood grouping:
i. **False positive:** It means that though there is no actual agglutination, there appears to be clumping. Formation of large rouleaux [this may happen if undiluted blood is used] may give a false impression of agglutination, but the cells will quickly disperse on tilting the slide a few times. Bacterial contamination of the antiserum or normal saline may also result in the appearance of agglutination in all tests or in all controls.
ii. **False negative:** The test fails to show agglutination when it should. This can occur if the antisera has lost its strength due to improper storage.
A control sample [red cells in saline] is always used to avoid these issues.)

18. *What is the zone phenomenon?*
(Ans. For agglutination to occur properly, the amounts of antigen [on red cells] and antibody (in serum) should be roughly equal. If there's too much of one compared to the other, agglutination might not happen. This is known as the zone phenomenon.)

19. *What is meant by autologous transfusion and predonation?*
(Ans. In addition to receiving blood from a donor, an individual may also receive their own stored blood [this might be done before a planned elective surgery]. In such cases, blood is collected and stored beforehand and then transfused during surgery. This is called **autologous transfusion.** The advantage of this procedure is that it avoids transmission of diseases such as AIDS and hepatitis and the risk of transfusion reaction.

   Predonation [Predeposit] is a form of autologous transfusion in which a course of iron tablets is given to the subject, after which two units of blood are collected (first unit 16 days before and second unit 8 days before surgery). An important technical innovation is the **cell-saver machine,** which sucks up blood from the wound during the operation, recycles it, and returns it to the patient's body.)

20. *What is blood doping ?*
(Ans. Blood 'doping' is the athletic malpractice in which one or two units of an athlete's blood [or red cells] are removed and stored two weeks before the athletic event. The blood is re-injected in two sessions just a few days before the event. Since oxygen delivery to active muscles is a limiting factor, increased red cell count enhances the person's performance in marathon events. This practice is banned by the International Athletic and Olympic Committees.)

21. *What is a suitable for blood substitute if a blood donor is not available?*
(Ans. When whole blood isn't available, fluids are given to maintain blood volume:
i. **Crystalloids** (like 6% glucose in 0.9% saline): Provide short-term volume but leave the bloodstream quickly.
ii. **Colloids** (like human albumin, plasma expanders): Stay longer and are better for volume replacement.
iii. **Blood substitutes** (like packed red cells, white cells, immunoglobulins, clotting factors): Used when only specific components are needed, reducing risks like fluid overload and reactions.)

22. *What is special about the Bombay blood group?*
(Ans. People with the Bombay blood group do not have the H antigen, so they lack A and B antigens too. Their plasma contains anti-A, anti-B, and anti-H antibodies, which means they can only receive blood from someone with the same Bombay group. It is very rare.)

23. *What are forward and reverse blood typing?*
(Ans. In blood grouping or typing, the red cells of a donor or a person whose blood type is to be determined are tested against anti-A and anti-B sera. This is called blood typing or **forward blood typing.**

   In **reverse blood typing** [also called serum typing or backward blood typing], the serum of the recipient is tested against red cells containing known antigens, i.e., red cells from persons with blood types A, B, AB, and O. If agglutination occurs with A and AB red cells, the blood type is B; if agglutination occurs with B and AB red cells, the blood type is A; if agglutination occurs with A, B, and AB red cells, the blood type is O, and if there is no agglutination in any RBCs, the blood type is AB. For blood transfusion in leukemic patients, serum typing is performed along with blood typing as an extra precaution, because in leukemias, the RBC antigens may become considerably weak. This is also performed in cases of pseudomonas infection, where RBCs become agglutinated by all antisera due to the unmasking of hidden antigens.)

24. *What is the MN system ? What is its clinical use?* (Ans. Refer to page 91, under 'Other Blood Group Systems', read 'MN System'.)

25. *Why does mismatching of blood of the Lewis system not cause hemolysis?* (Ans. Refer to page 91, under 'Other Blood Group Systems', read 'Lewis System'.)

26. *What is the clinical significance of the Ii system?* (Ans. Refer to page 91, under 'Other Blood Group Systems', read 'Ii System'.)

27. *What disease is closely associated with the Duffy system and why?* (Ans. Refer to page 91, under 'Other Blood Group Systems', read 'Duffy System'.)

28. *What is the clinical use of the Kell system?* (Ans. Refer to page 91, see 'Other Blood Group Systems', read 'Kell System'.)

29. *What are the different diseases associated with different blood groups?* (Ans. Refer to page 94, see 'Uses of blood grouping', point no. 4.)

16 | Osmotic Fragility of Red Cells

Learning Objectives

After completing this practical, you will be able to (MUST KNOW):
1. Describe the utility of this practical in clinical physiology.
2. Prepare saline solutions of different percentages.
3. Perform the osmotic fragility test.
4. Explain the mechanism of hemolysis when red cells are exposed to hypotonic solutions.
5. List the precautions taken for the osmotic fragility test.

6. Define and explain osmotic fragility.
7. List the conditions that alter the osmotic fragility of red cells.

You may also be able to (DESIRABLE TO KNOW):
1. Correlate the applicability of this practical in different clinical conditions.
2. Explain the physiological basis of alteration in osmotic fragility in different diseases of red cells.

PY2.12: Describe the tests for ESR, osmotic fragility, and hematocrit. Note the findings and interpret the test results.

INTRODUCTION

Osmotic fragility of red cells is defined as the **ease with which RBCs are ruptured** (hemolyzed) when they are exposed to hypotonic solutions. It assesses the integrity of the membrane of red cells.

Clinical significance: The osmotic fragility test helps in the **diagnosis of anemia** in which the physical properties of red cells are altered. This test detects whether or not red cells can be easily hemolyzed. The red cell membrane allows water to pass through while restricting solutes. This is called **osmosis**.

1. Red cells *shrink due to exosmosis* when they are placed in a solution that is more concentrated than the concentration of solute inside.
2. On the other hand, red cells absorb water by *endosmosis* when kept in a hypotonic solution like water. This results in hemolysis *due to swelling and rupture of the cells*.
3. In an isotonic solution, i.e., a solution of equal concentration as the red cell contents (e.g., 0.85% NaCl), the *red cells stay intact*.

Physiological significance: The test of osmotic fragility attempts to determine the concentration of solute inside the red cells by placing the cell in different concentrations of sodium chloride and observing hemolysis in a hypotonic solution. When red cells are introduced into a hypotonic solution of sodium chloride, they take up water and swell up until *a critical volume is reached, and then they rupture*. When the critical volume is reached, the cells become spherical. As cells take up water, they become more fragile.

1. Red cells that are *already spherical*, as seen in hereditary spherocytosis, have *increased osmotic fragility* in hypotonic solutions because they can swell only a little before they burst.
2. Conversely, cells that are **biconcave or flat** have **decreased osmotic fragility** in hypotonic solutions because they can swell considerably before they reach the spherical shape and burst.

Thus, osmotic fragility is a measure of the rate of hemolysis of red cells when exposed to hypotonic solutions of sodium chloride.

METHODS OF DETERMINING OSMOTIC FRAGILITY

Osmotic Fragility Test

Principle

When red cells are suspended in a hypotonic solution of sodium chloride, they take up water and swell until a critical volume is reached and hemolysis occurs. As cells take up water, they become increasingly fragile. Thus, the intracellular solute concentration, as reflected by red cell fragility, can be helpful in establishing the functional state of the red cells.

Requirements

▮ Apparatus
1. Clean test tubes
2. Test tube rack
3. Distilled water
4. 1% NaCl solution
5. Dropper

▮ Specimen

Freshly drawn **heparinized or defibrinated venous blood** is prepared for this test. The test should be carried out within two hours of blood collection. Heparin is frequently used as an anticoagulant because it causes less distortion of the red cells.

Procedure

1. Arrange the test tubes in the rack and number them serially from 1 to 12.
2. Prepare **solutions of increasing hypotonicity** by mixing the required number of drops of 1 per cent sodium chloride solution and distilled water in the test tubes serially from 1 to 12, as presented in Table 16.1. Use one dropper for all saline solutions and another for distilled water.

> **Note:** Note that the first tube contains saline, which is nearly isotonic and the last tube is filled with only distilled water (tonicity nil).

3. Shake the tubes thoroughly and add a drop of blood in each tube.
4. *Invert each tube gently* once to mix the blood with saline and then place them in the rack.
5. After 30 minutes, observe the tubes against a white background (or with a sheet of white paper behind) without disturbing the tubes. Note the number of the **first tube that shows partial hemolysis** and the number of the **tube in which hemolysis is complete**.
   i. A **tube with partial hemolysis** shows an upward supernatant fluid with pink colour proportionate to the degree of hemolysis and a lower layer of sedimented red cells at the bottom of the tube.
   ii. A **tube with complete hemolysis** shows a clear, uniformly pink solution in the absence of red cells at the bottom of the tube.
   iii. A **tube with no hemolysis** shows a clear, straw-coloured supernatant fluid with a few red cells settled at the bottom (Fig. 16.1).

Observation and results

1. Carefully observe each tube for the depth of the pink colour of the supernatant and the mass of red cells at the bottom.
2. Note the test tube number with beginning of hemolysis, i.e., onset of fragility (in per cent saline).
3. Note the test tube number in which hemolysis is complete (in per cent saline).
4. Report the result as follows: "Hemolysis began in __% saline and was completed in __% saline".
5. Report that: "Osmotic fragility of the given sample of blood ranges from __% saline to __% saline". Express the result as the range from the beginning of hemolysis to its completion.

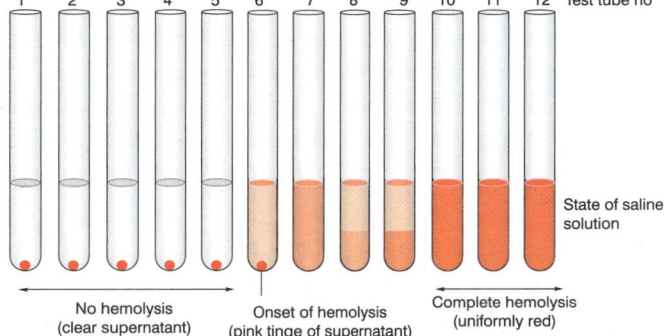

Fig. 16.1 Osmotic fragility test. Note that hemolysis starts in the sixth tube (slight pink tinge of the supernatant) and is completed in the tenth tube (solution is uniformly red). No hemolysis is observed in test tubes 1 to 5 (clear supernatant with red cell clumps at the bottom).

Normal value

Normally, osmotic fragility **begins at 0.45–0.50 and is completed at 0.30–0.33 per cent saline.**

Precautions

1. **Separate droppers** should be used for pouring drops of distilled water and 1% saline into the test tubes.
2. The **drops should be counted exactly** as recommended in Table 16.1.
3. A minimum **time of 30 minutes** should be allowed for hemolysis to occur.
4. Hemolysis should be **checked against a white background by** placing a sheet of white paper behind the tubes.
5. The **tubes should not be disturbed** while recording the observation.

DISCUSSION

When the rate of hemolysis of the red cell is increased, the osmotic fragility increases; when the rate of hemolysis is decreased, the osmotic fragility decreases. Increased osmotic fragility of red cells denotes decreased resistance of these cells to rupture.

1. Osmotic fragility is related to the **shape of red cells**. The shape of red cells is dependent on the volume, surface area, and functional state of the red cell membrane. As the resistance of the red cell membrane to rupture is related to its geometric configuration, red cells *that are spherical*

Table 16.1 Demonstration of osmotic fragility test of red cells

Test tube no.	1	2	3	4	5	6	7	8	9	10	11	12
Distilled water drops	3	9	10	11	12	13	14	15	16	17	18	25
1 per cent saline drops	22	16	15	14	13	12	11	10	9	8	7	0
% saline soln. obtained	0.88	0.64	0.60	0.56	0.52	0.48	0.44	0.40	0.36	0.32	0.28	0

(spherocytes) demonstrate increased hemolysis, while cells that are flat (sickle cell or target cells) demonstrate decreased hemolysis.

2. **Hypochromic red cells** (as seen in iron deficiency anemia) are very thin and contain less hemoglobin; therefore, they can swell to a greater extent before they rupture.

Conditions That Alter Fragility of RBCs

Diminished fragility
1. Iron deficiency anemia
2. Thalassemia
3. Sickle cell anemia
4. Obstructive jaundice
5. After splenectomy

6. A variety of anemias where target cells are seen in the peripheral blood
7. Chronic liver disease

Increased fragility
1. Hereditary spherocytosis
2. Congenital hemolytic anemia
3. Autoimmune hemolytic anemia
4. Deficiency of glucose-6-phosphate dehydrogenase (G6PD)
5. Toxic chemicals, poisons, and drugs (aspirin)
6. Other conditions in which spherocytes are found in the blood
7. The venom of cobras and some poisonous insects contains lecithinase, which dissolves lecithin in the cell membrane and makes them more fragile

VIVA

1. *What do you mean by osmotic fragility of red cells?* (Ans. Refer to page 98, under the heading 'Introduction'.)
2. *What do you mean by the terms 'red cell fragility' and 'hemolysis'?*
    (Ans. Red cell fragility refers to the susceptibility of red cells to be broken down either by osmotic effect [osmotic fragility] or by mechanical stress [mechanical fragility]. Hemolysis is the breakdown [rupture] of red cells resulting in the release of Hb into the surroundings.)
3. *What factors determine the osmotic fragility of red cells?*
    (Ans. The following factors affect osmotic fragility:
    i.   Shape of red cells—spherocytes demonstrate increased hemolysis. Flat cells [sickle or oval cells] demonstrate decreased hemolysis. Normal biconcave red cells have the least susceptibility to rupture.
    ii. Integrity of the membrane of red cell—membrane defects as seen in glucose-6-PD deficiency increases the fragility of red cells.
    iii. Hb content of red cell—hypochromic cells [lower Hb content as seen in IDA] can swell to a greater extent before they rupture.
    iv. Tonicity of the fluid in which red cells are suspended.)
4. *What is the principle of the osmotic fragility test of red cells?* (Ans. Refer to page 98, under the heading 'Method of determining...' and subheading 'Principle'.)
5. *What physical factors influence osmotic fragility?*
    (Ans. The following physical factors:
    i.   The final pH of blood in saline—decrease in pH increases fragility [a shift of 0.1 unit of pH is equivalent to change in saline concentration by 0.01 g%]
    ii. Relative volume of blood in saline
    iii. Temperature—a rise in temperature decreases fragility [rise in temperature by 0.05°C is equivalent to increase in saline concentration by 0.01 g/dL].)
6. *Define osmosis, osmotic pressure, and oncotic pressure. What is the osmotic pressure of blood? What is its significance?*
    (Ans. Osmosis is the process of movement of a solvent from a solution of lower concentration to one of higher concentration, when both the solutions are separated by a semipermeable membrane.
    i.   Osmotic pressure is the minimum pressure applied to the solution with higher solute concentration to prevent osmosis. Effective osmotic pressure is the portion of the total osmotic pressure of a solution that decides the propensity of the solvent to pass through the semipermeable membrane.
         The osmotic pressure of blood is approximately 7.65 atmospheres (atm) at 37°C (normal body temperature). This pressure is crucial for maintaining fluid balance and preventing cells from shrinking or swelling.
    ii. Oncotic pressure in body fluid is exerted by osmotically active substances dissolved in the fluid. The plasma proteins in the plasma are similar to a colloidal solution, and thus, the osmotic pressure due to these proteins is called colloidal osmotic pressure. The osmotic pressure of plasma is known as oncotic pressure, which is 25 mmHg.)
7. *What is osmolality? How does it differ from osmolarity? What is plasma osmolality?*
    (Ans. Osmolality of a solution refers to the number of osmoles [number of osmotically active particles] dissolved in a kilogram of water. Osmolarity refers to the number of osmoles in one litre of plasma.

Unlike osmolality, the value in osmolarity is affected by the volume of other solutes in the solution. Osmolarity is also affected by temperature. Though osmotic pressure is determined by osmolality, the difference between osmolality and osmolarity in normal conditions is negligible.

Plasma osmolality reflects the total concentration of particles in plasma, with over 90% due to NaCl. Plasma proteins contribute little despite their size. Normal plasma osmolality is ~290 mOsm/kg, with NaCl accounting for ~270 mOsm/kg.)

8. *What is tonicity? Give examples of isotonic, hypotonic, and hypertonic solutions.*
   (Ans. Tonicity refers to the osmolality of a solution in relation to plasma.
   i.   Isotonic: Solutions that have the same osmolality as plasma, like 0.9% NaCl, are said to be isotonic.
   ii. Hypotonic: Solutions with lower osmolality are said to be hypotonic.
   iii. Hypertonic: Solutions with higher osmolality than plasma are said to be hypertonic.)

9. *What is physiological saline? What is its importance?*
   (Ans. Normal saline [0.9% NaCl] is called physiological saline. It is used in treating volume depletion because it remains isotonic unlike other solutions. For example, a 5% glucose solution is initially isotonic, but becomes hypotonic as glucose is metabolised.)

10. *How do red cells behave in hypotonic and hypertonic solutions?*
    (Ans. 0.9% NaCl solution is isotonic. Therefore, red cells do not change their shape and size in this solution. In hypotonic solutions, red cells undergo osmotic lysis due to endosmosis, and in hypertonic solutions, cells shrink due to exosmosis.)

11. *Name some isotonic solutions.*
    (Ans. 1.5% Sodium bromide, 3.3% magnesium sulfate, 0.9% sodium chloride, 2.5% sodium nitrate, 5% dextrose, 10% sucrose, and 0.9% sodium bicarbonate.)

12. *What is the normal range of osmotic fragility of red cells?* (Ans. Refer to page 99, under the heading 'Normal Value'.)

13. *What is the effect of waiting 4–6 hours before recording observations?*
    (Ans. Delayed observation may show hemolysis in all hypotonic solutions. Without energy, the Na^+–K^+ pump fails, allowing NaCl influx, causing cells to swell and rupture.)

14. *In what conditions is there an increase in the osmotic fragility of red cells?* (Ans. Refer to page 100, under the heading 'Conditions that alter fragility of RBCs'.)

15. *In what conditions is there a decrease in the osmotic fragility of red cells?* (Ans. Refer to page 100, text under heading 'Conditions that alter fragility of RBCs'.)

16. *What is the physiological basis of the increased fragility of red cells in hereditary spherocytosis and decreased fragility in sickle cell disease?* (Ans. Refer to page 99, under the heading 'Discussion', point no. 1'.)

17. *Name a few hemolytic agents.*
    (Ans. Hypotonic saline, snake venom, drugs [aspirin is a common example], severe infection releasing septic toxins, and incompatible blood transfusion.)

18. *When does hemolysis occur in the body?*
    (Ans. Hemolysis can result from inherited red cell defects such as:
    i. **Unstable hemoglobins**, e.g., sickle cell anemia, thalassemia
    ii. **Enzyme deficiencies**, e.g., G6PD deficiency, pyruvate kinase deficiency.)

19. *What is the effect of 5% glucose, 10% glucose, urea solution, and urine on red cells?*
    (Ans. The effects are as follows:
    i.   5% glucose: Isotonic; no change in red cells.
    ii. 10% glucose: Hypertonic; cells shrink. Effect diminishes as glucose is metabolised.
    iii. Urea solution: Causes cells to swell and burst due to water influx.
    iv. Urine: Typically hypotonic, so cells swell. In concentrated urine, cells shrink.)

20. *Do all red cells in a sample of blood or in a person's body have similar osmotic fragility?*
    (Ans. Red cells in a sample of blood or in a person's body differ in age, hence their individual osmotic fragility will differ. Younger cells are more resistant than older cells to osmotic fragility.)

17 | Determination of Bleeding Time and Coagulation Time

Learning Objectives

After completing this practical, you will be able to (MUST KNOW):
1. Describe the importance of determining BT and CT in clinical physiology.
2. List the steps of blood coagulation.
3. Determine BT by the Duke method.
4. Determine CT by the capillary tube method.
5. Give the normal values of BT and CT.
6. List the precautions taken for the determination of BT and CT.
7. Name the diseases in which BT and CT are prolonged.

8. List the tests to determine platelet function and assess the efficiency of the intrinsic and extrinsic pathways of blood coagulation.

You may also be able to (DESIRABLE TO KNOW):
1. Explain the mechanism of intrinsic and extrinsic pathways of blood coagulation.
2. Describe the role of platelets in blood coagulation.
3. Explain the principle and clinical significance of different tests for the investigation of bleeding disorders.

PY2.11: Estimate Hb, RBC, TLC, RBC indices, DLC, blood groups, and BT/CT.

INTRODUCTION

Bleeding and clotting times are determined to assess the integrity of hemostatic mechanisms. **Hemostasis** is the stoppage of bleeding. It is a complex process that involves **three major steps** in sequence: (1) vasoconstriction, (2) platelet plug formation, and (3) coagulation or clot formation.

Bleeding time (BT) depends on the effectiveness of vasoconstriction and platelet plug formation, whereas clotting time (CT) mainly depends on the effectiveness of the clotting mechanism. BT is the time from the onset of bleeding till the stoppage of bleeding, and CT is the time from the onset of bleeding till clot formation.

Vasoconstriction

The immediate response of blood vessels to injury is vasoconstriction, which occurs due to the *contraction of smooth muscles* of the injured vessels. This **decreases the loss of blood** and assists in the process of platelet plug formation. It is *potentiated by the release of vasoconstrictors* like serotonin from the platelets aggregated at the site of injury.

The effectiveness of vascular response is detected by the **capillary fragility test**, but vascular response cannot be clearly separated from platelet response. Therefore, *determination of bleeding time and capillary fragility test* are necessary to *measure the integrity of both responses*.

Platelet Plug Formation

Platelet plug (**temporary hemostatic plug**) formation occurs due to *three properties* of platelets: **adhesion,**

aggregation, and release reaction (details in Chapter 18). The **effectiveness of platelets in hemostasis** can be assessed by the following: **i)** bleeding time, **ii)** platelet count, **iii)** platelet aggregation studies, **iv)** platelet adhesiveness test, **v)** clot retraction test, and **vi)** prothrombin consumption test.

Coagulation or Clot Formation

Blood coagulation occurs in **three stages: (1) activation of the Stuart–Prower factor, (2) formation of thrombin from prothrombin**, and **(3) formation of fibrin from fibrinogen** (Fig. 17.1). CT is the time from the onset of bleeding to the clot (definitive hemostatic plug) formation.

Activation of Stuart–Prower factor: The tissue extract (tissue thromboplastin or factor III) enters the blood through the site of injury and combines with factor VII and calcium (factor IV). This is called the **extrinsic system**. It originates outside the blood vessels and includes factors III, IV, and VII. In the meantime, there is activation of the **intrinsic system** when factor XII is activated by its contact with the negatively charged surface of the collagen fibres of the injured vessel walls. The intrinsic system originates inside the blood vessels and includes factors XII, XI, IX, VIII, and calcium (IV). Finally, both extrinsic and intrinsic systems follow a **common pathway**, which results in the formation of the active Stuart–Prower factor (Xa).

Any defect in the intrinsic system of stage 1 is recognised by the **activated partial thromboplastin time (APTT)**.
Formation of thrombin from prothrombin: In stage 2, prothrombin (factor II) is activated by Xa in the presence of Va, calcium, and platelet phospholipid, the end product of stage 1. This results in the formation of **thrombin**.

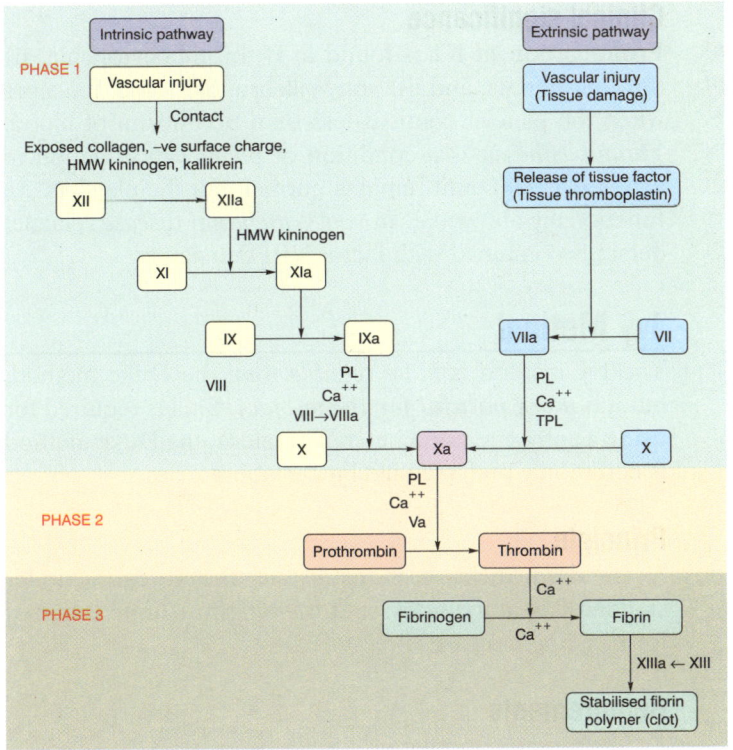

Fig. 17.1 Mechanism of blood coagulation. Note the three stages (phases) of blood clotting.

Any defect in this stage results in the prolongation of prothrombin time.

Formation of fibrin from fibrinogen: This is the final stage of the coagulation process. **Fibrin** is formed from fibrinogen by thrombin, the end product of stage 2. First, fibrin monomers are formed, then polymerisation of fibrin takes place with the help of activated factor XIII to form the fibrin clot. Thrombin time is prolonged if there is a defect in the formation of fibrin from fibrinogen.

METHODS OF DETERMINING BLEEDING TIME

Bleeding time (BT) is usually determined by two methods: **(1) Duke method and (2) Ivy method**.

Duke Method

The Duke method is the more frequently used method to determine BT in clinical laboratories as it is easy to perform and requires minimal equipment and laboratory skill.

Principle

A deep skin puncture is made, and the length of time required for bleeding to stop is recorded. This test determines the function of the platelets and the integrity of the capillaries.

Requirements

1. Equipment for sterile finger puncture
2. Blotting paper or filter paper
3. Stopwatch

Procedure

1. Assemble all the necessary materials and provide proper instructions to the subject (this can be done by the student).
2. Clean **the subject's fingertip or earlobe** with alcohol and allow the skin to dry completely.

Note: Though the earlobe is a good site for this test, the fingertip is more convenient.

3. Make a **deep puncture** (blood should flow freely to form a moderate-sized drop) with a sterile lancet and hold the finger firmly without squeezing hard or milking (Fig. 17.2).
4. Immediately start the stopwatch as soon as bleeding starts.
5. Blot the drop of blood coming out of the incision every 30 seconds using a blotting paper or circular filter paper (Fig. 17.3). Place each subsequent drop a little further along the side of the filter paper.

Note: Do not allow the filter paper to press on the bleeding spot. Note that the drops become progressively smaller.

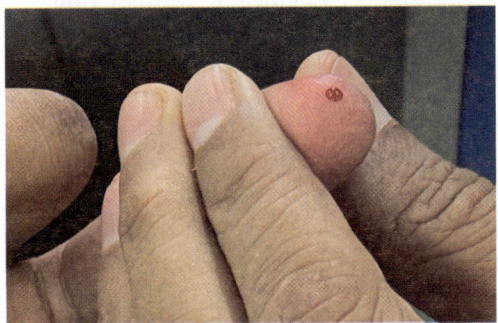

Fig. 17.2 Bleeding of the fingertip for estimation of bleeding time. Hold the finger firmly, but ensure that blood oozes spontaneously without squeezing. Wear gloves if you are bleeding an unknown subject or a patient.

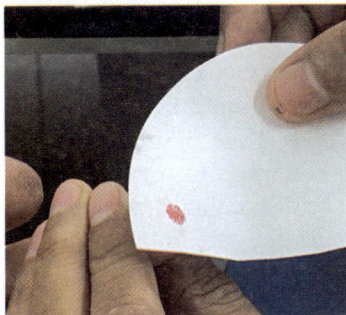

Fig. 17.3 Blotting of blood on the filter paper or blotting paper. Note that the blotting paper is just touched on the blood drop but not pressed on it.

6. Stop the stopwatch as soon as the bleeding ceases.
7. Count the **number of drops on the filter paper** and multiply it by 30 seconds, or the time can be noted on each drop of blood (Fig. 17.4). In some hospitals, blotting of drops of blood is done every 15 seconds; hence, noting the time on top of the marked spot of the blood drop is ideal.

> **Note:** If the bleeding does not stop in 10 minutes, discontinue the test and apply pressure to the spot to stop bleeding.

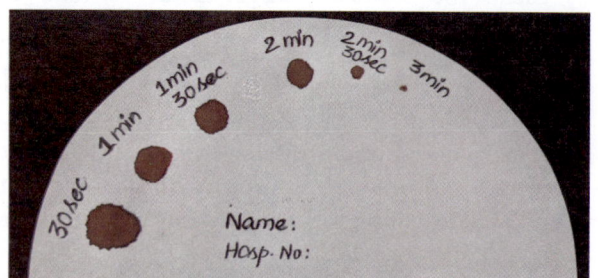

Fig. 17.4   Recording of bleeding time on the filter paper or blotting paper. Note that the size of the blood drop decreases gradually. The time can be written on top of each drop and the name of the subject/patient and the hospital number should also be noted.

Observation and results

1. Count the number of blood drops on the filter paper and multiply the number by 30 seconds. Also, note the time marked for each drop of blood.
2. Write the subject's name and hospital number on the blotting paper.
3. Report the result as follows: "The bleeding time of the subject _____ (name), male/female, aged _____ years is 03 minutes, as recorded by the Duke method (fingertip)."

Precautions

1. Gather all the necessary materials before starting the test.
2. Do not rub too much while cleaning the skin as rubbing increases blood flow and alters BT.
3. The skin should dry completely before pricking.
4. The **puncture should be deep** (about 4 mm).
5. The finger should not be squeezed. Blood **should flow freely**.
6. The blood should be blotted exactly every 30 seconds.
7. The *filter paper should not be pressed down on the bleeding spot* as it may interfere with bleeding.
8. If bleeding continues for more than 10 minutes, the test should be discontinued, and the subject should be asked to apply pressure to the wound.

Normal value

The normal range of BT by the Duke method varies from **1 to 5 minutes**.

Clinical significance

Prolongation of BT is found in **i)** thrombocytopenia, **ii)** thrombasthenia, and **iii)** von Willebrand disease. It occurs when the platelet count is less than 50,000/ml of blood. *Thrombasthenia* is a condition of platelet dysfunction in which platelet count remains normal, but the platelets are functionally abnormal. In *von Willebrand disease*, platelet defect is combined with factor VIII deficiency.

Ivy Method

The Ivy method is *more reliable* than the Duke method, but it is ***more painful for the subject***. Skill is required for using a sphygmomanometer. Therefore, the Duke method is commonly preferred in clinical laboratories.

Principle

A standard incision is made on the forearm under standardised conditions, and the length of time required for bleeding to cease is recorded.

Requirements

1. Sphygmomanometer
2. Sterile lancet capable of making an incision 1 mm wide and 3 mm deep
3. Blotting paper
4. Alcohol
5. Cotton wool

Procedure

1. Explain the procedure to the subject.
2. Tie the sphygmomanometer cuff on the subject's arm above the elbow.
3. **Raise the cuff pressure to 40 mmHg** and maintain it for the entire period.
4. Select an area approximately 5 cm below the cubital fossa on the anterior aspect of the forearm and clean it with alcohol.
5. Hold the skin tightly by grasping the underside of the forearm firmly and make ***two separate punctures*** 5 cm apart in quick succession using the sterile lancet.
6. Start the stopwatch.
7. *Blot the blood from each incision site* on a separate piece of blotting paper, every 30 seconds.
8. When the bleeding stops, stop the watch and release the pressure from the sphygmomanometer cuff.
9. Record the bleeding time of both the puncture sites. The ***longer of the two bleeding times is more accurate*** than the average of the two.
10. If the bleeding continues for more than 15 minutes, discontinue the test, apply pressure to the puncture to stop bleeding, and report the BT as more than 15 minutes.

Observation and results

1. Record the bleeding time of both the punctures.
2. Note the longer of the two bleeding times. Do not take the average of the two.
3. Report the result as follows: "Bleeding time of the subject _____(name), male/female, aged ____years is __minutes, as recorded by the Ivy method."

Precautions

1. The procedure should be explained to the subject beforehand.
2. The area selected for puncture should be properly cleaned.
3. *Two incisions* should ideally be made for the determination of BT by this method.
4. A constant *pressure of 40 mmHg should be maintained* throughout the procedure.
5. The incision should be made deep into the skin.
6. The *longer of the two bleeding times* (rather than the average) should be taken as the result.

Normal value

The normal range of BT by the Ivy method is **5–11 minutes**.

Clinical significance

The clinical significance is the same as that of the Duke method. Though the Duke method is commonly followed, the Ivy method should be the method of choice, as it is more reliable.

Simplate Method

In the Duke and the Ivy methods of bleeding time determination, it is not possible to control the depth of the wound made by a lancet for all individuals, though these tests are fairly reliable. Therefore, another technique is adopted, which uses a template or an automated scalpel to control the depth and length of the wound, i.e., usually 1 mm deep and 9 mm long. In this method, the blood pressure cuff is inflated to 40 mmHg to distend the capillary bed of the forearm. This is called the simplate method.

Normal BT: <7 minutes.

METHODS OF DETERMINING CLOTTING TIME

Clotting time (CT) is usually determined by two methods: **(1) the capillary tube method and (2) Lee–White (venipuncture) method**. The capillary tube method is routinely used in clinical laboratories to determine CT.

Capillary Tube Method

This is also called **Wright's capillary glass tube method**.

Principle

A standard incision is made into the subject's skin, and blood is collected in a capillary glass tube. The amount of time that it takes for the blood to clot (as detected by the appearance of fibrin string) is reported as CT.

Requirements

1. Materials required for sterile finger prick
2. Capillary tubing (10–15 cm in length and 1.5 mm in diameter) without anticoagulant

Procedure

1. Explain the procedure to the subject.
2. Make a sterile finger puncture using the lancet to a depth of 3 mm.
3. As soon as blood becomes visible, start the stopwatch.
4. Wipe off the first drop of blood. Allow the next drop of blood to form **a drop of larger size** (Fig. 17.5). Then allow the blood to flow into the capillary tube by introducing one end of the tube into the drop (Fig. 17.6). Usually, blood enters the capillary tube automatically by capillary action. If and if blood does not enter automatically, it can be done by holding the *other end of the capillary tube at a lower level* (Fig. 17.7). Blood enters the capillary tube by capillary action.

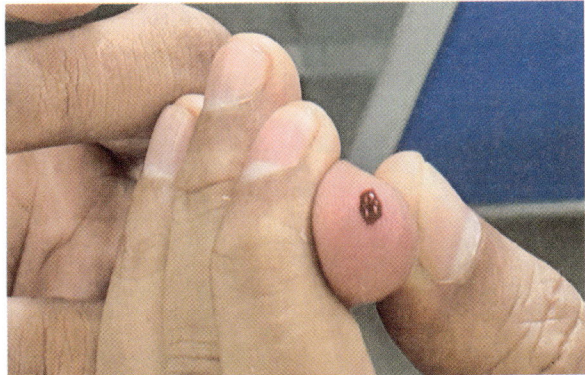

Fig. 17.5 Collection of blood drop from the fingertip for estimation of clotting time. Ensure that a large drop of blood forms so that blood enters a larger length of capillary tube in one go without an opportunity for air bubbles to enter.

Note: If the size of the blood drop is small, the blood may not be adequate to fill a larger length of the capillary tube, and doing it again may allow air bubbles to enter the tube.

5. Hold the capillary tube filled with blood between the palms so as to maintain it at body temperature.

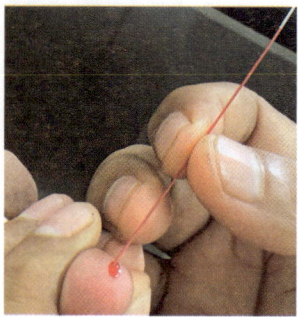

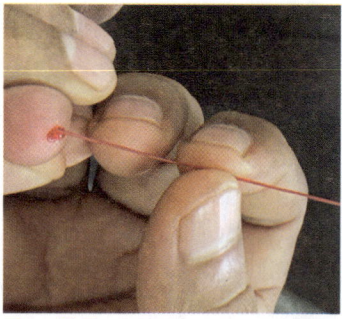

Fig. 17.6 Collection of blood in the capillary tube for estimation of CT. Note that blood enters the capillary tube automatically by capillary action.

Fig. 17.7 Collection of blood in the capillary tube by lowering the other end of the capillary tube.

6. After 2 minutes, **break off the capillary tubing 1–2 cm** from one end every 30 seconds and look for the appearance of a thread of fibrin.
7. When a **thin string of fibrin** is seen between the broken ends (Fig. 17.8), stop the watch and note the time.
8. In the report, mention the use of the capillary method.

Observation and results

1. When a thin string of fibrin is seen between the broken ends of the capillary tube, stop the watch and note the time.
2. Report the result as follows: "Clotting time of the subject _____(name), male/female, aged ____years, is __minutes, as recorded by the capillary tube method."

Precautions

1. The procedure should be explained to the subject beforehand.
2. The fingertip should be cleaned with alcohol before pricking.

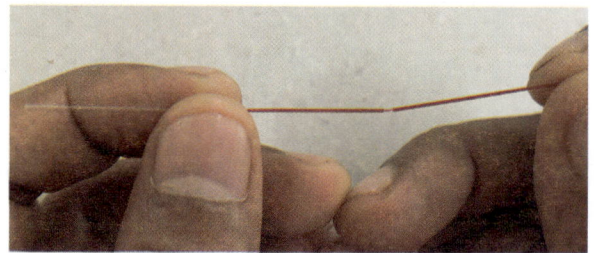

Fig. 17.8 Demonstration of fibrin string (thread of clot) by gently breaking the capillary tube and lightly separating the two broken ends. Note the thread of clot between the broken ends of the capillary tube.

3. The puncture should be sufficiently deep, and blood should flow spontaneously.
4. Immediately after filling, the capillary tube should be held between the palms to maintain its temperature (external temperature affects clotting).

5. With each break of the capillary tube, the appearance of the fibrin string should be looked for (Fig. 17.8).

Normal value

The normal range of CT by the capillary glass tube method is **2–8 minutes**.

Clinical significance

CT is prolonged in diseases in which **clotting factors are deficient**. If the CT is more than 10 minutes, the patient should be subjected to detailed investigations to identify the missing coagulation factors.

Lee–White Method

This is also called the **Lee–White test tube method**. It is **more reliable and sensitive** than the capillary method but needs special arrangements for venipuncture and a temperature-controlled water bath.

Principle

Venous blood is collected in a clean glass tube without any anticoagulant. The time taken by blood to clot at 37°C is noted as the clotting time.

Requirements

1. Materials for drawing blood by venipuncture
2. Test tubes
3. Water bath at 37°C
4. Stopwatch

Procedure

1. Explain the procedure to the subject.
2. Collect over **2 ml of venous blood** by making a sterile venipuncture.
3. Start the stopwatch as soon as the blood enters the syringe.
4. Remove the needle from the syringe and **fill each of the two tubes to the 1 ml mark**.
5. Plug the tubes with non-absorbent cotton wool and **place them in the water bath at 37°C**.
6. After 3 minutes, remove the first tube from the water bath and *tilt the tube gently to 45°* to check whether the blood has clotted. If not, return the tube to the water bath and *examine it every 30 seconds* to check for the appearance of a clot.
7. When blood clots, the tube can be tilted through an angle of 90° without spilling the contents.
8. As soon as the blood is clotted, examine the second tube. The blood in the second tube usually clots as soon as blood clots in the first tube.
9. Stop the stopwatch, and note the time.
10. The CT noted is the clotting time of the second tube.

Observation and results

1. Note the clotting of blood in both the tubes.
2. If there is a difference between the tubes, take the one with the longer time.
3. Report the result as follows: "Clotting time of the subject _____(name), male/female, aged _____years, is ___minutes, as recorded by the Lee–White method."

Precautions and sources of error

1. One important source of error is an inappropriate volume of blood taken for the test (less than 1 ml gives a shorter CT).
2. The temperature of the tubes should be maintained at 37°C.
3. While collecting blood, air bubbles should not enter the syringe. The presence of air bubbles shortens the CT.

Normal value

The normal range of CT by the Lee–White method is **5–12 minutes**.

Clinical significance

This method is **more reliable** than the capillary tube method. The clinical significance of this method is the same as that of the capillary tube method.

Single tube method and multiple tube method

In the Lee–White method, a single test tube can be used, which is called the **single test tube method**, or two or more test tubes of 8 mm diameter can be used, which is called the **multiple test tube method**.

OTHER TESTS FOR BLEEDING DISORDERS

Many other tests are performed to detect the nature and degree of various bleeding disorders. As these tests are not routinely carried out in physiology laboratories but may be asked in viva, the basic principle and clinical significance of each test are described in this section.

Capillary Fragility Test

Principle: This is also called the **capillary fragility test of Hess or the tourniquet test**. This test measures the ability of the capillaries to withstand increased stress. *Petechiae appear in the subject's forearm* when the blood pressure cuff in the arm is inflated to a maximum pressure of 100 mmHg for about 5 minutes.
Clinical significance: Normally, **0–10 petechiae appear**. More than 10 petechiae indicates capillary weakness or thrombocytopenia or both.

Platelet Aggregation Test

Principle: An aggregating agent is added to a suspension of platelets in plasma, and the response is measured *turbidometrically as a change in the transmission of light* by an instrument called the **aggregometer**.
Clinical significance: Measurement of platelet aggregation is an essential part of the investigation of any patient with suspected platelet dysfunction.

Platelet Adhesiveness Test

Principle: This test measures the *ability of platelets to adhere to a glass surface*. When anticoagulated blood is allowed to pass at a constant rate through a plastic tube containing glass beads, some platelets adhere to the beads. The **percentage difference between the platelet counts** before and after passing through the glass bead column indicates the functional status of platelets.
Clinical significance: The normal range is **75–95 per cent of platelet retention**. The platelet adhesiveness test is non-specific. The results are abnormal in several platelet functional disorders.

Clot Retraction Time

Principle: Blood clots when collected in a glass tube without any anticoagulant. The clot begins to retract (after blood has clotted) within 30 seconds and is about 50 per cent at the end of 1 hour. At the end of **18–24 hours, the clot should have retracted completely**.
Clinical significance: Abnormal clot retraction is reported when less than *50 per cent retraction occurs at 1 hour*. Clot retraction is primarily dependent on platelet function. *Hematocrit and fibrinogen levels* also affect it. Poor clot retractability is usually seen *when the platelet count is less than 1,00,000*.

Clot Lysis Time

Principle: Clots are lysed due to fibrinolysis, which is a natural process. Due to lysis, the clot becomes fluid, and red cells sink to the bottom of the test tube.
Clinical significance: The lysis time for a normal clot is **about 72 hours**. If lysis is seen within 24 hours, fibrinolysis is considered to be abnormal.

Prothrombin Consumption Test

Principle: This test determines the amount of prothrombin present in the serum after clot formation.
Clinical significance: Normally, in the coagulation process, *more than 95 per cent of prothrombin is used up* as it is converted to thrombin. The presence of more than **5 per cent of prothrombin in the serum** indicates a quantitative or qualitative platelet deficiency.

Prothrombin Time (PT)

Principle: A preparation of rabbit brain emulsion (which contains tissue thromboplastin) is added to plasma in the presence of calcium. This, in the presence of factor VII, triggers stage 2 of the coagulation mechanism. The clotting time is recorded after the addition of calcified thromboplastin to the plasma.

Normal value: The normal value is **12–16 seconds**.

Clinical significance: Prolonged PT suggests the possibility of **deficiency of factors II, V, VII, and X**. In stage 2, prothrombin is converted to thrombin, which triggers the transformation of fibrinogen to fibrin. Abnormal prothrombin time suggests a **stage 2 defect**.

Partial Thromboplastin Time (PTT)

Principle: The platelet substitute, in the form of partial thromboplastin, is prepared from rabbit brain as chloroform extract. When mixed with test plasma containing excess of calcium, it leads to clot formation.

Normal value: The normal value is **60–80 seconds**.

Clinical significance: PTT is prolonged when there is a deficiency of one or more **clotting factors XII, XI, IX, VIII, X, V, II, and I**. Abnormal PTT *indicates a stage 1 defect* and the *absence of one or more of the intrinsic factors*.

Activated Partial Thromboplastin Time (APTT)

Principle: A platelet substitute, in the form of partial thromboplastin, is prepared from rabbit brain and incubated with a contacting agent (kaolin) to provide *optimal activation of the intrinsic coagulation factors*. The clotting time is determined after the addition of an excess of calcium.

Normal value: The normal value is **25–40 seconds**.

Clinical significance: APTT is prolonged in **deficiencies of factors XII, XI, X, IX, and VIII**. APTT is a more reliable test than PTT. When used in conjunction with PT, it provides a simple method for *differentiating between stage 1 intrinsic defects and other factor deficiencies*. APTT is mainly determined in hemophilias that involve the deficiency of factors VIII, IX, or XI.

Thrombin Time (TT)

Principle: Thrombin (commercially available) is added to the plasma along with calcium, and the clotting time is determined.

Normal value: The normal value is **15–20 seconds**.

Clinical significance: Thrombin time detects the **effectiveness of stage 3 of coagulation**, in which fibrinogen is converted to fibrin. Prolonged TT is considered to be due to either a decrease in fibrinogen concentration or the presence of dysfunctional fibrinogen.

Plasma Recalcification Time (PRT)

Principle: When an excess of calcium is added to citrated plasma, clotting occurs. Because platelet factor III is also involved in clotting through the intrinsic pathway of coagulation, the clotting occurs in a shorter time in platelet-rich plasma than in platelet-poor plasma.

Normal values:
1. Platelet-rich plasma: **100–150 seconds**
2. Platelet-poor plasma: **135–240 seconds**

Clinical significance: This is an easy screening test that detects *deficiencies of the factors of the intrinsic pathway*, that is, factors XII, XI, IX, VIII, X, V, and II (all coagulation factors except VII and XIII).

DISCUSSION

Bleeding occurs when a blood vessel is injured and normally stops by a process called **hemostasis**. Abnormal bleeding occurs spontaneously or following trauma, due to the derangement of hemostasis, which warrants investigation. Patients prepared for surgery must be routinely checked for bleeding disorders to ensure normal hemostasis during the procedure.

Clinical Significance

Laboratory investigations for bleeding disorders are required for patients who have a history of spontaneous bleeding or excessive bleeding following injury or surgery. **Hemorrhagic disorders** are broadly classified into *inherited and acquired defects*. Acquired defects are more common than inherited defects and platelet defects are more common than coagulation defects. Deficiencies of factor VIII (hemophilia) and factor IX (Christmas disease) are more common inherited coagulation defects. The common **acquired defects** are thrombocytopenia, vitamin K deficiency, disseminated intravascular coagulation, and liver failure.

Bleeding time is prolonged in conditions in which platelets are defective or less in number, and the vascular response to injury is impaired. Clotting time is prolonged in conditions in which clotting factors are defective or deficient.

Conditions in which BT is prolonged, but CT is normal
1. Thrombocytopenia due to any cause
2. Thrombasthenia

3. Idiopathic thrombocytopenic purpura

Conditions in which CT is prolonged, but BT is normal
1. Hemophilia
2. Christmas disease
3. Any bleeding disorder in which clotting factors are deficient

Hemophilia

Hemophilia occurs due to the **deficiency of factor VIII**. It is an **X-linked recessive** bleeding disorder. The abnormality is located on the **X chromosome**. *Women are carriers* and usually do not suffer from the disease because they are protected by the second X chromosome, which is usually normal. The disease manifests with a bleeding tendency that usually appears in infancy, but, which in mild cases, may appear in adult life. ***Persistent bleeding from wounds*** is a characteristic symptom, which is usually slow and persists from days to weeks despite the presence of large clots. Bleeding may also occur spontaneously into the tissues, joints, and cavities of the body. The **patient is treated with fresh blood transfusions** because factor VIII is lost rapidly on storage. The better alternative is to administer a factor VIII concentrate.

Christmas Disease

Christmas disease occurs due to a **deficiency of factor IX**. It is clinically indistinguishable from hemophilia. Therefore, it is also called **hemophilia B**.

Purpura

Purpura refers to a group of diseases that occur **due to thrombocytopenia**. The two commonest forms of purpura are *idiopathic thrombocytopenic purpura (ITP)* and *drug-induced purpura* (which is also commonly seen in von Willebrand disease). Purpura *induced by a vascular defect* may be seen in vitamin C deficiency.

VIVA

1. *What are the methods of determination of BT and what are the normal values in these tests?* (Ans. Refer to page 103, under the heading 'Methods of Determination of BT' and 'Normal Values' on pages 103 and 104 respectively.)
2. *What are the precautions taken for determining BT by the Duke method?* (Ans. Refer to page 103, under the heading 'Duke method' and subheading 'Precautions'.)
3. *Which method is more reliable for determining BT and why?*
   (Ans. The Ivy method is more reliable, as it involves making a standard incision. Moreover, this method is more standardised and controlled. Two incisions are made, and the one having the longer duration of BT is noted.)
4. *What is the clinical significance of determining BT by the Duke method?* (Ans. Refer to page 104, under the heading 'Clinical Significance'.)
5. *What are the precautions taken for determining BT by the Ivy method?* (Ans. Refer to page 104, under the heading 'Ivy Method' and the subheading 'Precautions'.)
6. *What is the clinical significance of determining BT by the Ivy method?* (Ans. Refer to page 105, under the heading 'Clinical Significance'.)
7. *What are the methods of determination of CT and what are their normal values?* (Ans. Refer to page 106, under the headings 'Methods of Determination of CT' and 'Normal Values' on pages 105 and 106 respectively.)
8. *What are the precautions to be taken while determining CT by the capillary tube method?* (Ans. Refer to page 106, under the heading 'Capillary tube method' and the subheading 'Precautions'.)
9. *What are the precautions to be taken while determining CT by Lee–White method?* (Ans. Refer to page 107, under the heading 'Lee–White method' and the subheading 'Precautions'.)
10. *Which method of determination of CT is more reliable and why?*
    (Ans. The Lee–White method is considered more reliable and sensitive because it uses a standardised tube and follows a more controlled and consistent procedure. Additionally, the use of two tubes allows for comparative evaluation, with the longer clotting time being recorded.)
11. *What is the clinical significance of determination of CT by the capillary tube method?* (Ans. Refer to page 106, under the heading 'Clinical Significance'.)
12. *What is the clinical significance of determination of CT by Lee–White method?* (Ans. Refer to page 107, under the heading 'Clinical Significance'.)
13. *Why is CT normally more than BT?*
    (Ans. Bleeding time [BT] measures the time from the onset of bleeding until it stops, which reflects the formation of a temporary hemostatic plug. Clotting time [CT], on the other hand, measures the time required for the formation of a definitive fibrin clot. Since a stable clot takes longer to form than the initial platelet plug, CT is normally longer than BT.)

14. *What are hemostasis and homeostasis?*
(Ans. Hemostasis refers to the arrest of bleeding, while homeostasis is the maintenance of a constant internal environment [milieu intérieur]. Hemostasis contributes to homeostasis by maintaining blood volume and integrity.)

15. *What are the mechanisms of hemostasis?* (Ans. Refer to page 102, under the heading 'Introduction', read 'Hemostasis'.)

16. *What are the steps of blood coagulation, and how do you detect the defects in these steps?* (Ans. Refer to page 102-103, under the heading 'Coagulation or.....' and read 'three major stages'; to detect defects, refer to page 108, and read about PT, PTT, and APTT.)

17. *What are the tests to detect defects in the vascular response of hemostasis?* (Ans. Refer to page 107, under the heading 'Capillary fragility test'.)

18. *What are the tests to detect defects in platelets?*
(Ans. Defects in platelets can be detected by the following tests:
i.   Bleeding time
ii.   Platelet count
iii. Platelet aggregation studies
iv.   Platelet adhesiveness test
v.   Clot retraction test
vi.   Prothrombin consumption test)

19. *What is normal prothrombin time and what is its clinical significance?* (Ans. Refer to page 108, under the heading 'Prothrombin time'.)

20. *What is the normal partial thromboplastin time and what is its clinical significance?* (Ans. Refer to page 108, under the heading 'PTT'.)

21. *What is the normal value of activated partial thromboplastin time (APTT) and what is its clinical significance?* (Ans. Refer to page 107, under the heading 'APTT'.)

22. *What is normal thrombin time (TT) and what is its clinical significance?* (Ans. Refer to page 108, under the heading 'Thrombin Time'.)

23. *What is plasma recalcification time (PRT) and what is its clinical significance?* (Ans. Refer to page 108, under the heading 'PRT'.)

24. *What is hemophilia?* (Ans. Refer to page 109, under the heading 'Hemophilia'.)

25. *What is the simplate method of BT determination and what is its advantage?*
(Ans. In the Duke and Ivy methods, there is no precise control over wound depth, which affects the bleeding time [BT]. The simplate method uses an automated scalpel to create a standardised incision [1 mm deep, 9 mm long], providing consistent and reproducible results. See page 115 for details.)

26. *What are the factors that influence BT and CT?*
(Ans.
I. Factors influencing BT:
i.   Size (breadth and depth) of the wound
ii.   Degree of hyperemia of skin puncture site
iii. Number of platelets and their functional status
iv.   Functional status of the blood vessels
v.   Body temperature or temperature of the part to be pricked—if the skin is cold, there is less bleeding due to vasoconstriction; rubbing the part [hyperemia] promotes bleeding.
vi.   Environmental temperature—in cold weather, due to low temperature, BT is reduced [due to vasoconstriction]
II. Factors influencing CT
i.   Nature of contact surface—siliconised surface may prolong the CT.
ii.   Blood level of clotting factors
iii. Skin temperature—low temperature may prolong the CT)

27. *Name the conditions in which bleeding time is prolonged, but CT is normal.*
(Ans. *Prolongation of BT with normal CT* is seen in:
i.   Thrombocytopenia [decreased production of platelets or increased destruction of platelets]
ii.   Thrombasthenia [functional platelet defects]
iii. Drugs—aspirin, large doses of penicillin, corticosteroids, sulfa drugs.
iv.   von Willebrand disease
v.   Other diseases—uremia, cirrhosis, leukemia, etc.
vi.   Vessel wall defects [acquired, but may be inherited]
vii. Allergic purpura—there is damage to capillary wall by antibodies

viii. Infections—typhus, bacterial endocarditis, hemolytic streptococci, etc.

ix. Vitamin C deficiency—petechia, and bleeding from gums occur due to decreased intracellular substances and less stable capillary basement membrane

x. Senile purpura—in the elderly, small vessels rupture due to increased mobility of skin resulting from loss of elastic and connective tissues around blood vessels

xi. Connective tissue diseases

28. *How is the severity of bleeding linked to the level of platelet count?*

(Ans. The level of platelet deficiency is the main factor that contributes to severity of bleeding.

i. Above 100,000/mm^3: No clinical symptoms, bleeding is rare

ii. 50,000–100,000/mm^3: Bleeding may occur after major surgeries 20,000–50,000/mm^3: Bleeding occurs with minor trauma

iii. Below 20,000/mm^3: Spontaneous hemorrhages in urinary and GI tract, nose bleeds, etc.

iv. At <20,000/mm^3: Cerebral hemorrhages may occur)

29. *Give the causes of thrombocytopenia.*

(Ans.

I. Decreased production

i. Bone marrow suppression: Drugs [sulphas, chloramphenicol, cytotoxic drugs]; irradiation, toxemic conditions, and aplastic anemia.

ii. Bone marrow infiltration: Leukemias and secondary deposits of malignant disease.

iii. Periodic thrombocytopenic purpura [purpura hemorrhagica]

II. Increased destruction

i. Drugs: Thiazides, quinine, ethanol, estrogens, methyldopa, quinidine

ii. Idiopathic thrombocytopenic purpura

iii. Hypersplenism [Sequestration and destruction in spleen]

iv. Disseminated intravascular coagulation

v. Hemorrhage with severe transfusion)

30. *List the causes of thrombocytosis.*

(Ans.

i. *Primary thrombocytosis* [thrombocythemia]: It is a myeloproliferative disease involving megakaryocytes.

ii. *Secondary [or reactive] thrombocytosis:* Often occurs after removal of spleen or after severe hemorrhage.)

31. *What is the mechanism of clotting in the glass capillary tube in your experiment?*

(Ans. When blood comes in contact with the glass surface of the capillary tube [similar to the injury of blood vessel], it initiates intrinsic blood coagulation. The activation of platelets triggers the release of phospholipids [PPL]. The PPL, along with high-molecular-weight kininogens and kallikrein, convert factor XII to XIIa, which facilitates the intrinsic mechanism of clotting.)

32. *Give the causes of prolongation of clotting time.*

(Ans.

I. *Hereditary coagulation disorders*

i. Hemophilias A, B, C, D

ii. von Willebrand disease

iii. Afibrinogenemia and dysfibrinogenemia

iv. Deficiency of factor XIII

II. *Acquired coagulation disorders*

i. Vitamin K deficiency

ii. Liver diseases: There is a decrease of all clotting factors except VIII; there is also a reduced uptake of vitamin K, and abnormalities of platelet function

iii. Intravascular clotting: Clotting factors are used up and bleeding may occur

iv. Anticoagulant therapy: Patients receiving heparin or wafarin show an increased CT

v. Newborns: Premature babies have a tendency to bleed due to low levels of certain clotting factors in the plasma, especially prothrombin; usually, normal levels of the clotting factors are reached by the 2nd or 3rd week after birth)

33. *How is the fluid state of blood maintained in the body?*

(Ans. A balance between clotting and anticlotting mechanisms prevents intravascular clotting. In addition, the continuous nature of blood flow and endothelial factors contribute to fluidity of blood.

I. Continuous flow of blood [dynamic circulation]

II. *Endothelial factors:*
i.   Smoothness of endothelial surface [damage to endothelium causes this activation]
ii. The glycocalyx layer on the endothelium repels clotting factors and platelets
iii. Thrombomodulin removes thrombin as soon as it is formed
iv. Prostacyclin secreted by endothelium counteracts platelet aggregation
III. *Antithrombin action* of antithrombin III—Heparin complex and fibrin
IV. Fibrinolytic [plasmin] system

34. *Define thrombosis and embolism and give the causes for each.*
(Ans. **Thrombosis** is an intravascular clot. Generally, thrombosis develops due to two mechanisms:

i. *Local damage or roughness of endothelial surface of blood vessel:* This usually occurs at the site of atheromatous plaques [sites more prone are coronaries, carotid arteries, cerebral arteries], on damaged cardiac valves, or in veins of the lower limbs. At the site of atheromatous plaque, platelets aggregate, adhere and are activated, and slowly initiate the intrinsic system of clotting.

ii. *Slowing of blood flow [stasis]:* Decreased flow of blood in the pelvic and leg veins causes accumulation of clotting factors. This usually occurs in prolonged confinement to bed [fractures, major surgery, severe burns], during long flights in aeroplanes, as a complication of pregnancy, etc.

Emboli are small fragments of a thrombus that, after getting dislodged from thrombus, enter the downstream blood and block smaller vessels. This process is called embolism. Also, an embolus can be a blood clot, an air bubble, fat globules from broken bones, and a piece of tissue debris. Lodgment of emboli [embolism] in smaller arteries of any vital organ such as the heart, lung or brain could be life-threatening and should be treated with fibrinolytics and anticoagulant agents.)

18 | Platelet Count

Learning Objectives

After completing this practical, you will be able to (MUST KNOW):

1. Describe the importance of performing platelet count in practical physiology.
2. List the methods used to perform a platelet count.
3. Perform platelet counting by the Rees–Ecker method and the peripheral blood smear method.
4. List the precautions taken while performing the Rees–Ecker method and the sources of error.
5. State the normal value of platelet count.
6. List the functions of platelets.
7. Name the conditions that alter platelet count.

You may also be able to (DESIRABLE TO KNOW):

1. Explain the role of platelets in hemostasis (temporary hemostatic plug formation and blood coagulation).
2. Name the granules of platelets and list the chemicals present in these granules.
3. Describe the regulation of thrombopoiesis.
4. List the principle and advantages of platelet counting by the Brecher–Cronkite method.
5. Explain the causes of thrombocytopenia and thrombocytosis.

PY2.13: Describe the steps for reticulocyte and platelet count.

INTRODUCTION

Platelets are anuclear cytoplasmic fragments of megakaryocytes. They play an important role in **hemostasis** (the control of bleeding) and the **formation of clots** within the blood vessels.

Development of Platelets

Platelets develop from megakaryocytes, the giant cells in the bone marrow. The development of platelets is known as **thrombopoiesis.** The steps of thrombopoiesis are shown in Fig. 18.1.

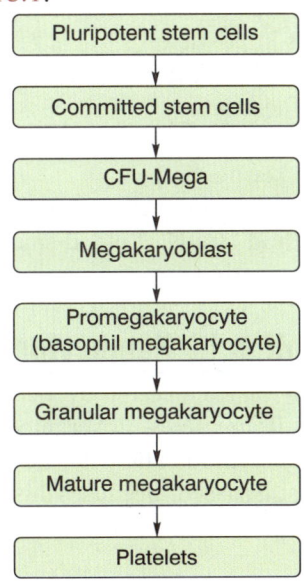

Fig. 18.1 Steps of thrombopoiesis.

Megakaryocytes form platelets by **pinching off bits of cytoplasm** and extruding them into the circulation. The production and release of platelets from the bone marrow normally remain constant. Production is depressed by the transfusion of platelets and enhanced by the removal of platelets from the blood (**thrombocytopheresis**). This indicates that there is a *feedback regulatory mechanism* for platelet production. **Thrombopoietin (TPO)**, a glycoprotein hormone produced by the liver, plays a crucial role in regulating platelet production by stimulating megakaryocyte growth and differentiation. Platelet production is also regulated by **cytokines** such as colony stimulating factors *(GM-CSF), IL1, IL3, and IL6.*

Life History

Platelets normally have a **half-life of about 4 days**. Their survival time in circulation is about 8–12 days. Aged platelets are removed from circulation by the reticuloendothelial system. The *spleen is an important site of sequestration and destruction* of platelets. Therefore, platelet count increases after splenectomy and decreases in hypersplenism.

Normal Count

In adults, the normal platelet count is **1.5–4 lakhs/mm³** of blood.

Structure

Platelets are small, anucleated, granulated, spherical or oval bodies, **2–4 μm in diameter**. They heavily contain *microtubules and microfilaments.* The cytoplasm contains **two types of granules: alpha and dense.**

The **alpha granules** contain PDGF (platelet-derived growth factor), platelet factor 3 (a phospholipid), fibronectin, plasminogen, platelet fibrinogen, proaccelerin (factor 5), thrombospondin, alpha-2 plasmin inhibitor, and hydrolases. The **dense granules** contain serotonin, ADP, and calcium ions.

Functions

Platelets perform **four main functions** in the body: **i)** temporary hemostasis (arrest of bleeding), **ii)** clotting of blood, **iii)** phagocytosis of small particles and organisms, and **iv)** storage and transport of chemicals.

Temporary hemostasis

The most important function of platelets is the **arrest of bleeding**. The quick formation of a hemostatic plug at the site of injury immediately stops bleeding. Since the hemostatic plug is formed by platelets, it is known as the **platelet plug**. The temporary hemostatic plug is formed by **three properties** of platelets: adhesion, aggregation, **and release reaction.**

1. **Platelet adhesion:** Platelets adhere to the exposed collagen of the lining of the damaged blood vessels. The *von Willebrand factor* facilitates platelet adhesion.
2. **Platelet aggregation:** Platelets have the tendency to stick to each other and to the damaged vessel wall. This phenomenon is called **platelet aggregation.** *Fibrinogen, thrombin, and PAF* (platelet activating factors) foster platelet aggregation.
3. **Platelet activation and release reaction**: The binding of platelets to collagen initiates platelet activation. Activation is also produced by *ADP and thrombin*. The activated platelets change their shape, put out pseudopodia, and discharge the contents of their granules. This is known as the *release reaction* of platelets or **platelet release**.

When platelets adhere to the collagen in the damaged vessel wall, ATP in the adhered platelets is converted to ADP. ADP and collagen *activate phospholipase A2*, which causes hydrolysis of membrane phospholipids to form arachidonic acid. Arachidonic acid is then converted to endoperoxides by cyclo-oxygenase. Endoperoxides, when acted upon by thromboxane synthase, form thromboxane A2. **Thromboxane A2** causes vasoconstriction and platelet aggregation and increases calcium influx into the platelets. Increased intracellular calcium brings about *contraction of microfilaments* that cause movement of granules to the canaliculi of the cells. Granules fuse with the canalicular membrane and finally *discharge their contents* to the exterior through the open canaliculi (**platelet release**).

Blood clotting

Platelets participate in the clotting process because **platelet factor 3** (platelet phospholipids) is needed for: i) *formation of Xa* (activation of the Stuart–Prower factor), ii) for the *conversion of prothrombin to thrombin* by factor Xa and Va, and iii) to *promote clot retraction*.

Clot retraction: This is the shrinkage of the clot, which depends on *metabolically active platelets*. It is produced by the contraction of attached platelet pseudopodia in the polymerised fibrin, which contains actin–myosin-like proteins. If the clot does not retract, it may not be stable and may disintegrate.

Phagocytosis

Carbon particles, immune complexes, and viruses undergo phagocytosis by platelets in circulation.

Storage and transport

Platelets take up 5-HT and synthesise, store, and transport serotonin. They also store and transport heparin.

METHODS OF COUNTING PLATELETS

Several **problems are encountered** in the counting of platelets because:

1. They are small and difficult to discern.
2. They have an adhesive character and attach readily to glassware, particles, or debris in the diluting fluid.
3. They clump easily.
4. They are not evenly distributed in the mixture of blood and diluting fluid.
5. They readily disintegrate in blood diluted with fluid, making it difficult to distinguish them from debris.

Therefore, unless carefully done, accurate counting of platelets becomes impossible.

Three types of methods are frequently used for platelet count. These are:

I.   **Direct method** (hemocytometry):
    i.   Rees–Ecker method
    ii. Brecher–Cronkite method
II. **Indirect method** (study of blood smear)
III. **Automated counting**

Platelet Counting by Hemocytometry

Two methods of platelet count by hemocytometry are frequently used: i) the Rees–Ecker method and ii) the Brecher–Cronkite method. The details of the Rees–Ecker method will be discussed because this is the method usually followed in our laboratories.

Rees–Ecker Method for Manual Platelet Counting

■ Principle

Whole blood is diluted with a solution of brilliant cresyl blue, which stains the platelets light blue. The diluent also prevents coagulation. No attempt is made to lyse the red cells. Platelets are then counted by hemocytometry.

■ Requirements

Equipment

1. Microscope
2. Hemocytometer (RBC pipette and **Spencer–Brightline counting chamber**): Instead of the Neubauer hemocytometer, a specially designed **Spencer–Brightline hemocytometer** is used for platelet counts. This uses the *Spencer–Brightline counting chamber*.
    i. The metallic surface of this chamber makes it easier to see the platelets.
    ii. The cell distribution also appears better, since the chamber's surface is smoother.
       If the Spencer–Brightline hemocytometer is not available, the Neubauer hemocytometer may be used.
3. Materials for sterile finger prick
4. Petri dish
5. Filter papers

Reagent

The diluent used for counting platelets must meet certain requirements:

1. Should provide fixation to reduce the adhesiveness of the platelets
2. Should prevent coagulation
3. Should prevent hemolysis
4. Should provide a low specific gravity so that the platelets settle in one plane
    The **Rees–Ecker fluid** meets all these requirements. 1% ammonium oxalate can also be used, but it is not as good as the Rees–Ecker fluid.

Composition of the Rees–Ecker fluid

1. **Sodium citrate**: Prevents coagulation, preserves RBC and provides the necessary low specific gravity
2. **Formalin**: Acts as a fixative
3. **Brilliant cresyl blue**: Identifies the diluent

Note: Brilliant cresyl blue does not stain the platelets, as it is not essential for counting. The dye is used only for the identification of the diluent.

4. Deionised water—Acts as a solvent

Note: The Rees–Ecker fluid must be stored in the refrigerator and **filtered before each use**.

Specimen

Though capillary blood (from a finger puncture) can be used, *venous blood gives more satisfactory results* because the *platelet count in capillary blood is usually less than that in venous blood*. This difference is due to the ***clumping of platelets at the site of the puncture*** when blood is collected by finger prick. The venous blood that is collected should be anticoagulated with EDTA ***because EDTA reduces the tendency of platelet clumping***. If venous blood is used, the test should be performed within 2 hours of collecting blood.

■ Procedure

1. Clean the RBC pipette and Neubauer chamber thoroughly.

Note: All glassware must be **scrupulously cleaned**. This is to prevent adhesion and aggregation of platelets. Anything in the pipette to which the platelets could adhere must be removed. 95 per cent ethanol should be used to clean the hemocytometer. A lint-free cloth should be used to wipe it.

2. Puncture the fingertip and suck blood exactly up to the 0.5 mark of the RBC pipette.
3. **Rapidly dilute** the blood with the Rees–Ecker fluid to the 101 mark of the pipette.
4. **Shake the pipette** immediately after dilution for at least 1 minute.
5. Discard 3–5 drops of the solution from the pipette.
6. Charge the Neubauer chamber.
7. Cover the charged chamber with a petri dish lined with moist filter paper and allow 15 minutes for the platelets to settle in the chamber.

Note: The chamber is covered to prevent evaporation.

8. After 15 minutes, count the platelets under a high-power objective.

Note: The platelets are bluish and must be distinguished from debris. Platelets are oval or round bodies, normally 2–4 μm in diameter and refractile in nature.

9. Count the platelets in all the **25 medium squares of the RBC square**, i.e., in 1 mm² area or 1/10 mm³ volume.
10. Enter the results in the squares drawn on paper.

■ Calculations

The cells are counted in 25 medium squares; each of these squares contains 16 smaller squares. The area covered by the 25 medium squares is 1 mm².

Platelet count / ml or mm^3 of blood

$$= \frac{\text{Number of platelets counted}}{\text{Volume of fluid}} \times \text{dilution}$$

The dilution is 200.

Volume of fluid in 1 mm² = $1 \times 1/10 = 1 \times 0.1$

$$= 0.1 \text{ ml or mm}^3$$

Platelet count/ml or mm³ of blood

= Number of platelets counted $\times 200/0.1$

= Number of platelets counted **(n) × 2000**

Observation and results

1. Draw 25 medium RBC squares in your notebook (as drawn below) and enter the number of cells counted in each (each medium RBC square has 16 small squares). Refer to Fig. 6.12 in Chapter 6 for the orientation of the platform of the Neubauer chamber and the squares.

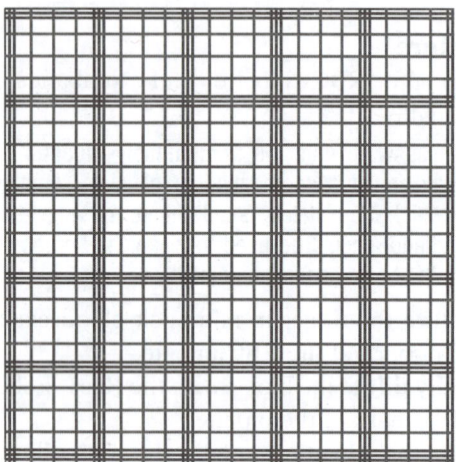

2. Total the number of cells counted; this is **expressed as n**.
3. Calculate the final result using the formula given above (**n × 2000 = __**).
4. Report your results as follows: "The TLC of the given blood sample is __/mm³ of blood."

Precautions and sources of error

1. The glassware must be **scrupulously cleaned**. Debris and dust are the main sources of error as they are easily mistaken for platelets.
2. The **diluting fluid must be filtered** just before use (to remove stained particles from the stain).
3. If venous blood is used, the platelets must be counted within 2 hours. Delay causes disintegration and clumping of platelets.
4. Blood should be **rapidly diluted**. This is essential because the platelets may form clumps.
5. Blood must be **thoroughly mixed with the diluent** by shaking the contents of the pipette for at least one minute. Inadequate mixing results in the clumping of platelets.
6. The charged chamber should be kept for **15 minutes under a petri dish** to prevent evaporation and for the cells to settle down.

7. Other precautions of hemocytometry (as described in Chapter 6) should also be followed.

Important notes

1. It is ideal to make a **duplicate count** to minimise errors. This is done by **charging both sides of the counting chamber simultaneously** and counting both sides separately.
2. A blood smear should be made and stained simultaneously to *check and compare the platelet count* by the blood smear method with the value observed in the direct method.
3. If the **count is low**, *the WBC pipette can be used* for dilution for recounting. The calculation can be made using the correct dilution factor.
4. If other hematologic tests are to be performed along with platelet count, and blood is used from the same puncture, it is necessary to *first draw blood for platelet count* and then proceed with drawing blood for other tests.
5. The finger should not be squeezed excessively to collect blood.
6. Despite all precautions, the error of platelet count in this method is 15–30 per cent.

Brecher–Cronkite method

Principle

The *other method* used is Brecher–Cronkite Method, which uses **phase-contrast microscopy**. **Ammonium oxalate** is one of the constituents of the diluent, which completely lyses the red cells. Platelets are then counted with a **phase-hemocytometer** and phase-contrast microscope to *enhance the refractility* of the platelets.

Advantages

1. Identification of platelets is easier.
2. The error involved is low (5–10 per cent).

Platelet Count by Study of Blood Smear

Principle

The principle is the same as that of making a blood smear.

Procedure

1. Place a **drop of 14% magnesium sulphate solution** on the tip of a finger and prick through this drop of solution.

Note: Magnesium sulphate prevents clumping of blood.

2. Make a blood smear and stain with Leishman stain.
3. Count platelets per 1000 red cells.

Normal count

The normal ratio of platelets to RBCs is 1:20.

Note: The total red cell count can be performed separately. If the red cell count is 5,000,000/mm³, and platelet count in the indirect method is 1:20, the indirect absolute count of platelets will be 250,000/mm³ of blood.

Platelet Count by Automated Method

Automated platelet counting is done with an **S Plus Coulter** counter, in which platelets and red cells pass through apertures. Particles that measure between 2 and 10 fL are counted as platelets. A platelet graph is also plotted according to the size distribution of the platelets counted.

DISCUSSION

Platelets participate in temporary hemostatic plug formation and coagulation of blood and are, therefore, associated with the hemostatic mechanisms of the body.

Clinical Significance

Platelet count is usually ordered as a part of the laboratory diagnosis of a bleeding disorder. When the platelet count increases in blood, the condition is known as **thrombocytosis**; when the count decreases, the condition is called **thrombocytopenia.**

Grades of thrombocytopenia

1. **Normal count**: 1.5 to 4 lakhs/mm³ of blood
2. **Low platelet count**: Count <1.5 lakhs/mm³ of blood (*prolonged bleeding time* is the hallmark of thrombocytopenia)
3. **Critical count**: Count <50,000 per mm³ of blood— this is called *critical count*, as the *risk of bleeding increases* manifold below this level
4. **Very low count**: Count <20,000/mm³ can lead to *spontaneous hemorrhage*

The **hemorrhagic tendency** is proportional to the degree of thrombocytopenia and is characterised by petechiae, ecchymoses, menorrhagia, and bleeding from mucous membranes into the central nervous system. To differentiate the causes of thrombocytopenia, *bone marrow examination* should be carefully done. If *megakaryocytes are absent* in the bone marrow, this implies *failure of platelet production*.

Conditions That Alter Thrombocyte Count

Thrombocytosis

1. Polycythemia vera
2. Chronic myeloid leukemia
3. Iron deficiency anemia
4. Splenectomy
5. Inflammatory disorders: Rheumatoid arthritis, inflammatory bowel disease
6. Following major surgery
7. Acute or chronic hemorrhage
8. Essential thrombocytosis

Thrombocytopenia

I. **Increased platelet destruction**
1. *Immune-mediated*
   i. Primary: Idiopathic thrombocytopenic purpura
   ii. Secondary:
      a. Autoimmune: SLE
      b. Allo-immune: Post-transfusion
      c. Drug-induced:
         • Quinidine
         • Sulfa compounds
         • Heparin
      d. Infection: HIV, cytomegalovirus
2. *Non-immune-mediated*
   i. DIC
   ii. Hemolytic-uremic syndrome
   iii. Thrombotic thrombocytopenic purpura
II. **Decreased production**
1. *Diseases of bone marrow*
   i. Aplastic anemia
   ii. Marrow infiltration
      a. Leukemia
      b. Disseminated cancer
   iii. Drug-induced
      a. Thiazides
      b. Cytotoxic drugs
      c. Alcohol
   iv. Infections: Measles, HIV
2. *Ineffective megakaryopoiesis*
   i. Megalobastic anemia
   ii. Myelodysplastic syndrome
III. **Sequestration of platelets**
1. *Hypersplenism*
   i. Portal hypertension
   ii. Lymphomas
   iii. Myeloproliferative disorders
2. *Hemodilutional*

VIVA

1. *Why does the platelet count produce inaccurate results unless performed very carefully?* (Ans. Refer to page 114, under the heading 'Methods of Counting'.)

2. *What are the different methods of platelet counting?* (Ans. Refer to page 114, under the heading 'Methods of Counting'.)

3. *What is the principle of the Rees–Ecker method?* (Ans. Refer to page 115, under the heading 'Rees-Ecker Method', read 'Principle'.)

4. *What are the advantages of using the Spencer–Brightline counting chamber for platelet counting?* (Ans. Refer to page 115, under the heading 'Rees-Ecker Method', read 'Requirements', 'Equipment'.)

5. *Why is the Rees–Ecker fluid an ideal diluent for platelet count?* (Ans. Refer to page 115, under the heading 'Requirements', read 'Reagent'.)

6. *What is the composition of the Rees–Ecker fluid? What are the functions of each constituent?* (Ans. Refer to page 115, under the heading 'Requirements', read 'Rees-Ecker fluid' under 'Reagent'.)

7. *Why is the Rees–Ecker fluid filtered before every use?* (Ans. Refer to page 116, under the heading 'Precautions', point no. 2.)

8. *Why is venous blood preferred over capillary blood for platelet count?* (Ans. Refer to page 115, under the heading 'Requirements', and subheading 'Specimen'.)

9. *Why is venous blood anticoagulated with EDTA?* (Ans. Refer to page 115, under the heading 'Requirements', read .....III. Specimen).

10. *Why is glassware cleaned thoroughly for platelet count?* (Ans. Refer to page 116, under the heading 'Precautions', point no. 1.)

11. *Why is diluting fluid filtered before use?* (Ans. Refer to page 116, under the heading 'Precautions', point no. 2.)

12. *Why is blood rapidly diluted and thoroughly mixed with the diluting fluid?* (Ans. Refer to page 116, under the heading 'Precautions', point no. 5.)

13. *Why is the charged chamber covered with a petri dish for 15 minutes?* (Ans. Refer to page 116, under the heading 'Precautions', point no. 6.)

14. *How do you identify platelets under the high-power objective?* (Ans. Refer to page 115, under the heading 'Procedure', point no. 8.)

15. *What are the sources of error in the manual method of platelet count?* (Ans. Refer to page 116, under the heading 'Precautions and sources of error'.)

16. *What is the other manual method of platelet counting using the principle of hemocytometry? What are its advantages?* (Ans. Refer to page 116, under the heading 'Brecher–Cronkite method'.)

17. *How is the indirect count of platelets performed?* (Ans. Refer to page 116, under the heading 'Platelet count by study of blood smear'.)

18. *Why is it ideal to perform a duplicate count for platelet counting?* (Ans. Refer to page 116, under the heading 'Important notes', point no. 1.)

19. *What are the special precautions/safeguards to be noted for platelet count?* (Ans. Refer to page 116, under the heading 'Important notes'.)

20. *What are the precursor cells for platelets?* (Ans. Refer to page 113, under the heading 'Development' and Fig. 18.1.)

21. *What are the factors that regulate the development of platelets?* (Ans. Refer to page 113, under the heading 'Development', read 'Thrombopoietin and cytokines'.)

22. *What is the lifespan of platelets and how are they removed from circulation?* (Ans. Refer to page 113, under the heading 'Lifes History'.)

23. *What is the normal platelet count?*
    (Ans. 1.5 to 4 lakhs/mm³ of blood in adults.)

24. *What are the properties of platelets? What are its functions?* (Ans. Refer to page 114, under the heading 'Temporary hemostasis'.)

25. *What are the causes of thrombocytosis and thrombocytopenia.* (Ans. Refer to page 117, under the heading 'Thrombocytosis and thrombocytopenia'.)

In addition to the questions given above, all the questions at the end of Chapter 17, especially the questions related to bleeding time, will apply to this chapter as well.

19 | Reticulocyte Count

Learning Objectives

After completing this practical, you will be able to (MUST KNOW):

1. Describe the importance of performing reticulocyte count in practical physiology.
2. State the normal value of reticulocyte counts in newborns and adults.
3. Identify reticulocytes in the smear prepared using supravital staining.
4. Perform reticulocyte counting by the manual method.
5. List the precautions and sources of error while performing the reticulocyte count.
6. Explain the meaning of supravital staining and name the supravital stains.
7. List the common causes of reticulocytosis and reticulocytopenia.

You may also be able to (DESIRABLE TO KNOW):

1. Explain the structure, function, and fate of reticulocytes.
2. Explain reticulocyte response.
3. Explain the physiological and clinical significance of reticulocyte counting.
4. Explain the physiological basis of reticulocytosis in different conditions.
5. Describe the method of performing the absolute reticulocyte count.
6. State the principle and advantages of reticulocyte count by the automated method.
7. Explain the phenomenon of punctate basophilia.

PY2.13: Describe the steps for reticulocyte and platelet count.

INTRODUCTION

Reticulocytes are juvenile red cells that pass into the bloodstream from the bone marrow. During the process of development, the nuclei are lost, but not the cytoplasmic RNA. Therefore, reticulocytes do not possess nuclei, but contain a **network of reticulum** in the cytoplasm, which represents the **remnants of the basophilic cytoplasm** (*remnants of RNA and ribosomes*) of the precursor cells.

1. On **vital staining** with cresyl blue, the reticular network appears in the form of a heavy wreath, or clumps of small dots, or a faint thread connecting two small nodes (Fig. 19.1).
2. The ribosomal and cytoplasmic remnants of reticulocytes pick up a **supravital stain** when the stain is allowed to penetrate the cells while in the living condition.
3. Supravital stains may also reveal **basophilic stippling**.
   - In pathological conditions, the stained basophilic materials present in the form of **clumps in the cytoplasm appear** as *discrete blue particles* (**punctate basophilia**).
   - Basophilic stippling represents the **precipitation of RNA in the cytoplasm**. Such stippling is seen **in red cells in toxic conditions** such as heavy metal poisoning, especially lead poisoning.

Reticulocyte Production

Reticulocytes are developed (produced) in the bone marrow **from late (orthochromatic) normoblasts**. The nucleus is extruded from the late normoblast to form reticulocytes. These reticulocytes lose their mitochondria, ribosomes, and basophilic tint to form mature erythrocytes. With the release of young red cells into circulation, a few reticulocytes are also released. When the bone marrow sends out red cells at an increased rate, more reticulocytes are released. Thus, the **number of reticulocytes in peripheral blood** is an index of erythropoiesis (production of red cells). As reticulocytes are the immediate precursors of red cells, whenever the demand for red cells in circulation increases, reticulocyte formation and release are also accentuated.

Lifespan

Reticulocytes **stay in circulation for about 24 hours** before they mature into erythrocytes. Most reticulocytes are present in the bone marrow, where they actually mature into red cells.

Normal Counts

1. **In adults**, the count is **0.5–2%** of the red cells (average 1%).
2. **In newborns**, the count is **2–6%**. The number falls during the first week to less than 1 per cent and then, the level is maintained throughout life.

Absolute reticulocyte count: Direct count by hemocytometry is not possible. The indirect absolute count is **25,000–75,000 cells/mm³** of blood.

METHODS OF COUNTING RETICULOCYTES

Reticulocyte counting can be done by **manual methods** and **automated methods**.

Manual Methods of Reticulocyte Counting

The **manual method** includes the following:

1. A *relative count* is taken against the number of red cells and then expressed as a percentage of red cells.
2. An *absolute count* is taken against the relative count and the total RBC count.

Relative count

▮ Principle

The RNA content of reticulocytes can be detected by exposing the living cells to a supravital stain. In **supravital staining**, *living blood cells are mixed with the stain* as opposed to the differential leucocyte count, where the smear is made before staining. *In one method*, the stain is sprayed on the slide, and blood is added to the stain. *In the other method*, the stain is mixed with a drop of blood and covered with a coverslip. The mixture is sealed on the slide and viewed in liquid form under the microscope.

▮ Requirements

1. Supravital stains
2. Glass slides
3. Watch glass
4. Filter paper
5. Microscope
6. Equipment for sterile finger puncture

Supravital stains

These are dyes that are used for **staining living cells in vitro** (outside the body). Usually in practice, living cells are stained (for diagnostic purposes) outside the body. *Vital stains* (also called, *intravital stain*) are used for staining living cells *in vivo* (rarely used nowadays). Therefore, *supravital stains* (not vital stains) are commonly used for staining *in vitro*, outside the body.

Brilliant cresyl blue stain

1. *Brilliant cresyl blue*: Stains the RNA of reticulocytes
2. *Sodium citrate*: Prevents coagulation
3. *Sodium chloride*: Provides isotonicity

   Brilliant cresyl blue is prepared as a *1% solution in isotonic saline* or methyl alcohol.

New methylene blue stain

1. *New methylene blue*: Stains the RNA of reticulocytes
2. *Sodium oxalate*: Prevents coagulation
3. *Sodium chloride*: Provides isotonicity

   New methylene blue is prepared as a *1% solution in isotonic saline* and then diluted to 100 ml with *3.8% sodium citrate*. New methylene blue is chemically different from methylene blue, which is a poor reticulocyte stain. It is preferred over brilliant cresyl blue as it *deeply stains the filamentous net-like structures* (reticulum) present in the cytoplasm of reticulocytes so that they are easily identified.

▮ Procedure

1. Clean the glass slides thoroughly.
2. Take *a drop of stain* on a clean slide.
3. Make a sterile finger prick to get a drop of blood.
4. Add the *drop of blood* to the stain.
5. *Mix the blood gently* with the help of the blunt edge of a slide without touching the specimen slide.
6. Cover the slide with a watch glass lined with *moist filter paper for 15 minutes* to prevent evaporation.
7. Select a spreader.
8. After 15 minutes, place the edge of the spreader on the mixture, transfer the portion of the mixture sticking to the spreader to another slide, and *immediately make a thin smear*.
9. Make a minimum of 2–3 such smears.
10. Allow the smear to dry.
11. First, examine the smear *under a low-power objective* and locate a thin portion of the smear where the red cells are evenly distributed.
12. Carefully change to the *oil-immersion objective*. Focus sharply and try to locate an area in which there are approximately 100–150 red cells visible in the oil-immersion field.
13. *Identify reticulocytes* and red cells.

Note: Reticulocytes are identified by the fine, deep violet filaments and granules arranged in a network. Red cells stain pale blue and are slightly smaller in size than reticulocytes (Fig. 19.1).

14. Enumerate the *reticulocytes and red cells* in each field. **Count a minimum of 1000 cells** (minimum of 10 fields).

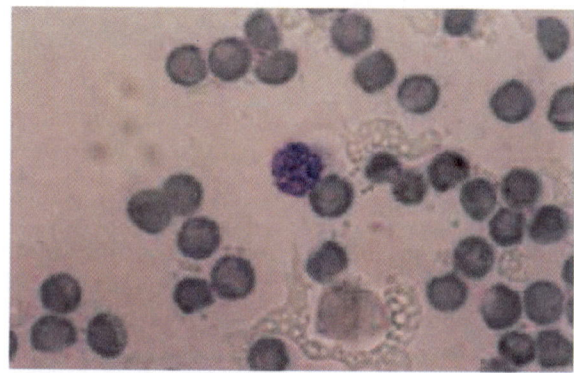

Fig. 19.1 Reticulocyte (supravital staining). Note the single reticulocyte in the field and appreciate the reticulin network in that cell.

Note. Counting is easier if the size of the microscopic field is reduced. This can be done by placing, in the eyepiece of the microscope, a small circular piece of black paper in which a hole of 5 mm diameter has been made with a puncher.

15. Enter your observations in a tabular form, as shown in Table 19.1.

Table 19.1 Observations of the reticulocyte count.

Field no.	Number of reticu-locytes (1)	Number of RBCs (2)	Total number of cells (1+2)
1			
2			
3			
4			
…			
…			
15			

■ Calculation

$$RC = \frac{\text{Number of reticulocytes counted} \times 100}{\text{Total number of cells counted}}$$

Where RC is the reticulocyte count (per cent).

For example, let us assume the total number of cells counted (reticulocytes + RBCs) to be = 1500. Number of reticulocytes seen (in 15 fields) = 15.

$$\text{Reticulocyte count (\%)} = \frac{15 \times 100}{1500} = 1 \text{ per cent}$$

■ Observation and results

1. Count 15 fields and enter the number of platelets and RBCs in their respective boxes for each field as shown in Table 19.1.
2. Total the number of cells counted to the number of reticulocytes seen.
3. Using the formula for the calculation described above, find out the reticulocyte count in %.
4. Report the result as follows: "The reticulocyte count of the given sample of blood (or of the person) is __%."

■ Precautions and sources of error

1. A **fresh specimen** should be used.
2. The **staining time** should not be less than 10 minutes.
3. **Mixing** of blood with the stain should be done *gently but thoroughly* before making the smear. This is important because reticulocytes have a lower specific gravity than mature red cells, and therefore, settle on top of the red cells in the mixture. Thus, an unmixed or poorly mixed blood specimen will not give the correct result.
4. Reticulocytes should be *properly identified*. Red cells showing highly refractile areas may be confused with reticulocytes. These artefacts in the red cells possibly occur due to moisture in the air and poor drying of the smear.
5. Careful focusing of the microscope is essential in the reticulocyte count. Stained platelet granules and leucocyte granules must not be mistaken for reticulocytes. Precipitated stains might also be mistaken for reticulum within the erythrocytes. To minimise this possibility, the *dye must be filtered immediately before use*. *Immediate drying* of the smear also prevents the formation of crystalline bodies that sometimes appear in the red cells.

6. Supravital stains also stain other **red cell inclusions** in addition to staining the RNA in the reticulocytes.. These include Howell–Jolly bodies, Heinz bodies, and Pappenheimer bodies. These bodies are present in different pathological conditions. While performing a reticulocyte count, if these bodies are present, they should be counted separately.

7. *Equal volumes of staining fluid and blood specimen* should be used. In case of low hematocrit value (anemia), a large proportion of blood should be used. When the hematocrit is high (polycythemia), a smaller volume of blood should be used. This variation in dilution helps in the spreading out of 100–150 red cells per microscopic field, making it easier to count cells. Therefore, the **hematocrit or hemoglobin content** of the blood should be determined *before performing the reticulocyte count*. At least the lower palpebral conjunctiva should be examined to clinically assess the hemoglobin status of the subject.

Absolute count

A direct absolute count of reticulocytes by hemocytometry is not possible. Instead, an **indirect absolute count** is taken against the number of red cells and expressed as *a percentage of red cells*. This relative value can be converted to an absolute value by performing the **total RBC count** of the same sample of blood.

Absolute count of reticulocytes / ml of blood

$$= \frac{RC\,(\%) \times RBC \text{ count / ml of blood}}{100}$$

Where RC is reticulocyte count (per cent).

Normal value: The normal value is **25,000–75,000/mm³** of blood.

Automated Method of Reticulocyte Counting

With the use of automated techniques, the process of counting reticulocytes has become easier. It is done by the **principle of flow cytometry**.

Principle

Cells are stained with a **fluorochrome dye** that preferentially stains RNA. The cells are counted using the **fluorescence technique**. The RNA-containing reticulocytes fluoresce when exposed to ultraviolet light, and the instrument used can count thousands of reticulocytes in just a few seconds.

Advantages
1. The process of counting is made easy.
2. It takes very little time.
3. It is an accurate method of counting reticulocytes.

DISCUSSION

Physiological Significance

The number of reticulocytes in circulation indicates the magnitude of bone marrow activity. When the marrow is very active, the reticulocyte count increases; when the marrow is suppressed, the reticulocyte count decreases. Therefore, the number of reticulocytes in the peripheral blood is a good *index of bone marrow activity,* especially erythropoiesis. Reticulocyte count is *proportionate to the red cell production.*

Clinical Significance

Reticulocyte response

The reticulocyte count is performed as a follow-up for *therapeutic response for anemias* in which the patient is deficient in one of the substances essential for the synthesis of red cells. When therapy begins, new red cells are formed and released rapidly into the circulation before the cells are fully matured. *Many reticulocytes are released* with the release of young red cells. The corresponding increase in reticulocyte count is called reticulocyte response. Reticulocyte response indicates a *favourable response to treatment.* This is typically observed in the **treatment of pernicious anemia and iron deficiency anemia.**

1. When *vitamin B12 is administered as part of the treatment of pernicious anemia,* the number of reticulocytes increases in the blood in the initial phase of the treatment. This indicates that the patient is responding well to the treatment.
2. Similarly, the reticulocyte count increases in the blood when iron is given in the treatment of *iron deficiency anemia.*

Thus, the reticulocyte count is performed to assess the response of the patient to the treatment in pernicious and iron deficiency anemia.

Detection of types of anemia

The **reticulocyte count** may provide useful information about the type of anemia. It is typically *elevated in conditions* in which the erythroid precursors can increase the production of red cells in response to an increase in the demand for them. This is commonly seen in **hemolytic anemia** in which erythropoietic activity remains unimpaired. It is also seen in **blood-loss anemia.**

Conditions That Alter Reticulocyte Count

An increase in reticulocyte count is known as **reticulocytosis**, and a decrease in reticulocyte count is known as **reticulocytopenia**.

Reticulocytosis
Physiological
1. Newborns and infants
2. High altitude
3. Pregnancy (may be high)

Pathological
1. **Hemolytic anemia**
2. **Acute hemorrhage**
3. During **treatment of deficiency anemias** (reticulocyte response)
4. Any condition that **stimulates the bone marrow** to produce red cells
5. *After splenectomy* (reticulocytes tend to increase initially, reflecting the body's increased demand for RBCs as the spleen is no longer removing aged or damaged red cells)
6. *Erythroblastosis fetalis* (as the bone marrow attempts to compensate for the destruction of red cells)
7. **Drugs:** Erythropoietin (used for treatment of anemia), anabolic steroids and performance-enhancing drugs, certain antibiotics like cephalosporins, levofloxacin, phenazopyridine (pyridium), phenytoin, and carbamazepine, and drugs that cause hemolytic anemia (cephalosporin, levodopa, nitrofurantoin, quinidine, methyldopa, etc.)

Reticulocytopenia
1. **Bone marrow failure** (aplastic anemia, pure red cell aplasia, bone marrow infiltration)
2. **Anemia** (autoimmune hemolytic anemia and untreated iron deficiency anemia can cause reticulocytopenia)
3. **Myxedema** (hypothyroidism can cause anemia and reticulocytopenia)
4. **Hypopituitarism**
5. *Transient erythroblastopenia of childhood* (TEC)
6. *Diamond–Blackfan anemia* (congenital red cell aplasia characterised by macrocytic anemia and reticulocytopenia)
7. **Leuko–erythroblastic anemia:** The leuko-erythroblastic blood picture is used to describe the presence of myeloid and erythroid precursors in the peripheral blood often associated with anemia as a consequence of a disturbance of bone marrow architecture by abnormal tissues (infiltration). It is seen in secondary carcinoma of the bone (metastatic cancer), primary myelofibrosis, multiple myeloma, etc.

8. Exposure to **toxic chemicals** (exposure to substances like benzene or pesticides can suppress the bone marrow and cause reticulocytopenia)
9. **Transcobalamin II deficiency** (a condition that can lead to failure to thrive, megaloblastic anemia, pancytopenia, and reticulocytopenia)
10. **Chronic kidney disease** (reduced erythropoietin production from the kidney can cause anemia and reticulocytopenia)

11. **Medications:** Antibiotics (penicillin and its derivatives, chloramphenicol, sulfas), anticonvulsants (diphenyl-hydantoin, and phenobarbital), immunosuppressants (azathioprine, cyclophosphamide, and fludarabine), and others (isoniazid, ribavirin, allopurinol, penicilla-mine, diclofenac, dapsone, sulfathiazole, tolbutamide, captopril, rituximab, phenothiazine, hydralazine, es-trogen, cytotoxic cancer drugs, NSAIDs, etc.)

Physiological: There is no physiological reticulocytopenia.

VIVA

1. *What is the normal reticulocyte count in adults and in newborns? At what age does it reach the adult value?* (Ans. Refer to page 119, under the heading 'Normal Count'.)
2. *What are the indications for reticulocyte count?*
   (Ans. i. Reticulocyte count is performed primarily to assess the degree of effective erythropoiesis and the functionality of the bone marrow in various clinical conditions in which bone marrow activity is compromised. ii. Reticulocyte count is also performed to assess an individual's response to treatment in deficiency anemias like pernicious anemia and iron deficiency anemia [reticulocyte response]. iii. In hemolytic anemias, it is performed to determine the severity of the condition and the marrow status.)
3. *What are the methods of reticulocyte counting?* (Ans. Refer to page 118-119, under the heading 'Methods of Counting'.)
4. *Define 'supravital stain' with examples. How does it differ from a vital stain?* (Ans. Refer to page 120, under the heading 'Supravital Stains'.)
5. *What is the composition and function of each constituent of brilliant cresyl blue stain?* (Ans. Refer to page 120, under the heading 'Supravital Stains', read 'Brilliant cresyl blue'.)
6. *What are the sources of error in the manual method of reticulocyte counting?* (Ans. Refer to page 121, under the heading 'Precautions and sources of error'.)
7. *What happens when blood is not properly mixed with the stain?* (Ans. Refer to page 121, under the heading 'Precautions', point no. 2.)
8. *How do you identify reticulocytes in the smear?* (Ans. Refer to page 121, text under the heading 'Precautions', point no. 3.)
9. *Why should equal volumes of staining fluid and blood be used for the reticulocyte count?* (Ans. Refer to page 121, under the heading 'Precautions', point no. 6.)
10. *How do you perform absolute reticulocyte count?* (Ans. Refer to page 121, under the heading 'Manual method [absolute count]'.)
11. *What is the principle of the automated method of reticulocyte counting and the advantages of this method?* (Ans. Refer to page 121, under the heading 'Automated Method'.)
12. *What is the lifespan and fate of reticulocytes?* (Ans. Refer to page 120, under the heading 'Lifespan'.)
13. *How do reticulocytes develop in the bone marrow?* (Ans. Refer to page 120, under the heading 'Lifespan'.)
14. *What is the physiological significance of the reticulocyte count?* (Ans. Refer to page 122, under the heading 'Reticulocyte Production'.)
15. *What is the clinical significance of the reticulocyte count?* (Ans. Refer to page 122, under the heading 'Lifespan'.)
16. *What is reticulocyte response? What is its significance?* (Ans. Refer to page 122, under the heading 'Clinical Significance'.)
17. *What are the physiological causes of reticulocytosis?* (Ans. Refer to page 122, under the heading 'Reticulocytosis – Physiological'.)
18. *What is the cause of reticulocytosis at high altitudes?*
    (Ans. At high altitudes, hypoxia stimulates the bone marrow for the production of a greater number of red cells, which results in physiological polycythemia. Increased bone marrow erythropoietic activity results in reticulocytosis.)
19. *What are the pathological conditions of reticulocytosis?* (Ans. Refer to page 122, under the heading 'Reticulocytosis – Pathological'.)
20. *What are the conditions of reticulocytopenia?* (Ans. Refer to pages 122-123, under the heading 'Reticulocytopenia'.)
21. *What is punctate basophilia? In what conditions is it seen?* (Ans. Refer to page 119, under the heading 'Introduction'.)

20 | Determination of Specific Gravity of Blood

Learning Objectives

After completing this practical, you will be able to (MUST KNOW):

1. List the methods of determining the specific gravity of blood.
2. State the principle of determination of specific gravity of blood by Philips and Vanslyke's copper sulphate method.
3. List the factors that affect the specific gravity of blood.
4. List the conditions in which the specific gravity of blood is altered.

INTRODUCTION

The specific gravity of blood is the *ratio of the weight of blood to the weight of an equal volume of water at 4°C*. It depends on the **hematocrit, plasma proteins, and water content** of blood. The specific gravity of blood gives an idea of the *solute and water content of blood*.

1. Under normal conditions, specific gravity is a **good index of the hemoglobin content of blood**.
2. It has proved to be useful in *screening blood donors* and in *emergency cases of burns* that need repeated transfusion.
3. This method was extensively used during World War II in *assessing battle casualties requiring blood transfusion*.

METHODS OF DETERMINING THE SPECIFIC GRAVITY OF BLOOD

Specific gravity of blood can be determined by **direct** and **indirect methods**.

Direct Method

Equal volumes of blood and water are taken in two capillary tubes called **pyconometers** and the liquids are weighed. The **ratio of the weights of the liquids** gives the specific gravity of blood.

Indirect Method

There are two indirect methods of determining the specific gravity of blood: Hammar Schlag's method, and Philips–Vanslyke's copper sulphate method.

Hammar Schlag's method

In this method, the specific gravity of blood is determined by **equalizing the density of two miscible liquids** like chloroform (specific gravity 1.470) and benzene (specific gravity 0.880) to that of blood.

Philips–Vanslyke's copper sulphate method

Principle

Two miscible liquids of known but different specific gravities are *mixed in varying proportions* to give a *number of solutions* covering the expected range of specific gravity. A drop of blood is then allowed to fall in each of the solutions and the behaviour is studied. The specific gravity of blood is **compared with solutions of copper sulphate** of known specific gravities.

Requirements

1. Stock solution of copper sulphate of specific gravity 1.100
2. Distilled water
3. Test tubes
4. Dropper

Procedure

1. Prepare **copper sulphate solution** (10 ml) of specific gravities ranging from **1.050 to 1.068** by mixing distilled water with a stock solution of copper sulphate in different test tubes as presented in Table 20.1.
2. Mix the solution in each tube properly.
3. Pour a drop of blood into each tube from a height of about 1 cm above the solution with the help of a pipette.
4. Observe the behaviour of the blood drop in the solution of each tube (Fig. 20.1).

Table 20.1 Copper sulphate solutions in a range of specific gravities.

Test tube	1	2	3	4	5	6	7	8	9	10
Copper sulphate solution (ml)	4.9	5.1	5.3	5.5	5.7	5.9	6.1	6.3	6.5	6.7
Distilled water (ml)	5.1	4.9	4.7	4.5	4.3	4.1	3.9	3.7	3.5	3.3
Specific gravity of solution	1.050	1.052	1.054	1.056	1.058	1.060	1.062	1.064	1.066	1.068

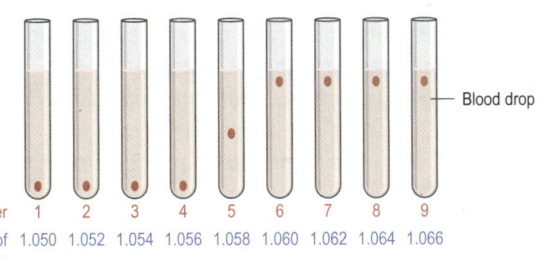

Test tube Number   1   2   3   4   5   6   7   8   9
Specific gravity of 1.050 1.052 1.054 1.056 1.058 1.060 1.062 1.064 1.066
CuSO₄ solution

Fig. 20.1 Position of blood drop in tubes containing copper sulphate solutions of varying specific gravities, which are mentioned below the number of each tube. Note that in tube no. 5 (specific gravity 1.058), the blood drop is suspended in the middle of the solution, which indicates the specific gravity of that sample of blood.

Note: The blood drop will travel for some distance because of momentum and then either sink (if it is heavier than the solution) or float on the surface or the solution (if it is lighter).

5. Note the tubes (specific gravity of the solution) in which the **blood drop remains suspended at the center** of the solution for 15–20 seconds. This gives the specific gravity of the blood sample.

Note: The blood drop floats in copper sulphate solution due to the covering of the copper proteinate layer, which is stable for about 15–20 seconds.

Observation and results
1. Note the number of the tube in which the blood drop remained suspended for about 15 seconds.
2. Record the specific gravity of copper sulphate solution in that tube. This is reported as the specific gravity of the blood sample.
3. Report as follows: "The specific gravity of the supplied blood sample is ___."

Normal values
The normal range of specific gravity of blood varies from **1.048–1.066.**
1. Average value in males: 1.057
2. Average value in females: 1.053

Precautions
1. While preparing the solution, the ratio of water in copper sulphate must be measured accurately.
2. The blood should be dropped into the copper sulphate solution from a height of about 1 cm from the upper level of the solution.
3. The reading should be taken within 10–15 seconds.

DISCUSSION
Physiological Significance
The specific gravity of blood may be altered by an **alteration in the solute content, water content, or cell content** of the blood.
1. Any condition that **leads to hemoconcentration**, like diarrhea, vomiting, and excessive sweating, **increases the specific gravity** of blood.
2. Any condition that **causes hemodilution**, like excessive saline infusion, pregnancy and so on, **decreases the specific gravity**.

Specific gravity indicates the solid and water content of blood.

Factors that affect the specific gravity of blood
1. The number of RBCs in the blood
2. Hemoglobin content of the blood
3. Plasma protein concentration
4. Water content of the blood

Clinical Significance
Conditions that affect the specific gravity of blood
Conditions that increase specific gravity
Physiological
1. High altitude
2. Newborns and infants
3. Excess sweating

Pathological
1. Diarrhea
2. Vomiting
3. Dehydration
4. Polycythemia

Conditions that decrease specific gravity
Physiological
1. Pregnancy
2. Excess water intake

Pathological
1. Different conditions in which there is overhydration (increased water content of blood), for example, nephritic syndrome

VIVA

1. *Define specific gravity of blood.* (Ans. Refer to page 124, under the heading 'Introduction'.)
2. *What is the importance of the determination of specific gravity of blood?* (Ans. Refer to page 124, under the heading 'Introduction'.)
3. *What are the methods of determining the specific gravity of blood?* (Ans. Refer to page 124, under the heading 'Methods'.)
4. *What is the principle of Philips–Vanslyke's copper sulphate method?* (Ans. Refer to page 124, under the heading 'Principle'.)
5. *Why is copper sulphate preferred over other mixtures?*
    (Ans. Copper sulphate is cheap and not hygroscopic. Moreover, its temperature coefficient of expansion is about the same as that of blood. Hence, no correction factor for temperature is required if copper sulphate is used.)
6. *What are the precautions to be taken while performing the Philips–Vanslyke's copper sulphate method?* (Ans. Refer to page 125, under the heading 'Precautions'.)
7. *What is the clinical significance of estimation of specific gravity of blood?* (Ans. Refer to page 125, under the heading 'Clinical Significance'.)
8. *What is the clinical significance of determining the specific gravity of serum, plasma, and blood?*
    (Ans. The specific gravity test is a quick and apparently good method for the estimation of **serum and plasma protein concentration, blood Hb concentration,** and **hematocrit.** It is primarily used as a preliminary test in the screening of blood donors, mass surveys for anemia, and in handling emergency cases of burns requiring repeated transfusions of plasma, plasma expanders, or blood. The method was extensively used during World War II for assessing battle casualties requiring blood transfusions.)
9. *What are the factors that affect specific gravity of blood?* (Ans. Refer to page 125, under the heading 'Factors that affect specific gravity'.)
10. *Is the specific gravity test used in blood banks?*
    (Ans. Yes, the specific gravity test is used in blood banks for selecting potential donors. A working solution [specific gravity = 1.053] is prepared by adding 48 ml of distilled water to 52 ml of stock solution of copper sulphate, as described in the section on methodology. A drop of blood is allowed to fall into the solution from a height of 1 cm. **i.** If the drop sinks, the **Hb in that sample is > 12.5 g%,** and the potential donor is considered for blood donation. **ii.** If the drop floats for more than 15 seconds, the Hb level is **less than 12.5 g%** and the donor is not preferred for blood donation.)
11. *List the conditions in which the specific gravity of blood is altered.* (Ans. Refer to page 125, under the heading 'Conditions that affect specific gravity'.)

21 | Stethography

Learning Objectives

After completing this practical, you will be able to (MUST KNOW):
1. Define stethography.
2. Tie the stethograph at the proper position around the subject's chest.
3. Record respiratory movements (normal and following different maneuvers).
4. List the precautions taken during stethographic recordings.
5. Define breaking point.

6. List the factors that affect the breaking point.
7. Define and give examples of periodic breathing.

You may also be able to (DESIRABLE TO KNOW):
1. Explain the effects of exercise and hyperventilation on respiration.
2. Explain the differences in breath-holding time following inspiration and expiration.

INTRODUCTION

Stethography is the method of recording **respiratory movements** using a stethograph. It is useful in assessing the **breath-holding time** (BHT) following inspiration and expiration and in response to different stimuli. Physiologically, BHT is a *determinant of the respiratory capacity* of the individual. This can be used as a tool to assess respiratory fitness.

METHOD OF USING A STETHOGRAPH

Principle

The stethograph is tied around the subject's chest. Movements of the chest cause changes in the air pressure in the stethograph, which are recorded on a moving drum.

Requirements

1. **Stethograph** (Fig. 21.1A and B): This instrument consists of a **corrugated rubber tube** with a stopper at each end and an **air outlet pipe** connected to the tambour.
2. **Marey's tambour**: It is a **metallic cup with a side tube** and a **rubber diaphragm** mounted at the top (Fig. 21.2A and B). A **writing lever** is attached to a small metal disc, which rests on the rubber diaphragm. The side tube of the metal cup is connected to the stethograph by a rubber tube.
3. Kymograph
4. A glass of drinking water

Procedure

1. Ask the subject to sit comfortably on a stool with his back towards the recording apparatus.
2. Tie the stethograph around the **mid-chest level** of the subject—preferably at the **level of the fourth intercostal space** (roughly corresponds to the level of the nipples) and connect it to the tambour (Fig. 21.3).

A)
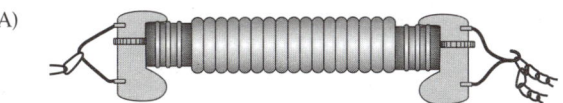

B)
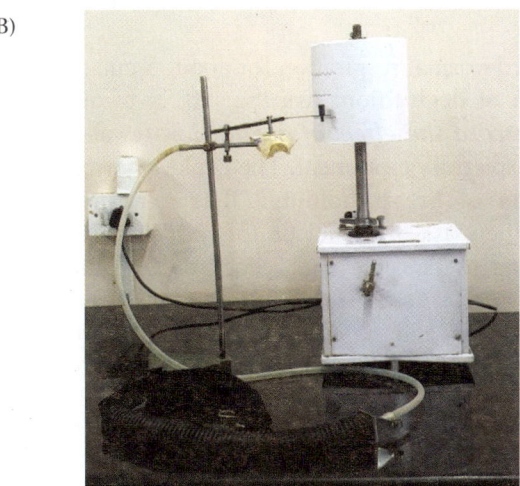

Fig. 21.1 Stethograph: (A) Schematic picture of a stethograph and (B) actual photograph of the stethograph setting. Note that the stethograph is connected through rubber tubing to the Marey's tambour, which is further connected to the kymograph recording.

A)
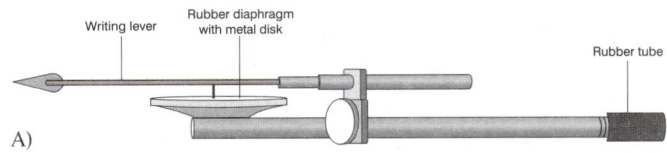

B)
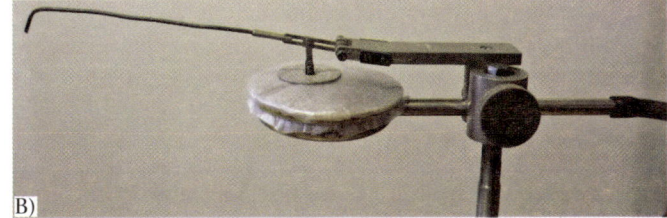

Fig. 21.2 Marey's tambour: (A) Diagrammatic representation and (B) a photograph.

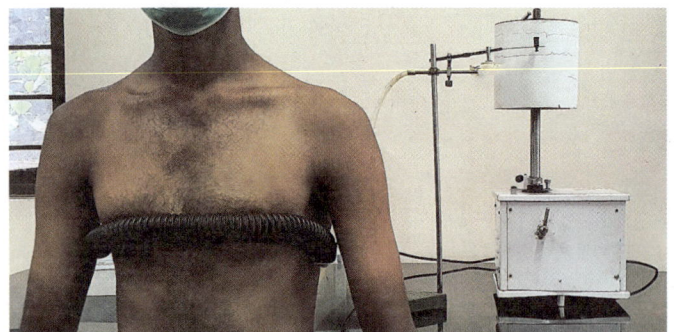

Fig. 21.3   Placing and tying the stethograph around the subject's chest at the level of the fourth intercostal space, which corresponds to the level of the nipples.

> **Note:** Check that when the stethograph is connected to the tambour, the pressure change in the stethograph is transmitted to it. This is confirmed by movements of the lever corresponding to movements of the chest.

3. Bring the writing lever in contact with the kymograph paper and set the drum to move at a slow speed (2.5 mm/s; Fig. 21.4).
4. Record normal respiration for about 5 cm.
5. **Effect of deglutition:** Ask the subject to drink water and ***record the effect of deglutition*** (swallowing) on the respiratory movement. Then, take a normal tracing.
6. **Effects of breath-holding:** Take a normal tracing and then ask the subject to ***hold his breath*** for as long as possible and record the effects after: i) *quiet inspiration*, ii) *expiration*, iii) *following deep inspiration*, and iv) *following deep expiration*. Take normal tracings after each type of breath-holding.

> **Note:** The effects of all these respiratory maneuvers should be recorded separately. Normal tracings should be recorded before and after each recording.

7. **Effects of modified respiratory movements:** Ask the subject to voluntarily cough, sneeze, and talk, and record the effects of these maneuvers.
8. **Effects of hyperventilation:** Record normal respiration and stop the drum. Ask the subject to take ***deep breaths as rapidly as possible*** for one and a half minutes. Immediately after hyperventilation, start the drum and record the effect on respiratory movements.
9. **Effects of exercise:** Record normal respiration. Disconnect the stethograph from Marey's tambour and ask the subject ***to exercise*** (moderate spot-jogging) for two minutes. Immediately after exercise, connect the stethograph to the kymograph and record the effect of exercise on respiratory movement.

Precautions

1. The subject should sit comfortably and in an erect posture.

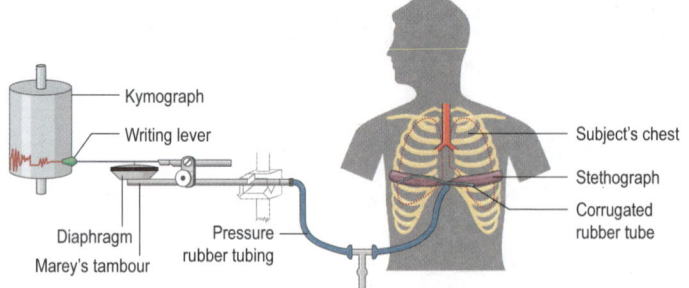

Fig. 21.4   Schematic diagram of stethographic recording.

2. The tambour should be tied at the level of the fourth intercostal space because expansion of the chest is maximum at this level.
3. Before and after the recordings for each maneuver (for example, swallowing water, coughing, etc.), normal tracings should be taken.
4. Recordings should not be made during the act of hyperventilation but immediately after.
5. The stethograph must be disconnected from the tambour during exercise, and the recording should be made immediately after exercise.
6. For BHT, the recording should be made after quiet inspiration and quiet expiration and forceful inspiration and forceful expiration.

Observation and Results

1. Note that ***downstroke is inspiration*** and ***upstroke is expiration***.
2. **Effect of deglutition:** Note that there is a temporary stoppage of breathing during deglutition, called ***deglutition apnea*** (Fig. 21.5).
3. **Effect of BHT:** Study the ***duration of BHT*** following normal and deep inspiration and expiration. Note that BHT is significantly higher after inspiration as compared to expiration. Observe that after a variable interval of 30 to 70 seconds or more, the subject 'tries' to make respiratory movements but can still hold his breath. However, within a few seconds, breath can no longer be held, and a deep breath is taken; this point is called the '**breaking point**'.
    Note the following:
    i.   Duration of breath-holding (after a deep inspiration) = _____ sec.
    ii. Duration for which breathing remains high after the breaking point = ___ sec.
4. **Effects of hyperventilation:** Observe the breathing pattern following hyperventilation, and note the periodic breathing.
5. **Effects of exercise:** Observe the breathing pattern following exercise (Fig. 21.5).

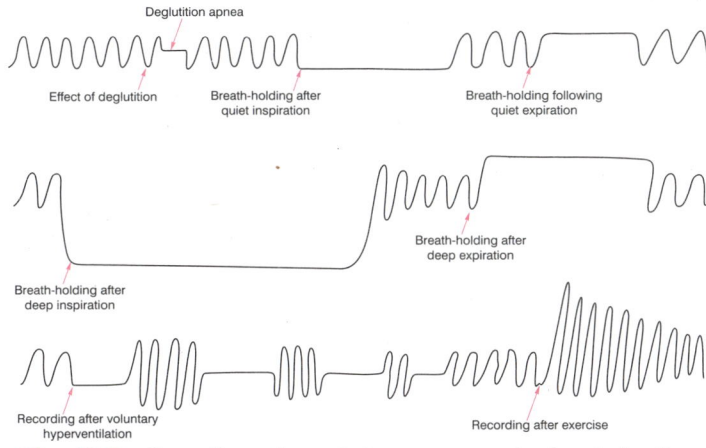

Deglutition apnea

Effect of deglutition   Breath-holding after   Breath-holding following
                          quiet inspiration   quiet expiration

Breath-holding after
deep expiration

Breath-holding after
deep inspiration

Recording after voluntary
hyperventilation   Recording after exercise

Fig. 21.5 Recording of respiratory movements to study the effects of deglutition, voluntary hyperventilation, and exercise and to determine the breath-holding time (BHT).

DISCUSSION

Deglutition Apnea

During deglutition (drinking of water), respiration stops temporarily. This is called **deglutition apnea**. It occurs due to the **closure of the glottis**, which helps in the passage of food or water through the esophagus and prevents the entry of food materials into the respiratory tract.

Breath-Holding Time (BHT)

BHT is the maximum time for which a subject can hold his breath. BHT is higher following inspiration than expiration. Respiration can be voluntarily held for some time, but eventually, voluntary control is overridden.

Breaking point: The point at which **breathing can no longer be voluntarily inhibited** is called the breaking point. It occurs due to a **rise in arterial pCO$_2$** and the **fall in pO$_2$** as body tissues continue to utilise oxygen and produce carbon dioxide. These changes stimulate central and peripheral chemoreceptors, which stimulate respiration. Generally, the breaking point is reached *at an alveolar pO$_2$ of 56 mmHg and alveolar pCO$_2$ of 49 mm Hg*. It has been suggested that proprioceptive impulses from respiratory muscles and joints may be involved in the breaking point.

Factors affecting breaking point

1. **Breathing 100 per cent oxygen** increases BHT. Breathing 100 per cent oxygen before holding the breath increases alveolar pO$_2$, thereby delaying the breaking point.
2. **Hyperventilation** at room air increases BHT. This is because hyperventilation removes CO$_2$ from the blood and thereby delays the breaking point.
3. **Psychological factors** play a role. Encouragement delays the breaking point.

Hyperventilation

Periodic breathing occurs following voluntary hyperventilation. There will be **apnea followed by a brief period of hyperpnea**. Apnea occurs due to the removal of carbon dioxide during hyperventilation, as a result of which respiration stops temporarily. This causes an accumulation of carbon dioxide, which stimulates respiration; as a result, there is hyperventilation. This phenomenon is seen **physiologically** in sleep (especially in infants), at high altitudes, and following voluntary hyperventilation.

Cheyne–Stokes respiration is a pathological form of periodic breathing (waxing and waning amplitude of flow or tidal volume) characterised by a crescendo–decrescendo pattern of hyperventilation between central apneas or central hypopneas.

Exercise

During exercise, **hyperventilation occurs** due to the stimulation of the respiratory centres by increased discharge from the proprioceptors in the joints, ligaments, and muscles. Though the increase in respiration is proportionate to the increase in oxygen consumption, the role of oxygen in the stimulation of hyperventilation is still not clear. **Increased body temperature, increased K$^+$ level, and increased lactic acid concentration** play a role in hyperventilation. However, since the exercise is mild to moderate in this practical, hyperventilation is chiefly due to *increased proprioceptive information from the exercising muscles and joints*.

Hyperventilation persists after intense exercise due to *increased arterial H$^+$ concentration*, which occurs due to lactic acidemia. Sometimes, a pattern of periodic breathing is also observed following exercise.

VIVA

1. *What is stethography?* (**Ans.** Refer to page 127, under the heading 'Introduction'.)
2. *Why is the stethograph tied at the mid-chest level (fourth intercostal space)?* (**Ans.** Refer to page 127, under the heading 'Precautions', point No. 2.)
3. *What are the precautions taken for stethography?* (**Ans.** Refer to page 128, under the heading 'Precautions'.)
4. *During recording, why should the subject not look at the recording?*
   (**Ans.** Respiratory movements during the recording are conscious movements. Therefore, the subject's chest movements and the act of recording are likely to be affected by him looking at the recordings. The result may not represent the true effects of various maneuvers in such cases.)

5. *What is deglutition apnea? Describe its mechanism and physiological significance.*
    (Ans. **Definition:** Apnea refers to a temporary stoppage of breathing during the act of swallowing [deglutition].
    Mechanism: It is a reflex phenomenon that occurs automatically whether one swallows—whether a sip of a liquid or a glass of water. During the pharyngeal stage of deglutition, which may last for 0.5 seconds or more, the food or fluid stimulates the tactile sensory nerve endings in the mucosa of the pharynx. Afferent nerve impulses are set up and relayed along the 5th, 9th, and 10th cranial nerves, via the deglutition centre. This results in the inhibition of the respiratory center and stops the breathing at any point of inspiration or expiration. Simultaneously, there is closure of the glottis, the opening between the vocal cords.
    Physiological significance: The stoppage of breathing and closure of the glottis prevents the entry of food or fluid into the upper respiratory passages, which would otherwise cause aspiration of food, choking, or other serious complications, resulting in **aspiration pneumonia.** Whenever a particle of food or fluid enters the respiratory passages, there is a strong bout of coughing till the offending particle is expelled, which happens reflexively.)

6. *What is the breaking point? What are its causes?* (Ans. Refer to page 129, under the heading 'BHT – Breaking Point'.)

7. *What are the factors that affect breaking point?* (Ans. Refer to page 129, under the heading 'Factors affecting Breaking Point'.)

8. *How can the breath-holding time be prolonged?*
    (Ans. The breath-holding time can be increased by: i. hyperventilating before holding breath, as this will decrease the arterial PCO_2 and raise PO_2 a little and ii. breathing pure oxygen before holding breath.)

9. *What are the causes of periodic breathing that occurs following voluntary hyperventilation?* (Ans. Refer to page 129, under the heading 'Hyperventilation'.)

10. *What is meant by eupnea, tachypnea, bradypnea, hyperpnea, hypercapnia and hypocapnia, hypoxia, and asphyxia?*
    (Ans. **Eupnea** means normal breathing; **apnea** is the stoppage of respiration [which occurs temporarily]. **Tachypnea** and **bradypnea** refer to increased and decreased rate of respiration respectively. **Hyperpnea** refers to increased ventilation [hyperventilation], usually with deep breathing and increased rate of breathing. **Hypercapnia** and **hypocapnia** refer to increased and decreased CO_2 in the body, i.e., retention and washing out of CO_2. **Hypoxia** refers to decreased oxygen supply at the tissue level, and **asphyxia** refers to an excess of CO_2 and lack of oxygen in the body.)

11. *Define hyperventilation. What are its mechanisms and effects? What will happen if it continues for a long time?*
    (Ans. Hyperventilation refers to increased breathing in terms of rate, depth, or both, resulting in an increased volume of air moving into and out of the lungs per unit time. Generally, it can result from:
    i) **Voluntary effort:** The main stimulus for increasing ventilation.
    ii) **Muscular exercise:** This is the second most important respiratory stimulus.
    iii) **Chemical stimuli:** Hyperventilation can occur due to high PCO_2, low PO_2, or increased H^+ ion concentration, resulting from lung and heart diseases.
    Voluntary hyperventilation can achieve an increase in the rate of ventilation from the resting level of 6–8 litres/minute to over 200 litres/minute, at least for a short period. Chemical stimuli can increase the ventilation to about 80–90 litres/ minute.
    Effects of voluntary hyperventilation: Hyperventilation results in periodic breathing, i.e., apnea followed by a brief period of hypernea. When a person hyperventilates for 1–2 minutes and then allows respiration to continue on its own, there is a short period of apnea, which is followed by a few rapid breaths and then another period of apnea followed by a few breaths. The cycle may last for a while before returning to normal rhythm. This apnea occurs due to the washing out of CO_2 (hypocapnia). As CO_2 accumulates, breathing resumes. It is to be noted that though CO_2 is a waste product of metabolism, it is a stronger stimulus for respiration. Thus, while a high PCO_2 stimulates breathing, a low PCO_2 inhibits it until the blood PCO_2 returns to normal.
    Harmful effects of chronic hyperventilation: A single act of hyperventilation will have no ill effects. However, repeated or chronic hyperventilation, as seen in neurotic patients, may produce adverse effects. The arterial PCO_2 may fall from the normal level of 40 mmHg to 15–20 mmHg (**hypocapnia**), which can produce vasoconstriction of cerebral blood vessels. As CO_2 is a strong vasodilator, hypocapnia causes vasoconstriction. **Cerebral ischemia** causes dizziness and light-headedness, and the **constriction of retinal blood vessels** may cause blurring of vision. A more serious effect of chronic hyperventilation and associated hypocapnia is **alkalosis** which causes precipitation of ionic calcium. If the serum calcium is already low in the subject, **tetany** may be triggered; this manifests as tetanic spasms of the skeletal muscles, especially in the limbs and larynx.)

12. *What are the effects of exercise on respiratory movement?* (Ans. Refer to page 129, under the heading 'Exercise'.)

13. *What are the causes of increased ventilation during exercise?*
    (Ans. The following factors are involved in increasing ventilation during exercise.)

    i. **Psychic stimuli:** Ventilation often increases in anticipation of the exercise, which happens before exercise starts. Soon after exercise begins, and before blood PCO_2, PO_2, and H^+ ions have time to change, there is a sudden and large increase in ventilation due to proprioceptive inputs and cortical inputs, as mentioned below.

    ii. **Impulses from proprioceptors:** Body movements, especially those of the limbs, stimulate the proprioceptors in the active muscles, tendons, ligaments, joints, etc. These excitatory impulses are also relayed to the respiratory centre.

    iii. **Impulses from motor cortex:** The motor cortex sends impulses through the corticospinal tracts to the motor neurons of active muscles and excitatory impulses through the collaterals of the tracts to the respiratory centre. The result is a sudden increase in ventilation.

    iv. **Chemical stimuli:** The increased ventilation supplies extra O_2 to the active muscles and removes excess CO_2 produced without causing any significant change in arterial PO_2 and PCO_2, especially in trained athletes. In fact, the PO_2 may be higher and PCO_2 lower than the normal. Thus, the established fact of low PO_2 and high PCO_2 stimulating ventilation cannot explain the chemical cause of respiratory stimulation during exercise. However, in the later stages of severe exercise, it is the chemical stimuli that increase the ventilation. Although there may be no change in the level of gas in the blood, the sensitivity of the respiratory centre to the normal levels may be involved.

    v. **Other factors:** Other factors such as increased body temperature, increased blood K^+, lactic acidosis, and hypoxia in exercising muscles stimulating the sensory nerve endings, and fluctuations in blood gases may increase the ventilation.)

14. *Why do ventilation and oxygen utilisation remain high after the end of exercise?*
(Ans. During moderate to severe muscular exercise, muscles obtain their energy from anaerobic metabolism of glucose [i.e., in the absence of O_2], which results in the formation of lactic acid. The buffering of lactate liberates more CO_2, which further stimulates respiration. After exercise, ventilation and O_2 utilisation remain high until the oxygen debt incurred during anaerobic glycolysis is repaid, i.e., the lactate is converted back to pyruvate when O_2 supply is restored after exercise. Therefore, the cause of increased ventilation after exercise is not high PCO_2 [which is rather normal or low] or low PO_2 [which is normal or high], but the increased arterial H^+ ion concentration due to lactic acidemia.)

15. *What is periodic breathing? Give examples.* (Ans. Refer to page 129, under the heading 'Hyperventilation – Periodic breathing'.)

16. *What is Cheyne–Stokes respiration? In which conditions does it occur?* (Ans. Refer to page 129, under the heading 'Hyperventilation – Cheyne-Stokes respiration'.)

17. *Is respiration an automatic process or a voluntary act? How is normal respiration maintained and controlled?*
(Ans. Respiration is both an involuntary and a voluntary process. Most of the time, we are not consciously aware of our breathing, whether we are awake or asleep, and it occurs automatically and spontaneously. However, we can voluntarily control our breathing whenever we choose — by becoming aware of it, we can consciously increase, decrease, or even temporarily stop breathing for a few minutes.

    Spontaneous or automatic breathing: The alternate contraction and relaxation of respiratory muscles rhythmically stimulated by impulses in their motor nerve supply (for example, for the diaphragm, the phrenic nerve is the chief muscle of inspiration) causes breathing. These motor nerves have no activity of their own but are activated by a rhythmic discharge of impulses from the medullary rhythmicity area, which is a part of the respiratory centre in the brainstem. Thus, the medullary rhythmicity area sets up the basic rhythm of inspiration and expiration.

    Voluntary control of respiration: Voluntary control over breathing is exerted via the corticospinal (pyramidal) tracts that control voluntary muscle activity throughout the body. The axons of these tracts, as upper motor neurons descend from the cerebral motor cortex, bypass the brainstem respiratory centre and end on phrenic and other neurons in the spinal cord that innervate respiratory muscles.

    Maintenance and control of respiration: Respiration is maintained by the rhythmic discharge of impulses from the medullary respiratory areas. The activity of medullary center is controlled by inputs from cerebral cortex, hypothalamus [emotions affect our respiration], central and peripheral chemoreceptors, baroreceptors, stretch receptors in the lungs, and muscles, joints, and ligaments.)

18. *Briefly explain the effects of pO_2, pCO_2, and H+ on respiration.*
(Ans. The hydrogen ion concentration and respiratory gas composition of the arterial blood profoundly influence respiration. In general, breathing activities are directly related to PCO_2 and H^+, and inversely related to arterial blood PO_2.

    i. The **two sets of receptors** that detect these chemical changes in blood are **peripheral and central chemoreceptors**.

    ii. Hypoxia, hypercapnia, and acidosis **stimulate respiration** that in turn raise PO_2, lower PCO_2, and raise pH.

    iii. **Responses to carbon dioxide and blood pH** depend mainly on the central chemoreceptors that are located in the brainstem, and **responses to hypoxia** depend mainly on peripheral chemoreceptors that are located in carotid and aortic bodies.

22 | Vitalography and Effect of Posture on Vital Capacity

Learning Objectives

After completing this practical, you will be able to (MUST KNOW):
1. Define vital capacity.
2. Record the effect of posture on vital capacity.
3. List the precautions taken during the recording.
4. State the normal value of vital capacity.
5. List the factors that affect vital capacity.

You may also be able to (DESIRABLE TO KNOW):
1. Explain the variations in vital capacity in different conditions.
2. List the reasons for alteration in vital capacity with changes in posture.
3. Explain the physiological significance of vital capacity.
4. Explain the prediction of VC with reference to height, body weight, BSA, age, and gender.

PY6.8: Demonstrate the correct technique to perform and interpret spirometry.

INTRODUCTION

Vital capacity (VC) is the maximum volume of air that can be expired from the lungs by forceful effort following a maximal inspiration. VC is computed as the sum of tidal volume, inspiratory reserve volume, and expiratory reserve volume. VC in a healthy adult is **3–5 litres**. The **average value of VC is 4.5 litres in males and 3.3 litres in females**. **Vitalography** is the process of measuring lung volumes and capacities, especially the vital capacity using a spirometer.

Factors Affecting Vital Capacity

Physiological factors
1. **Posture:** VC is greater in an erect posture than in the sitting and lying postures (for explanation, see 'Discussion').
2. **Age:** VC is high in young adults and low in children and old people. As age advances, compliance of the lungs and chest wall decreases, and consequently, vital capacity decreases.
3. **Gender:** VC is greater in males because the size of the chest is larger and muscle power is more.
4. **Height:** Taller individuals tend to have higher VC.
5. **Physical build:** VC is low in obese and very thin persons, and high in individuals with higher fat-free mass and well-built persons. Vital capacity depends on chest size, muscle power, and the body surface area of the individual.

6. **Pregnancy:** VC is low during pregnancy because chest expansion decreases as abdominal size increases.
7. **Physical training:** VC is higher in trained athletes than in untrained individuals. It is even higher in swimmers and divers.
8. **Ethnicity:** Caucasians (Europeans, Middle Eastern, and North African ancestry) tend to have higher VC than Asians, Africans, and Americans. Caucasians have larger chest dimensions and longer chests, and hence have comparatively higher VC.

Pathological factors
1. VC decreases in **diseases of the chest wall** (e.g., kyphoscoliosis), **lungs** (e.g., emphysema, asthma, fibrosis, and pulmonary edema), and **pleura** (e.g., pleural effusion and pneumothorax).
2. VC decreases in **diseases of the abdomen** in which lung expansion is restricted, as seen in abdominal tumors and ascites.

METHODS OF DEMONSTRATING THE EFFECT OF POSTURE ON VC

Principle
Change in posture affects the ability to exert physical effort and the ventilatory capacity of the lungs. Therefore, posture affects vital capacity.

Requirements
1. **Student's spirometer**; also called **vitalograph**, vitalometer, and simple spirometer (Fig. 22.1A and B)
2. Mouthpiece

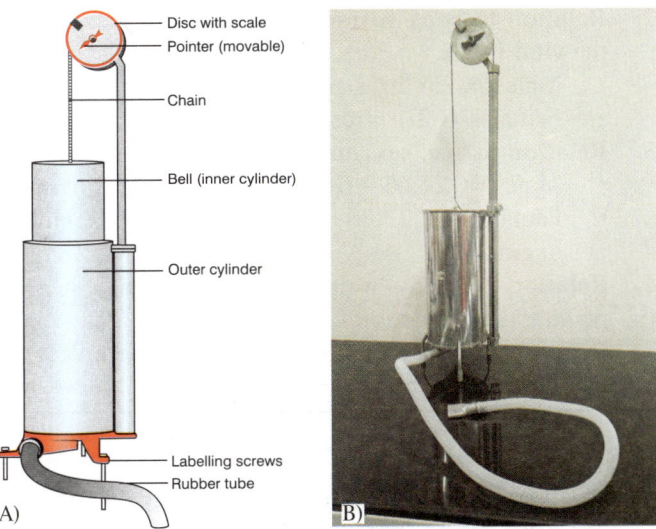

Fig. 22.1 Student's spirometer (vitalograph): (A) Schematic diagram and (B) photograph.

Procedure

1. Adjust the reading of the vitalometer to the zero mark.
2. Ask the subject to **lie down comfortably** on a couch.
3. Connect the mouthpiece of the vitalometer to the subject's mouth.
4. Ask the subject to **exhale forcefully to their maximum capacity** after taking a deep inspiration.
5. Record the vital capacity from the scale of the vitalometer (Fig. 22.2).
6. Change the position of the arrow to zero and ask the subject to repeat the maneuver.
7. Record vital capacity **three times**, with a gap of at least two minutes between recordings, and **note the best reading**.
8. Ask the subject to **sit on a stool** with his spine erect.
9. Record vital capacity (as described above) three times and record the best reading.
10. Ask the subject to **stand up**.
11. Record the vital capacity three times and note the best reading.
12. Compare the vital capacities recorded in the three positions.

Observation and Results

Note that the vital capacity is maximum in the erect posture and minimum in the supine posture. Report your result in the format given below.

Name: _____; **Age:** _____ years
Sex: _____; Date of recording: _____
Weight: ____ kg; **Height:** _____ cm
1. Rate of respiration: ____/min
2. Vital capacity:
    a. Standard method _____
    b. Two-stage method _____
3. **Effect of posture on VC:** _____

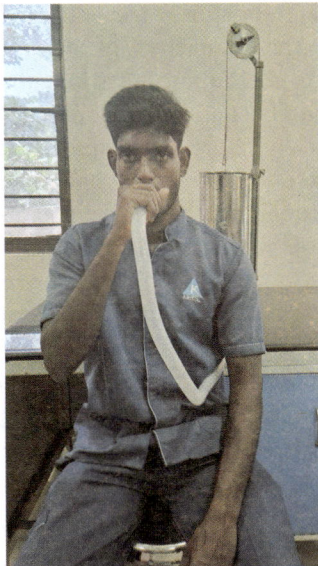

Fig. 22.2 Recording of vital capacity using student's spirometer. Note the change in the position of the pointer (red arrow) from the zero mark after the maneuver.

Recordings

Position	First recording	Second recording	Third recording
Standing			
Sitting			
Supine			

Calculate the vital capacity

Per kg body weight: _____
Per cm height: _____
Per m² BSA (vital index): _____
(Consult the nomogram for body surface area calculation)

Precautions

1. Each time, before recording vital capacity, the arrow mark of the scale should be adjusted to zero.
2. In the sitting and standing postures, the **subject's spine should be erect**.
3. The subject should be trained and encouraged to exert the maximum effort possible.
4. A minimum of three attempts should be made in all the postures, and the best of the three should be taken.
5. The gap between two attempts should be a minimum of one to two minutes.
6. The test should not be performed on a full stomach.

DISCUSSION

Vital capacity (VC) ranges between **3.0 to 5.0 litres**. It is more in males and about 20% lower in females. VC is **higher in the erect posture** than in supine and sitting postures for the following reasons:

1. **More physical (muscular) effort** is applied in the erect posture.

2. In the **erect posture**, the diaphragm descends. Therefore, the **capacity of the thoracic cage increases**. In the **supine position**, the diaphragm is pulled upward because the abdominal viscera push the diaphragm. Therefore, the **capacity of the thoracic cage decreases**. Hence, vital capacity is greater in the erect posture than in the supine position.

3. In the **supine position**, due to the elimination of the effect of gravity, the **blood flow to the lungs increases**. This decreases vital capacity. In the **standing posture**, blood is pooled in the lower extremities, and so, venous return decreases, which **decreases pulmonary blood flow**. Thus, vital capacity increases on standing.

Two-stage vital capacity: This is defined as the **sum of the inspiratory capacity (IC) and expiratory reserve volume (ERV),** measured separately with the help of a spirometer.

Physiological Significance

Vital capacity is routinely assessed as a **fitness test for recruitment** into the military, paramilitary, and police forces. VC indicates **the strength of the respiratory muscles**. The maximum inspiratory and expiratory effort possible for an individual can be assessed by determining vital capacity. VC is higher in trained individuals such as athletes, runners, swimmers, and divers.

Prediction of Vital Capacity

Various formulas have been introduced to predict VC in individuals based on their race, ethnicity, age, and gender. Various respiratory disorders are diagnosed by comparing the actual value (recorded value) with the **predicted value**. In general, VC is 20% lower in females. The vital capacity (and other volumes and capacities) is generally higher in males, taller persons, and younger adults.

As VC depends on age, sex, body build, occupation, etc., various formulae have been devised to predict and correct VC in an individual. Various disorders may then be diagnosed by comparing the actual (determined) values with the predicted normal values for one's age and gender. The vital capacity is high in athletes, swimmers, divers, etc., but is low in persons who have sedentary habits.

Prediction of VC to the height, age, gender, body weight, and BSA

1. **Relation to height:**
   - Males = Height in cm × 25
   - Females = Height in cm × 20
   - Athletes = Height in cm × 29

2. **Relation to body surface area (BSA):** This is called the **vital index**.
   - Males = 2.5 litres/m² BSA
   - Females = 2.1 litres/m² BSA

3. **Relation to age, sex, and height:**
   - Males = [27.63 − (0.112 × Age)] × Height in cm
   - Females = [27.78 − (0.101 × Age)] × Height in cm

4. **Relation to body weight:** For an average healthy person, the prediction formula is:
   Vital capacity (in ml) = W0.72/0.690, where W is the body weight in grams.

OSPE

I. Determine the vital capacity of the given subject in the sitting posture by using the student's spirometer.

Steps

1. Adjust the zero reading of the vitalometer.
2. Ask the subject to sit comfortably on a stool.
3. Instruct him to put in the maximum effort during recording.
4. Connect the mouthpiece of the vitalometer to the subject's mouth.
5. Ask the subject to exhale forcefully to their maximum capacity after taking a deep inspiration and note the reading.
6. Ask the subject to repeat the procedure three times and record the best reading.

II. Record the effect of standing up (from lying down posture) on the vital capacity of the given subject.

Steps

1. Adjust the zero reading of the vitalometer.
2. Ask the subject to lie down comfortably on a couch.
3. Instruct the subject to put in maximum effort during the recording.
4. Connect the mouthpiece of the vitalometer to the subject's mouth.
5. Ask the subject to exhale forcefully and maximally following a deep inspiration and record the reading on the vitalometer scale.
6. Ask the subject to stand erect.
7. Adjust the zero reading of the vitalometer.
8. Ask the subject to exhale forcefully and maximally following a deep inspiration and record the reading on the vitalometer scale.
9. Compare the two readings and report the findings.

VIVA

1. *Define vital capacity.* (Ans. Refer to page 132, under the heading 'Introduction'.)
2. *What is the normal value of VC in males and females?* (Ans. Refer to page 132, under the heading 'Introduction'.)
3. *What are the factors that affect vital capacity?* (Ans. Refer to page 132, under the heading 'Factors Affecting VC'.)
4. *What are the precautions to be taken while recording vital capacity?* (Ans. Refer to page 133, under the heading 'Precautions'.)
5. *Why is the vital capacity greater in the standing posture than in the sitting and supine postures?* (Ans. Refer to page 133, under the heading 'Discussion'.)
6. *What is the physiological significance of VC?* (Ans. Refer to page 134, under the heading 'Physiological Significance'.)
7. *What is two-stage vital capacity?* (Ans. Refer to page 134, under the heading 'Physiological Significance' and subheading 'Two-stage VC'.)
8. *What is the importance of the prediction of VC? How is the prediction done for height, BSA, body weight, age, and gender?* (Ans. Refer to page 134, under the heading 'Prediction of VC'.)
9. *What is slow vital capacity (SVC)? What is its importance?*
   (Ans. Slow vital capacity is the volume of air exhaled after a **maximal inhalation during a slow, unforced expiratory effort without any time constraint.** It is primarily used to assess lung volume and evaluate lung function. A reduced SVC may indicate restrictive lung disease.)
10. *What is forced vital capacity (FVC)? What is its importance?*
    (Ans. Forced vital capacity is the largest volume of air a person can expel from the lungs with maximum effort after first filling the lung fully with the deepest possible inhalation. SVC is more than SVC in patients with airway obstruction.)

23 | Pulmonary Function Tests and Spirometry

Learning Objectives

After completing this practical, you will be able to (MUST KNOW):

1. Describe the importance of performing this practical in clinical physiology.
2. Classify pulmonary function tests (PFTs).
3. Record the lung volumes and capacities and FEV$_1$ by spirometry.
4. Define lung volumes and capacities.
5. State the normal values of all PFTs.
6. Explain the differences between patterns of FEV$_1$ in obstructive and restrictive lung diseases.
7. State the importance of FVC and FEV$_1$ in the diagnosis of respiratory diseases.
8. Name the common conditions that alter the result of PFTs.

You may also be able to (DESIRABLE TO KNOW):

1. Explain the significance of all PFTs.
2. Explain the disturbances in pulmonary circulation, diffusion, and ventilation–perfusion ratio in the pathophysiology and diagnosis of respiratory diseases.

PY6.8: Demonstrate the correct technique of performing and interpreting spirometry.

INTRODUCTION

The important functions of the lung—to ensure adequate tissue oxygenation and to prevent the accumulation of carbon dioxide in excess in the body—are accomplished by **ventilation, diffusion, and perfusion**. Pulmonary function tests (PFTs) aim to assess different aspects of these three processes.

Classification of PFTs Based on Lung Function

From the physiology point of view, PFTs are best classified by categorising them to assess ventilation, ventilation–perfusion relationship and diffusion, and to measure dead space, compliance, airway resistance and pulmonary blood flow and pressure.

Parameters to assess ventilation

A. **Static lung volumes and capacities**
  1. Lung volumes
     - Tidal volume
     - Inspiratory reserve volume
     - Expiratory reserve volume
     - Residual volume
  2. Lung capacities
     - Vital capacity
     - Inspiratory capacity
     - Functional residual capacity
     - Total lung capacity

B. **Mechanics of breathing** (dynamic lung volumes and capacities)
  - Timed vital capacity
  - Maximum mid-expiratory flow rate
  - Maximum voluntary ventilation
  - Peak expiratory flow rate
  - Maximum expiratory flow–volume curve
  - Closing volume

Study of ventilation–perfusion relationship

Uniformity of ventilation is assessed by:
1. Nitrogen washout method (breath nitrogen test)
2. Radioactive xenon method

Assessment of diffusion

1. Measurement of pO$_2$ and pCO$_2$ in arterial blood
2. Measurement of diffusing capacity of O$_2$ and CO$_2$

Determination of pulmonary blood flow and pressures

Measurement of mean pulmonary artery pressure, pulmonary capillary wedge pressure, pulmonary blood flow, and pulmonary vascular resistance.

Assessment of Ventilation

Ventilation is the process of movement of air in and out of the gas exchanging units of the lung, i.e., the alveoli. Its adequacy depends on the lung volumes and capacities and the mechanics of breathing. Various **lung volumes and capacities are indices of static dimensions** of the lung at various stages of inflation (Fig. 23.1).

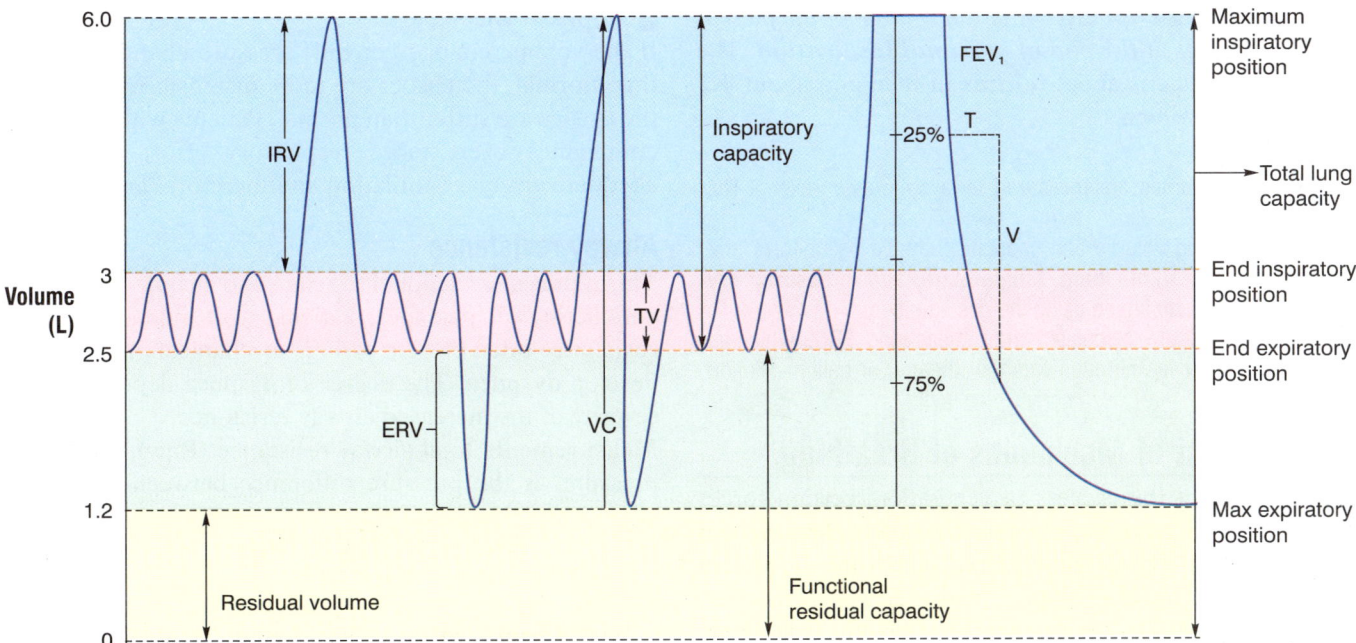

Fig. 23.1   Lung volumes and capacities (TV: tidal volume; IRV: inspiratory reserve volume; ERV: expiratory reserve volume; VC: vital capacity; VC = IRV + ERV + TV; FEV$_1$: Forced expiratory volume in first second). To calculate the FEF$_{25-75\%}$, note T as time and V as volume as drawn from the FEV$_1$ curve.

The mechanics of breathing deal with static as well as dynamic mechanical properties of the respiratory apparatus.

Lung volumes

1. **Tidal volume (TV):** This is the *volume of air inspired or expired* **during quiet breathing**. This is **500 ml** in adults. About 150 ml of this volume occupies the upper airways up to the respiratory bronchioles. This amount does not take part in gas exchange. This is called the **anatomical dead space**. The remaining volume, that is, 350 ml, is available for alveolar ventilation.

Minute ventilation (MV): This is the volume of air that can be **breathed in or out of the lung in one minute**.

MV = TV × respiratory rate per min.

This is also called **resting minute volume (RMV)** or **pulmonary ventilation (PV)**. The normal value of MV is **6 litres/min.**

> **Note:** Since the anatomical dead space volume of 150 ml is fixed, any decrease in resting ventilation (decrease in tidal volume) decreases the volume of air available for alveolar ventilation, which in turn, decreases the tissue oxygenation. Anatomical dead space is measured by single breath N$_2$ curve.

2. **Inspiratory reserve volume (IRV):** This is the *volume of air inspired* with a **maximal inspiratory effort in excess of the tidal volume**. The normal value of IRV is about **3 litres in men** and **2 litres in women**. Inspiratory muscles should be used to the maximum when measuring IRV.

3. **Expiratory reserve volume (ERV):** This is the *volume of air that can be expired* with a **maximum expiratory effort after passive expiration**. The normal value of ERV is about **1 litre in men** and **0.7 litre in women**. Expiratory muscles should be used to the maximum when measuring ERV.

4. **Residual volume (RV):** This is the *volume of air left in the lung* **at the end of a maximal expiratory effort**. The normal value of RV is **1.2 litres in men** and **1.1 litres in women**.

Lung capacities

1. **Vital capacity (VC):** This is the maximum amount of air that can be *expired forcefully after a maximal inspiratory effort*. The normal value of VC is about **4.5 litres in men** and about **3 litres in women**.

2. **Forced vital capacity (FVC):** It is the total volume expired forcefully with greatest force and speed after a maximal inspiration. FVC differs very little from VC in the normal subject but is proportionately more reduced when there is airway obstruction with air trapping.

3. **Inspiratory capacity:** This is the *maximum amount of air that can be inspired from the resting expiratory level*. Inspiratory capacity = **IRV+TV**. It is about **3.5 litres**.

4. **Functional residual capacity (FRC):** This is the amount of air *remaining in the lungs at the end of a normal expiration* at rest. FRC = ERV+RV.

5. **Total lung capacity:** It is the *volume of air present in the lungs* at **the end of maximal inspiration**. The normal value is about **6 litres in men** and about **4.2 litres in women**.

> **Note:**
> 1. All static volumes are measured by a spirometer, except RV, FRC, and TLC.
> 2. Values of lung volume and capacities should be uniform and converted with **standard temperature and pressure, dry (STPD)** for comparison using the gas equation.
> 3. RV and TLC are calculated after measuring FRC, which is performed by the nitrogen-washout method or helium dilution technique.

Assessment of Mechanics of Breathing

In carrying out the process of ventilation, certain forces are required to overcome the elastic recoil of the lung and thorax, the non-elastic resistance caused by the movement of tissues during breathing, and the airway resistance. Thus, assessment of the mechanics of breathing is aimed at assessing compliance and airway resistance.

Compliance

Compliance measures the relative stiffness and distensibility of the lungs and thorax. The elastic recoil of the lung, which is measured under static conditions, is called compliance.

Compliance (C) is defined as the **change in lung volume (ΔV) per unit change in transpulmonary pressure (ΔV)**. It is the difference between esophageal or intrapleural pressure and mouth pressure.

$$C = \Delta V / \Delta P$$

1. *Total respiratory compliance* (combined compliance of lung and chest wall), i.e., lung inside the thoracic cavity; normal value is 0.13 l/cm H_2O.
2. *Pulmonary compliance* (lung only), i.e., lung outside the chest wall; normal value is 0.22 l/cm H_2O.

■ Measurement of total compliance

Total respiratory compliance can be measured by the pressure–volume curve of the respiratory system, which can be obtained by spirometry (Fig. 23.5).

■ Static and specific lung compliance

1. *Static compliance* of any system depends on the size, which is the mass of functional lung tissue.
2. *Specific compliance* is the lung compliance *at relaxation volume*, i.e., the volume at the end of tidal expiration, which is the functional residual capacity (FRC). The compliance is *corrected for the lung volume*, which is referred to as the specific compliance and expressed as litres/FRC. For example, if FRC is 2.2 litres, specific compliance of both intact lungs will be 0.22/2.2 = 0.1 l/cm of water.

■ Application

If the volume change per unit pressure change is higher than normal, the tissues are more distensible; if it is less, the tissues are stiffer than normal. Patients with decreased compliance exert more respiratory effort to achieve adequate alveolar ventilation and therefore, are dyspneic.

Airway resistance

This represents frictional resistance to airflow through the conducting air passages. Patients with increased **airway resistance** often present serious mechanical problems and develop **dyspnea**. The degree of dyspnea depends on the severity of the increased airway resistance.

Measurement: Total airway resistance (Raw), the driving pressure, is the pressure difference between the mouth (P_{mouth}) and the alveoli (P_A).

$$Raw = \frac{P_{mouth} \quad P_A}{V}$$

The ***normal value*** in healthy adults is 1 to 3 cm of H_2O/litre per second.

Dynamic lung volumes and capacities

Dynamic lung volumes and capacities give a fair idea of the mechanics of breathing.

1. **Timed vital capacity:** This is also called ***forced expiratory volume in the first second*** (FEV1). This is defined as the fraction of the vital capacity expired in the specified time, for example, **FEV1**, that is, the fraction of vital capacity expired in the first second. This test measures the vital capacity in relation to time and yields the portion of the vital capacity expired in a specified time. This is an index of airflow rate. In normal conditions, **80–85 per cent of the forced vital capacity is expired in the first second**, 95 per cent in two seconds (FEV_2), and 97–100 per cent in three seconds (FEV_3). It is one of the most useful tests to detect generalised airway obstruction. It is a relatively insensitive indicator of small airway obstruction.

2. **Maximum mid-expiratory flow rate (MMEFR):** This is the *maximum flow achieved* during the **middle third of the total expired volume**. It is expressed as forced expiratory flow at 25–75 per cent of the lung volume ($FEF_{25-75\%}$).

   $FEF_{25-75\%}$ indicates the patency of the small airways. The measurement of flow rate between 200 and 1200 ml ($FEF_{200-1200\ ml}$) in litres per second indicates the patency of the larger airways.

3. **Maximum voluntary ventilation (MVV):** This is also called ***maximum breathing capacity*** (MBC). MVV is the maximum volume of air that can be breathed out per minute by maximal voluntary effort. The normal value of MVV is 150 l/min in adult males and 125 l/min in adult females.

i. *Breathing reserve (BR)*: BR is the difference between MVV and peak exercise ventilation (VEmax), i.e., **MVV–VEmax**. Normally, it is **11 litres/min**, or more than 15%. BR indicates how much a person can increase his ventilation during exercise compared to the MBC at rest. Decreased BR indicates reduced ventilatory capacity during exercise.

ii. *Dyspneic index (DI)*

$$DI = \frac{BR}{MVV} \times 100$$

Normally it is 90%. When **DI is <60%, dyspnea occurs at rest**. DI is also known as **breathing reserve ratio (BRR)**.

4. **Peak expiratory flow rate (PEFR)**: It is the *maximum velocity in litres per minute* with which *air is forced out of the lungs*. PEFR can be read directly from the dial of the peak flow meter. The normal value of PEFR is **400–600 l/ min or 6–10 l/sec**.

5. **Maximum expiratory flow–volume curve (MEFVC)**: Because of the limitation of FEV_1, certain other tests are performed to detect airway obstruction in its early phase. These include V_{max} **75 per cent**, response of maximum expiratory flow–volume curve to the inhalation of helium, and **closing volume**.

- In **MEFVC**, flow is plotted against the volume exhaled.
- V_{max} **75%** is the volume achieved after exhaling 75 per cent of the total FVC.
- **Flow–volume curve** : The *flow rate is plotted against the lung volume* to obtain a flow–volume curve (Fig. 23.2A) and a **flow-volume loop** (Fig. 23.2B). The subject expires maximally and forcefully to residual volume following a deep inspiration (TLC). The flow rate quickly reaches

a maximum and then falls slowly. In **obstructive diseases,** the volume is greater because of air trapping, and the flow rate is less in airway obstruction.

6. **Closing volume (CV)**: This test detects **small airway obstruction** by measuring the *volume of gas remaining in the lung after closure of small airways* in the gravity-dependent lung areas.

Ventilation–Perfusion Relationship

The inspired air is not distributed evenly even in normal conditions. When in the **erect posture**, resting ventilation per unit volume of the lung is *greater at the bases than at the apices*. The difference in values is less pronounced when **lying down** and during exercise. In disease states, the distribution becomes more uneven, resulting in hypo- and hyperventilated areas. Such non-uniform distribution of inspired gas leads to decreased oxygen tension in the arterial blood.

Nitrogen washout method

The **uniformity of distribution** of inspired air is measured by the nitrogen washout method.

1. *After 7 minutes of breathing oxygen*, an **alveolar gas sample** normally contains *less than 2.5 per cent of nitrogen*.
2. The *higher the percentage of nitrogen* in the alveolar sample, the **greater the degree of non-uniformity** of distribution of inspired gas.

Diffusion

Diffusion is the physical process by which gas moves across a membrane from a region of higher partial pressure to a region of lower partial pressure. In the lungs, oxygen

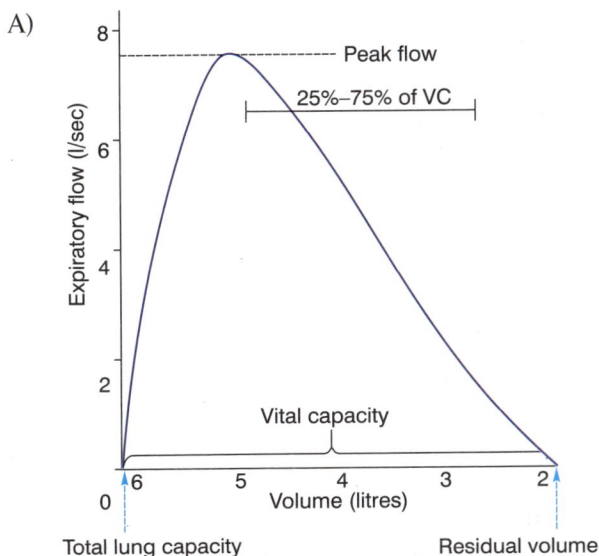

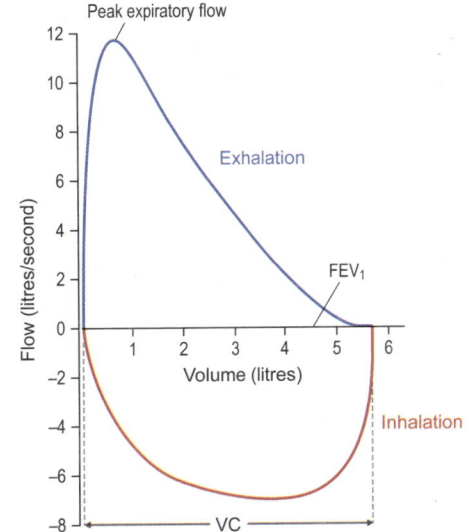

Fig. 23.2 (A) Expiratory flow–volume curve and (B) normal flow–volume loop.

moves from the alveoli to the pulmonary capillaries, and carbon dioxide moves in the opposite direction. The *diffusion capacity of carbon dioxide* **is twenty times** that of oxygen. Therefore, diffusion problems usually **do not produce carbon dioxide retention**.

PaO_2 and $PaCO_2$ depend on the diffusion of gases through the alveolocapillary membrane. It is difficult to measure the **diffusing capacity (DC)** of gases. Therefore, *measurement of the arterial blood gas tension, respiratory gases, and their DC/transfer factor* for gases are essential in the evaluation of pulmonary functions.

Arterial blood gas tension

Arterial blood gas (**ABG**) analysis is a valuable diagnostic tool for measuring O_2, CO_2, and pH in the arterial blood. An arterial blood sample is analysed in an automated AVG machine.

The normal values are as follows:
PaO_2: 85–100 mmHg
$PaCO_2$: 35–45 mmHg
pH: 4.35 to 7.45

Measurement of respiratory gases

Medical **gas analysers** rapidly and accurately provide specific and continuous measurements of respiratory gases. These instruments are used extensively in the diagnosis of lung disorders, and for monitoring patients under critical care anesthesia. Details of respiratory gas analysis are provided under the heading '**Procedures**' below.

DC/Transfer factor for gases

As it is technically difficult to measure the diffusing capacity (DC) of the lungs, depicted as **transfer factor (TF)** for O_2 directly, **CO is used for the purpose**. A small amount of CO and helium mixture is inhaled and breath held for 10 seconds. A *sample of expired air* is then analysed, and the **TF for CO** is read from the computer, which is about 17 ml/min/mmHg.

1. **DC for O_2:** Since the diffusing coefficient for *O_2 is 1.23 times that for CO*, the diffusing capacity for O_2 is = 17 × 1.23 = 21 ml/min/mmHg. Since the time-integrated pressure gradient for O_2 across the respiratory membrane is 11 mmHg, a normal resting person picks up about 21 × 11 = 230 ml of O_2 per minute.

2. **DC for CO_2:** Since the *TF for CO_2 is about 20 times that for O_2*, diffusion problems commonly affect O_2 but not CO_2 (i.e., uptake of O_2 is decreased while there is no CO_2 retention).

Pulmonary Blood Flow and Pressure

Measurement of pressures, vascular resistance, blood volume, and distribution of blood flow in the pulmonary circulation help in detecting vascular occlusion and decreased pulmonary capillary volume.

The pulmonary vasculature accommodates 5 l/min of right ventricular output. The **normal mean pulmonary artery pressure is 15 mmHg**. In an erect posture, the arterial pressure is lowest at the apex and highest at the lung bases. Details of the assessment of pulmonary blood flow and vascular resistance are provided in the section on '**Procedures**' below.

METHODS OF PERFORMING PFTS

PFT Using Spirometers

Spirometry is a method of performing pulmonary function tests (PFTs) using a device called a **spirometer**. PFTs have been recorded in the past using *recording spirometer*, which is presently **not in use**. Currently, PFTs are performed **using a computerized spirometer**.

Principle

The subject exhales forcefully into the instrument, and this is used to detect different parameters that reflect various lung functions.

Requirements

1. **Recording spirometer** (Fig. 23.3A): This is a spirometer with a **recording kymograph**. The spirometer consists of a hollow double-walled vessel. The space between the two walls contains water; making it airtight. In the space between the two walls, an inverted hollow cylindrical bell of 9 l capacity is placed. The bell is attached to a counterbalance with a chain that passes over a pulley. The counterbalance carries a pen for writing on the kymograph paper. The kymograph operates at speeds of 60 and 1200 mm/min. The spirometer records the volume and capacities of the lung.

   Computerised spirometer: Nowadays, lung functions are assessed by using a computerised spirometer (Fig. 23.3B) rather than the recording spirometer.

2. **Wright's peak flow meter**: This is a simple portable device for measuring ventilatory functions (Fig. 23.4). It has a mouthpiece which is connected to a body piece that contains a calibrated scale with a marker. The calibrations are from 60–800 litres per minute.

3. **Douglas bag**: This is a bag that collects air when a person breathes into it. It is used for determining MVV.

4. Gas volume meter

Procedures

■ **Lung volumes and capacities**

1. Fill three-fourths of the bell of the spirometer with air or 100 per cent oxygen.

2. Ask the subject to sit comfortably and relax.

A)

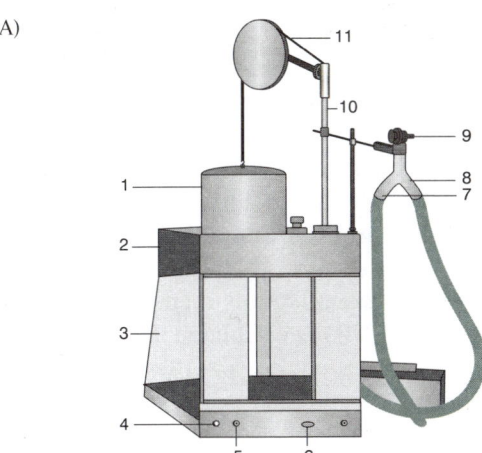

B)

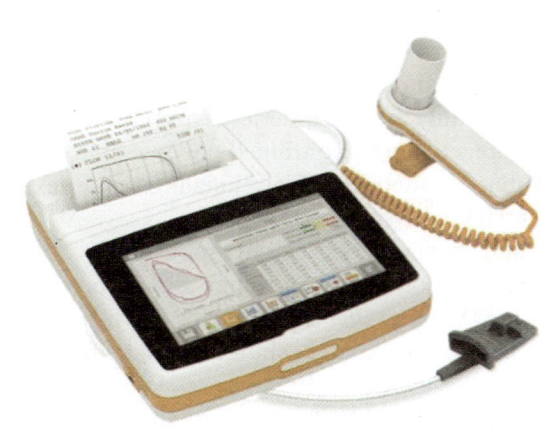

Fig 23.2 **(A)** Recording spirometer (expirograph) (1. Bell of the spirometer; 2. Paper speed selector; 3. Paper; 4. Pilot lamp; 5. On–off (power) switch; 6. Writing pen holder; 7. Expiratory valve; 8. Inspiratory valve; 9. Bidirectional valve tap; 10. Bell supporter; 11. Pulley) **(B)** computerised spirometer (Spirolab). Note that the mouthpiece is connected to the spirometer, which has a display screen and auto-printing facility.

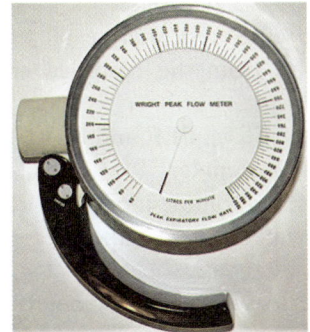

Fig. 23.4   Wright's peak flow meter

3. Adjust the speed of the spirometer at 60 mm/min.
4. Place a sterilized mouthpiece in the subject's mouth in such a way that the mouthpiece remains fitted between the teeth and the lips.

5. Connect the mouthpiece to the spirometer.
6. Close the nostrils with the help of a nose clip.
7. Ask the subject to breathe in and out normally through the mouth; this is the **tidal volume**.
8. Ask the subject to breathe in as much as possible after a normal expiration, this is the **IRV**. Then, also record a few normal breaths after that.
9. Ask the subject to exhale as much as he can after a normal inspiration to record **ERV** and record a few normal breaths afterwards.
10. Ask the subject to breathe out forcefully with maximum effort after taking a deep inspiration. This records **VC**.
11. Calculate TV, IRV, ERV, VC, and IC from these recordings (height 1 mm = 30 mL) as depicted in Fig. 23.1.

Timed vital capacity (FEV$_1$)

1. Ask the subject to sit comfortably and place the mouthpiece and nose clip as described above.
2. Record a few normal tidal respirations by asking the subject to take quiet breaths at 60 mm/min speed of the spirometer.
3. Ask the subject to **take maximum inspiration** and hold his breath. Immediately change the speed of the spirometer to 1200 mm/min and ask him to exhale as rapidly and as forcefully as he can to record timed vital capacity.
4. Repeat the procedure three times and note the best reading.
5. Calculate FEV$_1$ from the obtained recording.

Calculation of FEV$_1$: To calculate FEV$_1$, draw a vertical line from the top of the beginning of the curve, and take 20 mm (=1 sec) from its base to the right to check at what percentage it intersects the curve (Fig. 23.6). Similarly, calculate FEV$_2$, FEV$_3$, and FEV$_4$ by intersecting the curve with vertical lines at every 20 mm.

Calculation of FEF$_{25-75\%}$: Divide the FEV$_1$ curve (Fig. 23.1) into four equal parts. Draw a horizontal line from the 25% mark and a vertical line from the 75% mark and mark the point where the two lines intersect. The horizontal limb denotes time (T), and the vertical limb denotes volume (V).

Maximum voluntary ventilation

1. Ask the subject to sit comfortably.
2. Connect the mouthpiece of the Douglas bag to the subject's mouth.
3. Ask the subject to breathe as deeply (inhale to maximum) and as rapidly as he can **for 15 seconds** into the Douglas bag.
4. Measure the air collected in the Douglas bag with the help of a gas volume meter and multiply the volume by 4 to derive the MVV.

Alternative method: MVV can also be calculated by recording FEV1 in a spirometer and multiplying the value by 38. This gives an approximate value of MVV.

Peak expiratory flow rate

1. Ask the subject to sit comfortably.
2. Connect a Wright's peak flow meter to the subject's mouth.
3. Ask the subject to inhale maximally and then blow out as fast as he can into the flow meter.
4. Note the reading from the dial of the flow meter.
5. Repeat the procedure a minimum of three times at a gap of two minutes each and take the value of the best performance.

Using computerized spirometer: Entire functions are assessed using a computerised spirometer (Fig. 23.3B).

1. Ask the subject to comfortably sit up straight, keeping his feet flat on the floor.
2. Turn on the spirometer switch and ensure that the display screen is visible.
3. Enter the subject's personal data (name, age, gender, height, weight, hospital number) into the spirometer system.
4. Attach a new disposable mouthpiece to the hose/tube of the spirometer.
5. Place the mouthpiece in the subject's mouth in such a way that it remains well-fitted between the teeth and the lips.
6. Close the subject's nostrils with the help of a nose clip.
7. Ask the subject to breathe in maximally and then breathe out forcefully with the maximum effort possible. The expiration be at least for six seconds.
8. Repeat the maneuver three times.
9. Note all lung volumes and capacities **with the predicted values.**

Gas sampling and analysis

Respiratory gas analysis: Gas analyzers show the partial pressure of different gases. Samples of **inspired air** (atmospheric air), **mixed expired air** (from the **Douglas bag**), and **alveolar air** (collected by the Haldane–Priestley method) are taken for the analysis of partial pressure of oxygen, carbon dioxide, and nitrogen.

Blood gas analysis: The oxygen content of blood is determined using **Haldane's gas analysis apparatus.** Arterial and venous blood are collected and sent for analysis by computerised **automated ABG analyzers.** The oxygen-carrying capacity of blood is estimated by the **Van Slyke gasometry method.** The partial pressure of carbon dioxide is also determined with the help of gasometers.

Pulmonary blood flow

Assessment of pulmonary circulation depends upon **measuring pulmonary vascular pressures and cardiac output.** These are usually measured in **intensive care units** with facilities for invasive monitoring. With a flow-directed pulmonary arterial (Swan–Ganz) catheter, the **pulmonary arterial and pulmonary capillary wedge pressures** are measured directly. The **cardiac output** is obtained by the thermodilution method. **Pulmonary vascular resistance (PVR)** is calculated as follows:

$$PVR = \frac{80\,(PAP - PCW)}{CO}$$

Where PAP = mean pulmonary arterial pressure in mmHg, PCW = pulmonary capillary wedge pressure in mmHg, and CO = cardiac output in l/min.

Precautions

1. The subject should be comfortable and relaxed.
2. The apparatus should be sterilised and cleaned properly.
3. The subject should be trained adequately to perform different maneuvers like inhaling and exhaling maximally, and so on.
4. The subject should sit with his spine erect.
5. A minimum of three recordings should be taken for FEV1, MVV, and PEFR at a gap of two minutes each, and the best of the three should be taken for the final reading.
6. For recording of FVC and FEV1, the subject should be encouraged to put his maximum effort to exhale fast and to the maximum extent possible.

Observation and results

Nowadays, all PFT parameters such as lung volumes and capacities, FEV_1, including the flow-volume curve, etc., are recorded by computerised spirometers. Also, **predicted values** are displayed in the screen for comparison of the recorded values with the standard one *matched for age and gender.*

1. Carefully observe and analyse all the lung volumes and capacities from the recorded spirometry graph (Fig. 23.5).
2. Note the FVC, FEV_1, PEF, and FEV_1/FVC, in addition to other PFT parameters.
3. Analyse the flow-volume loop (Fig. 23.5).
4. Provide a printed copy of the recorded PFTs in the subject's hospital case sheet.
5. **Report the results of spirometry** with all the pulmonary function test parameters including all lung volumes and capacities, the expiratory flow–volume curve, and the flow–volume loop, stating whether they are within normal limits (Table 23.1).

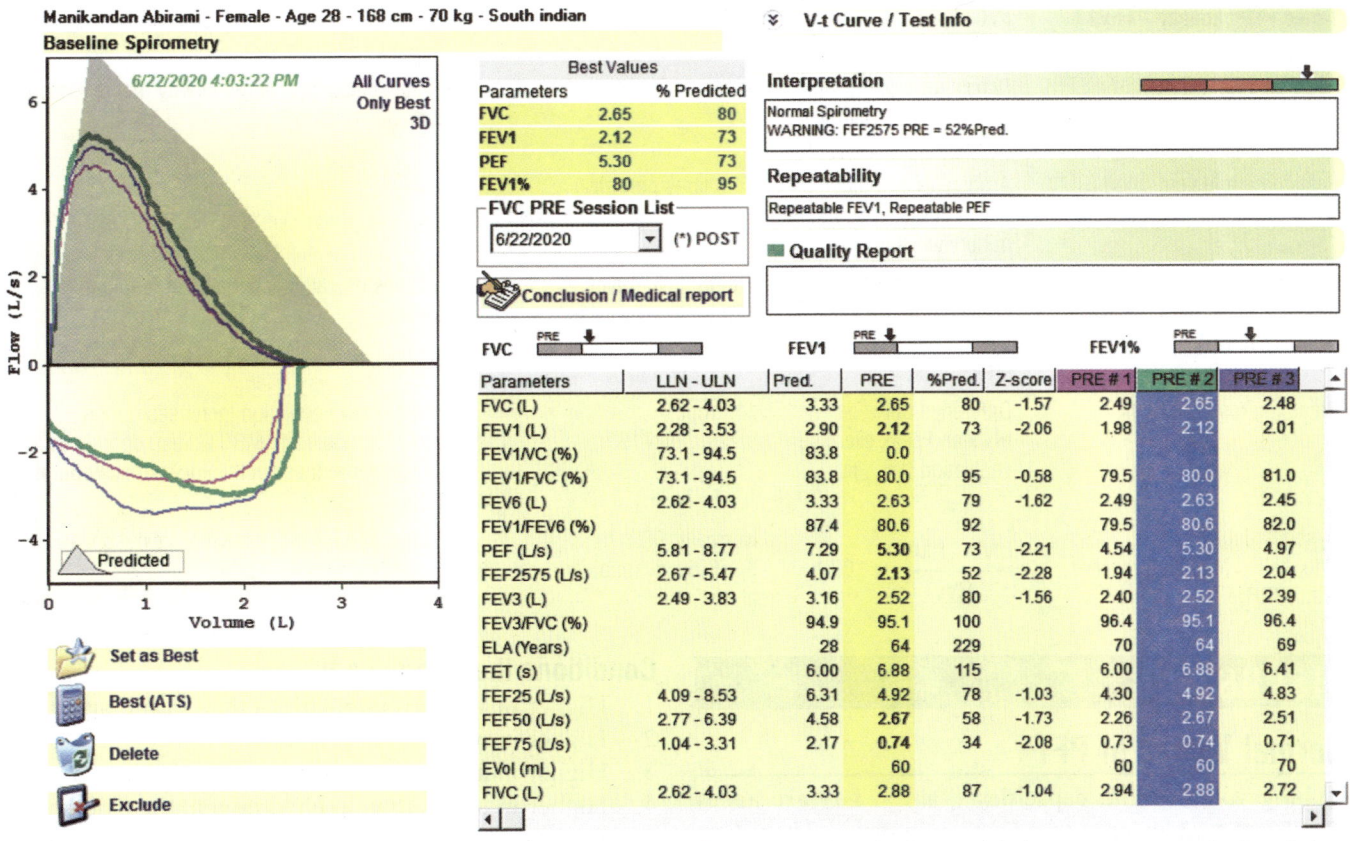

Fig. 23.5   5 PFT parameters recorded by computerised spirometer. Note that the predicted values and their percentages are displayed along with the recorded values.

Table 23.1   Normal values of PFT parameters.

Lung volumes and capacities	Meaning and definition	Normal value	Importance
Tidal volume (TV)	Volume inspired or expired during quiet breathing	500 ml	Represents magnitude of normal breathing; helps in rate calculation
Inspiratory reserve volume (IRV)	Volume maximally inspired above TV	About 3 litres (2.5–3.2 litres)	Lung reserve for utilisation during active efforts such as exercise
Expiratory reserve volume (ERV)	Volume maximally expired after tidal expiration	1.0–1.2 litres	Lung reserve is utilised during deep breathing exercises such as *pranayama*
Residual volume (RV)	Air left in lungs after maximal expiration	1.2 litres	Maintains gas exchange; prevents collapse
Inspiratory capacity	TV + IRV	2.5–3.7 litres	Exercise reserve
Vital capacity (VC)	TV + IRV + ERV	About 4.8 litres in males and 3.2 litres in females	Major PFT parameter for assessing overall respiratory strength; used for recruitment into police, army, etc.
Functional residual capacity	RV + ERV	2.3–2.5 litres	Improves by pranayamic breathing; improves gas exchange
Total lung capacity	VC + RV	About 6 litres	Represents overall lung dimensions, functional lung mass, and respiratory capacity
Forced vital capacity (FVC)	Total volume expired forcefully with greatest force and speed after maximal inspiration	It is almost the same as VC in healthy persons	Reduced in cases of airway obstruction with air trapping

Timed vital capacity – FEV1	FVC expired in first second	>80% of FVC	Detects generalised airway obstruction
Peak expiratory flow rate (PEFR)	Maximum velocity with which air is forced out of lungs	400–600 lit/min	Indicates patency of larger airway; decreases in airway obstruction.
Resting minute ventilation (RMV)	Amount of air breathed in or out of the lungs in one minute while at rest	5–8 litres per min	
Maximum voluntary ventilation (MVV) or maximum breathing capacity (MBC)	Maximum volume of air breathed out per minute by maximum voluntary effort	150 l/min in males 125 l/min in females	Expresses overall functionality of respiratory apparatus
Breathing reserve (BR)	Difference between MVV and peak exercise ventilation (VE_{max})	11 l/min; greater than 15%	Indicates how ventilation increases during exercise compared to MBC at rest; decreased BR indicates reduced ventilatory capacity during exercise
Dyspneic index (DI) also, called breathing reserve ratio (BRR)	$\dfrac{MVV - RMV}{MVV} \times 100$	Normally, 90% If <60%, dyspnea occurs at rest	Indicates presence and severity of dyspnea

DISCUSSION

Normal Values of PFT

All lung volumes and capacities (Table 23.1) are about 15–25 per cent lower in females than in males. The values may be higher in athletes and tall persons and lower in non-athletes and asthenic persons.

Lung volumes and capacities

Lung volumes and capacities show a wide range of values in the normal population depending on the age, sex, and height of the subject. The Indian population shows significantly lower values than their Western counterparts. *Predicted normograms* are available based on these variable factors (Fig. 23.5). Deviations up to 20% from the predicted value for a given age, sex, and height are commonly seen in normal subjects (Table 23.1).

Vital Capacity

Conditions that decrease VC

1. Loss of functioning lung tissue
   - Interstitial pulmonary fibrosis
   - Chest deformity
   - Neuromuscular disease
   - Thickened pleura
2. Loss of distensibility of lung tissues or pleura
   - Atelectasis
   - Consolidation
   - Pulmonary edema
   - Pulmonary resection

Conditions that increase VC

1. Higher in Western populations than in Indians
2. Higher in males
3. Higher in athletes compared to non-athletes
4. Higher in adults than in children and the elderly
5. Increases in the standing posture as compared to the supine and sitting postures; there is no pathological condition in which VC increases

Mechanics of Breathing

Static lung compliance

Static lung compliance decreases in:
1. Pulmonary edema
2. Chronic pulmonary congestion
3. Kyphoscoliosis
4. Fibrothorax
5. Interstitial fibrosis
6. Atelectasis

Patients with decreased compliance have to put in more respiratory muscular effort to achieve adequate alveolar ventilation. Therefore, they are very often dyspneic.

Airway resistance

Airway resistance increases in the following conditions:
1. Bronchial asthma
2. Chronic bronchitis
3. Emphysema
4. Other diseases that are characterised by airway obstruction

Patients with increased airway resistance are often dyspneic, and dyspnea depends on the severity of airway obstruction.

Forced vital capacity (FVC)

FVC decreases in conditions in which there is obstruction to the airways resulting in air trapping, e.g., bronchial asthma.

Timed vital capacity (FEV$_1$)

FEV$_1$ is the single most useful test to **detect generalised airway obstruction**. However, it should be performed properly, as it is effort-dependent. FEV$_1$ is not specific for small airway obstruction. It **decreases in obstructive diseases** of the lung, e.g., bronchial asthma.

Obstructive lung diseases: Obstructive lung diseases are characterised by *reduction in airflow*, which manifests as **reduced FEV$_1$** and FEV$_1$/FVC less than the 5th percentile of the predicted value. FEV$_1$ decreases in asthma, emphysema, chronic bronchitis, bronchiectasis, and cystic fibrosis.

Restrictive lung diseases: Restrictive lung diseases are characterised by **reduction in lung volume**, specifically TLC less than the 5th percentile of the predicted value. **Both FEV$_1$ and FVC are low.** FEV$_1$/FVC is normal or increased. Restrictive lung diseases occur due to the following:

1. **Extrapulmonary causes** of restrictive lung diseases are severe obesity, kyphoscoliosis, and neuromuscular disorder.
2. **Interstitial lung diseases** causing restrictive lung disease include acute respiratory distress syndrome (ARDS), pneumoconiosis, sarcoidosis, and idiopathic pulmonary fibrosis.

The **severity** of spirometric abnormalities based on FEV1 (FEV$_1$ interpretation of % predicted) is as presented in Table 23.2.

Table 23.2 Severity of spirometric abnormality based on FEV$_1$

FEV$_1$ % pred	Degree of severity
>70%	Mild obstruction
60–69%	Moderate obstruction
50–59%	Moderately severe obstruction
<35–49%	Severe obstruction
<35%	Very severe obstruction

FEV$_1$/FVC

The ratio of FEV$_1$/FVC is approximately **0.75–0.80**. This is a more *sensitive indicator* of airway obstruction than FVC or FEV$_1$ alone.

Interpretation of absolute value of FEV$_1$/FVC:

1. 80 or higher—Normal
2. 79 or lower—Abnormal

MMEFR (FEF$_{25–75\%}$)

This is one of the **most sensitive indicators of patency of the small airways**. It slows down in diseases that cause small airway obstruction.

FEF$_{200–1200\ ml}$

This is the flow rate between 200 and 1200 ml of FVC. FEF$_{200–1200\ ml}$ is one of the most **sensitive indicators of patency of the larger airways**. It is slower in diseases that cause large airway obstruction.

PEFR

As it measures peak expiratory flow rate during peak expiration, PEFR **decreases in airway obstruction**. MMEFR and FEF200–1200 ml are better indicators and more sensitive than PEFR.

MVV

The normal value is about **150 l in adult males and 125 l in adult females**. However, these values can be fallacious if the patient does not cooperate and fails to exert the maximum possible effort to perform the test. MVV decreases in patients with **subjective dyspnea.**

Ventilation–perfusion relationship

Perfusion is affected in diseases like pulmonary embolism and diseases with destruction of lung tissue. The arterial blood gas tension is primarily affected by the relationship of ventilation with perfusion. The normal **ventilation–perfusion ratio is 0.8**. Alteration in this ratio affects PaO$_2$ more than PaCO$_2$.

Diffusion

The **pulmonary diffusing capacity decreases** during the following circumstances:

1. When the total *surface area of the alveolar capillary membrane is reduced*, as in:
   - Emphysema
   - Pulmonary embolism
   - Thrombosis of pulmonary capillaries
   - Following surgical removal of lung tissues
2. When there is a *defect in the membrane* (thickening of the membrane), as in:
   - Asbestosis
   - Sarcoidosis
   - Progressive systemic sclerosis
   - Collagen diseases
   - Interstitial edema
   - Interstitial fibrosis
   - Diffuse metastatic lesions of the lung

The **pulmonary diffusing capacity increases** in exercise.

Disturbance in Pulmonary Circulation

Pulmonary vascular resistance (PVR) is *increased by different mechanisms:*

1. Pulmonary arterial or arteriolar vasoconstriction in response to alveolar hypoxia increases PVR.
2. Intraluminal thrombi in pulmonary vessels decrease the luminal cross-sectional area and increase PVR.

3. Proliferation of the smooth muscle within the vessel wall decreases the luminal cross-sectional area and increases PVR.

4. Destruction of small pulmonary vessels either by scarring or by loss of alveolar wall, decreases the total cross-sectional area of the pulmonary vascular bed and increases PVR.

When PVR increases, the pulmonary arterial pressure rises; this decreases the right ventricular output.

PVR increases in the following conditions:

1. Cardiac conditions that elevate left atrial pressure, such as mitral stenosis
2. Chronic pulmonary hypoxemia
   - COPD (chronic obstructive pulmonary diseases)
   - Interstitial lung disease
   - Chest wall diseases, e.g., kyphoscoliosis
   - Obesity hypoventilation
   - Sleep apnea syndrome
3. Diseases affecting pulmonary vessels
   - Recurrent pulmonary embolism
   - Scleroderma (occludes small pulmonary arteries and arterioles)

Restrictive and Obstructive Lung Diseases

Commonly, two major patterns of abnormal ventilatory functions of the lung are encountered—restrictive and obstructive lung disease. In **obstructive diseases**, the hallmark of dysfunction is the **decrease in expiratory flow rates**, particularly the MMEFR and FEV_1/FVC. The hallmark of **restrictive diseases** is the **reduction in FVC** (Fig. 23.6).

In **obstructive diseases**, FEV_1 decreases as there is **obstruction to the outflow** of air from the lung, but TLC remains normal (TLC may increase due to air trapping).

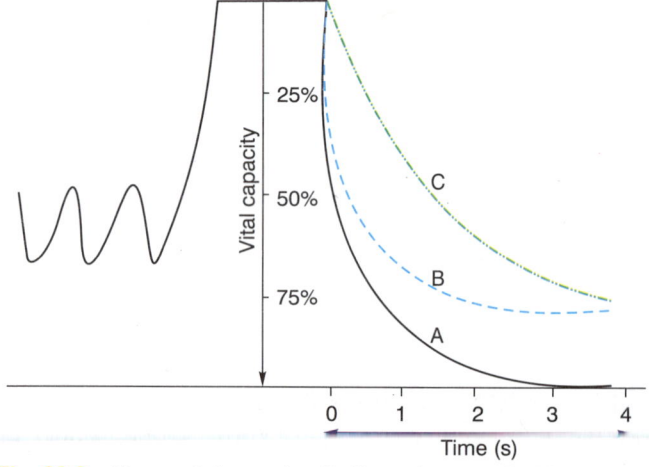

Fig. 23.6   Times vital capacity (**A:** Normal pattern [>80% expired in first second}; **B:** Restricted pattern [total vital capacity is less, but FEV_1 as per cent of FVC is normal]; **C:** Obstructive pattern [FEV_1 is grossly reduced, even FEV_4 is less than 80%])

In **restrictive lung diseases**, TLC is decreased as there is a **problem in lung expansion** but FEV_1 remains normal (as per cent of FVC) as there is no obstruction to the outflow of air from the lung.

Obstructive diseases

The **features of a restrictive pattern** are:
1. TLC is normal or increased.
2. RV is elevated due to trapping of air during expiration.
3. Ratio of RV/TLC is increased.
4. VC is frequently decreased (not due to decreased lung volumes but due to increased RV).
5. FEV_1 is less than 80 per cent of FVC.
6. FEV_1/FVC decreases.
7. MMEFR decreases.

In the early phase of obstruction, which originates in the small airways, FEV_1/FVC may be normal, but **decrease in MMEFR** and an *abnormal configuration* in the terminal portion of forced expiratory flow–volume curve may indicate the presence of the disease.

Restrictive diseases

The **hallmarks of a restrictive pattern** are:
1. Decreased TLC
2. Decreased VC
3. Decreased RV
4. Normal preservation of forced expiratory flow rates, especially *FEV_1 expressed as percentage of FVC.*

The restrictive diseases can be broadly subdivided into **parenchymal and extraparenchymal** disease. Extraparenchymal dysfunction is again of two kinds—extraparenchymal dysfunction in inspiration and extraparenchymal dysfunction in inspiration plus expiration.

■ Restrictive parenchymal dysfunction
1. Decreased TLC
2. Decreased RV
3. Decreased VC
4. Normal or increased FEV_1/FVC

■ Restrictive extraparenchymal dysfunction
1. **Inspiratory dysfunction:** In extraparenchymal inspiratory dysfunction, which usually occurs due to *inspiratory muscle weakness* or a *stiff chest wall*, the adequate distending forces are prevented from being exerted on an otherwise normal lung. Therefore, **TLC is reduced but RV is not affected,** and expiratory flow rates are preserved.
2. **Inspiratory plus expiratory dysfunction:** This usually occurs in *expiratory muscle weakness* or *due to a deformed chest wall,* which is abnormally rigid at lung volumes below FRC. Therefore, **RV is**

often significantly elevated. The ratio of FEV_1/FVC may be affected depending on the strength of the expiratory muscles.

Simple Bedside PFTs

Some lung function tests can be performed at the bedside of the patient. These include: i) chest expansion, ii) breath holding time, iii) respiratory endurance test, iv) expiratory blast test, and v) Snider test.

1. **Chest expansion:** With the help of a measuring tape, measure the chest expansion at the mid-level of the chest, just below the level of the nipples. Normally, the chest expands by 5–10 cm following a deep inspiration taken after a forceful expiration.

2. **Breath-holding time:** Ask the subject to hold their breath after a deep inspiration and note the breath-holding time. Refer to Chapter 21 for details.

3. **Respiratory endurance test:** Disconnect the rubber tube from the blood pressure apparatus. Ask the subject to take a deep breath, pinch his nostrils, and exhale into the tube, *raising the pointer to 40 mm level and to hold it* there for as long as possible. This is also called the **40 mmHg test.**
    Normal value: 40–70 seconds or more.

4. **Expiratory blast test:** Using the same procedure as the respiratory endurance test described above, ask the subject to take a deep breath and then raise the *pointer column to as high a level as possible*. A healthy person can raise the pointer column to 55–100 mm or more during a single forceful expiration.

5. **Snider's test:** Hold a *burning matchstick* about 12 inches in front of the subject's face and **ask him to blow it** out with a single forceful expiration. If he succeeds, his lung functions are normal.

Special PFTs

Apart from spirometry, the following special tests are conducted to detect lung problems.

1. **Lung volume test:** This is also called **body plethysmography**. It is the *most accurate way* to measure the amount of air a person's lungs can hold. It also measures the amount of air that remains in the lungs after the subject exhales as much as he can.

2. **Lung diffusion capacity test:** This test measures how the lungs deliver oxygen to the blood from the air inhaled.

3. **Exercise tests:** There are different types of tests that measure how well the lungs work when a person is most active, including:
    *   Six-minute walk test
    *   Cardiopulmonary (heart and lung) exercise test (CPET)

4. **Plain chest X-ray:** Very useful in providing the integrity of lung parenchyma and its general vascularity.

5. **Bronchoscopy:** Under local anesthesia support, a fibreoptic (flexible) bronchoscope is introduced through the nose or mouth, through the larynx and the trachea, into the bronchial tree. This allows direct visualisation of the insides of the trachea and lower bronchial passages. A biopsy of any growth inside can also be obtained through bronchoscopy.

6. **Other special tests:** Tests like computerized axial tomography (CAT, or CT scan), magnetic resonance imaging (MRI), methacholine challenge test, pulmonary hypertension tests, etc., are also used to determine lung function.

Uses of PFTs

1. Assist in the diagnosis of respiratory diseases.
2. Help in monitoring the efficiency of treatment.
3. Help in monitoring the progress of the disease.
4. Help in monitoring the efficacy of physical training.
5. Help in studying the prevalence of respiratory diseases in the community or respiratory industrial hazards.
6. Help in evaluating the respiratory fitness of the patient for general anesthesia prior to surgery.
7. Assist in medicolegal cases to decide fitness or amount of compensation.
8. Used in the evaluation of lung functions in research.

OSPE

I. Record the vital capacity of the given subject by using recording spirometer.

Steps

1. Ask the subject to sit comfortably with an erect spine.
2. Check that the bell of the spirograph is filled up to three-fourths of its capacity with air.
3. Adjust the speed of the spirometer at 60 mm/min.
4. Place the mouthpiece in the subject's mouth in such a way that it remains between the teeth and the lips.
5. Connect the mouthpiece to the spirometer.
6. Instruct the subject to breathe in and out quietly through the mouth to record tidal volume.
7. Ask the subject to exhale as much as he can immediately following a deep inspiration.

II. Record the FEV_1 of the given subject and report your findings.

Steps

1. Ask the subject to sit comfortably with an erect spine.
2. Check that the bell of the spirograph is filled up to three-fourths of its capacity with air.
3. Adjust the speed of the spirometer at 60 mm/min.
4. Place the mouthpiece into the mouth of the subject in such a way that the mouthpiece remains between the teeth and the lips.

5. Connect the mouthpiece to the spirometer.
6. Instruct the subject to breathe in and out quietly through the mouth to record a few tracings of tidal volume.
7. Ask the subject to take a deep breath and hold it.
8. Immediately change the speed of the spirometer to 1200 mm/min and ask the subject to exhale to the maximum and as rapidly as possible.
9. Switch off the spirometer as soon as FEV_1 is recorded.

VIVA

1. *What are the uses of pulmonary function tests?* (Ans. Refer to page 147, under the heading 'Uses of PFTs'.)
2. *Classify PFTs and name different PFTs under each category.* (Ans. Refer to page 136, under the heading 'Classification of PFTs'.)
3. *What are lung volumes and capacities? Define each and give their normal values.* (Ans. Refer to Table 23.1, on page 143.)
4. *Define vital capacity. What is the normal value of vital capacity in males and females and why is there a difference?* (Ans. Refer to page 137, see 'Lung capacities'.)
5. *Define residual volume. What is its normal value?* (Ans. Refer to page 137, under the heading 'Lung volumes', point no. 4.)
6. *What is the significance of functional residual capacity? How is it determined? In what condition is it altered?*
   (Ans. FRC maintains a constant RV and at the same time, allows continuous exchange of gases in both phases of respiration. It checks any sudden fall in partial pressure of gases in the blood. It is measured by the helium dilution and nitrogen washout methods. FRC increases in conditions in which air trapping occurs, such as asthma, emphysema and so on.)
7. *What are the tests that determine the mechanics of breathing (compliance and airway resistance)?* (Ans. Refer to page 138, under the heading 'Assessment of mechanical Breathing' and the subheadings 'Compliance' and 'Airway resistance'.)
8. *What is timed vital capacity and what is its significance?* (Ans. Refer to page 138, under the heading 'Dynamic lung volumes and capacities', read point no. 1.)
9. *What is maximum mid-expiratory flow rate (MMEFR) and what is its significance?* (Ans. Refer to page 138, see 'Dynamic lung volumes and capacities', point no. 2.)
10. *What is maximum voluntary ventilation (MVV) and what is its normal value?* (Ans. Refer to page 138, see 'Dynamic lung volumes and capacities', point no. 3.)
11. *What is breathing reserve and what is its significance?* (Ans. Refer to page 139, under the heading 'Dynamic lung volumes and capacities', point no. 3.)
12. *What is dyspneic index and what is its significance?* (Ans. Refer to page 139, under the heading 'Dynamic lung volumes and capacities', no. 3. MVV, read 'Dyspneic index'.)
13. *Define peak expiratory flow rate (PEFR) and give its normal value.* (Ans. Refer to page 148, no. 4, PEFR.)
14. *Draw the maximum expiratory flow–volume curve (MEFVC) and flow-volume loop and explain their significance.* (Ans. Refer to page 148, see no. 5, MEFVC.)
15. *Name the tests to assess diffusion. Give the normal values of arterial tension of oxygen and CO_2.* (Ans. Refer to page 139, under the heading text under the heading 'Diffusion'.)
16. *What are the precautions for recording of PFTs?* (Ans. Refer to page 142, see 'Precautions'.)
17. *Why are most of the parameters of PFT recorded at least three times and the best of three noted?*
    (Ans. Most of the recording of PFTs are effort-dependent; maximal effort should be applied by the subject during the maneuvers. Adequate instructions are given to bring out the maximum effort from the subject. Hence, recordings are taken at least three times, and the best of them is considered.)
18. *Name the conditions in which vital capacity decreases and increases.* (Ans. Refer to page 144, see 'Vital capacity'.)
19. *Name the conditions in which FEV1 decreases.* (Ans. Refer to page 145, under the heading 'Timed Vital capacity'.)
20. *Why is the ratio of FEV1/FVC a better indicator of obstruction than the FEV1 and FVC alone?*
    Ans. The ratio of FEV1/FVC is a better indicator of airway obstruction than FVC or FEV1 alone. Therefore, FEV1/FVC is calculated for the purpose. FEV1/FVC of 80 or above is normal.
21. *What are the differences between restrictive and obstructive lung diseases? How do you differentiate between these two patterns?* (Ans. Refer to page 145, under the heading 'Restrictive and obstructive lung disease', and the subheadings 'Obstructed disease' and 'Restrictive disease'.)
22. *What are the diagnostic hallmarks of obstructive lung disease?* (Ans. Refer to page 145, under the heading 'Obstructive disease'.)
23. *What are the two subcategories of restrictive extraparenchymal dysfunction? Name one test to differentiate between these two dysfunctions.*

(Ans. The two subcategories of restrictive extraparenchymal dysfunctions are inspiratory dysfunction and inspiratory plus expiratory dysfunction. In extraparenchymal **inspiratory dysfunction**, due to **inspiratory muscle weakness**, adequate distending forces are prevented from being exerted on an otherwise normal lung. Therefore, TLC is **reduced but RV is not affected**, and expiratory flow rates are preserved. In **inspiratory plus expiratory dysfunction**, due to **expiratory muscle weakness or due to deformed chest wall**, which is abnormally rigid at lung volumes below FRC, **RV is often significantly elevated**. The ratio of FEV1/FVC may be affected depending on the strength of the expiratory muscles. Therefore, recording of **residual volume mainly differentiates** these two restrictive extraparenchymal dysfunctions.)

24. *Name the tests to detect the abnormalities of pulmonary circulation.* (Ans. Refer to page 145, under the heading 'Pulmonary blood flow'.)
25. *What are the mechanisms of increased pulmonary vascular resistance?* (Ans. Refer to page 145, under the heading 'Disturbance in pulmonary circulation'.)
26. *Name the diseases in which pulmonary vascular resistance increases.* (Ans. Refer to page 146, under the heading 'Disturbance in Pulmonary Circulation' and the subheading 'PVR increases in...'.)
27. *What are the lung volumes and capacities that cannot be recorded by a simple spirometer?*
    (Ans. RV, FRC, and TLC cannot be recorded by a simple spirometer.)
28. *What is the breathing reserve ratio? What is its clinical significance?* (Ans. Refer to page 139, under the heading subheading '3. MVV', and the point on 'Breathing reserve ratio'.)
29. *What is minute ventilation? What is its normal value?* (Ans. Refer to page 138, under the heading 'Lung volumes' and subheading '1. Tidal volume', read 'Minute ventilation'.)
30. *What is $FEF_{200-1200}$ ml? What is its significance?* (Ans. Refer to page 138, see 'Dynamic lung volumes and capacities', and the subheading '2. MMEFR.... $FEF_{200-1200}$ ml'.)
31. *Name the bedside PFTs. Explain the Snider Test.* (Ans. Refer to page 147, under the heading 'Simple bedside PFTs'... the last one is Snider Test).
32. *Name the Special PFTs. Explain the importance of body plethysmography.* (Ans. Refer to page 147, under the heading 'Special PFTs' and the subheading 'Lung volume test'.)
33. *What is effort independent expiratory flow, and what is its significance?*
    (Ans. The term effort-independence was coined to describe the phenomenon of **expiratory flow limitation**. It states that there is a limit to maximal expiratory flow at a given lung volume, such that pressures in excess of the lowest pressure necessary to produce maximal flow do not increase the flow. As the lung volume decreases, airways start to narrow, and a point is reached where even greater effort from expiratory muscles does not lead to higher air flow. Thus, flowrate is also a function of lung volume rather than only the effort exerted.)

24 | Cardiopulmonary Resuscitation

Learning Objectives

After completing this practical, you will be able to:

1. Explain the meaning of cardiopulmonary resuscitation (CPR).
2. List the indications for CPR.
3. List the objectives of CPR.
4. List the measures for basic life support.
5. Describe the procedure for mouth-to-mouth breathing and external cardiac massage.
6. List the measures for advanced life support.

PY11.14: Demonstrate basic life support in a simulated environment.

INTRODUCTION

Cardiopulmonary resuscitation (CPR) is the **supportive and specific treatment given immediately to patients in whom, for some reason, the cardiac and the ventilatory activities**. CPR is given in an acute medical emergency that requires adequate life-saving procedures to restart and preserve circulation and ventilation. Therefore, CPR should be carried out by a well-trained and experienced team.

Cardiopulmonary cerebral resuscitation: CPR is also called as **CPCR** (cardiopulmonary cerebral resuscitation) because its primary aim is not only the *re-establishment of circulation and respiration*, but also the **preservation of neurologic function**, especially the brain function, following an arrest. Since its inception in the late 1800's, CPCR has saved the lives of countless human and veterinary patients. However, low overall survival rates following CPCR indicate that there is still much room for improvement in these practices.

Objectives of CPR

1. To **provide adequate pulmonary ventilation** so that the partial pressure of oxygen in the arterial blood is maintained.
2. To **facilitate the pumping of the heart** so that effective circulation is maintained.

Indications for CPR

CPR is indicated in **conditions of cardiorespiratory arrest**. The common situations that can lead to cardiorespiratory arrest include:

1. Primary cardiac arrhythmias
2. Arrhythmias associated with acute myocardial infarction
3. Electric shock
4. Poisoning
5. Trauma
6. Drowning
7. Pulmonary embolism
8. Muscular relaxation during surgery
9. Anaphylactic shock
10. Head injury
11. Cardiac surgery
12. Cardiac tamponade
13. Acute pulmonary edema
14. Chronic lung disease (rare)

The chief mechanisms responsible for **cardiac arrest** or cessation of heart action are ***cardiac asystole and ventricular fibrillation***.

Diagnosis of Cardiac Arrest

The following are the characteristic features of cardiac arrest:

1. Absence of pulsation of the large arteries
2. Absence of heart beats
3. Gasping movements followed by total arrest of respiration
4. Blood pressure not recordable
5. Dilated pupils, not responding to light
6. Pallor (pale and cold skin) and cyanosis
7. Unconsciousness

METHOD OF PERFORMING CPR

General Plan for CPR

CPR can be divided into two broad supportive measures: **emergency measures and definitive treatments**.

Classically, they are described as **A B C D E F G H I**, administered in two phases (**phase I and phase II**).

A: Airways
B: Breathing
C: Circulation
D: Drugs
E: ECG monitoring
F: Fibrillation treatment (with defibrillator)
G: Gauging for restoration of breathing and circulation
H: Hypothermia
I: ICU Management

The **two phases** of management are:
1. **Phase I:** Emergency measures (basic life support), which consists of **A, B, and C**.
2. **Phase II:** Definitive treatment (advanced life support), which consists of **D, E, F, G, H, and I**.

Phase I: Basic life support

Basic life support should be started immediately. A clear airway and presence of breathing are essential parts of successful resuscitative measures. Unless **adequate ventilation** is achieved, attempts to restore circulation become futile. The following are the **steps to achieving adequate ventilation**:

1. *Assess the responsiveness* of the patient by gently shaking him.
2. *Position the patient* on a firm, flat surface.
3. *Open the mouth* and *remove vomitus, mucus, or debris* if visible.
4. **Head tilt–chin lift maneuver**—to extend the neck, place the palm of one hand on the patient's forehead and apply firm pressure to tilt the head backwards. At the same time, place the palm of the other hand under the chin to support it (*head tilt–chin lift maneuver*). This *raises the tongue* away from the spine and **opens up the airway**.

   To **ventilate the lungs**, perform any of the following *three maneuvers: mouth-to-mouth* breathing, which is performed on adults; *mouth-to-nose* breathing, which is preferred for infants and children; and the *Holger Nielsen method*, which is usually not performed unless there are respiratory problems as seen in drowning.
5. **Mouth-to-mouth respiration** (Fig. 24.1):
   - Clear the airway.
   - Extend the neck.
   - Close the patient's nostrils by pinching the nose with the thumb and the index finger of the right hand.
   - Take a deep breath.
   - Apply your mouth close to the patient's mouth and exhale forcefully into the subject's mouth.
   - Look for chest expansion and abdominal distension.

   - Repeat and maintain the breathing at a rate of 10–15 breaths per minute.
6. **Mouth-to-nose respiration:** This method is most **suitable for children**. The steps are the same as those of mouth-to-mouth respiration except that the patient's mouth is closed and the rescuer breathes into the patient's nostrils.
7. **Manual manipulation of the thorax (Holger–Nielsen method** or back pressure–arm lift method):
   - Lay down the patient in prone position.
   - Abduct the arms at the shoulder and flex the elbows.
   - Turn the head to one side so that it is resting on the hands.
   - Kneel down with one knee near the patient's head.
   - Hold the patient's arm and straighten yourself to raise the subject's arm until resistance is felt. The details are demonstrated in Fig. 24.2A–C.

> **Note:** During this maneuver, the patient's thorax expands, intrathoracic pressure drops, and inspiration takes place.

   - Then, gently drop the patient's arm.
   - Place your hands with fingers spread apart on the patient's back, in the midaxillary space, and slightly compress to produce expiration (Fig. 24.2D and E).
   - Repeat the whole cycle 10–12 times per minute.
   - Palpate the carotid pulse.

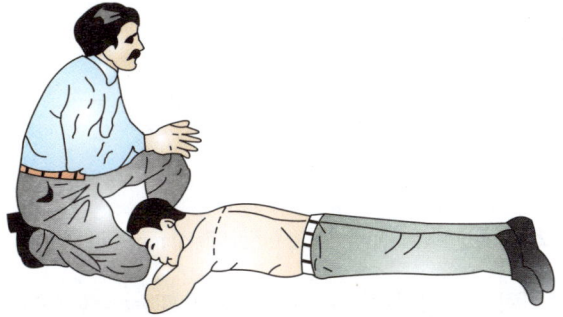

(A) Place the patient face down, elbows bent, one hand on the other with the face turned to one side.

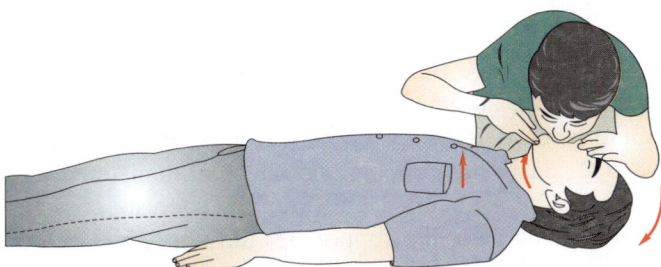

Fig. 24.1   Proper method of opening the airway with the head tilted and chin lifted to administer mouth-to-mouth respiration.

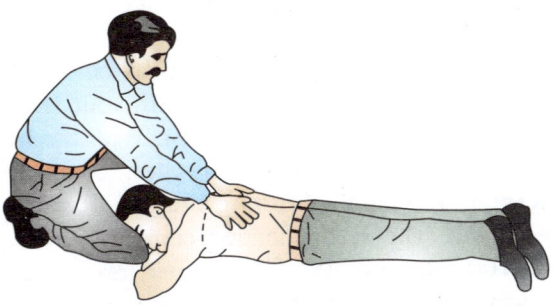

(B) Place your hands, thumbs touching, just below a line running between the armpits.

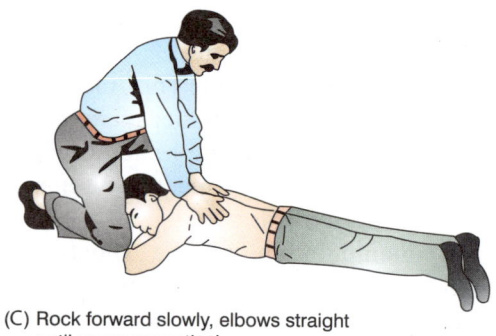

(C) Rock forward slowly, elbows straight until arms are vertical.

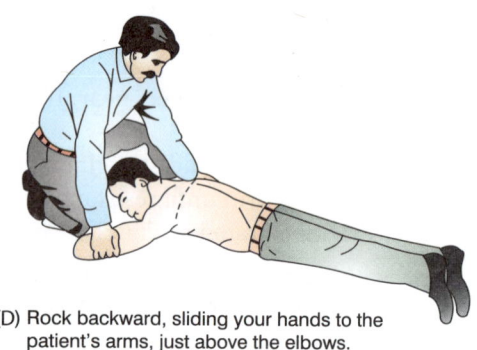

(D) Rock backward, sliding your hands to the patient's arms, just above the elbows.

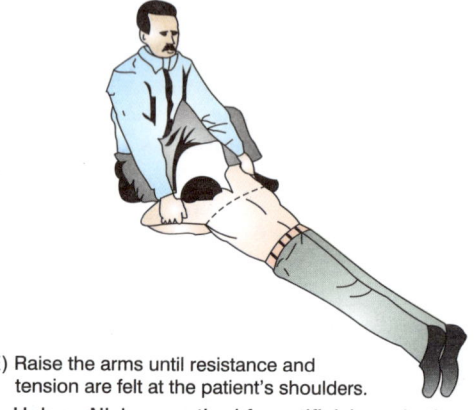

(E) Raise the arms until resistance and tension are felt at the patient's shoulders.

Fig. 24.2 Holger–Nielsen method for artificial respiration.

Note: Palpation for at least 10 seconds is recommended to ensure that slow, irregular, or very weak pulses are not missed.

8. **External cardiac massage:** If the carotid pulse is not felt, perform external cardiac massage (Fig. 24.3). If the patient is in bed, place a hard board under him. Position the patient's hands about 3 cm above the xiphoid process and to the left, with your shoulders vertically above the patient's chest. With the **heel of the hand** and the fingers on the chest, **compress the sternum 4–5 cm** by thrusting straight down towards the spine. The recommended **compression rate is 80–100 per minute**. The rescuer responsible for airway management should assess the adequacy of

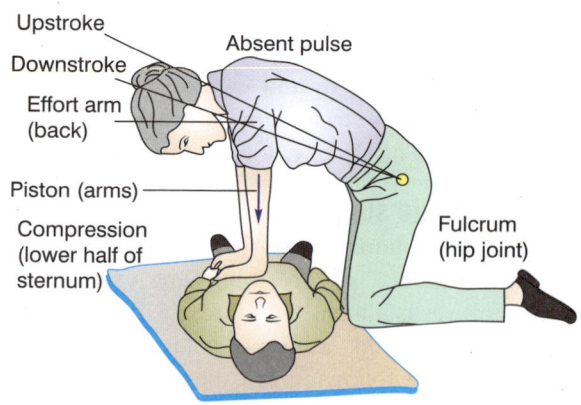

Upstroke
Downstroke
Effort arm (back)
Absent pulse
Piston (arms)
Compression (lower half of sternum)
Fulcrum (hip joint)

Fig. 24.3 Proper technique for chest compressions (uses the principle of a lever). Note that the forearm and arm are straight (elbows extended). The recommended compression is 80–100 per minute. Fifteen chest compressions are performed before ventilating twice when there is a single rescuer. The carotids are palpated to detect a pulse every two minutes.

compression by periodically palpating for the carotid pulse. The **compression–ventilation ratio is 5:1**.

9. If pulse returns, ventilation should be continued as required.

Phase II: Advanced life support

Advanced life support comprises **primary and adjunctive therapies**.

▌Primary therapies

Primary therapies for advanced life support include:

1. Defibrillation
2. Airway management and oxygen therapy

Defibrillation: This is one of the ***most important modalities*** of treatment under CPR. It should be started as early as possible. The time between the onset of the arrest and the successful defibrillation is the major determinant of survival in cardiac arrest **due to ventricular fibrillation**. A fibrillating heart cannot pump blood because effective contractions do not occur. Defibrillation ***converts a fibrillation into a flutter or normal rhythm*** so that effective ventricular contractions occur and the heart pumps blood. ***Adrenaline*** (0.5 ml of 1:1000 adrenaline) and ***sodium bicarbonate*** (100 ml of 8% sodium bicarbonate) are administered intravenously.

Airway management and oxygen therapy: ***100% O_2*** should be administered and endotracheal intubation should be carried out by a qualified individual as soon as possible. Basic life support should be administered and continued by a qualified individual as soon as possible. However, the basic life support should not be delayed or interrupted for more than 30 seconds for intubation.

■ Adjunctive therapies

1. **Self-induced cough:** When the arrest is detected before loss of consciousness, *self-induced vigorous coughing* can produce minimum blood flow to the brain, which is required to maintain consciousness temporarily until definitive treatment is initiated.

2. **Precordial thump:** A quickly applied solitary precordial thump may convert ventricular fibrillation or asystole to a normal rhythm.

3. **Atropine sulphate:** Atropine sulphate (**0.5 mg**) is injected *intravenously every 5 minutes* for the treatment of bradycardia. It may also help in the treatment of cardiac asystole.

4. **Sodium bicarbonate:** It is given as *1 mEq/kg intravenously every 10 minutes* for the treatment of cardiac arrest due to hyperkalemia or acidosis.

5. **Pacemakers:** These help patients with problems with abnormal impulse formation. Packing is carried out early during resuscitation in conditions of refractory bradyarrhythmias or persistent asystole (Fig. 24.4 and 24.5).

DISCUSSION

There are different methods to assist ventilation in CPR: the **Sylvester–Brosche method, Drinker's method, Paul–Bunnel method, and Rocking method**, but these are not routinely followed. Despite resuscitative efforts, a patient in a state of cardiac arrest may not recover and regain spontaneous ventilation and circulation. Persistent deep unconsciousness and absence of respiration, reflex response, and pupillary reaction to light suggest cerebral death. In this condition, resuscitative efforts are unproductive.

BCLS training for all: The survival rate after CPR given to patients out of hospital conditions as seen in heart attacks in a public place, road traffic accidents, etc., is very poor. This is chiefly due to delay in institution of CPR and CPR given by unskilled individuals. Therefore, proper basic cardiac lifecare support (BCLS) training that includes CPR should not only be given to the doctors, but also *to all nursing staff, other paramedical staff* like physiotherapists, to *all students, interns and residents* of medical, nursing, and paramedical (Allied Health Science) courses.

Open Chest CPCR

Open chest cardiopulmonary cerebral resuscitation (CPCR) is performed when cardiac arrest is caused by or in association with **pleural space disease** (pneumothorax, pleural effusion, diaphragmatic hernia), **pericardial effusion**, **penetrating injury** resulting in cardiac arrest, or **failure of external cardiac massage or CPR**. Perform external CPCR for 5 minutes and then open the chest if there is little or no evidence of effective circulation. Open chest CPCR has the advantage of allowing the clinician to directly compress the heart and improve stroke volume (**internal cardiac massage**). In addition, opening the chest makes assessment of ventricular filling feasible, aiding in the decision of volume delivery. Open chest CPCR is usually performed in advanced veterinary centres for animals (e.g., pet dogs) having cardiorespiratory arrest.

Other Methods of CPR

1. **Sylvester–Brosche method:** The clinician holds the patient's wrists and lifts the arms upward while bending backwards. This movement expands the chest and induces inspiration. Then, bending forward, the clinician presses the patient's arms firmly against the chest, promoting expiration.

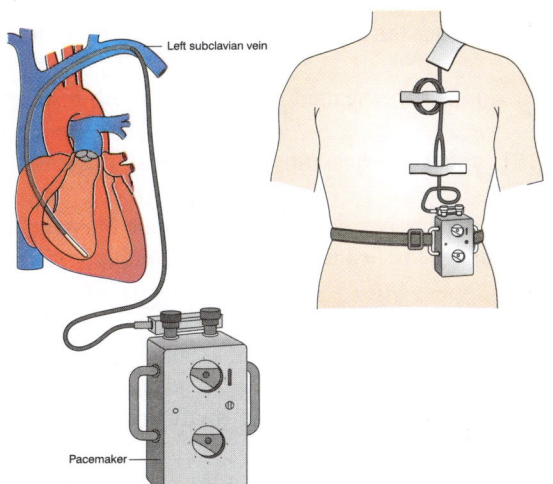

Fig. 24.4 Temporary pacemaker. The transvenous catheter electrode is attached to a battery-powered external pacemaker. The catheter is wedged in the apex of the right ventricle.

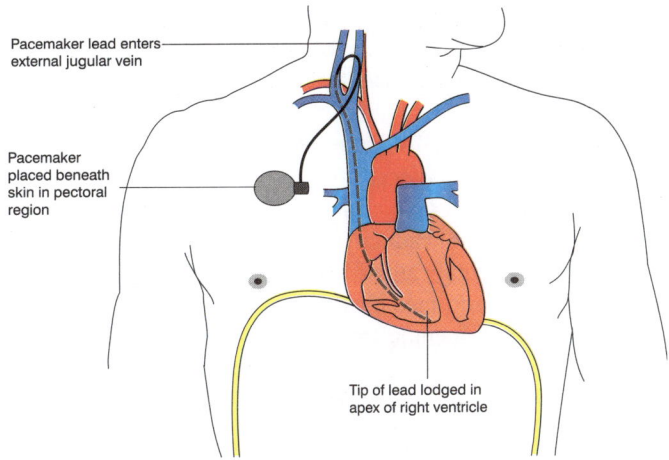

Fig. 24.5 Permanent pacemaker.

2. **Heimlich maneuver:** This maneuver is performed when there is respiratory arrest (choking) caused by an object lodged in the upper respiratory passage. A **person can perform the maneuver on themselves if** they are alone. One hand is rolled into a fist and placed just below the ribcage and about two inches above the navel (thumb side in); the fist is then grasped with the other hand. Then, five quick, forceful inward and upward thrusts are applied through the fist. The thrusts are repeated until the object is dislodged. **When performed on someone else,** the rescuer stands behind the patient, wraps his arms around their abdomen, and delivers sharp upward thrusts below the rib cage to expel the obstruction.

3. **Drinker's method:** Invented in 1929, the **Drinker and Shaw tank-type ventilator** was one of the first *negative-pressure machines* widely used for mechanical ventilation. Better known as the iron lung, this **metal cylinder** completely engulfed the patient up to the neck.

4. **Sahlin's jacket model and Brag–Paul pulsator:** These mechanical ventilators have undergone many modifications. They are *inelastic chest jackets* in which pressure can be increased and decreased at intervals.

5. **Rocking method:** In this technique, the **patient is placed on a stretcher mounted on a central pivot.** The *rhythmic tilting of the stretcher up and down* causes the abdominal organs to shift and helps move the relaxed diaphragm, thereby facilitating inhalation and exhalation.

CPR in Drowning

CPR in cases of drowning requires more expertise and experience. As soon as the patient is brought out of the water, check their carotid pulse and breathing.

1. If **both pulse and breathing are present but the patient is unconscious:** Press on the lower abdomen to expel water from the stomach. Then, place the patient in the 'recovery position', i.e., *partial supine position*, with the head turned to one side, left arm under the left thigh, right arm above the head, and right leg bent.

2. If the **pulse is present, but the victim is not breathing:** Immediately start *mouth-to-mouth breathing* or Holger–Neilson method of artificial respiration.

3. If **both pulse and breaching are absent:** Quickly *start* CPR and continue it until the victim patient recovers or is shifted to the hospital.

VIVA

1. *What is the meaning of cardiopulmonary resuscitation and CPCR?* (Ans. Refer to page 150, under the heading 'Introduction'.)
2. *What are the causes of cardiorespiratory arrest?* (Ans. Refer to page 158, under the heading 'indications'; the list of indications also includes the causes of CPA.)
3. *What are the indications for CPR?* (Ans. Refer to page 150, under the heading 'Indications'.)
4. *What are the signs of cardiac arrest?* (Ans. Refer to page 150, under the heading 'Diagnosis of Cardiac Arrest'.)
5. *What are the objectives of CPR?* (Ans. Refer to page 150, under the heading 'Objectives of CPR'.)
6. *What measures constitute basic life support?* (Ans. Refer to page 151, under the heading 'Basic Life Support' and subheading 'Phase I: ABC of CPR'.)
7. *How is mouth-to-mouth respiration carried out?* (Ans. Refer to page 151, under the heading 'Mouth-to-mouth respiration' and Fig. 24.1.)
8. *How is mouth-to-nose respiration carried out?* (Ans. Refer to page 151, under the heading 'Mouth-to-mouth respiration' and read the subheading 'Mouth-to-nose respiration'.)
9. *What is the Holger–Nielson method of CPR?* (Ans. Refer to page 151, under the heading 'Holger-Nielson Method' and Fig. 24.2.)
10. *How is external cardiac massage carried out?* (Ans. Refer to page 152, under the heading 'External Cardiac Massage'.)
11. *What are the advanced life support measures?* (Ans. Refer to page 152, under the heading 'Advanced Life Support'.)
12. *What is the physiological basis of use of defibrillation in cardiac arrest due to ventricular fibrillation?* (Ans. Refer to page 152, under the heading 'Defibrillation'.)
13. What is internal cardiac massage?
    (Ans. It is performed if cardiac arrest occurs during cardiac surgery or in case of failure of CPR in an advanced centre with provision of opening the chest for internal cardiac massage. The heart is directly compressed rhythmically at a rate of 80/min.)
14. *What is the Paul–Bunnel method of CPR?*
    (Ans. This is an alternative method to assist ventilation. Air tubes are wrapped around the chest and the thorax is rhythmically compressed by forcing air in and out of the tubes.)

15. *What is the rocking method of CPR?*
    (Ans. The patient is laid and strapped down on a stretcher. The stretcher is then rocked up and down 10 times per minute. The movements of the diaphragm stimulate respiration.)
16. *What is the Heimlich maneuver? How is it performed?* (Ans. Refer to page 154, under the heading 'Other Methods....' And subheading 'Heimlich maneuver'.)
17. *What is Drinker's method? What is it used for?* (Ans. Refer to page 154, under the heading 'Other Methods...', and subheading 'Drinker's method'.)
18. *What is the Sylvester–Brosche method? How is it performed?* (Ans. Refer to page 153, under the heading 'Other Methods...' and subheading 'Sylvester–Brosche method'.)
19. *What is open-chest CPCR?* (Ans. Refer to page 153, under the heading 'Open-chest CPCR'.)
20. *How is the CPR performed in cases of drowning?* (Ans. Refer to page 154, under the heading 'CPR in Drowning'.)
21. What are the potential causes of failure of CPR?
    (Ans. Despite best efforts, CPR may sometimes be unsuccessful. Common reasons for failure include:
    1. **Severe injury to vital organs:** Extensive trauma to the heart or lungs—such as a penetrating chest injury—may be too severe to reverse.
    2. **Delayed arrival at the hospital:** When patients reach the emergency unit too late, serious complications like acid-base imbalance (e.g., lactic acidosis) and electrolyte disturbances may have progressed to an irreversible stage.
    3. **Improper CPR at the scene:** Inadequate or incorrect CPR administered at the site of the incident or during transportation can significantly reduce the chances of successful resuscitation.
    4. **Limited resources:** The lack of trained personnel or essential equipment—especially during mass casualty situations—can hinder effective resuscitation efforts.)

25 | Body Composition Analysis, Assessment of BMR, and Energy Cost of Work

Learning Objectives

After completing this practical, you will be able to (MUST KNOW):
1. Understand the importance of assessing body composition and metabolism.
2. State the principle of BIA for the assessment of body composition and metabolism.
3. Define BMR.
4. State the normal value of BMR in males and females.

5. List the conditions necessary for the measurement of BMR.
6. Enumerate the factors that affect the BMR.

You may also be able to (DESIRABLE TO KNOW):
1. Say why measurement of BMR by BIA is a better one.
2. Explain the clinical importance of assessment of body composition and BMR.

BODY COMPOSITION ANALYSIS

INTRODUCTION

Body mass index (BMI), waist circumference (WC), waist-to-hip ratio (WHR), waist-to-height (WhtR), and skin fold thickness have been reported as the predictors of cardiovascular (CV) risk. However, ***body fat (BF) mass, body lean mass,*** and ***body fat mass index*** (BFMI) are better predictors of CV risks.

Body composition is determined by **bioelectrical impedance analysis (BIA)**, a method that involves the measurement of **bioelectrical resistive impedance** (R). This method is regarded as safe and reliable, and based upon the principle that the electrical conductivity of the fat-free tissue mass is far greater than that of fat. Measurements at 5/50/100/200 kHz are obtained using the multiple frequency BIA instrument Bodystat. BIA includes BF, lean body mass, body cell mass (BCM), total body water (TBW), intracellular water (ICW) and extracellular water (ECW). The current range of 50–100 kHz displays BF, BF%, BF mass index (BFMI), lean body mass, basal metabolism (BM), and activity metabolism (AM).

METHODS OF ASSESSING BODY MASS COMPOSITION

Principle

Bioimpedance analysis is based on the principle that the **volume of a conductor** (in the human body, it is the highly conductive body water) is ***proportional to its length and inversely proportional to its electrical resistance***, as defined by the following formula:

$$\text{Volume} = \frac{\rho L^2}{R}$$

Where ρ is the resistivity (ohm cm) of the conductor, L is the conductor length (cm, for whole body measurements in humans; stature is used as a surrogate for unknown true conductive length), and R is the electrical resistance of the conductor (ohm).

BIA devices determine the body composition by **measuring the electrical impedance** of an imperceptible electric current passing through the body. Impedance is a vector composed of two frequency-dependent parameters, **resistance and reactance**. Reactance is a measure of body cell mass and resistance reflects total body water.

Requirements

Equipment: Bodystat Quad Scan 4000, with its accessories (Fig. 25.1)
Accessories: Body stat electrodes
Software: Quad scan 4000 software

Preparation of the subject

1. The subject is instructed to avoid eating or drinking for 4 h prior to the test and to avoid exercise and alcohol for 24 h prior to the test.
2. The subject's hydration status is assessed by clinical examination.
3. It should be ensured that the subject is not wearing any metal objects.

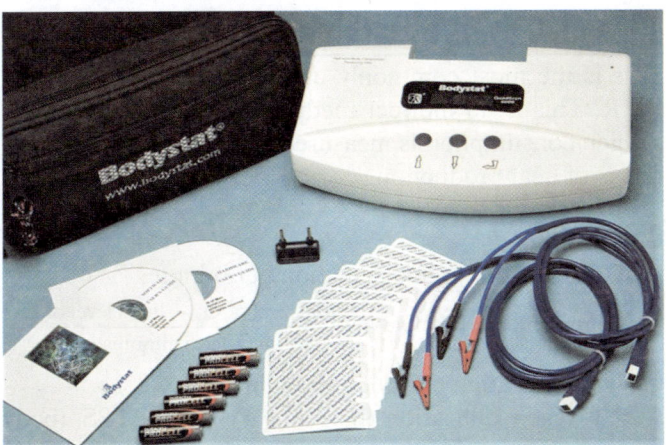

Fig. 25.1   BIA equipment.

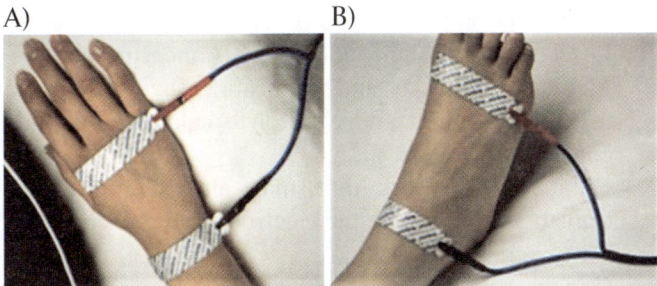

Fig. 25.2   Electrode placements: (A) On the arm and (B) on the leg.

4. The subject is placed in the supine position with no part of the body touching another for at least 10 minutes in standardised conditions (quiet environment and ambient temperature).
5. The electrodes are placed on the dorsal surfaces of the hand and foot, proximal to metacarpal–phalangeal and metatarsal–phalangeal joints respectively.

Laboratory temperature

A thermo-neutral temperature must be maintained in the lab throughout the procedure.

Procedure

1. Obtain the subject's consent.
2. Record his height, weight, and waist and hip circumference as per standard methods (this data to be fed into the machine for analysis).
3. Check that there is sufficient battery power in the machine before starting the procedure by switching on the machine and checking the battery indicator (series of bars on the left of the display).
4. Assess the physical activity of the participant using the International Physical Activity Questionnaire (IPAQ).
5. Clean the area with spirit and cotton before electrode placement.
6. Let the subject lie down in the supine position for 10 minutes. The arms should be abducted from the trunk and both legs should be abducted by placing a rolled blanket or towel (to separate the legs 30° to 40°).
7. Place two signal-introducing electrodes—on the right side on the dorsum of the hand and foot, close to the metacarpal-phalangeal and metatarsal-phalangeal joints respectively (Fig. 25.2A and B).
8. Apply two voltage-sensing electrodes in the pisiform prominence of the wrist and between the medial and lateral malleolus of the ankle (the distance between the electrodes should be 5 cm (Fig. 25.2).

9. Feed all the anthropometric details measured from the subject into the machine.
10. Apply a current of 500 to 800 microamperes with 50 KHz frequency to the body via the cables of the BIA equipment.
11. By measuring the impedance and applying the predictive equations used in the hardware unit, the machine estimates the body composition, and the results are displayed on the LCD screen and stored in the apparatus.

Results

BIA is a simple, inexpensive, quick and non-invasive technique for measuring many body composition parameters. The following results (various parameters) are noted from the LCD screen of the equipment:

1. Body weight (kg)
2. Body cell mass (kg)
3. Body cell mass (%)
4. Extracellular mass (kg)
5. Fat-free mass (%)
6. Body fat (kg)
7. Body mass index (BMI)
8. Body fat mass index (BFMI)
9. Fat-free mass index (FFMI)
10. Phase angle
11. Total body water
12. Extracellular water
13. Intracellular water
14. Third space water
15. Nutritional index
16. Basal metabolism (BM)
17. Active metabolism (AM)
18. BM/BW
19. BM/BF

FACTORS INFLUENCING BIA PARAMETERS

1. Weight and height
2. Position of the body and limbs

3. Consumption of food and beverages
4. Level of physical activity before BIA measurements
5. Medical conditions and medication that are known to influence fluid and electrolyte balance and body composition
6. Cutaneous diseases that may alter the electrical transmission between the electrode and the skin
7. Environmental conditions
8. Gender, age, and skin temperature
9. Ethnicity
10. Technical fault—non-adherence of electrodes, use of wrong electrodes, loosening of cable clip, interchanging of electrodes

BASAL METABOLIC RATE (BMR)

INTRODUCTION

The total energy expenditure of the body is the sum of the energy required to carry out various body activities. Basal metabolism is the lowest level of energy production. Body metabolism is directly linked to **the production of body heat**. The **measurement of heat production under basal conditions is called basal metabolic rate (BMR).** It is measured as kcal/h/m² body surface area (BSA).

For measurement of BMR, the following **basal conditions are required**:
1. Minimum 12 hours of fasting
2. Complete physical and mental rest
3. Comfortable, ambient temperature (about 25°C).

BMR is estimated by measuring the oxygen consumption of the subject for 6 minutes under basal conditions.

Normal values of BMR (in adults)
1. **Males:** 40 kcal/h/m² BSA
2. **Females:** 37 kcal/h/m² BSA
   ±10% is considered to be normal.

METHODS OF MEASURING BMR

BMR is measured by measuring oxygen consumption in the basal state. Oxygen consumption can be measured by three methods: the open-circuit method, the closed-circuit breathing method, and the BIA method.

Open-circuit Method

Expired air is collected in a Douglas bag and then analyzed for carbon dioxide and oxygen content. The difference in the composition of the atmospheric air and the total expired air, when computed, indicates the total oxygen consumption.

Closed-Circuit Breathing Method

This is the most commonly used method for measuring BMR. This is an indirect method in which the subject's oxygen consumption is measured and then translated into forms of heat production.

Calculation

Calculation of oxygen calculation per minute:

$$O_2 \text{ Consumption per minute} = \frac{\text{Initial level of } O_2 - \text{Final level of } O_2}{6 \text{ (after 6 minutes)}}$$

Oxygen utilization per hour (60 min), i.e.,

A = Oxygen utilization in 6 min × 10 at BTPS (body temperature, ambient pressure, saturated with water vapour)

Oxygen utilization at STPD (B) = A × Correction factor

(C) = B × 4.82*

Hence, BMR of the subject = (B × 4.82)/BSA in kcal/h/m²

Refer to the appendix for the BSA nomogram and Du Bois nomogram.

BIA Method

The bioelectrical impedance analysis (BIA) for body composition measures **basal metabolism and active metabolism** and provides the ratio of metabolism to body weight and body fat (BM/BW, BM/BF), which **are more accurate methods** of estimating body metabolism. Presently, BMR is assessed by the BIA method, as described in detail under the heading 'Assessment of Body Composition'.

DISCUSSION
Physiological and Clinical Significance

1. Body composition is required for assessing the **cardiovascular risk** of an individual in many clinical and research settings.
2. Body metabolism and composition are needed for **diagnosing various pathological conditions**, e.g., hypothyroidism and hyperthyroidism.
3. It helps in understanding the **effects of nutrition on the BMR**, which in turn, may help in preparing a dietary plan for a patient.

Factors That Affect the BMR
Factors That increase BMR
1. Obesity
2. Greater muscle mass
3. Greater height (more surface area)
4. Children and young adults

5. Elevated levels of thyroid hormone
6. Stress
7. Fever, illness
8. Male gender
9. Pregnancy and lactation
10. Certain stimulants such as caffeine and tobacco

Factors That Decrease BMR

1. Old age
2. Lower lean body mass
3. Lower height
4. Depressed levels of thyroid hormone
5. Fasting and starvation
6. Female gender

ENERGY COST OF WORK

BACKGROUND

The energy cost of work depends on the number of muscles involved, the duration of the activity, the speed or rate of movement, and the total strength exerted.

Metabolic energy cost of work: Energy cost of work is also called metabolic energy cost of work as metabolism is a major determinant of the energy expenditure or gain. The energy utilised for the basal metabolism of an individual contributes to the energy expenditure during activity.

Energy is continuously utilised in the body. The **rate of energy utilisation** is influenced mainly by **three factors**: i) *basal metabolic rate* (BMR), ii) *physical activity* and iii) the *specific dynamic action of food*.

Measurement of energy cost of work: The *extra amount of oxygen consumed during the performance of work of reasonable severity* is a measure of the energy cost of work.

To assess the energy utilised during a specific activity, it is necessary to know the energy utilized for basal metabolism. **Energy of basal metabolism subtracted from the total energy utilised is calculated from the spirometric record of oxygen consumption obtained after the steady state has been reached during exercise.**

Basic Principle

Metabolic requirements: The metabolic requirements of the body at rest or during exercise are met with by *supplying oxygen to tissues and by removing carbon dioxide* from them. These mechanisms, which operate to maintain metabolic requirements, are primarily *governed by the respiratory system and the cardiovascular system*. In order to operate these mechanisms maximally, i.e., to supply adequate oxygen and remove CO_2 effectively, the *large muscle groups should essentially be engaged* during exercise. Therefore, **treadmills or bicycle ergometers are** most commonly used because they enable a known power output, which is used for analysis.

Steady-state power output: In a steady-state power output or constant-power output test, a power output is maintained constant for long enough for most variables to reach relatively constant steady-state values. Increase in oxygen consumption and carbon dioxide output occurs rapidly in the first 2 to 4 minutes at a given workload, and thereafter the changes occur in small quantities. Thus, after 4 to 5 minutes of exercise at a constant work rate, steady state is assumed to have been reached for the measurement of cardiorespiratory responses.

METHODS OF MEASURING ENERGY COST OF WORK

In the past, for the estimation of energy consumption of work, a **spirometer** was used to record BMR and O_2 utilisation, and the work output was calculated using the formula. But, as spirometry has now become almost obsolete, the entire process is done by **computerised bicycle ergometry**.

The modern **computerised ergometer** has provisions for recording the distance travelled, speed, respiratory frequency, ventilation, O_2 uptake (through a digital oximeter sensor attached), respiratory exchange ratio, calories spent, rate of metabolism, pulse rate, blood pressure, blood lactate level, ECG, and work done (Fig. 25.3). In a more **advanced** ergometer, mitral valve dynamics, VO_2max, and systolic pulmonary artery pressure (SPAP) are measured. Leg cycling is usually calibrated between **50 to 200 watts** (300 and 1200 kg/min).

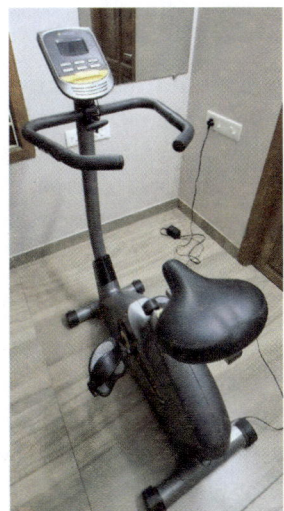

Fig. 25.3 Bicycle ergometer with digital facilities. Note the display of many parameters, and sensors beneath the handle of the ergometer to detect the changes in functions.

Bicycle Ergometry

Procedure

1. Keep the bicycle ergometer ready for the test.
2. Ask the subject to sit on the bicycle ergometer.
3. Adjust all basal parameters to zero and set the metronome.
4. Instruct the subject to pedal the bicycle at the rate of 50 times per minute, which is equivalent to approximately 130 revolutions per minute (rpm) at

the wheel. Note the exact rpm of the wheel from the revolution counter attached to the bicycle screen.

5. Calculate/observe the oxygen consumption per minute during the period of exercise, as displayed on the bicycle recording screen.

6. Also, note the other respiratory and cardiovascular parameters (pulse and heart rate) from the same record.

7. Allow the subject to recover and note his heart rate, respiratory rate, and blood pressure at one-minute intervals during the recovery period.

8. Calculate the energy cost of work.

Observation and Results

1. In a tabular format, note the pre- and post-exercise values of all the parameters, especially the distance travelled, O_2 uptake, calories spent, rate of metabolism, pulse rate, blood pressure, and the work done.

2. Alternatively, calculate the energy cost of work, the work done, and the mechanical efficiency of work as described below.

■ Calculation of energy cost of work

The oxygen consumption measured before and during the performance of moderately severe work is the energy cost of work. Energy cost is expressed either as: i) litres of oxygen consumed for one minute or ii) calories spent per minute.

■ Calculation of work done (W)

Work done (W) in kpm/minute =

[Distance]×[Force] = [Wheel circumference × rpm]×[Tension(kg)]

Here, kpm (kilopond meter) is the unit of work, whereas power is the rate at which work is done. Therefore, kpm may be converted to power output (watts) by multiplying with a factor of 0.1635 (since kpm/min × 0.1635 = watt).

■ Calculation of mechanical efficiency

$$\text{Mechanical efficiency} = \frac{\text{Output} \times 100}{\text{Input}}$$

Output = Work done in kpm/min
          (426.7 kpm per minute = 1 kcal)
Input = O_2 consumption in l/min (1 litre of O_2 consumed at STPD gives out 5 kcal)

$$\text{Thus, mechanical efficiency} = \frac{W\,(kpm/min)\,/\,426.7 \times 100}{O_2\ \text{consumption(l/min)} \times 5}$$

DISCUSSION

The calculation of energy cost of work is essential in *obesity management and maintaining cardiorespiratory fitness*. We spend energy while walking, cycling, jogging, and doing routine household activities. If we know how much the energy cost of work is, we can schedule our routine and professional activities accordingly.

Physiological Significance

Energy requirement: Energy is a basic human requirement for the maintenance of life, growth, and physical outputs. Like other animals, human beings obtain their energy from food in which it exists in chemically bound forms in the molecules of carbohydrates, proteins, and fats. This energy from food is liberated through dynamic biochemical oxidative reactions in the body and is utilised in the **following functions**:

1. Maintenance of basal metabolic processes and promoting growth
2. Regulation of body temperature
3. Performance of various physical activities

The amount of energy available to different categories of people varies widely. It is dependent primarily on the physical, mental, and economic status of the person.

Energy costs of household tasks: To work out well-balanced energy-spending patterns, homemakers need to know the energy costs of various activities. Household tasks are roughly divided into three classes: i) *light work*, such as knitting, darning, and sewing by hand or with a motor-driven machine, etc.; ii) *moderate work*, such as ironing clothes, dressing infants/children, washing dishes, and sewing with a foot-driven machine, etc.; and iii) *strenuous work*, such as washing clothes, sweeping the floor, etc. People have no knowledge of energy cost of these tasks. The energy cost of these tasks should be available to the general population, which will motivate them to perform these activities.

Clinical Significance

Obesity management: While walking (locomotion) and performing other activities, muscles use metabolic energy to produce mechanical work. Thus, calorie (energy) utilisation is the energy used by the body. The more is the activity, the more are the calories utilised. This forms the basis of reduction of body weight and obesity management. Morning walks, yoga (*surya namaskar*) and routine household tasks are the best ways of reducing calories and body fat, which can be practiced by everyone to maintain good health and to manage obesity.

VIVA

1.   *What is the importance of assessing body composition?* (Ans. Refer to page 156, under the heading 'Introduction'.)
2.   *What is the principle of BIA?* (Ans. Refer to page 156, under the heading 'Methods...', read 'Principle'.)
3.   *What is BMR?* (Ans. Refer to page 158, under the heading 'BMR'.)
4.   *What is the normal value of BMR?* (Ans. Refer to page 158, under the heading 'BMR', see 'Normal Values'.)
5.   *What are the basal conditions necessary for the measurement of BMR?* (Ans. Refer to page 158, under the heading 'BMR'.)
6.   *What are the factors that affect the BMR?* (Ans. Refer to page 158-159, under the heading 'Factors that affect BMR'.)
7.   *Why is the measurement of BMR by BIA a better method?* (Ans. Refer to page 158, under the heading 'BIA Method'.)
8.   *What is the meaning of energy cost of work? What is its importance?* (Ans. Refer to page 159, under the heading 'Introduction'.)
9.   *How is the energy cost of work calculated by bicycle ergometry?* (Ans. Refer to page 160, under the heading 'Methods'.)
10. *What is the physiological and clinical significance of knowing the energy cost of work?* (Ans. Refer to page 160, under the heading 'Physiological and Clinical Significance'.)

26 | Electrocardiography

Learning Objectives

After completing this practical, you will be able to (MUST KNOW):
1. Define ECG.
2. Classify ECG leads.
3. Handle the ECG machine properly.
4. Record ECG.
5. List the precautions taken while recording ECG.
6. List the uses of ECG.
7. Identify the different waves and complexes of ECG.
8. State the cause of production of the P wave, QRS complex, and T wave.
9. Calculate the heart rate and mean QRS axis.
10. Define and state the normal duration and significance of PR interval, QRS complex, and QT interval.

You may also be able to (DESIRABLE TO KNOW):
1. Explain the physiological significance of different waves, complexes, and intervals.
2. List the conditions that cause alteration in different waves, complexes, and intervals.
3. Explain the physiological basis of such alterations.

PY5.13: Record and interpret normal ECG in a volunteer or simulated environment.

INTRODUCTION

Electrocardiography is the method of recording an electrocardiogram (ECG). **ECG** is the recording, and the **electrocardiograph** is the machine that records the ECG. It is one of the most important and commonly ordered diagnostic tests in clinical practice.

ECG is the *graphic recording of the electrical activities* of the heart. The body is a volume conductor, that is, body fluids are good conductors of electricity. Therefore, electrical changes occurring in the heart with each heartbeat are conducted throughout the body and can be picked up from the body surface. The record of these electrical fluctuations during the cardiac cycle is called an **electrocardiogram**. Thus, the ECG recorded at the body surface represents the **algebraic sum of the action potential of the individual cardiac muscle fibres**.

Uses of ECG

An ECG is useful in the diagnosis of many heart diseases. It is regularly recorded before any surgical intervention to assess the cardiac status of the patient. ECG may be completely normal in a patient with organic heart disease or may show some non-specific abnormalities in a normal subject. Therefore, it must be interpreted with the clinical features of the patient and correlated with the findings of other investigations.

Usually, ECG investigation is performed for the following:
1. Anatomical orientation of the heart
2. Relative size of the chambers of the heart
3. A variety of *disturbances of rhythm and conduction*

4. To detect *ischemia of the myocardium*, if present
5. The location, extent and progress of *myocardial infarction*
6. The effects of *altered electrolyte concentration*
7. The influence of certain drugs like digitalis
8. Evaluation of electronic pacemaker function
9. For special assessments like *HRV studies*, Holter monitoring, etc.
10. In *health and fitness assessments* and exercise testing

ELECTROCARDIOGRAPHY—METHOD

Principle

Electrical activities generated with each beat are conducted from the heart to the body surface, which are picked up and recorded by the electrocardiograph.

Requirements

■ 1. ECG machine

In modern electrocardiography, two types of ECG apparatus are used: *the string galvanometer and the radio-amplifier*. The apparatus should be sensitive to potential changes of the order of microvolts and have a frequency response of 50–100 Hz. The use of the string galvanometer needs experience. This apparatus is not used in routine practice because the photographic paper used for recording needs to be developed. At present, the **transistor amplifier and cathode ray tubes** are used for this purpose.

The ECG machine has a **main switch** which regulates the power supply; a **lead selection switch** which selects various leads; a **calibration/sensitivity switch** used for calibration, and a **start–stop switch** to regulate the paper speed (Fig. 26.1A).

2. Electrodes and electrode jelly

Limb electrodes are *flat metal plates* that are kept in position by plastic flat-clip type of clamps, usually red, *yellow, green, and black* in colour. **Chest electrodes** are *metal cups* that are kept in position by suction produced by rubber bulbs, usually *blue in colour* (Fig. 26.1B). **Electrode jelly** (also known as cardiac jelly) is a specially made paste that contains *fine sand or glass particles* used for placing electrodes on the body surface. It helps in *establishing proper contact* between the electrode plates and the body.

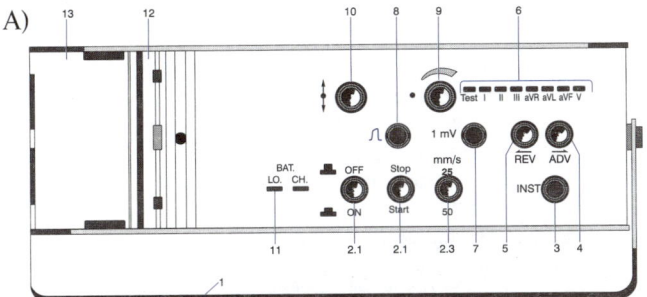

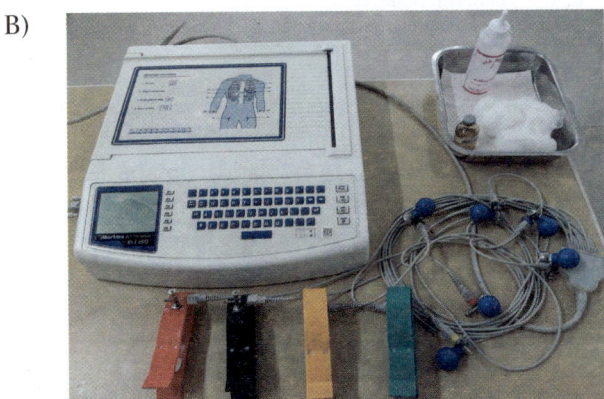

Fig. 26.1 **(A)** Schematic diagram of the front view of an ECG machine (1: Handle; 2.1, 2.2, and 2.3: Control switches; 3: Stylus adjuster; 4 and 5: Lead positioners; 6: Lead selection button; 7: Voltage selection; 8: Filter A/C; 9: Gain; 10: Stylus deflector; 11: Battery strength indicator; 12 Stylus protector; 13: Table for guiding paper movement); **(B)** ECG machine, electrodes, and jelly (Courtesy: Cardidat 108T/MK-VI; BPL Ltd.).

3. ECG paper

This is a strip of graph paper that has vertical and horizontal lines drawn 1 mm apart. The horizontal axis represents time, and the vertical axis denotes amplitude. There is a heavy line every 5 mm in both the planes. Thus, there are small squares of 1 mm × 1 mm, and big squares of 5 mm × 5 mm. The ECG paper is a heat-sensitive, plastic-coated paper. The ECG is inscribed on this paper by a hot stylus.

Paper speed: Conventional ECG is taken at a **speed of 25 mm/s**. One small square (1 mm) corresponds to 0.04 seconds, while the big square (5 mm) is equivalent to 0.20

seconds (Fig. 26.2). When the ECG paper runs through 5 big squares, it means that a one-second recording has been taken.

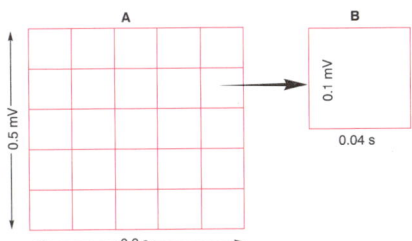

Fig. 26.2 Squares of the ECG paper: **(A)** Large square and **(B)** small square. Time depicted in the figures represents the time at a paper speed of 25 mm/s.

Sensitivity: Voltage is measured along the vertical axis. Usually, a *10 mm deflection is equivalent to 1 mV*. There is provision to change the sensitivity in special circumstances, for example, when **ECG complexes are too small**, the sensitivity can be doubled so that a 1 mV deflection is equivalent to 20 mm. When **ECG complexes are too large**, sensitivity may be reduced to half of the original so that 1 mV is equivalent to 5 mm. The **process of determination of sensitivity** is called **standardization**. It is displayed by pressing the calibration button before and after an ECG is recorded.

4. ECG leads

The ECG leads are broadly classified into **two categories: direct and indirect** (Fig. 26.3). A lead or an electrode is a **metal plate** (flat discs of dimension 7.5 × 5 cm, non-corrosive) applied snugly over an appropriate body part. For better contact between the leads and the body, ECG jelly is applied after the skin surface is cleaned thoroughly.

1. **Direct leads:** Leads applied *directly to the surface of the heart* to record ECG are called direct leads. These leads are used to record cardiac activities during cardiac surgery or during an experiment.

2. **Indirect leads:** Leads applied away from the heart to record cardiac activities are called indirect leads. The different indirect leads are **limb leads, chest leads, and esophageal leads**.

i. **Limb leads** are of *two types*, **bipolar and unipolar**.

• **Bipolar limb leads** (I, II, and III): These are the original leads designed by Einthoven to record electrical potential on the frontal plane. In this method, two similar electrodes are placed on the body surface, and the potential difference between the two electrodes is recorded. The electrodes are attached to the *right arm, left arm, and left foot* as depicted in the Einthoven triangle (Fig. 26.4). Another electrode is applied to the **right leg**, which acts as a ground wire to prevent external disturbances during recording.

Types of ECG Leads

```
                              ECG Leads
                                  |
          +-----------------------+-------------------+
          |                                           |
    Indirect Leads                               Direct Leads
          |                                           |
  +-------+----------------------+--------------------+        Applied directly
  |                   |                      |                 to the surface of
Limb Leads       Chest Leads        Esophageal Leads           the heart
  |                   |                                         (during cardiac
+-------+      +------+------+                                  surgery or
|       |      |            |                                  experiments)
Bipolar Unipolar Bipolar  Unipolar
```

Bipolar	Unipolar	Bipolar (not used nowadays)	Unipolar	Positioned in esophagus close to heart.
Standard limb leads (Lead I, II, III)	Augmented leads (aVR, aVL, aVF)	Special chest lead (Lewis lead for ECG recording in atrial arrhythmia)	Precordial leads (V1-V6). However, V7-V9 also used sometimes	E_{15-25}: Used for recording the activity of the right atrium E_{25-35}: Used for recording the activity from the AV groove region. E_{40-50}: Used for recording the activity from the posterior surface of the left ventricle. (Representing distance of electrode in cm from incisor teeth)

Fig. 26.3   Classification of ECG leads.

Lead I: Between the right arm (negative electrode) and the left arm (positive electrode).

Lead II: Between the right arm (negative electrode) and the left leg (positive electrode).

Lead III: Between the left arm (negative electrode) and the left leg (positive electrode).

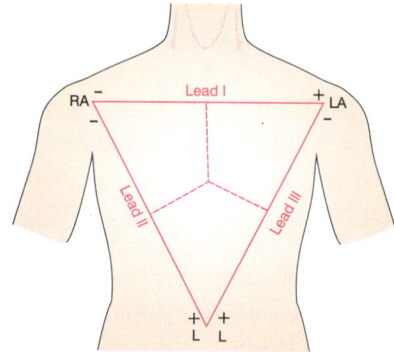

Fig. 26.4   Einthoven's triangle (RA: right arm; LA: Left arm; LL: Left leg). Note that perpendiculars drawn from the midpoint of each limb of the triangle intersect at the centre of electrical activity.

• **Unipolar limb leads:** In this method, *one electrode is active* while the other is indifferent. There are three unipolar limb leads: **aVR, aVL, and aVF**. Here 'a' stands for augmented leads. The potential recorded in aVL is one-and-a-half times that recorded in VL, and similarly for aVR and aVF. Therefore, these leads are called augmented leads. 'V' stands for voltage, and **R, L, and F** indicate that the exploring (active) electrode is on the right arm, left arm, and left foot respectively. The other (indifferent) electrode is connected to the remaining two leads through a high-resistance coil. For example, while recording from lead aVL the active electrode is placed on the left arm, the *indifferent electrode* is connected through a high resistance to the other two electrodes placed on the left foot and right arm.

aVR: Between the right arm (positive electrode) and left arm + left leg (negative electrode).

aVL: Between the left arm (positive electrode) and right arm + left leg (negative electrode).

aVF: Between the left foot (positive electrode) and right arm + left arm (negative electrode).

Vector of augmented limb lead = 3/2 vector of unaugmented limb lead.

$$aVR = VR - \frac{VL + VF}{2}$$
$$2aVR = 2VR - (VL + VF)$$
Since VR + VL + VF = 0 (Einthoven triangle),
$$VR = -(VL + VF)$$
$$2aVR = 2VR + VR$$
$$aVR = \frac{3}{2}VR$$

ii.   **Chest leads** are of two types, bipolar and unipolar.
• ***Bipolar chest leads:*** These leads were used before the discovery of unipolar chest leads. They record differences of potential between any given position on the chest and on one extremity. Bipolar chest leads are no longer used because the potential in the extremity appreciably alters the pattern of the chest leads.

Lewis lead: This is a special bipolar chest lead used for recording ECG in atrial arrhythmias. It amplifies the waves of atrial activity.

- **Unipolar chest leads:** There are six chest leads used routinely: **V1 to V6.** Three other chest leads are used less often (V7–V9). The chest leads employ an exploring electrode on the chest surface. The reference electrode is connected to the right arm, left arm, and left leg through a high resistance called **Wilson's terminal,** which is maintained at zero potential. The right leg is connected with a grounding electrode to avoid electrical interference. The position of the chest electrodes (positive electrodes) on the chest surface in different leads are as follows:

    V1: In the right fourth intercostal space at the right border of the sternum.

    V2: In the left fourth intercostal space at the left border of the sternum.

    V3: At the midpoint between V2 and V4.

    V4: In the left fifth intercostal space on the midclavicular line.

    V5: In the left fifth intercostal space on the anterior axillary line.

    V6: In the left fifth intercostal space on the midaxillary line.

    V7: In the left fifth intercostal space on the posterior axillary line.

    V8: In the left fifth intercostal space on the posterior scapular line.

    V9: In the left fifth intercostal space on the back just left to the spine.

iii. **Esophageal leads** have an electrode fixed on the tip of the esophageal catheter, which is positioned in the esophagus, close to the heart chambers. The leads are designated as E18, E20, and so on. In this, E stands for 'esophageal', and the number indicates the distance of the electrode from the incisor teeth expressed in centimetres.

- E_{15-25}: Used for recording the activity of the right atrium.
- E_{25-35}: Used for recording the activity from the AV groove region.
- E_{40-50}: Used for recording the activity from the posterior surface of the left ventricle.

Procedure

1. Ask the subject to lie down on a couch comfortably.
2. Clean the skin thoroughly with alcohol around the left and right wrists and left and right leg just above the ankle joint and apply jelly.
3. Connect the electrodes in these positions.
4. Switch on the machine and keep the stylus at the centre of the paper.

5. Adjust the sensitivity to get a standard calibration of 1 cm/1 mV by pressing the 'CAL' button 3–4 times.
6. Adjust the lead selector knob to record ECG of the 12 leads in the following order: I, II, III, aVR, aVL, and aVF.
7. Place the chest electrodes in an appropriate position on the chest after thorough cleaning and application of jelly and record the ECG from V1 to V6.
8. Again, take the standard calibration.
9. Tear out the paper from the machine and label the record.
10. Write the name and age of the subject and the date of the recording.
11. Calculate heart rate and QRS axis as described in the 'Discussion'.
12. Study and interpret the ECG as described under 'Results' and 'Discussion - Systematic Interpretation of ECG'.

Observation and Results

Observe the ECG for a moment for a general impression on the quality of recording, magnitude of ECG waves, sharpness of tracings, and any gross abnormality in the ECG. Immediately note the following parameters:

1. **Heart rate:** It can be determined by any of the following two methods:
    a. By dividing 1500 by the number of small squares between two successive R waves (1500 small squares represent 1 minute)
        For example, number of small squares between 2 R waves = 21
        Heart rate = 1500/21 = 70 per minute
    b. By dividing 60 by the RR interval in seconds
        For example, number of small squares between 2 R waves = 20
        RR interval = 20 × 0.4 = 0.80
        Heart rate = 60/0.80 = 75 per minute
2. **Rhythm:** Check for normal sinus rhythm or whether irregularities are present.
3. **Mean cardiac vector:** Determine the mean cardiac vector as described later in this chapter.
4. Carefully study the **morphology of various waves, intervals, and segments.**
5. Assess the ECG as described below in 'Discussion' (Features of good ECG/Normal ECG/Interpretation of ECG).
6. Report your major findings and concluding remarks.

Precautions

1. The subject should be totally relaxed.
2. The skin at the area where the electrodes are connected should be *thoroughly cleaned,* and **jelly should be applied** to decrease skin resistance.

3. The right foot should be connected for **grounding**.
4. Ensure that the leads are properly applied at the appropriate places and are in good contact with the body surface.
5. Before starting the recording, ensure that the ***required voltage is available*** at the mains and that the instrument is **properly earthed**.
6. **Standardization** should be done before and after the recording, to ensure that the proper standard was maintained throughout the recording.
7. A minimum of three ECG complexes should be recorded for each lead.
8. The stylus should be adjusted so that it records at the centre of the paper.
9. The recording of the 12 leads should be performed in ***proper sequence*** as I, II, III, aVR, aVL, aVF, and V1 to V6.

DISCUSSION

Features of a Good ECG

1. Optimal standardization of the calibration signal forms rectangles. The corners of the signal form a right angle.
2. The baseline is stable.
3. It contains a minimum of three complexes of each lead.
4. It contains a long strip of II and V1 if arrhythmia is suspected or present.
5. There is no interference by alternating current.
6. ECG complexes are recorded at the centre of the paper and do not overshoot the margins.

Normal ECG

The ECG tracing shows different waves, intervals, and segments (Fig. 26.5).

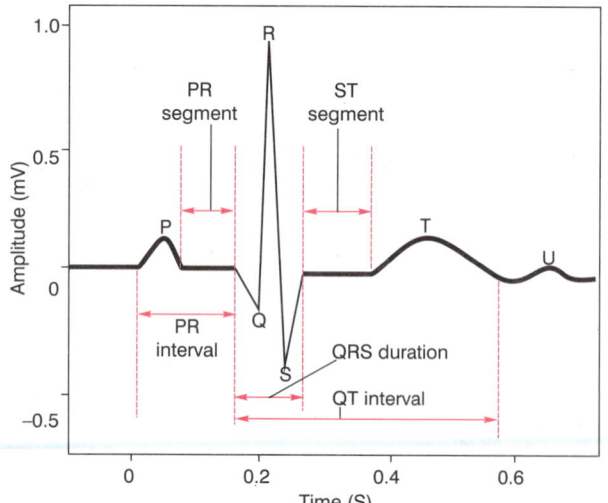

Fig. 26.5 Normal ECG showing different waves, segments, and intervals.

Waves

1. **P wave:** This is the deflection produced by atrial depolarization.
2. **QRS complex:** This consists of Q, R. and S waves. The QRS complex is the deflection produced by ventricular depolarization.
3. **Q wave:** This is the initial negative deflection in the QRS complex.
4. **R wave:** This is the positive deflection in the QRS complex.
5. **S wave:** This is the second negative deflection in the QRS complex.

      QS complex is the term used when the entire QRS complex is negative, without any positive deflection.
6. **T wave:** This is the positive deflection produced by ventricular repolarization.
7. **U wave:** This is the final positive deflection in the ECG. This wave is not always present normally. It occurs due to slow repolarization of the papillary muscle.

Segments

1. **PR segment:** This lies between the end of the P wave and the beginning of the QRS complex.
2. **ST segment:** This lies between the end of the QRS complex and the beginning of the T wave. The point where the QRS complex ends and the ST segment begins is called **the J point**. There is no *electrical activity* at the J point. **Elevation of the J point** (even 1 mm from the base) suggests *myocardial ischemia*.

Intervals

▮ PR interval

Definition: This is the interval between the *beginning of the P wave to the beginning of the QRS complex.*

Normal duration: The range of PR interval is **0.12–0.20 seconds** (average 0.18 s). PR intervals shorten as the heart rate increases—from the average of 0.18 s at the rate of 70 to 0.14 s at the rate of 130.

Significance: The PR interval represents *atrial depolarization and conduction through the AV node.*

▮ QRS interval (QRS duration)

Definition: This is the interval of the QRS complex. It is measured from the *beginning of the Q wave (or R wave if the Q wave is absent) to the J point.*

Normal duration: The normal range is **0.08–0.10 seconds**.

Significance: The QRS interval represents *ventricular depolarization*. Atrial repolarization also occurs in this period.

QT interval

Definition: This is the interval of the QRS complex and T wave. It is measured from the *beginning of the QRS complex to the end of the T wave*.

Normal duration: The normal range is **0.40–0.43 seconds**.

Significance: The QT interval *represents ventricular depolarization and ventricular repolarization*. It corresponds to the duration of electrical systole.

ST interval

Definition: This is the interval *between the J point and the end of the T wave*. It is calculated by deducting the QRS interval from the QT interval.

Normal duration: The average duration is **0.32 seconds**.

Significance: This *represents ventricular repolarization*.

PP interval

Definition: This is the interval measured *between either the peaks or the beginnings of two successive P waves*.

Significance: The PP interval is *measured for calculating the atrial rate*.

RR interval

Definition: This is the *interval between two successive R waves*. It is measured between the peaks of two successive R waves.

Significance: The RR interval is measured for *calculating the heart rate* (the ventricular rate).

The duration, amplitude, causes, and significance of ECG components are summarized in Table 26.1.

Table 26.1 Waves, intervals, and segments of ECG

Waves, intervals, and segments	Duration and amplitude	Cause	Significance
P wave	Duration: 0.08–0.10 sec Amplitude: Usually <2.5 mm in lead II	Due to atrial depolarization	If duration >0.10 sec, indicates left atrial enlargement If amplitude >2.5 mm, represents right atrial enlargement
QRS complex	Duration: 0.08–0.10 sec Amplitude is quite variable from lead to lead	Due to ventricular depolarization	If duration >0.10 sec, may indicate bundle branch block
T wave		Represents ventricular repolarizations	Normal T wave is usually in the same direction as the QRS complex in right precordial leads T wave is always upright in lead I, II, and V3-6 and always inverted in lead aVR.
U wave		Slow repolarization of papillary muscles	
PR segment	Isoelectric	Extends from the end of P wave to the start of QRS complex	
PR interval	Isoelectric Duration: 0.12-0.20 sec Average: 0.18 sec	Beginning of P wave to the start of QRS complex It includes the conduction delay in the AV node	PR interval is measured for calculating atrial rate; it shortens as the heart rate increases
QT interval	QT interval: 0.39 sec at a heart rate of 60/min Duration of QTc: 0.35-0.43 sec	Onset of Q wave to the end of the T wave Represents ventricular depolarization + repolarizations and corresponds to the duration of electrical systole	Shortens with tachycardia and lengthens with bradycardia so it must be corrected for the effect of the associated heart rate (QTc)
ST segment	Isoelectric	Extends from the J point to the onset of T wave	Convex or straight upward ST segment elevation (e.g., in lead II, III and aVF) is abnormal and suggests transmural injury or infarction ST segment depression is always abnormal, though often non-specific

ST interval		End of S wave to the end of T wave	
RR interval	Duration of the cardiac cycle		RR interval is measured for calculating heart rate (ventricular rate)

Normal 12-lead ECG

The deflection of waves in a particular lead is governed by the following basic laws:

1. A **positive (upward) deflection** is seen in any lead if electrical depolarization spreads towards the positive pole of that lead.

2. A **negative (downward) deflection** is seen if depolarization spreads towards the negative pole of the lead.

3. An **isoelectric or biphasic deflection** is seen when the depolarization starts in the SA node and spreads downwards to the subject's left (towards the positive pole of lead II and away from the positive pole of lead aVR).

The **P wave is always positive** in lead II and negative in lead aVR (Fig. 26.6). The ventricular septum depolarizes from the left to right (towards lead V1 and away from lead V6). This produces a **small q wave** (septal q wave) in V6 and a **small r wave** (septal r wave) in lead V1.

During ventricular depolarization, because the left ventricular mass is more than the right ventricular mass, the net direction of depolarization is towards the left chest leads (Fig. 26.7). This produces **tall 'R' wave** in leads V5

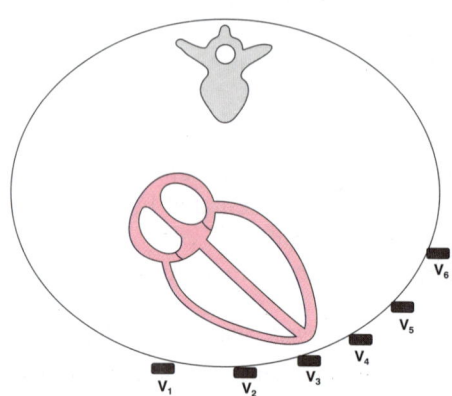

Fig. 26.7 Diagram of orientation of precordial ECG leads. Leads V1 and V2 overlie the right ventricle. Leads V3 and V4 are transitional leads between the right and left ventricles, and leads V5 and V6 overlie the left ventricle .

and V6 and a **deep s wave** in leads V1 and V2. Chest leads between these two positions show a transitional pattern.

In the **extremity leads**, the QRS complex varies depending on whether the heart is more horizontal or vertical. When the heart is more vertical, *leads II, III, and aVF* show a **qR pattern** and when the heart is more horizontal, leads I and aVL show a **qR pattern**. The T wave normally follows the direction of the QRS complex deflection.

In the **chest leads**, the *T wave is positive in left-sided leads* (and also in V2). In V1, the T wave may be positive or negative.

Systematic Interpretation of ECG

Routine screening of the ECG requires step-by-step examination of the ECG to answer the following questions:

1. What is the **heart rate**? What is the atrial rate and what is the ventricular rate?

2. Is the **rhythm** regular or irregular?

3. What is the **mean cardiac vector**?

4. Are the **P waves** normal? Do the P waves have a fixed relation to the QRS complexes?

5. What is the **PR interval**? What is the voltage duration and configuration of the QRS complex?

6. Is the **ST segment** isoelectric?

7. Are the **T waves** normal?

8. What is the **QT interval**? Is the **QTc** appropriate for the heart rate? (QTc is the QT interval corrected for the rate.)

9. Is the **J point** on the isoelectric line?

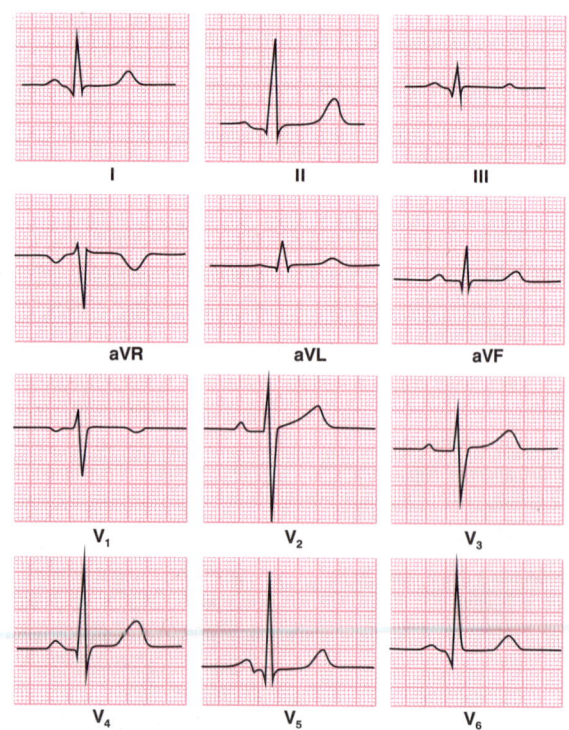

Fig. 26.6   Normal 12-lead ECG.

Rate

The heart rate should be calculated first. The comment should be made on **both atrial and ventricular rates.** Usually, the heart rate means the ventricular rate.

At a paper speed of 25 mm/s:

$$\text{Atrial rate / min} = \frac{1500}{\text{PP interval in mm}}$$

$$\text{Ventricular rate / min} = \frac{1500}{\text{RR interval in mm}}$$

Normally, the RR interval is equal to the PP interval. Sometimes, however, the ventricular rate may be different from the atrial rate.

When the RR interval is irregular, as in atrial fibrillation, the number of QRS complexes are counted over 5 seconds in the rhythm strip, and this number is multiplied by 12 to provide the number of QRS complexes in 60 seconds (1 minute). This enables the measurement of the average ventricular rate.

The normal heart rate is **60–100 per minute.**

Rhythm

It is obtained by calculating successive cycle lengths (RR intervals). Normally, the rhythm is regular. However, there may be minor variations of rhythm. A variation up to 10 per cent in the adjacent cycle length is considered normal.

Mean QRS axis (cardiac vector)

Cardiac vector can be calculated roughly and accurately.

■ Rough estimation

1. **Normal:** For rough estimation of cardiac vector, QRS complexes in lead I and aVF are noted. When the QRS complexes are predominantly upright (i.e., there is a *dominant R in both leads*), the axis is normal.
2. **Right axis deviation:** If the QRS complex in lead I is predominantly negative (i.e., *dominant S in lead I*), while it is predominantly positive in aVF (i.e., *dominant R in aVF*), there is right axis deviation.
3. **Left axis deviation:** If the QRS complex is predominantly positive in lead I but negative in aVF, left axis deviation is present.

When the QRS complexes in both lead I and aVF are predominantly negative, the axis is intermediate.

■ Accurate estimation

The vector at any given moment in the two dimensions of the frontal plane can be calculated from any *two standard limb leads*. The height of QRS complexes in mm in lead I, II, and III are measured and an Einthoven's triangle is drawn (Fig. 26.8A).

1. In each lead, **distances equal to the height** of the R wave minus the height of the largest negative deflection in the QRS complex are measured. These distances are *drawn from the midpoint to the side* of the triangle representing that lead.
2. **Perpendicular lines** are drawn from the midpoint of the arms of the triangle to the centre and from the end of the QRS complexes drawn on the triangle.
3. An **arrow is drawn** from the centre of the triangle to the point of intersection of the perpendiculars extended from the distances measured on the sides. This arrow represents the *magnitude and direction of the mean QRS vector*.

The normal direction of the mean QRS vector is generally said to be **−30 to +110 degrees** (Fig. 26.8B). If the axis falls to the left of −30°, *left axis deviation* is present; if the axis falls to the right of +110°, *right axis deviation* is present.

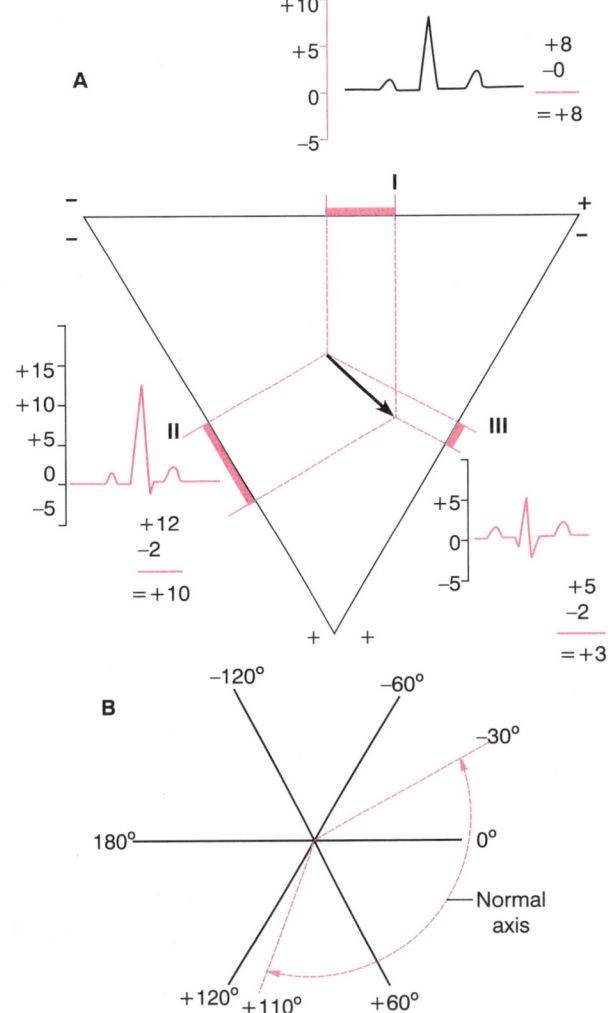

Fig. 26.8 Mean QRS axis: (A) Determination; (B) normal value in a hexaxial system (Cabrera system).

Waves and intervals

▌P wave

Duration and amplitude: Normal P wave duration **does not exceed 0.10 s**. P waves are not more than 2.5 mm tall.
Configuration: Usually, P waves are **upright** in lead I to aVF, and V3–V6; **inverted** in aVR; and **upright, inverted,** or **biphasic** in lead III, aVL, and V1, and V6. P wave morphology is best studied in lead II and V1.

▌PR interval

The normal PR interval is **0.12–0.20 seconds**, that is, 3–5 small squares. Normally, there should not be any variation in PR intervals.

▌QRS complex

Amplitude: In the limb leads—I, II, III, aVR, aVL, and aVF—the total amplitude of QRS should be 5 mm or more. In the chest leads, the amplitude of QRS complex *should be 10 mm or more*.
Duration: The normal duration of the QRS complex **does not exceed 0.11 seconds**.
Configuration: Normally, the **R wave is dominant** in leads I, II, V4–V6, and the **S wave is dominant** in aVR, V1, and V2. Either R or S wave may be dominant in lead III, aVL, aVF, and V3 depending on the position of the heart.

▌Q wave

Normally, Q waves are small in leads I, aVL, V5, and V6. A **QS complex** is commonly found in aVR. There may be **deep Q waves** in lead III alone in normal individuals, which may become less prominent on deep inspiration. Occasionally, a deep Q wave is found in V1 and V2. The depth of a Q wave is **less than 25 per cent** of the height of the ensuing R wave in most leads and may be up to 50 per cent in aVL. Any Q wave with **greater amplitude is considered pathological**.
J point: The J point occurs at the end of QRS complex. At this point, the entire ventricular muscle is depolarized. Normally, the J point is **on the isoelectric line,** but it is displaced up or down by the current of **injury resulting from myocardial ischemia or infarction**.

▌ST segment

The normal ST segment is **isoelectric**. ST depression less than 0.5 mm is not abnormal. **ST elevation** up to 1 mm in the limb leads and in V5 and V6 and 2 mm in V1–V4 may be normal.

▌T wave

T waves are **upright** in leads I, II, and V4–V6; **inverted** in aVR; and **upright, inverted, or biphasic** in lead III, aVL, aVF, and V1–V3.

▌QT interval

The upper limit of a normal QT interval is **0.42 s in males and 0.43 s in females**. QT intervals should be measured in the lead where the end of the T wave is most discernible. QT interval varies with the heart rate. Therefore, **corrected QT interval (QTc)** is measured by using **Bazett's formula**.

$$QTc = \frac{QT}{\sqrt{RR}}$$

(Where QT is the QT interval and RR is the RR interval in seconds.)

Abnormal ECG

Abnormalities of heart rate

The physiological basis for alteration in heart rate has been described in Chapter 27.

▌Bradycardia

1. Sinus bradycardia
   - Athletes
   - Sick sinus syndrome
   - Drugs (e.g., beta-blockers)
   - Obstructive jaundice
   - Raised intracranial pressure
   - Myxedema
2. Junctional (nodal) rhythm
3. Complete heart block

▌Tachycardia

1. Sinus tachycardia
   - Anxiety
   - Fever
   - Hypoxemia
   - Thyrotoxicosis
   - Cardiac failure
   - Acute carditis
2. Ectopic (re-entrant) tachycardia
3. Atrial premature beats
   - Anxiety
   - Excess tea or coffee intake
   - Viral infections
   - Rheumatic heart disease
   - Digitalis toxicity
   - Cardiomyopathies
4. Paroxysmal supraventricular tachycardia
5. Atrial fibrillation
   - Rheumatic heart disease with mitral stenosis
   - Coronary artery disease
   - Cardiomyopathies
   - Thyrotoxicosis
6. Atrial flutter
   - Rheumatic heart disease
   - Coronary artery disease

7. Ventricular premature beats
8. Ventricular tachycardia

Abnormal axis deviation
Right axis deviation
1. Right ventricular hypertrophy
2. Left posterior hemiblock
3. WPW syndrome
4. Dextrocardia

Left axis deviation
1. Left ventricular hypertrophy
2. Left anterior hemiblock
3. WPW syndrome
4. Inferior myocardial infarction
5. Obstructive airway disease

P wave abnormalities
P wave may be abnormal due to atrial enlargement and intra-atrial conduction abnormalities. Atrial enlargement results in tall and peaked P waves.

Abnormal PR interval
Short PR interval
1. WPW syndrome
2. Nodal rhythm
3. Atrial premature beats

Long PR interval (first-degree AV block)
1. Rheumatic carditis
2. Digitalis effect
3. Coronary artery disease

Abnormalities of QRS Complex
Amplitude
1. Low amplitude
   - Marked emphysema
   - Myxedema
   - Pericardial effusion
   - Cardiomyopathy
2. High amplitude
   - Ventricular hypertrophy

Pathological Q waves
Depth of the Q wave of more than **>25 per cent of the height of the ensuing R wave** or **more than 0.04 s in duration** is considered pathological. Common causes are:
1. Acute or old myocardial infarction
2. Unstable angina
3. Dilated cardiomyopathy
4. Hypertrophic cardiomyopathy

Abnormalities of ST Segment
ST elevation
1. Acute myocardial infarction
2. Acute pericarditis

ST depression
Commonly seen in myocardial ischemia.

Abnormalities of T Wave
Tall T wave
1. Hyperkalemia
2. Acute myocardial infarction

Inverted T wave
1. Physiological
   - Young children
   - Deep inspiration (occasionally)
   - After a heavy meal (occasionally)
2. Pathological
   - Ventricular hypertrophy (due to strain)
   - Bundle branch block
   - Digitalis effect
   - Myocardial ischemia

Abnormal QT Interval
Prolonged QT interval
1. Hereditary
2. Antiarrhythmic drugs like quinidine
3. Hypokalemia
4. Acute myocardial infarction

Shortened QT interval
This is of less clinical significance and may be seen in hypercalcemia.

Special Uses of ECG
1. **ICU ECG monitoring:** In case of cardiac arrest or severe arrhythmia or in critical conditions in which patients are shifted from the general ward to the ICU, continuous ECG recording and special monitoring are required.
2. **Ambulatory ECG monitoring (Holter):** Patients with episodic palpitation and dizziness or unstable angina are given a Holter monitor to wear for 12–24 hours. The analysis of the recorded tape often identifies the cause of the condition.
3. **HRV recording:** ECG is recorded continuously for 5 to 10 minutes for **short-term HRV recording** in AFT/HRV labs and for 12–24 hours for **long-term recording**, for assessment of autonomic dysfunction for diagnostic purposes and for research.

4. **Exercise ECG monitoring:** The ECG recorded during exercise (treadmill test, TMT), as per Bruce protocol in otherwise normal. Arrhythmias and ST segment changes are more likely to be detected during TMT.

VIVA

1. *Define ECG.* (Ans. Refer to page 162, under the heading 'Introduction'.)
2. *What are the uses of ECG?* (Ans. Refer to page 162, under the heading 'Introduction'.)
3. *What are the types of ECG machines used to record ECG in the laboratories?* (Ans. Refer to page 162, under the heading 'ECG Machine'.)
4. *How does the stylus write on the ECG paper? What should be the usual paper speed?* (Ans. Refer to page 163, under the heading 'ECG Paper', and subheading 'Paper speed'.)
5. *What is the need for standardization before and after the recording of ECG?* (Ans. Refer to page 163, under the heading 'ECG Paper', and subheading 'Sensitivity'.)
6. *What are the types of ECG leads?* (Ans. Refer to page 163, under the heading 'ECG Leads'.)
7. *What is Einthoven's triangle? What is its significance?* (Ans. Refer to page 164, under the heading 'Bipolar Leads', Fig. 26.4.)
8. *Where should the different chest leads be placed?* (Ans. Refer to page 164-165 under the heading 'Chest Leads'.)
9. *What is the use of esophageal leads?* (Ans. Refer to page 165, under the heading 'Esophageal Leads'.)
10. *What are the precautions taken during recording of ECG?* (Ans. Refer to page 165, under the heading 'Precautions'.)
11. *Why is the right leg connected during ECG recording?* (Ans. Refer to page 166, under the heading 'Precautions' read point no. 3.)
12. *How is the main line frequency interference kept free from the ECG recording?*
    (Ans. Main line frequency disturbance is kept free by keeping electrode resistance below 10,000 ohms using a single grounding electrode from the subject and keeping all AC cords away from the subject.)
13. *What are the features of good ECG?* (Ans. Refer to page 166, under the heading 'Features of good ECG'.)
14. *What does a QRS complex represent?* (Ans. Refer to page 166, under the heading 'Normal ECG' Waves – QRS Complex.)
15. *What do the P, QRS, T, and U waves represent?* (Ans. Refer to page 167, under the heading 'Normal ECG' ...Waves, Table 26.1.)
16. *What is ST segment and what is its significance?* (Ans. Refer to page 167, under the heading 'Normal ECG' Segments – ST segment, Table 26.1.)
17. *What is the 'J' point? What is its significance?* (Ans. Refer to page 166, under the heading 'Normal ECG' Segments – ST segment)
18. *How do you calculate the PR interval? What is its normal duration and its significance?* (Ans. Refer to page 166, under the heading 'Normal ECG' Intervals – PR Interval.)
19. *How do you calculate the QRS interval? What is its normal duration and its significance?* (Ans. Refer to page 166, under the heading 'Normal ECG' Intervals – QRS Interval.)
20. *How do you calculate the QT interval? What is its normal duration and its significance?* (Ans. Refer to page 167, under the heading 'Normal ECG' Intervals – QT Interval.)
21. *How do you calculate the ST interval? What is its normal duration?* (Ans. Refer to page 167, under the heading 'Normal ECG' Intervals – ST Interval.)
22. *How do you calculate the PP interval? What is its significance?* (Ans. Refer to page 167, under the heading 'Normal ECG' Intervals – PP Interval.)
23. *How do you calculate the RR interval? What is its significance?* (Ans. Refer to page 167, under the heading 'Normal ECG' Intervals – RR Interval)
24. *Why is T wave repolarization positive? What is its significance?*
    (Ans. This wave is due to ventricular repolarization. Normally, it is in the same direction as the QRS complex because repolarization follows a path that is opposite to that of depolarization, i.e., from the epicardium to the endocardium. As the endocardial areas have a longer period of contraction, they are slow to repolarize. A vulnerable period occurs during the down slope of T wave when the ventricle is partially repolarized and the cardiac muscle fibres are in a state of relative refractoriness An ectopic stimulus in the ventricles due to myocardial damage may bring on extrasystoles or fibrillation.)
25. *How do you calculate the heart rate?* (Ans. Refer to page 169, under the heading 'Rate'.)
26. *How do you calculate ventricular rate when the RR interval is irregular?* (Ans. Refer to page 169, under the heading 'Rate'.)
27. *How do you determine the QRS axis (cardiac vector)?* (Ans. Refer to page 169, under the heading 'Mean QRS Axis'.)
28. *What do you mean by right and left axis deviation? Give examples.* (Ans. Refer to page 169, under the heading 'Mean QRS Axis'.)
29. *What is Bazett's formula? What is it used for?* (Ans. Refer to page 170, under the heading 'QT Interval', and subheading 'Bazett's formula'.)

30. *What are the causes of tachycardia?* (**Ans.** Refer to page 170, under the heading 'Abnormalities of Heart Rate', and subheading 'Tachycardia'.)

31. *What are the causes of bradycardia?* (**Ans.** Refer to page 170, under the heading 'Abnormalities of Heart Rate', and subheading 'Bradycardia'.)

32. *What are the causes of short and long PR intervals?* (**Ans.** Refer to page 171, under the heading 'Abnormalities of PR Interval'.)

33. *What are the causes of high and low amplitudes of QRS complex?* (**Ans.** Refer to page 171, under the heading 'Abnormalities of QRS Complex'.)

34. *When does a Q wave become pathological? What are the conditions of pathological Q wave?* (**Ans.** Refer to page 171, under the heading 'Abnormalities of QRS Complex', and subheading 'Pathological Q waves'.)

35. *What are the conditions of ST depression and ST elevation?* (**Ans.** Refer to page 171, under the heading 'Abnormalities of ST Segment'.)

36. *What are the causes of tall T wave?* (**Ans.** Refer to page 171, under the heading 'Abnormalities of T wave'.)

37. *What are the causes of inverted T wave?* (**Ans.** Refer to page 171, under the heading 'Abnormalities of T wave'.)

38. *What are the causes of prolonged QT interval?* (**Ans.** Refer to page 171, under the heading 'Abnormalities of QT Interval'.)

39. *What are the special uses of WCG?* (**Ans.** Refer to page 171, under the heading 'Special Uses of HRV'.)

40. *How is ECG recording done for HRV studies?* (**Ans.** Refer to page 171, under the heading 'Special Uses of HRV', and subheading 'HRV recording'.)

27 | Examination of Radial Pulse, Demonstrations of Pulse Tracing, and Other Vascular Phenomena

Learning Objectives

After completing this practical, you will be able to (MUST KNOW):

1. Outline the importance of examining radial pulse in clinical physiology.
2. Define arterial pulse.
3. List the parameters to be considered for the clinical examination of radial pulse.
4. Examine radial pulse properly (with proper sequence and procedure).
5. List the common causes of tachycardia, bradycardia, irregular pulse, high and low volume pulses, water hammer pulse, pulsus paradoxus, and pulsus alternans.
6. Name the waves observed in an arterial pulse tracing and list the causes of production of these waves.
7. Understand the importance of carotid sinus reflex.

8. Explain the concept of venous blood flow and venous pressure
9. Define the triple response and name its components and mechanisms.

You may also be able to (DESIRABLE TO KNOW):

1. Define and describe different abnormal pulses.
2. Explain the causes of variation of different parameters of the arterial pulse.
3. State the physiological basis of the changes in the different parameters of the arterial pulse in different conditions.
4. Explain the mechanism of genesis of tachycardia, bradycardia, irregular pulse, high and low volume pulse, water hammer pulse, pulsus paradoxus, and pulsus alternans in different conditions.
5. Explain the importance of carotid sinus reflex, venous blood flow, venous pressure, and triple response.

PY5.12: Record blood pressure and pulse at rest and in different grades of exercise and postures in a volunteer or simulated environment.

PY5.16: Record arterial pulse tracing using finger plethysmography in a volunteer or simulated environment.

INTRODUCTION

Examination of the radial pulse is an important and essential part of the clinical examination of a patient. It is not only important for the assessment of the cardiovascular system but also for any systemic examination, because arterial pulse is one of the **vital signs** that must be checked along with the general examination of every patient.

Definition: Arterial pulse is defined as the palpable rhythmic expansion of the arterial wall due to transmission of pressure waves along the walls of the arteries which are produced during each systole of the heart.

Importance of arterial pulse examination: Examination of the arterial pulse provides physiological information regarding:

1. The working of the heart
2. The circulatory state and hemodynamics (blood volume, blood pressure, etc.)
3. The condition of the blood vessels
4. The state of autonomic activity in the body at that moment
5. The mental state of the subject
6. The state of body metabolism and temperature

The Radial Pulse

Clinically, **radial pulse is preferred** for the examination of arterial pulse for the following reasons:

1. Clinically, it is easily accessible, given its peripheral location in the upper limb.
2. It is easy to palpate as it lies over the radial bone.
3. It is ideal for assessing the condition of the arterial wall (to roll the artery against the bone).

Arterial Pulse Tracing

The pulse tracing recorded using a sphygmograph or student's physiograph from the radial artery shows the **following waves** (Fig. 27.1). The pulse wave has **an upstroke and a downstroke**.

1. The 'p' wave (**percussion wave** or tidal wave) occurs due to *ejection of blood from the ventricle* during systole.
2. The 'd' wave (**dicrotic wave**) occurs due to the *rebound of blood against the closed aortic valve* during diastole.
3. The 'n' (**dicrotic notch**) represents the *closure of the aortic valve*.

Sometimes, in the upstroke of the pulse wave, a small 'a' or **anacrotic wave** is seen due to a *change in the velocity of ejection* of blood from the ventricle towards late systole.

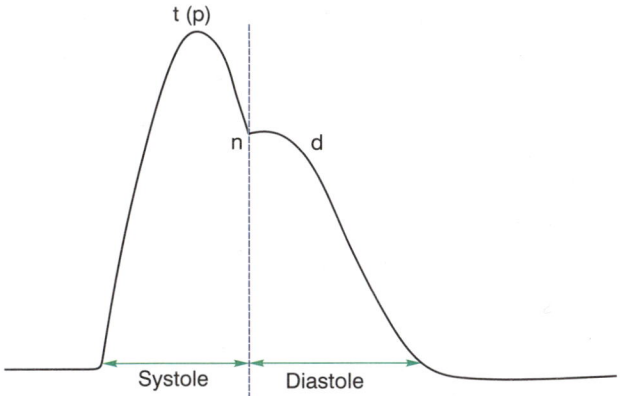

Fig. 27.1   The radial pulse tracing (t: tidal [percussion: p] wave; n: dicrotic notch; d: dicrotic wave).

METHODS OF EXAMINATION OF RADIAL PULSE

Principle

With each ventricular contraction, not only is blood pumped into the aorta, but also, pressure waves that are transmitted along the walls of the vessels are generated. These pressure waves expand the arterial wall, and the expansion is palpated as a pulse.

Procedure

The arterial pulses are detected by gently compressing the vessel against the bone. The radial pulse is examined by compressing the radial artery against the head of the radius. For better elicitation of the pulse, the subject's *forearm should be semipronated, and the wrist slightly flexed* (Fig. 27.2A).

The **following aspects (parameters) of the pulse** are examined:

1. Rate
2. Rhythm
3. Volume (amplitude)
4. Character
5. Condition of the arterial wall
6. Radiofemoral delay (presence/absence of delay of the femoral pulses as compared to the radials)
7. Other peripheral pulses

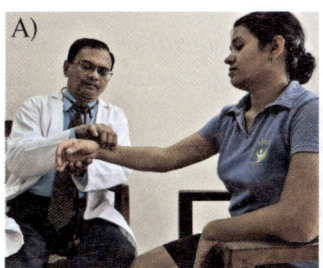
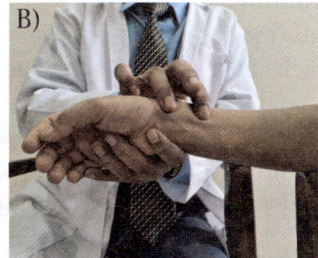
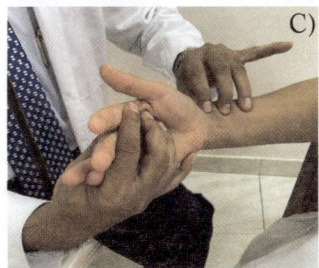

Fig. 27.2   (A) Examination of the radial pulse—note that the subject's hand is supported by the examiner's left hand, subject's forearm is semiflexed and semipronated, and the wrist is slightly flexed; **(B)** assessment of the condition of the arterial wall—first, the artery is fixed and emptied by index finger and ring finger and **(C)** then, with the help of the middle finger, the artery is rolled against the bone to feel the wall thickness.

Rate

Count the rate of the pulse, not immediately after placing the finger on the artery, but once the patient's nervousness subsides. Count the pulse completely for one minute.

> **Note:** Pulse rate should be counted only when the pulse resumes its normal rate. Therefore, it is advised to feel the radial pulse gently while eliciting the history of the patient. The pulse should be counted for a minimum of one minute. Counting for just 5 or 10 seconds and multiplying it by 12 or 6 to estimate the rate per minute often leads to inaccurate results, especially for beginners. Ideally, the pulse should be counted for two minutes, and the average of the two one-minute intervals may be used.

Pulse deficit: In conditions of irregularities of the heart, the counting of the radial pulse may not reflect the true ventricular contractions. In these conditions, the heartbeat should be counted by auscultating the apex. The *difference between the pulse rate and the heart rate* is called pulse deficit. It should also be noted that the pulse rate can never be more than the heart rate.

Rhythm

Rhythm is the *spacing order* at which successive pulse waves are felt. When the spacing between all the waves is constant, the pulse is said to be **regular**. When spacing is not constant, the pulse is said to be **irregular**. An irregular pulse may have a fixed pattern of irregularity (*irregular at regular intervals*) or it may not have any pattern (*irregularly irregular*).

Volume

It is the *degree of expansion of the arterial walls* during each pulse wave. Usually, in physiological conditions, the volume is normal and equal on both sides. Normal volume may not be described but can be well appreciated by palpating the artery of a normal individual. The pulse volume gives an **indication of the stroke volume** of the left ventricle.

Character

Study the character of the arterial pulse waves. The character of a normal pulse is described as **'normal'** when no abnormalities are detected. **Abnormalities** may be seen in *rate, rhythm, or amplitude of the pulse*. Depending on these changes, various types of abnormal pulses are described. The character of the pulse may be better appreciated by palpating the carotid artery in the neck.

Condition of the arterial wall

Place **three middle fingers** on the artery to assess the condition of the arterial wall. *Obliterate the flow* of blood into the artery by pressing the index finger and *empty the vessel* by the ring finger (Fig. 27.2B). Then *palpate the artery* with the middle finger. *Roll the artery* against the bone to assess the thickness of the arterial wall (Fig. 27.2C).

Normally, the arterial wall is not palpable or is just palpable. But, in old age, it is well palpable (thickened) and may be tortuous.

Symmetry and delay (if any)

Compare with the **radial pulse of the opposite side** to assess the symmetry (both sides appear simultaneously). Also, compare the **appearance of the femoral pulse** with the appearance of the radial pulse, and **mark any delay** that is present between them. Normally there is **no radio-femoral delay**.

Other peripheral pulses

Palpate the **femoral, popliteal** (Fig. 27.3A), **posterior tibial** (Fig. 27.3B), **dorsalis pedis** (Fig. 27.3C), **brachial** (Fig. 27.3D), **superficial temporal** (Fig. 27.3E), **frontal branch of superficial temporal** (Fig. 27.3F) and **carotid** (Fig. 27.3G) arteries of both the sides as detailed in the caption of Fig. 27.3. Appreciate whether the pulses are well felt and appear simultaneously on both sides.

Observation and Results

1. After step-wise examination of the pulse as described above, note your observation on the following aspects of pulse:
   - Rate and rhythm: 82/min (for example), regular
   - Volume and character: Normal
   - Condition of the arterial wall: Neither thickened, nor tortuous
   - Bilateral symmetry and if any radio-radial or radio-femoral delay: Symmetrical, no radio-radial/radio-femoral delay
   - Impression on other peripheral pulses and carotid pulse: All are well-felt

2. Report your observations (as in the case of a normal pulse): The pulse **rate is 82 per min, regular in rhythm, normal in volume and character, arterial wall is neither thickened nor tortuous, bilateral symmetry is observed, no radio-femoral delay, and peripheral pulses are well felt**.

3. If any abnormality is observed in any of the above-mentioned parameters, make a note of the same and report noticeably.

Precautions

1. The subject should relax and rest for a minimum of five minutes before the examination.

2. The subject's forearm should be semipronated and the wrist should be *mildly semiflexed*.

3. • Pulse rate should be counted for a minimum of one minute. If *irregularity is detected*, the pulse should ideally be counted for three minutes and the average of the three should be taken as the pulse rate.

4. If the pulse is *irregularly irregular*, heartbeats must be auscultated to detect pulse deficit, if present.

5. Pulses of **both the sides** should be examined and compared.

6. The femoral artery should be examined simultaneously with radial artery to *detect radio-femoral delay*, if present.

7. The radial pulse should be examined with the **middle three fingers** to check the condition of the arterial wall. The index finger should be used to obliterate the flow of blood, the ring finger should be used to empty the vessel, and the middle finger should be used to palpate and roll the artery against the bone.

8. If the artery is thickened and tortuous, the *brachial artery* should be examined for locomotor brachii.

9. The condition of the *other peripheral pulses* should be assessed.

10. If alternating pulses appear to be strong and weak, *sphygmomanometry* should be performed to confirm the presence of pulsus alternans.

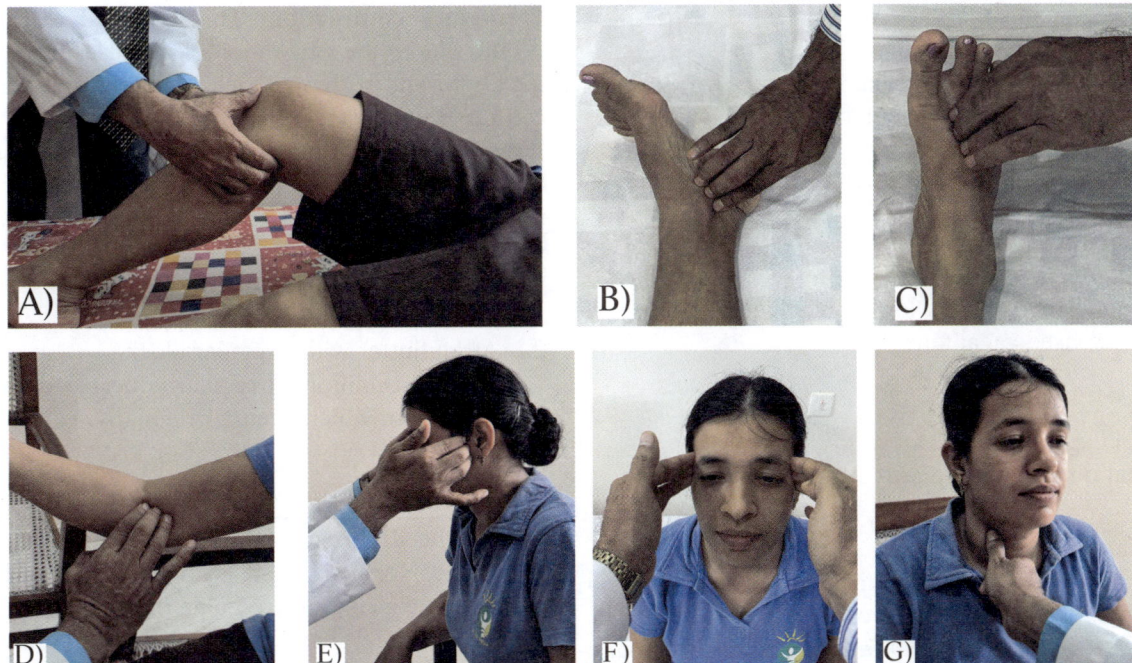

Fig. 27.3   Procedure of examination of other peripheral pulses and carotid pulse: **(A)** The popliteal artery is palpated in the popliteal fossa by flexing the knee joint to relax the popliteal fascia and hamstrings and by keeping the fingers of both hands from the two sides on the inferior part of the fossa; **(B)** the posterior tibial artery is palpated by placing the fingers just below the medial malleolus; **(C)** the dorsal pedis artery is palpated by keeping the fingers on the dorsum of the foot in the upper part of the groove between the big toe and the second toe; **(D)** the brachial artery is palpated in the antecubital fossa by partially flexing the elbow joint and by placing the fingers just medial to the insertion of the biceps tendon; **(E)** the superficial temporal artery is palpated by placing the fingers above the zygomatic arch in front of the tragus of the ear; **(F)** the frontal branch of the superficial temporal artery is palpated by placing the fingers on both sides of the face above the outer part of the orbit; **(G)** the carotid artery is palpated by firmly placing the tip of the thumb or index finger between the sternomastoid and trachea approximately at the level of the cricoid cartilage.

DISCUSSION

Pulse Rate

The normal pulse rate is **60–100 per minute**. The heart rate is primarily under the control of the autonomic nervous system, especially the vagal influence. The heart rate increases with increased sympathetic activity and decreases with increased parasympathetic activity. A heart rate of more than 100 is called **tachycardia**, and less than 60 is called **bradycardia**. Normally, the heart rate is higher in children and low in elderly people. The heart rate is higher during inspiration and lower during expiration.

Conditions That Alter Heart Rate
▌Tachycardia
Physiological
1. Exercise
2. After eating
3. Anger
4. Emotion and excitement
5. Infants and children
6. Pregnancy
7. High environmental temperature

During exercise, the heart rate increases due to **sympathetic stimulation** and due to *increased body temperature*. Increased sympathetic discharge to the SA node causes tachycardia. It also occurs **after eating** due to *increased body metabolism*, which increases body temperature. The heart rate increases during heightened emotional states like **anger and excitement** due to increased sympathetic activity. Tachycardia **in pregnancy** occurs due to *increased blood volume*, *effects of progesterone,* and the ***need to pump more blood*** to meet the demands of growing the fetus and placenta.

Pathological
1. *Fever*: Increased body temperature causes tachycardia by directly stimulating the SA node.
2. *Anemia*: Tachycardia occurs in anemia as a compensatory mechanism to improve blood (oxygen) supply to the tissues.
3. *Thyrotoxicosis*: Thyroxine increases the number of beta receptors in the heart and also increases the sensitivity of beta receptors to catecholamines.
4. Beriberi
5. Paget's disease

6. Arteriovenous fistula
7. Heart failure
8. Paroxysmal atrial tachycardia
9. Ventricular or supraventricular tachycardia
10. Other tachyarrhythmias
11. Shock as seen in hemorrhage

▮ Bradycardia
Physiological
1. **Athletes:** Heart rate is lower in athletes because of their increased vagal tone
2. Fear
3. Grief
4. Very old age
5. Meditation and *pranayama*

Pathological
1. *Myxedema:* In hypothyroidism, the number and sensitivity of beta receptors to catecholamines decreases.
2. *Increased intracranial pressure, as in brain tumours:* Increased intracranial pressure decreases heart rate by activating Cushing's reflex.
3. *Obstructive jaundice:* The concentration of bile salt increases in the blood. The toxic effect of bile salt inhibits the SA node, thereby producing bradycardia.
4. Different types of heart block.
5. *Drugs like propranolol and digitalis:* **Propranolol** is a non-selective beta blocker. It produces bradycardia by inhibiting beta receptors on the SA node. **Digitalis** produces bradycardia by **slowing AV nodal conduction** and by **causing vagal stimulation** (by stimulating the receptors of nodose ganglion, which is the sensory ganglion of the vagus nerve located just below jugular foramen in the skull base, and by activating the central vagal nucleus in the medulla).

Rhythm

The normal rhythm is regular. Irregular rhythms may be regularly irregular or irregularly irregular. **Irregular rhythm** may be due to *sinus irregularity* or *premature contraction.*
Sinus irregularity: This is a physiological phenomenon, also called **sinus arrhythmia,** of the normal variation of heart rate with the phases of respiration. In the normal sinus rhythm (respiratory sinus arrhythmia), the pulse rate increases in inspiration and decreases in expiration, which is primarily due to alterations in the vagal tone. In expiration, there is more vagal activity, which decreases the heart rate. In inspiration, there is less vagal activity, which increases heart rate. However, the sinus arrhythmia may be more intense and associated with symptoms (non-respiratory sinus arrythmia), which can be due to sick sinus syndrome, certain medications, heart block, etc.

Premature contraction: This is called **extrasystole.** It occurs due to the generation of impulses from an ectopic focus present in the ventricle. Therefore, it is also called **ectopic beat.**
Irregularly irregular pulse: This is commonly seen in **atrial fibrillation.** In this condition, irregularity occurs not only in the interval between the beats, but also in the volume of the beats.
Irregularity associated with heart blocks:
1. Partial heart block with dropped beat
2. Atrial flutter with irregular block
In these conditions, irregularity occurs due to a block in conduction, which occurs irregularly.

Pulse Deficit

This is the **difference between the pulse rate and the heart rate.** Normally, there is no pulse deficit. However, in conditions causing an irregular rhythm, some heartbeats may be weak. The heart may beat, but the contraction may not be sufficient enough to generate pressure waves in the walls of the arteries. Therefore, the pulse rate may be less than the rate of heart contraction. Pulse deficit is usually seen in **atrial fibrillation** in which the deficit is more than ten. Pulse deficit seen in other types of heart blocks is usually less than ten.

Volume

The volume of the pulse indicates the amplitude or strength of the pulse, which is determined by the volume of blood ejected from the ventricle with each heartbeat, i.e., the stroke volume. Thus, the volume of the pulse chiefly reflects the stroke volume.

When the volume of the pulse decreases, the pulse is called a **low-volume pulse** (**weak pulse**) and when the volume increases, the pulse is called **high-volume pulse** (**strong pulse**).

Conditions that alter the volume of the pulse
▮ Low-volume pulse
A low-volume pulse is also known as **pulsus parvus** (Fig. 27.4D). It occurs when the stroke volume of the heart decreases or when the pulse pressure decreases. Pulsus parvus is seen in:
1. Aortic stenosis
2. Obstructive cardiomyopathy
3. Pericardial effusion
4. Constrictive pericarditis
5. Pulmonary stenosis
6. Tight mitral stenosis
7. Shock due to any cause—the pulse becomes **thready** (low volume and increased rate)

High-volume pulse

The high-volume pulse is called **pulsus magnus** (Fig. 27.4E). It is seen in conditions in which the stroke volume is greater and there is *widening of the pulse pressure*. Pulsus magnus is seen in:

1. Aortic incompetence
2. Thyrotoxicosis
3. Patent ductus arteriosus
4. Beriberi
5. Anemia
6. Fever
7. Old age (due to increased pulse pressure)
8. Exercise

Bounding pulse: This is a very strong and forceful high-volume pulse, often felt as a **water-hammer pulse**. It is commonly seen in anxiety, hyperthyroidism, and aortic regurgitation. The pulse pressure is very high.

Character

The character of a pulse is described as normal when no abnormalities are detected. Different types of abnormal pulses are described in various clinical disorders. Common among these are the anacrotic pulse, dicrotic pulse, water hammer pulse, pulsus bisferiens, pulsus paradoxus, and pulsus alternans.

Anacrotic pulse

This is also called an **anadicrotic pulse**, which means two upbeats. A secondary wave occurs in the upstroke of the pulse. It is commonly *found in aortic stenosis*. The upstroke is slow and sloping (Fig. 27.4A). The *anacrotic wave* is exaggerated and has *two upbeats*. Therefore, this pulse is called anacrotic pulse.

Dicrotic pulse

A better name for this is 'twice-beating pulse'. The dicrotic wave is prominent in this pulse and gives the *impression of two beats*. Therefore, this is called dicrotic pulse (Fig. 27.4B). It is commonly seen in *febrile states*, especially in *typhoid fever*.

Water-hammer pulse

This is also called **collapsing pulse** or **Corrigan's pulse**. This is typically seen in *aortic regurgitation*. The collapsing pulse is characterized by a **rapid upstroke and a rapid downstroke** (descent) of the pulse wave. A dicrotic notch is usually absent (Fig. 27.4C). The rapid upstroke is due to greatly increased stroke volume and the *rapid descent* is due to the collapse of the pulse. Therefore, the **pulse pressure is very high**; sometimes, as high as 100 mmHg.

Causes

1. Common causes
   - Aortic incompetence/regurgitation (AR)
   - Patent ductus arteriosus (PDA)
2. Less common causes
   - Arteriovenous fistula (AVF)
   - Ventricular septal defect (VSD)
   - Hyperkinetic circulatory states, e.g., thyrotoxicosis, severe anemia, and beriberi

Note: The collapsing pulse is better appreciated when the patient's arm is elevated and the wrist is grasped with the palm (of the examiner's hand) against the palmar surface of the wrist of the subject (Fig. 27.5).

Physiological basis

The collapsing pulse occurs due to *rapid upstroke and rapid downstroke* of the pulse wave. The **rapid upstroke** is due to a forceful, high-amplitude, and steep-rising percussion wave, which gives a sharp tap to the palpating hand and the **rapid downstroke** is due to a rapid fall of the descending limb of the pulse wave, which results in sudden disappearance of the pulse from the palpating hand.

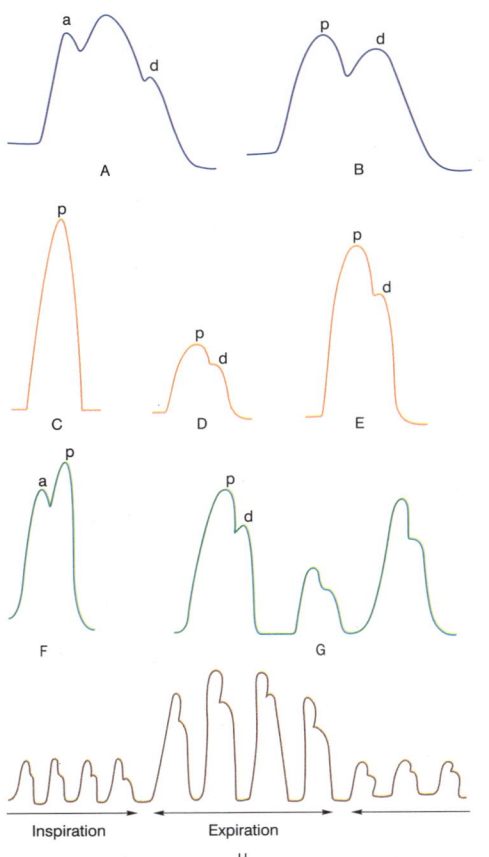

Fig. 27.4 Abnormal pulses: (A) Anacrotic pulse (note that the anacrotic wave is prominent); (B) dicrotic pulse (note that the dicrotic wave is abnormally large); (C) collapsing pulse (dicrotic notch absent); (D) pulsus parvus; (E) pulsus magnus; (F) pulsus bisferiens; (G) pulsus alternans; and (H) pulsus paradoxus.

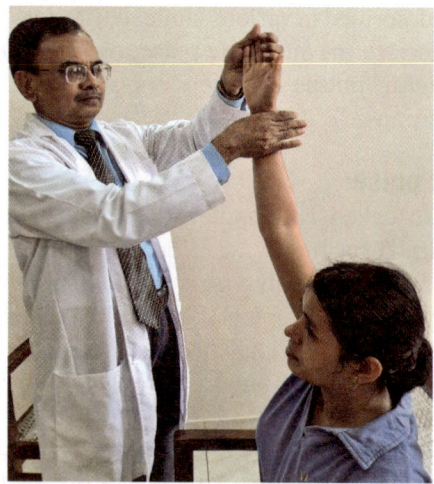

Fig. 27.5 Method of eliciting water-hammer pulse. Note that the collapsing pulse is better appreciated with the patient's arm elevated and the examiner's palm placed firmly against the surface location of the radial artery in the wrist.

Mechanism in AR: The **steep rise of the ascending limb** of the pulse wave is due to *increased end diastolic volume* (EDV) of the left ventricle, which causes forceful ejection of blood during systole. This is because, during diastole, in addition to the ventricular filling from the left atrium, *filling also occurs from the aorta through the incompetent aortic valve*. The aortic valve does not close completely, and so blood from the aorta enters the left ventricle during diastole, aiding the normal diastolic filling. This **increases the total EDV** of the left ventricle. Thus, during systole, the force of contraction of the left ventricle increases due to the **Frank–Starling mechanism**. Therefore, there is a *steep rise in the percussion wave* during systole.

The **steep fall of the descending limb** of the pulse wave is due to the *collapse* (sudden disappearance) of the pulse wave from the palpating hand. This occurs due to *two factors*:

1. *Diastolic run-off of blood* into the left ventricle due to incompetence of aortic valve
2. *Rapid run-off of blood* into the periphery because of decreased systemic vascular resistance

> **Note:** When the pulse pressure is greatly increased, as observed in AR, pulsations can be visible in the capillaries. Applying pressure on the nailbed or on the mucosa of the lip with a glass slide will make the alternate pulsatile flushes visible.

Pulsus Bisferiens

Pulsus bisferiens is a **combination of low-rising pulse** (anacrotic pulse) and the *collapsing pulse* (Fig. 27.4F). This is typically seen in *aortic stenosis associated with aortic incompetence*.

Pulsus Paradoxus

This is a misnomer since there is nothing paradoxical in this type of pulse. Actually, pulsus paradoxus is an accentuation of the normal phenomenon, where the volume of the pulse decreases during inspiration and increases during expiration. In pulsus paradoxus, **during inspiration, the volume of the pulse is grossly decreased** or may be absent in severe cases (Fig. 27.4H).

Causes

1. Common causes
   * Constrictive pericarditis
   * Pericardial effusion
2. Less common causes
   * Emphysema
   * Asthma (in the acute phase of severe asthma)
   * Massive pleural effusion
   * A mass in the thorax
   * Advanced right ventricular failure

Mechanisms (physiological basis)

1. **During inspiration**, the *intrathoracic pressure becomes more negative*. Blood pools in the pulmonary vascular bed. This **decreases venous return** to the left atrium. So, *left atrial filling decreases*, which results in **decreased left ventricular stroke volume**. Therefore, the volume of the pulse decreases during inspiration. This is more accentuated in the above conditions.
2. **In pericardial effusion and constrictive pericarditis,** during inspiration, the *intrapericardial pressure normally increases* due to traction from the attachments referred to the pericardium. This *decreases venous return* to the heart and results in *low stroke volume*. This is **accentuated in** pericardial effusion and constrictive pericarditis.
3. **In constrictive pericarditis and pericardial effusion**: The filling of the atria and ventricles decreases due to restriction to the expansion of the heart chambers. The limitation in the diastolic filling of the atria and the ventricles during inspiration results in lowering of left ventricular stroke volume.
4. In **advanced stages of right ventricular failure**, increase in lung volume in inspiration accommodates more blood than normal due to **much decreased pulmonary vascular resistance**. There is as such *decreased right ventricular output*. Therefore, these **two factors** result in *decreased left ventricular stroke volume* (due to decreased venous return to left atrium).
5. In **acute and severe bronchial asthma**, the increased respiratory effort makes *intrathoracic pressure*

more negative during inspiration. So, there is more pooling of blood in the pulmonary veins, which results in *decreased left ventricular stroke volume*.

Pulsus Alternans

The pulse is regular, but **alternate beats are strong and weak** (Fig. 27.4G). It is difficult to appreciate pulsus alternans by palpating the artery. Diagnosis is **confirmed while measuring blood pressure**. There will be a *difference of 5–20 mmHg in the systolic pressure* between two alternate beats. When the mercury is being lowered, the stronger beats are heard first. On further lowering, the weaker beats also become audible, thus suddenly doubling the number of audible beats.

Causes

1. *Left ventricular failure*—this is the commonest cause of pulsus alternans
2. Toxic carditis

Physiological basis: In left ventricular failure, because of the **decreased myocardial contractility**, the left ventricular **stroke volume decreases**. This results in **low pulse volume**. Therefore, the amount of blood left in the ventricle at the end of systole (end systolic volume of the left ventricle) increases. Consequently, prior to the next ventricular contraction, the **ventricular volume (EDV) is increased**. This increases the force of contraction of the left ventricle in the next beat due to the Frank–Starling mechanism. Hence, the *second beat becomes stronger*. Likewise, *strong beats alternate with weak beats*.

Condition of the Arterial Wall

Normally, in young individuals, the arterial wall is soft and elastic or may not be palpable. In the elderly, it is palpable and hard and may be tortuous. This is due to thickening of the arterial wall by atherosclerosis. In such a condition, the brachial and temporal arteries may be quite prominent and tortuous. The brachial artery may exhibit a typical dancing movement with each beat, called **locomotor brachii**.

Bilateral Symmetry and Delay

Normally, there is no delay between the appearance of pulse on both sides and in the radial and femoral arteries. **Radiofemoral delay** is typically seen in **coarctation of the aorta** (especially when the constriction is present distal to the origin of the left subclavian artery).

Other Peripheral Pulses

In the absence of any pathology, all the peripheral pulses are well felt and appear simultaneously on both sides. Peripheral pulses may not be felt properly in peripheral vascular diseases.

Pulse tracing is usually not done in clinical practice as physicians can diagnose cardiovascular problems by performing a clinical examination of the arterial pulses. It is used more for physiological and research purposes.

DEMONSTRATION OF OTHER VASCULAR PHENOMENA

Arterial Pulse Tracing

Arterial pulse tracing is done mainly to study the difference between central and peripheral pulses. The peripheral pulse tracing is recorded by a sphygmograph or student's physiograph from the radial artery. The pulse tracing records a percussion eave and dicrotic wave (see Fig. 27.1).

The recording of the **arterial pulse from a central artery** like the aorta is characterized by a fairly rapid rise to a somewhat rounded peak. The anacrotic shoulder present on the ascending limb occurs at the time of the peak rate of aortic flow, just before the maximum pressure is reached. The less steep descending limb is interrupted by a sharp downward deflection synchronous with aortic valve closure, called **incisura. Recording from the peripheral artery** shows a steep upstroke, less apparent anacrotic shoulder and replacement of incisura by a smoother dicrotic notch (Fig. 27.6).

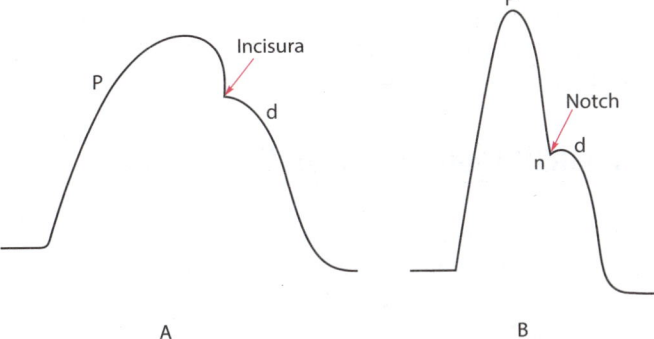

Fig. 27.6 Arterial pulse recorded from: (A) a central artery and (B) a peripheral artery (P: percussion wave; d: dicrotic wave; n: dicrotic notch).

Demonstration of Carotid Sinus Reflex

Baroreceptors are present in the walls of carotid sinuses, close to the surface of the anterior surface of the neck. These can be stimulated by **massaging them or by exerting pressure on them** from the anterior surface of the neck.

Procedure

1. Ask the subject to lie down in supine position on the bed or the examination couch.
2. Expose the subject's neck and ask him to turn his head slightly to the left. Stand to the right of the subject.

3. Place your hand on the right-side anterior part of the neck and locate the anterior edge of the sternomastoid muscle.
4. Feel the pulsation of the common carotid artery, which lies deeper and medial to the anterior edge of the sternomastoid muscle.
5. Locate the upper border of the thyroid cartilage, and feel the pulsation in the carotid sinus, which lies just below the angle of the jaw.
6. Palpate the radial artery with your left hand and with the thumb of your right hand, press the carotid sinus against the vertebral bodies for 2 seconds only. The pulse can be felt at this site as well as in the redial artery.

> Note: **Do not compress both carotids** simultaneously.

Effects: Compressing the carotid sinus stimulates the carotid baroreceptors. Impulses are transmitted in the 9th cranial nerve to stimulate the cardioinhibitory centre (nucleus tractus solitarius, nucleus ambiguous, and motor nucleus of the vagus) in the medulla, which in turn, inhibits the vasomotor centre and the sympathetic output. This results in *reflex slowing of the heart and decrease in peripheral resistance* due to inhibition of the tonic discharge in the vasoconstrictor nerves supplying the arterioles.

> **Important Note:** As activation of this reflex results in the slowing of the heart, stimulation of the carotid sinus for more than two seconds or simultaneous stimulation bilaterally (both sides in the neck) could *result in temporary stoppage of the heart*, which may even be life-threatening. Therefore, extreme care should be taken not to compress both carotids simultaneously or stimulate it for a long time.

Demonstration of Venous Blood Flow

The **flow of blood through the veins** of the forearms and the **presence of the valves** in these veins can be demonstrated by the following experiment.

1. Ask the subject to sit on a stool with his arm placed on a table.
2. Tie the BP cuff of an aneroid sphygmomanometer in his upper arm and inflate it to 40 mmHg.
3. Keep the **pressure at 40 mmHg** for a short while and note that the superficial veins of the forearm become prominent.
4. Place the tip of your right index finger over one of the veins (mark it as 'R') and mark the position of the valve (mark it as 'V') above it using a ball pen.
5. Keeping the finger 'R' in the same position and using your left index finger, squeeze out the blood from this vein toward the elbow. Note that the segment of the vein between points 'R' and 'V' remains collapsed

and that there is no backflow of blood. However, the vein above the valve 'V' is distended, and the valve becomes prominent.
6. Keeping the finger 'R' in position, place the left index finger downward toward the finger 'R'. You will notice that the blood cannot be forced backward across the valve 'V' unless pressure is applied, which will be enough to rupture the valve.

Recording of Venous Pressure

There is a pressure gradient from the arterial to the venous side of the circulation. The pressure gradient in the systemic circulation is about 95 mmHg (mean aortic pressure is 95 mmHg and right atrial pressure is 0–4 mmHg). The venous blood pressure can be demonstrated by the following simple experiment.

1. Ask the subject to sit on a stool with his right arm hanging downwards. Note that the veins of the arm will become distended within a few seconds.
2. While watching the veins on the back of the hand and the wrist, slowly and gently raise the subject's arm till these veins begin to empty out, and venous prominence disappears.
3. Measure the vertical distance between the wrist and the junction of third costal cartilage with the sternum, which is the level of entry of the superior vena cava into the right atrium.
4. The distance measured in cm is the approximate measure of the right atrial pressure.
5. Note that normally, the hand will be a few cm above the heart when the veins empty out completely.

Demonstration of Triple Response

The response of the skin to a mechanical injury, called the triple response or the Lewis' response, was described first by Sir Thomas Lewis in 1927. With a lighter injury produced by a pointed object, only a white line is seen across the path of the injury. However, with a stronger stimulus, all the three stages of the triple response will be seen, which can be demonstrated as follows.

With the help of a pointed object such as a forceps, draw a stronger line on the skin on the anterior aspect of the forearm with a little more force. Observe the changes in the skin that happen in three stages:

1. **The red line (red reaction):** A red line appears in about 10 seconds due to the relaxation of the precapillary sphincters resulting from the effects of histamine, kinins, polypeptides, etc., released locally from injured tissue. Passive capillary dilatation and increased blood flow cause the red line.

2. **The flare:** A reddish, mottled area surrounding the red line appears within a few minutes, which occurs due to dilation of arterioles resulting from the axon reflex. In this reflex, the impulse originating in the sensory axon is relayed antidromically (i.e., opposite to the normal direction) down other branches of the sensory nerve fibres that supply the arterioles. This is also an example of **antidromic conduction in a nerve fibre**.

3. **The wheal:** Within a few minutes, local edema (swelling) appears, which occurs due to the increased permeability of the capillaries and small venules, caused by the release of histamine from local mast cells, kinins, substance P, and other polypeptides.

OSPE

I.   **Examine the radial pulse of the given subject and report your findings.**

Steps

1. Stand on the right side of the subject and hold the subject's right hand in a semipronated and slightly flexed position. Support the limb.
2. Place your three middle fingers on the radial artery just above the wrist.
3. Count the pulse for 1 minute and check for volume and character of the pulse.
4. Check the condition of the arterial wall by obliterating the blood flow with one index finger, by emptying the vessel peripherally by the ring finger and palpating and rolling the artery on the bone by the middle finger.
5. Compare with the pulses of the opposite side.
6. Examine the femoral artery to check for radiofemoral delay.
7. Report your findings.

VIVA

1. *Define arterial pulse.* (**Ans.** Refer to page 174, under the heading 'Definition'.)
2. *What is the importance of examining the radial pulse in clinical medicine?* (**Ans.** Refer to Page 174, under the heading 'Importance'.)
3. *What are the precautions to be taken during examination of the radial pulse?* (**Ans.** Refer to page 176, under the heading 'Precautions'.)
4. *What are the different aspects of the pulse, which are examined during clinical examination of the radial pulse?* (**Ans.** Refer to page 175, under the heading 'Procedure'.)
5. *Why are the three middle fingers used for examining the radial pulse?* (**Ans.** Refer to page 176, under the heading 'Procedure' and the subheading 'Condition of the arterial wall'.)
6. *What is pulse deficit? What is its most common cause?* (**Ans.** Refer to page 175, under the heading, Rate – 'Pulse Deficit'.)
7. *What is the normal pulse rate and what is the main factor that regulates it?* (**Ans.** Refer to pages 177 and 178, under the heading 'Pulse Rate'.)
8. *What are the physiological conditions that cause tachycardia?* (**Ans.** Refer to page 177, under the heading 'Tachycardia')
9. *What is the cause of tachycardia in exercise?* (**Ans.** Refer to page 177, under the heading 'Tachycardia' and subheading 'Exercise'.)
10. *Why does tachycardia occur after eating?* (**Ans.** Refer to page 177, under the heading the text under 'Tachycardia' and the subheading 'Effects of eating'.)
11. *What are the causes of tachycardia in pregnancy?* (**Ans.** Refer to page 177, under the heading 'Tachycardia' and the subheading 'Pregnancy'.)
12. *Name the pathological conditions in which tachycardia occurs.* (**Ans.** Refer to page 177-178, under the heading 'Tachycardia' and the subheading 'Pathological'.)
13. *What is the cause of tachycardia in thyrotoxicosis?* (**Ans.** Refer to page 177, under the heading 'Tachycardia' and the subheading 'Pathological'.)
14. *What is the cause of tachycardia in anemia?* (**Ans.** Refer to page 177, under the heading 'Tachycardia' and the subheading 'Pathological'.)
15. *What is the cause of bradycardia in trained athletes?* (**Ans.** Refer to page 178, under the heading 'Bradycardia' and the subheading 'Athletes'.)
16. *Why is the heart rate reduced during sleep?*
    (**Ans.** Sympathetic activity decreases and parasympathetic activity increases during sleep. Therefore, the heart rate is lower in sleep than in the awake state.)
17. *What is the cause of bradycardia in increased intracranial pressure?*
    (**Ans.** When intracranial pressure increases as seen in a brain tumour, the blood flow to the vasomotor centre [VMC] in the medulla decreases because of the compression of intracranial blood vessels. This causes local hypoxia and hypercapnia, and stimulates VMC, which results in intense vasoconstriction. This is called Cushing's reflex. Vasoconstriction increases

blood pressure, which stimulates baroreceptors, and the activation of baroreceptor reflex results in bradycardia. Therefore, bradycardia rather than tachycardia is one of the important clinical features of raised intracranial pressure.)

18. *What is the relationship between pulse rate and blood pressure?*
(Ans. Pulse rate is inversely proportional to the blood pressure but not vice versa. This is called Mary's law. When blood pressure increases, the baroreceptors present in the arterial side of the circulation are stimulated. This activates the baroreceptor reflex, which results in bradycardia and hypotension. Conversely, when blood pressure decreases, there is tachycardia. Therefore, heart rate is inversely proportional to the blood pressure. But, blood pressure may not change with change in heart rate.)

19. *What is sinus arrhythmia?* (Ans. Refer to page 182, under the heading 'Rhythm' and the subheading 'Sinus Irregularity'.)

20. *What are the causes of high-volume and low-volume pulses?* (Ans. Refer to page 178, under the heading 'Volume' read subheading 'Conditions that ...'.)

21. *What is the physiological significance of examining the volume of the pulse?* (Ans. Refer to page 178, under the heading the text under 'Volume'.)

22. *What do you mean by the collapsing pulse and what is its physiological basis?* (Ans. Refer to page 179, see the text under 'Water-Hammer Pulse'.)

23. *What is pulsus paradoxus and what are the conditions that produce it?* (Ans. Refer to page 180, see 'Pulsus Paradoxus'.)

24. *What is the physiological basis of pulsus paradoxus in constrictive pericarditis and pericardial effusion?*
(Ans. In constrictive pericarditis and in pericardial effusion, the filling of the atria and ventricles decreases due to restriction to the expansion of the heart chambers. The limitation in the diastolic filling of the atria and the ventricles during inspiration results in lowering of left ventricular stroke volume.)

25. *What is pulsus alternans and what is the physiological basis of this pulse?* (Ans. Refer to page 181, under the heading 'Pulsus Alternans'.)

26. *What is the significance of examining the femoral artery simultaneously with the radial artery?* (Ans. Refer to page 181, under the heading 'Radio-femoral Delay'.)

27. *What are the differences between central and peripheral pulses as recorded by arterial pulse tracing?* (Ans. Refer to page 181, under the heading 'Pulse Tracing'.)

28. *What are the waves observed in an arterial pulse tracing? How are they caused?* (Ans. Refer to page 181, under the heading 'Pulse Tracing'.)

29. *What is carotid sinus reflex? How is it elicited? What is its clinical significance?* (Ans. Refer to page 181-182, under the heading 'Demonstration of Carotid Sinus Reflex'.)

30. *How do you demonstrate venous blood flow? What is its physiological significance?* (Ans. Refer to page 182, under the heading 'Demonstration of Venous Blood Flow'.)

31. *How do you demonstrate venous pressure? What is its physiological significance?* (Ans. Refer to page 182, under the heading 'Demonstration of Venous Pressure'.)

32. *What is triple response? What are the components?* (Ans. Refer to page 182, under the heading 'Demonstration of Triple Response'.)

33. *What is the function of the sinoaortic reflex?*
(Ans. Sinoaortic baroreceptor reflex is a robust short-term mechanism for the regulation of BP. The impulses along the sinus and aortic nerves [buffer nerves] are relayed to the CIC in the medulla, which in turn, are projected to the VMC, which control sympathetic discharge and BP. This is described in detail in Chapter 28.)

34. *What is the practical significance of carotid sinus reflex?*
(Ans. Stretching or exerting pressure on the carotid sinus—e.g., by hyperextension of the head, carrying heavy shoulder loads, and wearing tight collars—may decrease the HR and BP to cause carotid sinus syncope. The person may faint due to inappropriate stimulation of carotid baroreceptors. Massaging of the carotid sinus is useful to slow the HR in cases of paroxysmal atrial tachycardia [PAT].)

35. *What are the normal venous pressures?*
(Ans.
   i.   The pressure in the venules is 12–16 mmHg. The peripheral venous pressure in the forearm (at the heart level) is 6–8 mmHg and in the great veins near the heart is 3–4 mmHg, though it varies with respiration.
   ii. The pressure in the dural sinuses [with the head upright] is sub-atmospheric [i.e., negative] because these venous channels are rigid and cannot collapse.)

36. *When does the peripheral venous pressure increase?*
(Ans. It occurs in right heart failure [congestive heart failure]. The failure of the right ventricle causes back pressure to increase in the systemic veins. Increased pressure in the portal veins causes exudation of fluid, a condition called **ascites**. In the limb veins, the back pressure increases the capillary hydrostatic pressure, which leads to edema in the dependent parts of the body.)

28 | Measurement of Blood Pressure

Learning Objectives

After completing this practical, you will be able to (MUST KNOW):

1. Define blood pressure and define systolic, diastolic, mean arterial, and pulse pressure.
2. State the normal values of systolic, diastolic, mean arterial, and pulse pressure.
3. Tie the BP cuff properly around the subject's arm.
4. Raise and decrease the mercury column of the sphygmomanometer at the required speed during BP recording.
5. Detect the appearance and disappearance of sounds by placing a stethoscope on the brachial artery while measuring blood pressure.
6. Record BP by palpatory and auscultatory methods, and list the precautions of recording BP.

7. List the physiological variations of blood pressure.
8. Define hypertension and hypotension.
9. Name the reflexes involved in regulation of BP.
10. State the importance of baroreceptor reflex.

You may also be able to (DESIRABLE TO KNOW):

1. List the merits and demerits of different methods of measuring blood pressure.
2. Explain the mechanism of alteration in blood pressure in different physiological conditions.
3. Explain the physiological basis of different types of hypertension and hypotension.
4. Explain the mechanism of short-term and long-term regulation of blood pressure.
5. Correlate the changes in BP in common clinical conditions.

PY5.12: Record blood pressure and pulse at rest and in different grades of exercise and postures in a volunteer or simulated environment.

INTRODUCTION

Blood pressure (BP) is defined as the **lateral pressure exerted by the column of blood on the walls of the arteries**. Blood pressure usually means arterial pressure. The pressure in the arteries fluctuates during the systole and diastole of the heart.

Systolic BP

Definition: Systolic blood pressure (SBP) is defined as the **maximum pressure recorded during the cardiac cycle**. Because it is recorded during a systole, it is called systolic blood pressure.

Significance: SBP depends mainly **on the cardiac output**. Thus, SBP increases in conditions in which cardiac output is high.

Normal value: **100–119 mmHg** (120 to 139 mmHg in pre-hypertension; see Table 28.1).

Diastolic BP

Definition: Diastolic blood pressure (DBP) is defined as the **minimum pressure recorded during the cardiac cycle**. It is recorded during a diastole. Therefore, it is called diastolic pressure.

Significance: DBP depends mainly **on peripheral resistance**. Thus, DBP changes in conditions in which

there is a change in the peripheral resistance. Peripheral resistance depends chiefly on the **diameter of the blood vessels** and **viscosity of the blood**.

Normal value: 60–79 mmHg (80–89 mmHg in pre-hypertension).

Pulse Pressure

Definition: Pulse pressure (PP) is the difference between systolic and diastolic blood pressures.

Significance: This is the pressure that maintains the normal pulsatile nature of the flow of blood in the vascular compartment. The pulsatile nature of the flow is required for the perfusion of the tissues.

Normal value: 20–50 mmHg.

Mean Arterial Pressure

Definition: Mean arterial pressure (MAP) or mean arterial blood pressure (MABP) is the **average pressure produced during the cardiac cycle**. It is calculated by adding one-third of the PP to the diastolic pressure.

MAP = DBP + 1/3 PP

Because the duration of a systole is less than the duration of a diastole, MAP is slightly lower than the value halfway between systolic and diastolic pressure. MAP also determines tissue perfusion.

Significance: MAP is the pressure that helps in the forward movement of blood in the lumen of the blood vessels. MAP also determines tissue perfusion.

Normal value: 75–105 mmHg.

Casual Blood Pressure

Blood pressure measured at any time of the day is called casual blood pressure.

Basal Blood Pressure

Blood pressure recorded in the basal state is called basal blood pressure. It is recorded following complete physical and mental rest for 15 to 20 minutes.

Table 28.1   Classification of BP by Joint National Committee (JNC-7).

Category	Systolic BP (mmHg)	Diastolic BP (mmHg)
Normal	100–119	60–79
Pre-hypertension	120–139	80–89
Stage I Hypertension	140–159	90–99
Stage II Hypertension	160 or above	100 or above

Factors Affecting BP

Blood pressure = Cardiac output × Peripheral resistance.

Thus, factors that affect cardiac output and peripheral resistance also affect blood pressure. Alteration in cardiac output mainly affects systolic pressure, whereas alteration in peripheral resistance mainly affects diastolic pressure.

Factors affecting cardiac output

Cardiac output = Stroke volume × Heart rate.

Therefore, any factor that affects stroke volume or heart rate alters cardiac output. Stroke volume is affected by **preload, afterload, and myocardial contractility**, and the heart rate is chiefly affected by **parasympathetic and sympathetic activities**.

1. Preload

Preload is the end diastolic volume (EDV), i.e., the amount of blood present in the ventricle at the end of the diastole. When the EDV increases, the cardiac output increases and conversely, when EDV decreases, the cardiac output decreases. This occurs due to the **Frank–Starling mechanism**. EDV depends on the venous return to the heart.

Factors that increase preload
1. Increased total blood volume
2. Increased venous tone
3. Increased pumping action of the skeletal muscle
4. Increased negative intrathoracic pressure
5. Increased atrial contraction

Factors that decrease preload
1. Decreased blood volume
2. Venodilation

3. Increased intrapericardial pressure
4. Decreased ventricular compliance

2. Afterload

Afterload is peripheral resistance. When peripheral resistance increases, as in hypertension, the cardiac output decreases; when peripheral resistance decreases, as in anemia, the cardiac output increases.

3. Myocardial contractility

The contractility of the myocardium exerts a major influence on the cardiac output. The strength of the cardiac contraction is called the **inotropic state of the heart**. The factors that increase the strength of contraction are said to be **positively inotropic** and the factors that decrease the strength of contraction are said to be **negatively inotropic**.

Factors that are positively inotropic
1. Sympathetic stimulation
2. Digitalis
3. Glucagon
4. Caffeine and theophylline

Factors that are negatively inotropic
1. Parasympathetic stimulation
2. Hypoxia, hypercapnia and acidosis
3. Loss of myocardium
4. Drugs like propranolol, quinidine and barbiturate

4. Heart rate

Increase in heart rate increases cardiac output and decrease in heart rate decreases cardiac output. However, a change in heart rate cannot significantly alter the cardiac output unless it is associated with a change in ventricular filling.

Factors affecting peripheral resistance

1. Diameter of blood vessels

Any decrease in vessel diameter (vasoconstriction) increases both peripheral resistance and blood pressure. Vasodilation decreases peripheral resistance and decreases blood pressure. The diameter of the blood vessels depends mainly on the **vasoconstrictor tone**, which is the *rate of discharge in the vasoconstrictor nerves (sympathetic tone)*. **Increase in vasoconstrictor tone** causes arteriolar constriction and increases blood pressure. Conversely, **decrease in vasoconstrictor tone** decreases blood pressure. When the wall of the blood vessel becomes stiff (**less compliant**), peripheral resistance increases and, therefore, blood pressure increases.

2. Viscosity

Viscosity of blood depends on the composition of plasma, the total number of cells in the blood, and resistance of the cells to deformation, and temperature.

Factors that increase viscosity
1. Polycythemia
2. Hyperproteinemia
3. Hereditary spherocytosis
4. Decreased temperature

Factors that decrease viscosity
1. Anemia
2. Hypoproteinemia
3. Increased temperature

METHODS OF MEASURING BP

Blood pressure is measured by two methods, **direct and indirect.**

Direct Method

Blood pressure is measured directly by **placing a cannula in the lumen of the artery** and connecting the cannula to a mercury manometer or a pressure transducer. This method is used for recording blood pressure in experimental animals. In humans, blood pressure can be measured directly during open thoracic surgeries. In clinical practice, blood pressure is measured by the indirect method.

Indirect Method (Sphygmomanometry)

The instrument used in this method is the **sphygmomanometer.** Therefore, the method of measurement is called sphygmomanometry.

A sphygmomanometer is an instrument used to measure blood pressure; it is also known as a **blood pressure meter/blood pressure gauge/blood pressure monitor.** The word sphygmomanometer is derived from the Greek word '*sphygmos*' meaning beating of the heart or the pulse and *manometer* meaning a device used for measuring pressure or tension. This instrument was invented by **Samuel Siegfried Karl Ritter von Basch** in the year 1881. But in the year 1896, **Scipione Riva-Rocci** introduced a simplified version of the sphygmomanometer.

Principle

The cuff of the sphygmomanometer is wrapped around the subject's arm. The bag is then inflated until the **air pressure in the cuff overcomes the arterial pressure** and obliterates the arterial lumen. This is confirmed by palpating the radial pulse, which disappears when the cuff pressure is raised above the arterial pressure. The pressure is then raised further by about 20 mmHg and then slowly reduced. When the **pressure in the cuff reaches just below the arterial pressure**, blood escapes beyond the occlusion into the peripheral part of the artery, and the pulse starts reappearing. This is detected by the **appearance of sounds** in the stethoscope and is taken *as the systolic pressure*. Subsequently, the quality of the sound changes and finally disappears. The level **where sound disappears** is taken as the *diastolic pressure*. The sound disappears because the flow in the blood vessels becomes laminar.

Requirements

1. Sphygmomanometer
2. Stethoscope

■ Sphygmomanometer

There are **three major types** of sphygmomanometers.

i. **Mercury sphygmomanometer:** In the past, the sphygmomanometer used was a mercury manometer consisting of a manometer that had a mercury reservoir, cuff, and air pump. However, since the manometer contains *mercury, a highly toxic material*, and there are possibilities of leakage of mercury from the mercury reservoir of the sphygmomanometer, its use has been banned in many countries. Recently, the use of the mercury sphygmomanometer has been prohibited in India.

ii. **Aneroid sphygmomanometer:** This apparatus is commonly used in practice, especially for teaching and training of medical and paramedical students and staff.

iii. **Automatic digital sphygmomanometer:** This apparatus is routinely used now-a-days for measurement of BP in hospital patients.

Aneroid sphygmomanometer

Aneroid means '**without fluid**'. In this instrument, there is no use of mercury and hence, the name. The aneroid sphygmomanometer uses a spring mechanism and dial gauge to display the BP reading without the use of mercury. It consists of a manometer gauge which is attached to the cuff. To convert the cuff pressure into gauge pressure, the gauge head has a mechanical part. The aneroid sphygmomanometer has three parts: a manometer gauge, cuff, and air pump (Fig. 28.1A and B).

1. **Aneroid manometer gauge:** The manometer is a round device, which is graduated from **0 to 300 mm**, with the smallest division being 2 mmHg (Fig. 28.2A and B). It has **a long needle**, which moves when the cuff is inflated or deflated to indicate the level of pressure. The manometer is connected to a rubber tube of the cuff, and has a **short, metallic or rubber tube** that connects to the air pump.

2. **Cuff:** In mercury manometers, the cuff is known as the *Riva–Rocci cuff*. In the aneroid manometer, the cuff consists of an inflatable rubber bag covered with non-distensible cotton fabric. Two tubes are attached to the bag, one transmits air pressure to the manometer and the other is connected to the air pump. The **width of the cuff is usually 12 cm.** The

length and width of the cuff are different for different age groups and body builds. Roughly, the length of the rubber bag should be two-thirds and the width should be one-third of the mid-arm circumference of the subject. On the cuff, there is a mark that says '**Artery**', which is the artery position indicator level, i.e., the cuff is tied around the arm in such way the 'Artery' remains anteriorly and approximately overlying the position of the artery.

The width of the cuff should be **12.5 cm for measuring BP in adults**, **8 cm for children** up to 8 years, **5 cm for children up to 4 years**, and **2 to 3 cm for newborns and infants**.

3. **Air pump (inflation bulb):** It is a hand-operated **rubber bulb** provided with a one-way valve at its free end and a leak valve arrangement at the other (Fig. 28.2B). A short **metallic tube** or a rubber tube connects the air pump to the manometer. The rubber bag is inflated by turning the screw clockwise and repeatedly compressing the bulb. The bag is deflated by turning the screw anti-clockwise. The pump has spoon-like **curved, metallic or plastic plate** to the right side, which provides stability to the pumping mechanism while inflating the cuff.

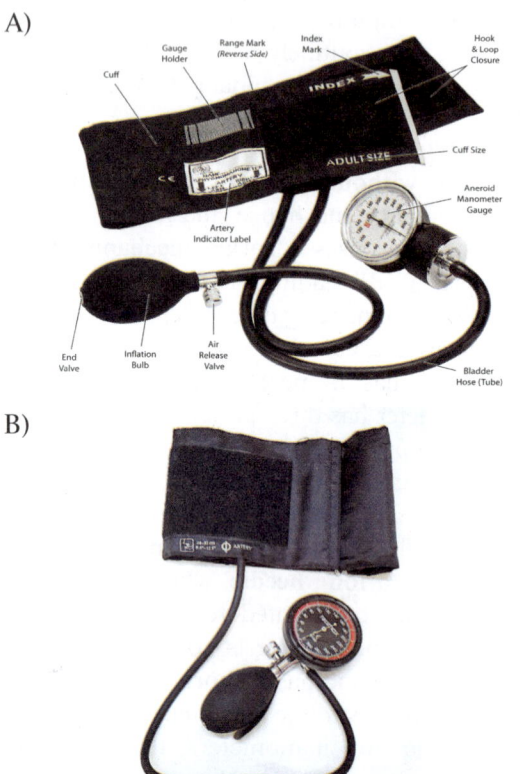

Fig. 28.1   Aneroid sphygmomanometer: (A) With detailed labelling of its three parts: manometer gauge, cuff, and air pump and (B) a variant of the aneroid sphygmomanometer, which is commonly used in current practice.

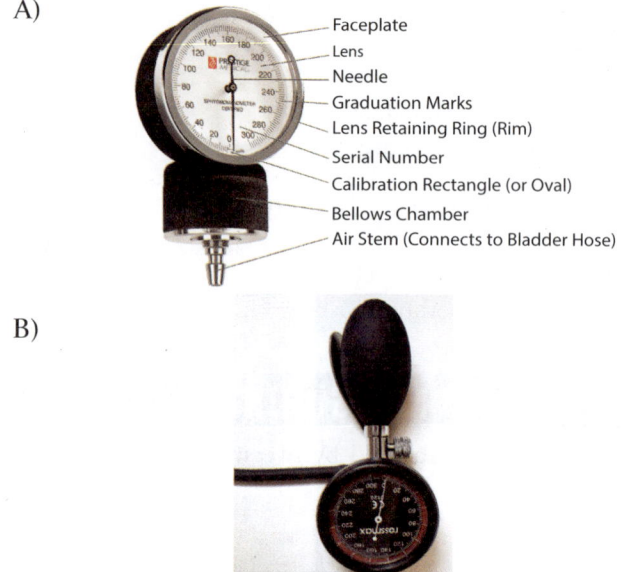

Fig. 28.2   Aneroid manometer gauge: (A) With detailed labelling and (B) manometer gauge (a variant) attached to the air pump, showing the metallic air release screw-valve on one side and the tube of the cuff on the other side.

Stethoscope

Stethoscopes (*steth*—chest; *scope*—to see or inspect) are of two types, the **bell type** and the **diaphragm type**. Modern stethoscopes are a ***combination of the bell and diaphragm types*** (Fig. 28.3A). The ***bell type chest piece*** detects low-pitched sounds like heart sounds, whereas high-pitched sounds such as aortic diastolic murmurs are better heard with the diaphragm of the stethoscope. For recording blood pressure, the ***diaphragm type chest piece*** is used (Fig. 28.3B).

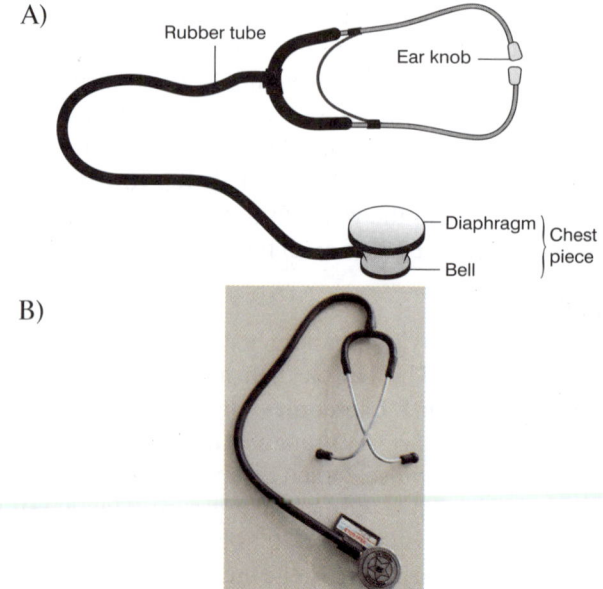

Fig. 28.3   Stethoscope: (A) Diagram showing the parts and (B) picture of a stethoscope.

Pre-recording instructions

Before recording blood pressure, the following conditions need to be satisfied:

1. The subject should be physically and mentally relaxed, free from excitement and apprehension.
2. The subject should lie down or sit comfortably.
3. The 'zero' of the sphygmomanometer and the cuff should be at the level of the heart.

   Blood pressure can be measured by three methods: palpatory, auscultatory, and oscillatory. Ideally, blood pressure should be measured *first by the palpatory and then by the auscultatory* method.

Palpatory method

▌Procedure

1. Check and ensure the needle of the gauge is leveled with the zero of the manometer calibration.

   Note: Before recording the blood pressure, it should be ensured that the needle in the manometer gauge coincides with the 'zero' of the manometer calibration.

2. Expose the subject's arm up to the shoulder.
3. The subject should lie down on a couch or sit comfortably in an armchair just next to the table.
4. Ask the subject to keep his forearm comfortably on the table or on the arm of the chair.
5. Wrap the cuff around the middle of the arm (so that the 'Artery' mark of the cuff lies over the brachial artery) in such a way that the lower edge of the cuff remains at a minimum distance of one inch above the cubital fossa.
6. Palpate the radial artery at the wrist by placing your middle three fingers over it.
7. Hold the rubber bulb in the other hand in such a way that your thumb and index finger remain free to manipulate the leak-valve screw.
8. Raise the pressure of the mercury manometer by repeatedly compressing the rubber bulb and continue to feel the radial pulse simultaneously. Note the level of the mercury in the manometer scale when the pulse disappears.
9. Raise the mercury column to about 10 mmHg above the point of disappearance of the pulse.
10. Reduce the pressure gradually by 2–4 mmHg per second. However, reduction in this pressure may be further slowed if there is significant bradycardia. Note the mercury level when the pulse reappears.

    Note: The pulse reappears at the same level where it had disappeared.

11. Reduce the pressure rapidly to the zero level.
12. Note your observation and express the result in mmHg.

    Note: The point of disappearance (or appearance) of the pulse is the blood pressure recorded by the palpatory method. This blood pressure is the systolic pressure.

▌Precautions

1. The subject should be mentally and physically relaxed.
2. The subject should lie down or sit comfortably with his forearm on the arm of the chair or on the table for a minimum of five minutes before the recording.
3. The pin of the gauge should level with the zero reading of the manometer calibration.
4. The subject's arm should be completely exposed and kept at heart level.
5. The cuff should be tied neither very tightly nor loosely around the arm.
6. The width of the cuff should be according to the circumference of the arm to overcome tissue resistance. The width of the cuff in adults is 12.5 cm. If a narrower cuff is used in adults, the recorded pressure will be falsely high. A narrower cuff is used for children.
7. The cuff and the equipment should be kept at the level of the heart to avoid the effect of gravity. The pressure in any vessel above the heart level is lower and in any vessel below the heart is higher.
8. The level of disappearance or reappearance of the pulse should be noted accurately.

▌Advantages

1. A stethoscope is not required for measuring BP.
2. As auscultation is not required, this method can be performed by less experienced medical personnel.
3. Recording is not time-consuming.
4. It gives a rough indication of the systolic pressure before recording BP by the auscultatory method.
5. An auscultatory gap, if present, is not missed in the auscultatory method when the blood pressure is first recorded by the palpatory and then by the auscultatory method.

▌Disadvantages

1. This method records only the systolic pressure. Diastolic pressure cannot be determined.
2. The systolic pressure recorded is about 2–5 mmHg less than the actual pressure.

Auscultatory method

▌Procedure

1. Record blood pressure by the palpatory method as described above.
2. Raise the pressure to 20 mmHg above the palpatory level, i.e., 20 mmHg above the level at which radial pulsation is no longer felt.
3. Place the diaphragm of the stethoscope lightly on the brachial artery in the cubital fossa, i.e., over the upper part of the forearm, medial to the tendon of the biceps (Fig. 28.4).

4. Lower the pressure at the rate of 2–4 mmHg per second. Note the appearance of the sound, the change in character of the sound, and finally the cessation of the sound, while the pressure in the cuff is progressively lowered.

5. Note the level at which the sounds are first heard as the systolic pressure, and the level at which the sounds cease as the diastolic pressure.

> **Note:** When pressure in the cuff is progressively lowered, the sounds undergo a series of changes in quality and intensity. These sounds are known as **Korotkoff sounds** (described by the Russian scientist Nikolai Sergeyevich Korotkov in 1905). These sounds are heard in five different phases (Fig. 28.5).

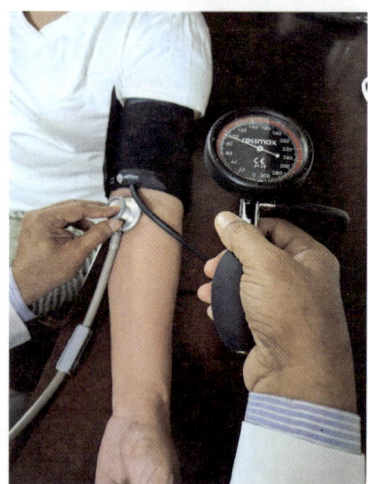

Fig. 28.4 Measurement of blood pressure by the auscultatory method using an aneroid sphygmomanometer. Note that the sphygmomanometer is held at the level of the heart.

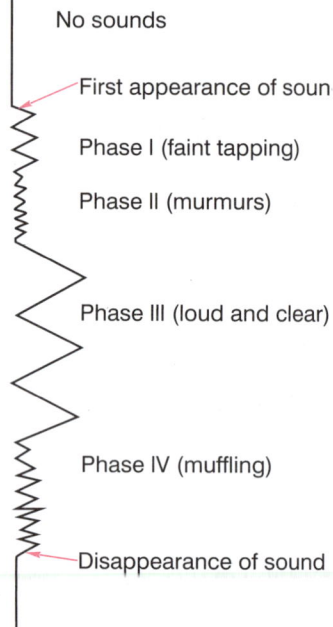

Fig. 28.5 Phases of Korotkoff sounds.

1. **Phase I:** Sudden appearance of faint tapping sounds, which become gradually louder and clearer during the succeeding 10 mmHg fall in pressure.

2. **Phase II:** The sound becomes murmurish in the next 10 mmHg fall in pressure.

3. **Phase III:** The sound changes a little in quality but becomes clearer and louder in the next 15 mmHg fall in pressure.

4. **Phase IV:** Sounds become muffled in character during the next 5 mmHg drop.

5. **Phase V:** Sounds completely disappear.

   The appearance of the sound is recorded as systolic blood pressure and the disappearance of sound is recorded as diastolic blood pressure. In persons with severe hypertension and in children, muffling rather than the disappearance of the sound is taken as the diastolic pressure.

▮ Observation and results

Report the BP of the subject as follows:

1. Note the systolic BP by palpatory method, recorded in the left arm and over three separate times.

2. Calculate the average of three values of systolic BP recorded by the palpatory method in the left arm.

3. Note the systolic and diastolic BP obtained by auscultatory methods, recorded in the left arm, and three times separately.

4. Calculate the average of the three values of both systolic and diastolic BP obtained by the auscultatory method in the left arm.

5. Note the systolic BP by the palpatory method, recorded in the right arm, recorded three times separately.

6. Calculate the average of three values of systolic BP recorded by the palpatory method in the right arm.

7. Note the systolic and diastolic BP obtained by auscultatory methods, recorded in the right arm, and three times separately.

8. Calculate the average of three values each of systolic and diastolic BP obtained by the auscultatory method in the right arm.

9. Express your result in a tabular column and calculate the average BP as depicted below in the tabular format.

Recording of systolic BP (mmHg) by the palpatory method

	Left arm	**Right arm**
1st recording		
2nd recording		
3rd recording		
Average of the three		

Recording of BP values by the auscultatory method (all values in mmHg)

	Left Arm		Right Arm	
	Systolic	*Diastolic*	*Systolic*	*Diastolic*
1st recording				
2nd recording				
3rd recording				
Average of three				

10. Calculate the mean arterial pressure (MAP) and pulse pressure (PP) from the final (average of three) result of systolic and diastolic pressure as noted in the above tables, and tabulate the observations presented in the tabular format below.

Recording MAP and PP

	Left arm (in mmHg)	Right arm (in mmHg)
Systolic BP		
Diastolic BP		
MAP		
PP		

11. Report your results with a comment saying whether the BP recorded is within the normal range, in the pre-hypertension stage, or the hypertension stage (1 or 2). If there is hypertension, comment whether it is only systolic or only diastolic hypertension or both.

▮ Precautions

1. The subject should be mentally and physically relaxed.

Note: When a subject visits the doctor's clinic for consultation and his BP is measured, it is usually found to be much more than the BP recorded in the same subject at home. This is termed as **white coat hypertension**. It is largely a result of the subject's apprehension while in the doctor's clinic. Ensuring physical and mental relaxation prior to BP recording decreases the impact of white coat hypertension.

2. The size of the cuff should be proportionate to the circumference of the subject's arm.
3. The zero reading of the manometer should be kept at the level of the heart.
4. Blood pressure should be detected first by the palpatory method before recording by the auscultatory method.
5. Pressure should be raised by 20 mmHg above the palpatory level. This is because the sensitivity of auscultatory method is more than the palpatory method. Sounds created by the beginning of blood flow into the artery will be heard at an earlier level of pressure level than the feeling of pulse by palpation.
6. The cuff pressure should be decreased to the zero level between successive trials.

7. While reading the manometer, the eye should be at the level of the manometer pin to avoid visual parallax.
8. If coarctation of the aorta is suspected, blood pressure should also be recorded in the thigh.

Note: A cuff of greater width (about 18 cm) is used for measuring blood pressure in the thigh. The patient lies face down, the cuff is applied above the knee, and auscultation is carried out over the popliteal artery.

9. Blood pressure should ideally be checked by the palpatory method before recording by the auscultatory method.

Note: Blood pressure is checked by the palpatory method before the auscultatory method to include the auscultatory gap in the pressure range. In severely hypertensive patients, after the appearance of the sounds, occasionally, the sounds disappear at a point below 200 mmHg for a range of 20–50 mmHg, and then reappear and finally disappear at the level of diastolic pressure. The period of the first (temporary) disappearance of sounds is called **silent gap** or **auscultatory gap**. The auscultatory gap is never missed if the pressure is measured first by the palpatory method because the auscultatory gap comes within the range of the systolic pressure recorded by the palpatory method. If the BP is directly measured by the auscultatory method, the auscultatory gap may be missed, and the systolic value maybe reported as lower than the actual value. The exact cause of the auscultatory gap is not known. It is thought to be due to the transient hyper-responsiveness of the vessel to compression.

10. The cuff and the equipment should be kept at the level of the heart to avoid the effect of gravity.

▮ Advantages

1. Gives accurate value for systolic pressure.
2. Detects diastolic pressure.

▮ Disadvantages

1. Unless followed by the palpatory method, the auscultatory method may miss the auscultatory gap.
2. Adequate experience needed for detecting quality of change in sounds by the stethoscope.

Special Note:
1. Diastolic pressure recorded in the sitting posture is about 5 mmHg more than in the supine posture.
2. Arm position above and below heart level yields lower and higher BP values, respectively.
3. If the BP values are different in the two arms, the higher value should be used.

Oscillatory method
▮ Procedure

The procedure is the same as that in the palpatory method, but instead of palpating the artery, the oscillations of the pin of the gauge in the sphygmomanometer are noted to record BP. The pressure in the cuff is raised, and the appearance and disappearance of oscillations of the manometer pin are observed while lowering the mercury column. The point of appearance of the oscillation gives the systolic pressure, and the point of disappearance of the oscillations gives the diastolic pressure. The oscillation of the pin is not as well appreciated in the aneroid sphygmomanometer as they are in the mercury column of the mercury sphygmomanometer. Therefore, the aneroid manometer is usually not preferred for measuring BP by the oscillatory method.

■ Disadvantages
1. This method does not yield accurate values for systolic and diastolic pressure.
2. Adequate experience is needed to detect the exact level of the appearance and disappearance of oscillation.

Using an automated digital monitor
The device used is called the **'automatic digital sphygmomanometer'** or **'automatic digital BP monitor'**. It is the most technologically advanced sphygmomanometer. The automated digital monitor consists of an **electronic sensor** to measure blood pressure and a **digital monitor**, on which the readings are displayed. In order to measure blood pressure, this instrument measures the fluctuations of arteries.

Parts: This automatic device has a **cuff** that connects through tubing to a **digital monitor** (a pressure gauge). The monitor has a **display screen** and a **start button**. The screen has three labels: i. 'Systolic (mmHg)'—which displays systolic pressure, ii. 'Diastolic (mmHg)'—which displays diastolic pressure and, iii. 'Pulse (per/min)'— which records the pulse or heart rate/min (Fig. 28.6). On the back of the monitor, there is *box-like compartment* for batteries (usually four) that supply power to the manometer; an arrow mark indicates how to open the battery-box.

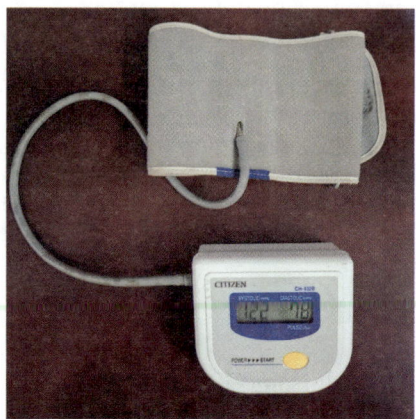

Fig. 28.6   Automatic digital sphygmomanometer.

■ Principle
When the 'Start' button is pressed, the cuff inflates and deflates automatically. When the cuff is tightened around the arm during inflation, it temporarily blocks blood flow in the artery of the arm. Loosening the cuff during deflation allows the blood flow to start again. Thus, the maximum and minimum pressures in an artery are detected.

■ Procedure
1. Ask the subject to sit comfortably in an armchair, with his arm on the arm of the chair (Fig. 28.7).
2. Tie the BP cuff around the arm as described in 'Measurement of BP using Aneroid Sphygmomanometer'.
3. Press the 'Start' button and note the inflation of cuff with a typical buzzing sound. The device senses automatically how much to inflate the cuff. It will become tight enough to hurt a little, but only for a few seconds.
4. Simultaneously, note the flashing of numbers that keep increasing in count. After reaching a peak, the sound stops, and the numbers keep decreasing.
5. When it is done (deflation is completed), the display shows the systolic and diastolic blood pressures and the pulse rate (the heart rate.

Note: Sometimes, the screen displays an **'E' (error)** message when there is a problem in the recording. This is usually due to old batteries that are exhausted. Exhausted batteries should be removed and replaced quickly.

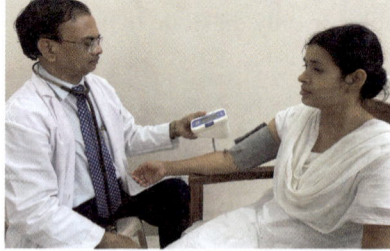

Fig. 28.7   Recording of BP using automatic BP monitor. Note that the cuff and the equipment are approximately at the level of the heart and the subject is seated on a wooden chair with her hand resting on the arm of the chair and her back upright against the back of the chair.

■ Advantages
The advantages of an automatic digital monitor are: **i)** it is a small device that is lightweight, portable; **ii)** it is easy to operate (no need of expertise of the use of a stethoscope); **iii)** when kept at home, recording can be done by the patient himself, without any assistance; **iv)** the pulse rate is measured automatically along with BP; **v)** in the 'Memory' of the device, the past few recordings will be available; **vi)** calibration is not an issue with this device; **vii)** recordings can be done much faster, and many measurements can be done; **viii)** it is easy to record BP at health camps or screening camps for a larger population.

■ Disadvantages

The disadvantages are as follows: **i)** the equipment should be manufactured by a good company, otherwise there will be many errors (Omron and Citizen, Japan, have been reported to be the relatively better ones); **ii)** BP measured by this equipment initially needs to be checked and standardised simultaneously with the BP recording using an aneroid sphygmomanometer (BP measured by digital sphygmomanometer is usually little lower than the BP values of aneroid sphygmomanometer); **iii)** since the monitor is battery operated, batteries need to be checked for their life, and exhausted batteries should be removed from the device early; and **iv)** the cost of frequent replacement of batteries at regular intervals could be a financial issue.

Continuous BP monitoring in an ICU

Continuous blood pressure (BP) monitoring in an ICU is done **invasively by intra-arterial cannulation**. This involves inserting a catheter into an artery, typically the radial or femoral, to directly measure blood pressure. This method provides a beat-by-beat record of BP, allowing for real-time tracking and management of hemodynamic stability. Though non-invasive methods like *oscillometric cuffs or finger sensors* are also used, **invasive monitoring is often considered the gold-standard** for accuracy, especially in critically ill patients.

Principle

The pressure transducer *translates the mechanical pressure* in the artery into an *electrical signal* that is displayed on the monitor. This allows for continuous measurement of BP, including beat-to-beat variations.

Procedure

Since this is an invasive technique, it requires expertise.

1. An arterial line is inserted into a suitable artery (e.g., radial, brachial, or femoral) by a trained medical professional.
2. A catheter is threaded into the artery, and a pressure transducer is connected to the catheter.
3. The transducer measures the pressure in the artery and transmits it to a monitor, displaying a continuous waveform.
4. The monitor displays systolic, diastolic, and mean arterial pressures, as well as the arterial waveform.

Advantages

i) *Continuous measurement*—It provides continuous BP readings, allowing for timely detection of changes in pressure and facilitating appropriate interventions; ii) *BP waveform tracings* are also recorded, which gives knowledge of magnitude of pressure pulse; iii) *Accuracy*—the invasive method is the most accurate method, especially in patients with severe hemodynamic instability; iv) *Clinical utility*— continuous BP monitoring is crucial in the ICU for managing hemodynamic stability, guiding fluid resuscitation, and adjusting medication dosages.

DISCUSSION

Clinical Significance

Physiological conditions altering BP

1. **Age:** Blood pressure increases with age.
   1. *In children*: Systolic pressure is 90–119 mmHg. Diastolic pressure is 50–79 mmHg.
   2. *In adults*: Systolic pressure is 100–119 mm Hg. Diastolic pressure is 60–79 mmHg.
   3. *In the elderly*: The upper limit of systolic may be considered to be 160 mmHg, but diastolic pressure of 90 mmHg or above is always considered abnormal.
2. **Gender:** BP is **lower in females** due to the effect of progesterone, which relaxes the smooth muscles of the blood vessels. Moreover, the *cardiac vagal drive is relatively higher in females* compared to males. Therefore, the heart rate is comparatively lower in females. Consequently, the systolic BP is lower in females than it is in males. This difference in females disappears after menopause.
3. **Food intake:** BP increases after a meal. This may be due to increased body metabolism, which increases circulation.
4. **Sleep:** BP is lower during sleep than in the waking state. This is because a human being is under constant stress in the waking state, and not during sleep.
5. **Emotion and excitement:** In emotional and excited states, increased sympathetic discharge increases blood pressure.
6. **Exercise:** During exercise, the **systolic pressure always rises** because of increased cardiac output due to sympathetic stimulation, which causes tachycardia and increased myocardial contractility. **Diastolic pressure** depends on the degree of exercise. Diastolic pressure increases in mild exercise due to vasoconstriction, usually remains unchanged (or slightly more) in moderate exercise, but may fall (or remain stable or slightly rise) in intense exercise because of metabolic vasodilation and increased body temperature. During exercise, a rise in diastolic BP by more than 15 mmHg above resting value is considered abnormal.
7. **Posture:** On standing up suddenly from a supine (lying down) posture BP decreases and then returns to normal or increases due to correction by the baroreceptor reflex.

8. **Temperature:** BP decreases in a hot environment due to vasodilation and increases in a cold environment due to vasoconstriction.

9. **Pregnancy:** Increase in cardiac output due to increased blood volume **increases systolic pressure** during pregnancy, but **diastolic pressure falls slowly** reaching a nadir around mid-pregnancy due to gradual decrease in peripheral resistance. Peripheral resistance decreases due to the effect of progesterone, which relaxes the smooth muscles of blood vessels (causes vasodilation). Therefore, pulse pressure increases in pregnancy. Then, diastolic pressure **increases slowly to normal level** by term.

Pathological conditions altering BP

Blood pressure increases (hypertension) and decreases (hypotension) in different pathological conditions.

Pathophysiology of Hypertension

Hypertension is defined as sustained elevation of systemic arterial pressure. Usually, hypertension means rise in diastolic BP. Hypertension is broadly classified as essential and secondary.

Essential hypertension

This is the commonest type of hypertension and is seen in 90 per cent of patients with hypertension. The cause of essential hypertension is not known. It is thought to occur due to a hereditary defect or unhealthy lifestyles that predispose a person to hypertension.

Secondary hypertension

This is hypertension secondary to a disease elsewhere in the body. The following are the causes of secondary hypertension.
1. Adrenocortical diseases
   1. Hyperaldosteronism
   2. Cushing syndrome
   3. Hypertensive form of congenital virilizing tumour
2. Renal diseases
   1. Glomerulonephritis
   2. Pyelonephritis
   3. Polycystic disease
   4. Tumours of the JG cells
3. Pheochromocytoma
4. Severe polycythemia
5. Oral contraceptives

Pathophysiology of Hypotension

Systolic pressure less than 90 mmHg in adults is known as hypotension. Clinically, there are three types of

hypotension: chronic hypotension, acute hypotension, and postural hypotension.

Chronic hypotension

Chronic hypotension is characterized by persistent low blood pressure. Usually, patients are asymptomatic, but sometimes, they complain of lethargy, weakness, and giddiness.

▮ Causes
1. Primary adrenocortical insufficiency
2. Hypopituitarism
3. Malnutrition and anemia
4. Chronic diarrhea
5. Prolonged bed rest

Acute hypotension

A sudden fall of blood pressure is called acute hypotension. Usually, if severe, it is associated with fainting.

▮ Causes
1. Acute hemorrhage
2. Acute diarrhea
3. Severe vomiting
4. Acute myocardial infarction
5. Excessive diuresis
6. Acute vasodilation

Postural hypotension

If systolic blood pressure falls by 20 mmHg or more when a subject assumes the erect posture (from the supine posture), the condition is called postural or orthostatic hypotension. This usually results from autonomic imbalance. It may be of the chronic or acute variety.

Acute postural hypotension: This is due to a temporary fall in blood pressure, which results in transient fainting. It is usually seen in the following conditions:
1. Prolonged standing
2. Rising from bed after a prolonged illness
3. Strenuous physical exercise

Chronic postural hypotension: It can be primary or secondary. Chronic primary postural hypotension is also called **idiopathic postural hypotension**. The cause of this type of hypotension is not known. It usually occurs in the elderly and may be due to the degeneration of peripheral autonomic nerves. Chronic secondary postural hypotension has the following causes:
1. Polyneuropathy as seen in diabetes, amyloidosis, and beriberi
2. Autonomic neuropathy as seen in syringomyella, tabes dorsalis, and subacute combined degeneration of the spinal cord
3. Patients receiving sympatholytic drugs
4. Surgical sympathectomy

Physiological Significance

Regulation of blood pressure

The mechanisms involved in the regulation of blood pressure can be divided into two broad categories: (1) short-term regulation and (2) long-term regulation. Short-term regulation is chiefly neural and long-term regulation is chiefly hormonal.

■ Short-term regulation

Baroreceptor reflex: Baroreceptors are present in the **carotid sinus and aortic arch** and respond to stretching. They detect changes in pressure in the vessels in which they are situated. **Increase in blood pressure** causes distension of the carotid sinus and aortic arch, which stretches the baroreceptors and increases the firing rate in the **afferent nerves (IX and X cranial nerves).** This leads to the *excitation of the NTS* (nucleus tractus solitarius) in the medulla, which in turn, *inhibits the VMC* (vasomotor centre) via interneurons. The inhibition of the vasomotor centre *decreases sympathetic discharge* and causes vasodilation, bradycardia, decrease in cardiac output, and *fall in blood pressure* (Fig. 28.8). The excitation of the NTS also **stimulates the vagus nerve,** which decreases the heart rate and cardiac output.

Conversely, **when blood pressure falls,** less distension of the carotid sinus and aortic arch inhibits the receptors and decreases the discharge rate in the afferent nerves. Due to decreased activity in the IX and X cranial nerves, NTS is inhibited, which in turn, causes *disinhibition (stimulation) of the VMC.* This results in **increased sympathetic output** (Fig. 28.9). Inhibition of NTS also inhibits the vagus nerve and finally results in vasoconstriction, tachycardia, increased cardiac output, and increase in blood pressure. The baroreceptor reflex regulates blood pressure in the **pressure range of 70–150 mmHg.**

Chemoreceptor reflex: Chemoreceptors are located in the **aortic and carotid bodies.** They respond to changes in the chemical composition of blood, which occur in conditions like **hypoxia, hypercapnia, and acidosis.**

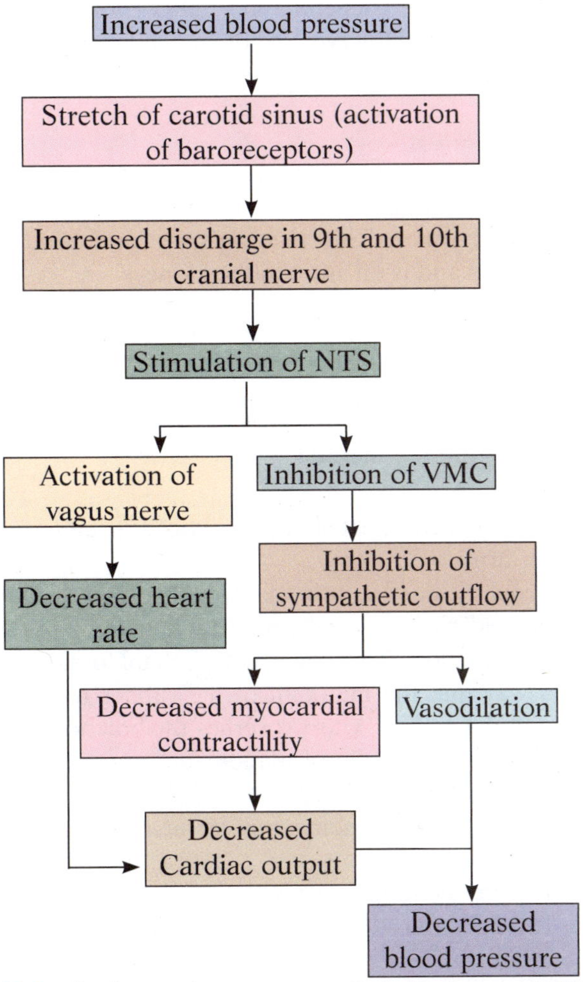

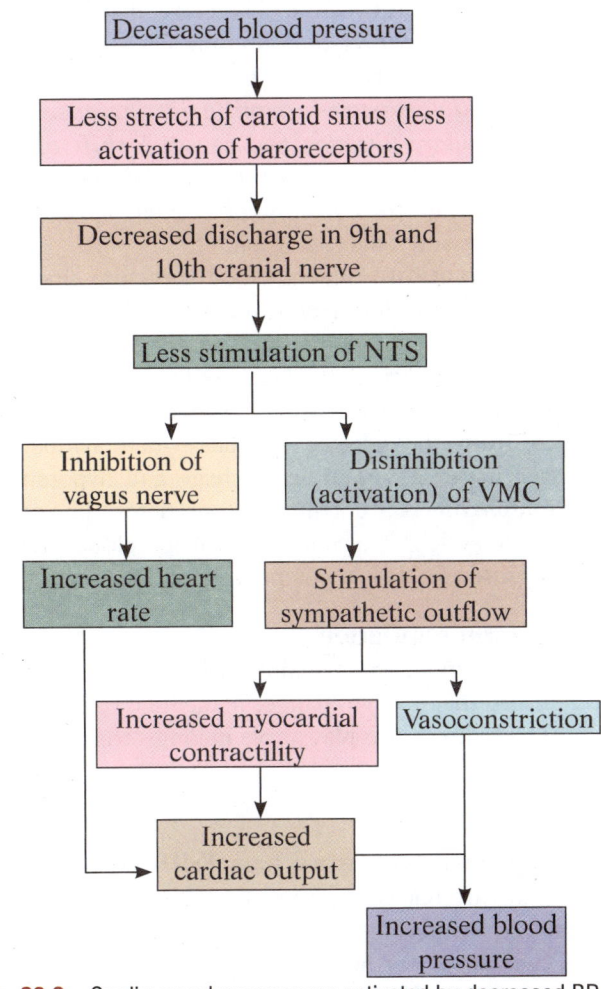

Fig. 28.8 Cardiovascular responses activated by increased BP that stimulates baroreceptors.

Fig. 28.9 Cardiovascular responses activated by decreased BP.

Stimulation of these receptors results in bradycardia and vasoconstriction. This also causes pulmonary hyperventilation and secretion of catecholamines from the adrenal medulla, which increase the heart rate. Therefore, the net effect of the stimulation of chemoreceptors is either no change in heart rate or mild tachycardia and hypertension. Chemoreceptors regulate blood pressure in the **pressure range of 40–70 mmHg**.

Cushing's reflex: In severe hypotension, blood flow to the brain decreases. Hypoxia and hypercapnia of the vasomotor centre occur. This causes stimulation of the vasomotor centre to the maximum, which results in intense vasoconstriction in order to bring the pressure back to normal. This response is called **CNS ischemic response** and is a life-saving mechanism when blood pressure falls below 40 mmHg.

When **intracranial pressure increases**, blood flow to the vasomotor centre decreases due to the compression of blood vessels. This stimulates the vasomotor centre and causes intense vasoconstriction, which results in increased blood pressure. This is called Cushing's reflex. The increase in blood pressure activates the baroreceptor reflex and causes bradycardia. Therefore, ***bradycardia is an outstanding feature*** of brain tumours.

Capillary fluid shift: When blood pressure increases, the ***hydrostatic pressure in capillaries increases***. This ***increases capillary filtration*** and causes a ***shift of fluid*** from the intravascular compartment to the extravascular space. As a result, the *circulating blood volume decreases* and blood pressure falls to normal.

Stress relaxation: When blood pressure increases suddenly, the ***smooth muscles of the blood vessels relax*** in response to the sudden stretching. This decreases the vascular tone and brings the pressure back to normal.

Hormonal mechanisms: Catecholamines are released from the adrenal medulla when sympathetic discharge increases, as in hemorrhage and hypotension. *Norepinephrine* is a potent vasoconstrictor. The renin–angiotensin system is also activated when blood pressure falls. *Angiotensin II* is a potent vasoconstrictor.

■ Long-term regulation

Long-term regulation is mainly achieved by hormonal mechanisms that involve changes in the fluid volume of the body. The kidneys also play a role in long-term regulation of BP.

Hormonal mechanism

1. **The renin–angiotensin system: Fall in blood pressure** trigger the release of renin from the JG cells of the kidney. Renin converts angiotensinogen to angiotensin I, which is further converted to angiotensin II. *Angiotensin II* causes vasoconstriction and increases blood pressure. It also increases the synthesis and secretion of aldosterone, which increases sodium and water reabsorption from the kidney, which in turn assists in the restoration of pressure.

2. **Vasopressin (ADH):** Decrease in extracellular fluid volume increases the release of ADH from the posterior pituitary. ADH increases water reabsorption from the kidneys and causes vasoconstriction.

3. **Catecholamines:** Stimulation of sympathetic fibres to the adrenal medulla causes the release of catecholamines. These hormones (especially norepinephrine) are potent vasoconstrictors.

4. **Nitric oxide (NO):** Endothelium-derived relaxing factor (EDRF) is the nitric oxide (NO) synthesized from arginine in the endothelial cells of blood vessels. NO produces ***relaxation of vascular smooth muscle*** and decreases blood pressure. In fact, NO mediates the action of many vasodilator substances.

5. **NO-dependent vasodilators:** *Histamine* (at H1 receptors), ***acetylcholine, bradykinin, VIP, and substance P*** depend on EDRF for producing vasodilation. However, ANP and adenosine *do not depend on EDRF* for their vasorelaxation effect.

Renal mechanism

When an alteration in blood pressure occurs, the kidneys try to restore the pressure by changing the excretion of sodium and water. This mechanism is independent of other factors and is intrinsic to the kidneys.

OSPE

I. **Record the blood pressure of the given subject by the palpatory method.**

Steps

1. Inform the subject about the procedure and expose his arm.
2. Properly tie the cuff of the sphygmomanometer around the subject's arm (not too tight nor too loose), about 2.5 cm above the cubital fossa in such a way that the midpoint of the rubber bag of the cuff marked as 'Artery' overlies the brachial artery.
3. Check that the pin of manometer gauge is leveled with the zero reading.
4. Keep the sphygmomanometer at the level of the subject's heart.
5. Palpate the radial artery.
6. Raise the pin of manometer by raising the pressure in the cuff.
7. Mark the level of the pin of the manometer for disappearance of the radial pulse.
8. Release the pressure in the cuff.

II. Record the blood pressure of the given subject by the auscultatory method.

Steps

1. Inform the subject about the procedure and expose his arm.
2. Properly tie the cuff of the sphygmomanometer around the subject's arm (neither too tight nor too loose) about 2.5 cm above the cubital fossa in such a way that the midpoint of the rubber bag of the cuff marked as 'Artery' overlies the brachial artery.
3. Check that the pin of manometer gauge is leveled with the zero reading.
4. Keep the sphygmomanometer at the level of the heart of the subject.
5. Palpate the radial artery.
6. Raise the pin of the manometer by increasing the pressure in the cuff and mark the level of disappearance of the radial pulse.
7. Raise the pin of the manometer about 30 mmHg above the palpatory level.
8. Place the diaphragm of the stethoscope medial to the tendon of the biceps where the pulsation of the brachial artery is felt.
9. Slowly lower the manometer pin by releasing the pressure in the cuff at the rate of 2–4 mmHg per second. While decreasing the pin of the manometer, auscultate for the appearance, change in quality, and disappearance of the sounds.
10. Note the appearance of the sounds as systolic and disappearance of the sounds as diastolic blood pressure.
11. Release the pressure from the cuff.

VIVA

1. *Define blood pressure.* (**Ans.** Refer to page 185, under the heading 'Introduction'.)
2. *Define systolic and diastolic blood pressure and give their normal values.* (**Ans.** Refer to page 185, under the headings 'Systolic BP' and 'Diastolic BP'.)
3. *What is mean arterial pressure? What is its significance?* (**Ans.** Refer to page 185, under the heading 'Mean Arterial Pressure'.)
4. *What is pulse pressure? What is its significance?* (**Ans.** Refer to page 185, under the heading 'Pulse Pressure'.)
5. *What are the methods of measuring blood pressure?* (**Ans.** Refer to page 187, under the heading 'Methods'.)
6. *What are the conditions that must be satisfied before recording blood pressure?* (**Ans.** Refer to page 189, under the heading 'Pre-recording Instructions'.)
7. *Why is the zero level of the sphygmomanometer and the cuff kept at the heart level of the subject while recording blood pressure?* (**Ans.** Refer to page 189, under the heading 'Procedure', read 'Note' under point no. 1.)
8. *Why is the blood pressure ideally recorded by the palpatory method before recording by the auscultatory method?* (**Ans.** Refer to page 191, under the heading 'Precautions', read the 'Note' under point no. 9.)
9. *What are the precautions for measuring blood pressure by the palpatory method?* (**Ans.** Refer to page 189, under the heading 'Precautions'.)
10. *Why is the pressure in the cuff raised by about 30 mmHg above the palpatory level for recording blood pressure by the auscultatory method?* (**Ans.** Refer to page 191, under the heading 'Precautions', read the 'Note' under point no. 8.)
11. *What is auscultatory gap? What is its significance?* (**Ans.** Refer to page 196, under the heading 'Precautions', read point no. 5.)
12. *What is the cause of the appearance, change in quality, and disappearance of sounds at various phases of blood pressure measurement?* (**Ans.** Refer to page 190, under the heading 'Procedure', read 'Korotkoff sounds'.)
13. *What are the ideal cuff sizes for different age groups?* (**Ans.** Refer to page 188, under the heading 'Requirements' and the subheading 'Cuff'.)
14. *How does using a large (oversized) or small (undersized) cuff affect the reading?*
    (**Ans.** BP reading will be higher if an undersized or oversized cuff is used, as more pressure will be required in the cuff to overcome the extra tissue resistance and to form a cone of pressure.)
15. *What would happen if the standard-sized cuff were to be used on an obese subject?*
    (**Ans.** If the standard cuff is used for an obese person, the reading will be higher than the actual because more cuff pressure will be required to overcome the extra tissue resistance, resulting in a falsely higher reading.)
16. *What would happen if the standard-sized cuff were to be used on an extremely thin subject?*
    (**Ans.** In a very thin person whose arm circumference is very small, using the standard cuff will yield a higher than actual reading due to the extra cuff pressure needed to overcome tissue resistance.)
17. *What are the precautions taken for recording blood pressure by the auscultatory method?* (**Ans.** Refer to page 191, under the heading 'Precautions'.)
18. *What is the oscillatory method of measuring blood pressure?* (**Ans.** Refer to page 191-192 under the heading 'Oscillatory Method'.)

19. *In which condition is the blood pressure measured in the lower limb? What is the size of the cuff used for this purpose?* (**Ans.** i. BP is measured in the lower limb, typically at the ankle, as an alternative when measurement of BP in the arm becomes challenging, e.g., due to injury or disability, or when there is a concern about peripheral vascular disease. It is also used in specific clinical situations like diagnosing hypertension when standard arm measurements are not possible. ii. For lower limb BP measurement, the cuff bladder should be at least 40% of the circumference of the limb being measured, and the length should be about 75–80% of that circumference. This means that the bladder should encircle at least 80% of the limb's circumference. For example, if a patient's thigh circumference is 40 cm, the cuff should have a bladder length of at least 32 cm (80% of 40 cm) and a width of at least 16 cm (40% of 40 cm). iii. When measuring BP in the lower limb, it is crucial to use the correct cuff placement and technique, as readings can differ from those in the arm. Ankle blood pressure measurements are generally preferred over those at the calf or thigh, and the cuff bladder should encircle 80% of the limb. Systolic BP reading is usually higher in the leg than the arm, while diastolic readings are similar in upper and lower limbs.)

20. *What is the principle of the digital sphygmomanometer? What are its advantages?* (Ans. Refer to page 192, under the heading 'By Using Digital Sphygmomanometer'.)

21. *What is the principle of BP measurement in the ICU? What are the advantages of this method?* (Ans. Refer to page 193, under the heading 'BP measurement in ICU'.)

22. *What are the factors that affect blood pressure?* (Ans. Refer to page 193, under the heading 'Physiological Conditions Altering BP'.)

23. *Why is blood pressure lower in females?* (Ans. Refer to page 193, under the heading 'Physiological Conditions Altering BP', read point no. 2.)

24. *Why is blood pressure lower during sleep?* (Ans. Refer to page 193, under the heading 'Physiological Conditions Altering BP', read point no. 4.)

25. *What is the mechanism of alteration of systolic and diastolic pressure during exercise?* (Ans. Refer to page 193, under the heading 'Physiological Conditions Altering BP', read point no. 6.)

26. *What happens to blood pressure on suddenly standing up from a supine position?* (Ans. Refer to page 193, under the heading 'Physiological Conditions Altering BP', read point no. 7.)

27. *What are the BP changes that occur during pregnancy?* (Ans. Refer to page 194, under the heading 'Physiological Conditions Altering BP', read point no. 9.)

28. *What is the baroreceptor reflex? How does it adjust BP when BP is decreased or increased?* (Ans. Refer to page 195, under the heading 'Regulation of BP' and the subheading 'Baroreceptor reflex'.)

29. *What is essential hypertension?* (Ans. Refer to page 194, under the heading 'Essential hypertension'.)

30. *What are the causes of secondary hypertension?* (Ans. Refer to page 194, under the heading 'Secondary hypertension'.)

31. *What are the causes of acute hypotension?* (Ans. Refer to page 198, under the heading 'Acute hypotension'.)

32. *What is postural hypotension? List the causes of postural hypotension.* (Ans. Refer to page 194, under the heading 'Postural hypotension'.)

33. *What are the mechanisms of short-term regulation of blood pressure?* (Ans. Refer to page 195-196 under the heading 'Regulation of BP' and the subheading 'Short-term regulation'.)

34. *Why is bradycardia a feature of raised intracranial pressure?* (Ans. Refer to page 196, under the heading 'Cushing reflex'.)

35. *What is the role of the renin–angiotensin system in hypertension?* (Ans. Refer to page 196, under the heading 'Long-term regulation' and the subheading 'Hormonal mechanisms'.)

36. *What is malignant hypertension?*
(**Ans.** Malignant hypertension is a severe and potentially life-threatening condition characterized by extremely high blood pressure and rapid organ damage. It is considered a hypertensive emergency requiring immediate treatment. A common definition includes both very high blood pressure (systolic >180 mmHg, diastolic >120 mmHg) and evidence of organ damage.)

37. *What is hypertensive crisis?*
(**Ans.** A hypertensive crisis is a medical emergency like malignant hypertension, characterized by blood pressure readings of 180/120 mmHg or higher that occurs rapidly and usually without warning. This sudden and severe elevation in blood pressure can cause serious organ damage and requires immediate medical attention.)

38. *What are the common complications of hypertension?*
(**Ans.** Uncontrolled and poorly managed hypertension can cause many long-term serious complications: i. hypertensive heart disease and heart attack, ii. stroke and paralysis, iii. heart failure, iv. kidney damage, v. eye problems, vi. metabolic syndrome, and vii. memory loss.

29 | Effect of Posture on Blood Pressure and Heart Rate

Learning Objectives

After completing this practical, you will be able to (MUST KNOW):

1. Record the effect of change in posture on heart rate and blood pressure (BP).
2. List the precautions to be taken while recording this effect.
3. Enumerate the changes in heart rate and BP response to standing.

You may also be able to (DESIRABLE TO KNOW):

1. Explain the compensatory mechanisms in response to standing.
2. Describe the physiological and clinical utility of this practical.

PY5.12: Record BP and pulse at rest and different grades of exercise and postures in a volunteer in a simulated environment.

INTRODUCTION

Change in body posture affects the functions of the cardiovascular system. The changes are more marked when a person suddenly stands up from the supine posture. The cardiovascular changes are different on immediate standing and on prolonged standing.

Cardiovascular Changes on Immediate Standing

Effects

When a person assumes an erect posture, blood is pulled to the lower parts of the body due to the effect of gravity. About **200–500 ml of blood** is immediately pulled in the capacitance vessels of the lower extremities. This **decreases venous return**, which results in **decreased cardiac output**. This is the cause of the **immediate fall in blood pressure** on standing. The effects of a change in posture are *especially marked if it is achieved passively* with the help of a tilt table because the muscular activity of the act of standing is minimal in passive tilt.

The **mean arterial pressure** in the feet in the standing posture is 180–200 mmHg and at the head level is 60–80 mmHg. The **venous pressure** at the level of the feet is 85–90 mmHg and at the head level is 0.

Compensatory mechanisms

The immediate compensatory mechanisms on standing are **vasoconstriction, tachycardia, and increased cardiac output**. These compensatory mechanisms are triggered by a fall in blood pressure and are mediated by the

baroreceptor reflex. Decreased pressure in the carotid and aortic sinus decreases the rate of discharge from the baroreceptors, which in turn decreases stimulation of nucleus tractus solitarius (NTS). This in turn, decreases vagal activity and increases sympathetic activity, which results in restoration of blood pressure (Fig. 29.1).

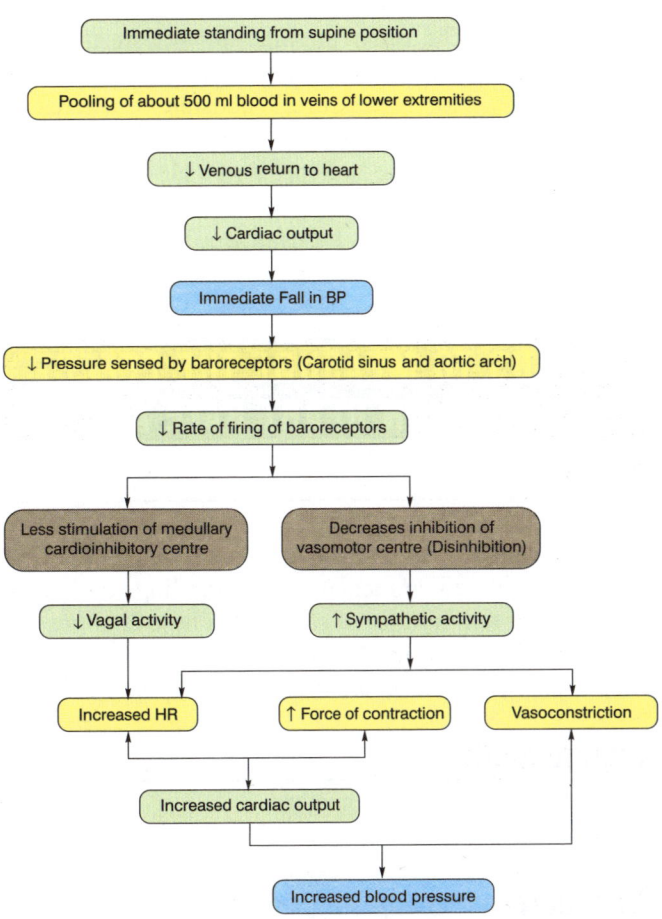

Fig. 29.1 Compensatory mechanisms activated by fall in BP in response to immediate standing from supine position.

Cardiovascular Changes on Prolonged Standing

Effects

If the individual does not move (stands still) for a long period, **more than 500 ml** of blood is pulled into the capacitance vessels of the lower extremities. This *increases the capillary hydrostatic pressure* in the lower limbs. The *fluid from the intravascular compartment* moves into the interstitial tissue spaces and accumulates there. As a result, *venous return to the heart significantly decreases*. This **decreases the stroke volume** by up to 40 per cent. Therefore, cardiac output is considerably reduced, which **decreases cerebral blood flow**. The subject may become unconscious and fall down. *Fainting is a homeostatic mechanism* to restore venous return, cardiac output, and cerebral blood flow in the horizontal position by automatic change of posture.

Compensatory mechanisms

The **baroreceptor reflex** restores blood pressure to normal. **Activation of sympathetic fibers** leads to the release of catecholamines from the adrenal medulla. Catecholamines increase heart rate, cardiac output, and blood pressure. The renin–angiotensin–aldosterone axis is also activated. Angiotensin II causes vasoconstriction and increases blood pressure. Aldosterone increases reabsorption of sodium and water from the kidneys and maintains blood volume and pressure. However, if the subject continues to stand for a much longer period, the compensatory mechanisms may fail, and the subject may develop features of hypotension.

METHODS TO MEASURE THE EFFECT OF POSTURE ON HEART RATE AND BP

Principle

On resuming an erect posture, changes occur in the cardiovascular function. Changes in heart rate and blood pressure are noted immediately on standing, and after two, five, and ten minutes of standing. These changes are compared with the heart rate and blood pressure recorded in the supine position before the change in posture.

Requirements

1. Aneroid sphygmomanometer
2. Stethoscope

Procedure

1. Ask the subject to **lie down in the supine position** on the couch, for a *minimum of 5 minutes*.

2. Properly tie the BP cuff at the correct position on the arm of the subject.
3. Record blood pressure and pulse rate in the supine position.
4. Do not remove the BP cuff; ask the subject **to stand up** and immediately record the pulse rate and blood pressure of the subject.

> **Note:** The subject should preferably stand with the support of the wall (leaning against the wall) to prevent the effect of the **muscle–heart reflex**. The increase in heart rate due to the contraction of skeletal muscles is known as **muscle–heart reflex**. If the subject stands without support, the muscles in the lower limb and trunk contract more, which affects the heart rate. Therefore, maximum possible relaxation should be achieved during the procedure by asking the subject to stand passively.

5. Record pulse rate and blood pressure **two, five, and ten minutes** after standing (alternatively, pulse and BP can also be recorded **every 2 minutes** for 10 minutes).
6. Calculate **pulse pressure, mean pressure, and rate pressure product** from the heart rate and blood pressure.
7. Enter your observations in a tabular form.
8. Ask the subject to *lie down again and rest for five minutes*. Then ask the subject to **sit up immediately** and record the BP and HR immediately, 2 minutes and 5 minutes after sitting.

Observation and Results

Enter your observation in a format as shown in Table 29.1.
1. Note that BP falls immediately on standing. Within 15–30 seconds, systolic pressure returns to normal (or remains slightly elevated), but diastolic pressure remains elevated, and tachycardia persists.

Table 29.1   Observations of effects of changes in posture.

Posture	PR	SBP	DBP	PP	MP	RPP
Supine (after 5 min)						
On standing:						
1. Immediate						
2. After 2 min						
3. After 5 min						
4. After 10 min						
Supine (after 5 min)						
On sitting:						
1. Immediate						
2. After 2 min						
3. After 5 min						
4. After 10 min						

PR = pulse rate; SBP = systolic blood pressure; DBP = diastolic blood pressure; PP = pulse pressure; MP = mean pressure; RPP = rate pressure product (RPP = systolic pressure × heart rate × 10^{-2}).

2. Note that changes in BP and HR on immediate sitting will be similar but of lesser magnitude than the effects of immediate standing.

Precautions

1. The subject should relax for 5 minutes before recording blood pressure and pulse rate in the supine position.
2. Pulse rate and blood pressure should be recorded as soon as the patient stands up (within 15 seconds, if possible).
3. The BP cuff should not be removed while changing the subject's posture.
4. The subject should stand passively (by leaning against the wall) or sit passively.

DISCUSSION

The immediate result of standing is that the cardiac output decreases due to the pooling of blood in the lower extremities. Therefore, a **fall in blood pressure** is noted immediately (if possible, **within 15 seconds**). The fall in pressure (through baroreceptor reflex) results in **tachycardia, increased cardiac output, and vasoconstriction**. Therefore, within 15–30 seconds, the blood pressure reverts to normal. However, because of vasoconstriction, the peripheral resistance increases, which in turn, increases the diastolic pressure. Heart rate increases and systolic pressure remains normal or slightly raised.

Physiological Significance

A change in posture initiates changes in cardiovascular function, which can be detected by various tests. These changes reflect the integrity of the autonomous nervous system because the compensatory mechanisms are dependent on the intactness of the reflex activities, especially the baroreceptor reflex. Therefore, the **heart rate and blood pressure response to standing is among the important tests to assess autonomic functions**. This test detects the efficiency of cardiovascular autonomic functions.

Clinical Significance

Postural hypotension

In some individuals, sudden standing causes a significant fall in blood pressure (fall in systolic pressure of more than 20 mmHg and fall in diastolic pressure of more than 10 mmHg), which results in fainting. This is called **postural** or **orthostatic hypotension**. It is usually seen in **people with autonomic neuropathy** like diabetes or syphilis. It also occurs in patients receiving sympatholytic drugs.

Postural hypotension is seen in primary autonomic failure and sometimes in primary hyperaldosteronism because the baroreceptor reflex is abnormal in these conditions.

Therapeutic uses

Acute changes of posture are part of different *asanas* practiced in *Hatha Yoga*. In fact, **asanas are different body postures**. There is enough scientific evidence that regular practice of changes of posture (*asanas*) **improves autonomic functions**. People who practice *asanas* regularly keep good health because doing so improves their cardiac, respiratory, neuromuscular, autonomic, mental, and physiological functions. For their beneficial effects, *asanas* have been recently included under **yoga therapy** in the treatment of metabolic disorders such as diabetes, hypertension, obesity, cardiorespiratory diseases, autonomic dysfunctions, psychiatric problems, cognitive deficits, etc. **Lying down in a prone position and *asanas* in prone posture** are known to facilitate the functions of the respiratory apparatus and improve oxygenation, and they were found to be of great help in improving respiratory functions in patients infected with COVID-19.

Problems faced by traffic personnel

Traffic police personnel stand in the traffic (without much activity) for hours together. This causes the accumulation of fluid in the lower parts of the body, and may cause **hypotension and pedal edema**; sometimes, it even results in **fainting (syncope)**. Therefore, instead of standing at one place, police personnel regulating traffic are advised to **walk around while regulating the traffic** so that the skeletal muscle pump activity increases the venous return and maintains cardiac output and blood pressure.

Apart from the effect of prolonged standing, fainting (syncope) also occurs in acute emotional distress, dehydration, heat stress, etc., due to decreased cardiac activity and vasodilation. Such syncopes are called **vasovagal syncope**. Usually, a person can be revived from vasovagal syncope if early interventions can be administered.

OSPE

1. **Record the effect of standing on the blood pressure of the given subject and report your findings.**

Steps

1. Give proper instructions to the subject.
2. Expose the subject's arm.
3. Tie the BP cuff properly (not very tight or very loose) on the arm of the subject in such a way that the middle of the cuff lies over the brachial

artery and the lower edge remains 1 inch above the cubital fossa.

4. Place the chest piece of the stethoscope on the brachial artery just below the cubital fossa, medial to the insertion of the biceps tendon; record systolic

and diastolic pressure by appropriately inflating and deflating the pressure in the cuff.

5. Ask the subject to stand up and immediately record systolic and diastolic pressure.

6. Report your findings.

VIVA

All the questions of the previous chapter are also applicable to this chapter.

1. *All the questions of the previous chapter are also applicable to this chapter.*

2. *What are the physiological changes that occur on suddenly standing up? Why do they occur?* (Ans. Refer to page 199, under the heading 'Cardiovascular Changes on Immediate Standing'.)

3. *What are the physiological changes that occur on prolonged standing and why?* (Ans. Refer to page 200, under the heading 'Cardiovascular Changes on Prolonged Standing'.)

4. *How does the baroreceptor reflex maintain BP following a change in posture from supine to standing?* (Ans. Refer to page 199, under the heading 'Compensatory Mechanisms' and Fig. 29.1.)

5. *Why should the pulse rate and blood pressure ideally be recorded within 15 seconds to record the immediate cardiovascular response to standing?* (Ans. Refer to page 201, under the heading 'Discussion'.)

6. *What is the muscle-heart reflex? How can the effect of this reflex be minimized while assessing the effect of posture on HR and BP?* (Ans. Refer to page 200, under the heading 'Procedure', the 'Note' under point no. 4.)

7. *What are the differences in the effect of changing of posture from supine to standing and vice versa?* (Ans. The transition from supine to standing causes a significant shift in blood volume toward the lower parts of the body due to gravity. This leads to a reduction in cardiac output [CO] and blood pressure [BP], which then triggers the baroreceptor reflex to restore circulatory stability, resulting in an increase in heart rate [HR]. In contrast, when changing posture from supine to sitting, the gravitational effect is less pronounced, so the resulting drop in CO and BP is smaller. Although the overall pattern of physiological responses—such as activation of the baroreceptor reflex—is similar in both cases, the magnitude of changes is noticeably less when moving to a sitting position compared to standing.)

8. *What is orthostatic hypotension? What are its common causes?* (Ans. Refer to page 201, under the heading 'Discussion' and the subjeading 'Clinical Significance' and 'Postural hypotension'.)

9. *What is vasovagal syncope? In what conditions does it happen?* (Ans. Refer to page 201, under the heading 'Discussion' and the subheading 'Problems faced by traffic personnel'.)

10. *What is the significance of rate pressure product (RPP)?* (Ans. Since RPP is the product of heart rate and systolic BP, it reflects the myocardial work load. RPP is the functional index of myocardial oxygen demand and myocardial work stress. Chronically elevated RPP, especially in the presence of high blood pressure, is a known cardiovascular risk. Increased RPP has been associated with CV morbidities and mortality.)

11. *What is the physiological usefulness of this practical?* (Ans. Refer to page 201, under the heading 'Discussion' and the subheading 'Physiological significance'.)

12. *What is the clinical utility of this practical?* (Ans. Refer to page 201, under the heading 'Discussion' and the subheading 'Clinical significance'.)

13. *How is posture important in practice of asana in Hatha Yoga?* (Ans. Refer to page 201, under the heading 'Discussion'.)

14. *How can traffic police personnel use the knowledge of the effects of posture to improve their health?* (Ans. Refer to page 201, under the heading 'Discussion' and the subheading 'Problems faced by traffic personnel.)

30 | Effect of Exercise on Blood Pressure and Heart Rate

Learning Objectives

After completing this practical, you will be able to (MUST KNOW):

1. Describe the importance of study of the effect of exercise on blood pressure and heart rate.
2. List the types and degrees of exercise.
3. List the differences between isotonic and isometric exercise.
4. Record the effect of exercise on heart rate and blood pressure.
5. List the precautions of recording this effect.

6. Explain the effects of exercise on heart rate and blood pressure.
7. List the cardiovascular changes following acute exercise.
8. List the benefits of regular exercise.

You may also be able to (DESIRABLE TO KNOW):

1. Explain the differences between isotonic and isometric exercise.
2. Describe and explain the various effects of acute and chronic exercise on different body systems.
3. State the therapeutic uses of exercise in the treatment of lifestyle disorders.

PY3.15: Demonstrate the effects of mild, moderate, and severe exercise, and record changes in cardiorespiratory parameters.

PY5.12: Record blood pressure and pulse rate at rest and in different grades of exercise and posture in a volunteer or in a simulated environment.

INTRODUCTION

The body's responses to exercise can be either short-term responses to acute exercise or long-term responses to regular exercise. Long-term response to regular exercise makes exercise easier and improves performance. The immediate response to acute exercise depends on the degree and type of exercise and the exercise training that the individual has received. The cardiovascular responses to exercise are different in trained and untrained individuals.

Degree of Exercise

Depending on the rate of oxygen consumption, work done, and rate of rise in heart rate, exercise is classified into three categories: mild, moderate, and severe. The **WHO's criteria for grading exercises** are presented in Table 30.1.

VO_2 max = Maximum oxygen consumption
MET = Oxygen consumption in multiples of basal oxygen consumption
RLI = Oxygen consumption as a percentage of VO_2 max

Mild exercise: In this grade of exercise, oxygen consumption is 0.5–1 litre per minute; work done is

150–350 watts; and the rise in heart rate is about 25 per cent, that is, if the basal heart rate is 80, the heart rate will increase to about 100 per minute.

Moderate exercise: In this type of exercise, oxygen consumption is 1–2 litres per minute; work done is 350–550 watts; and rise in heart rate is about 50 per cent, i.e., it rises from a basal heart rate of 80 to 120 per minute.

Severe exercise: Oxygen consumption is more than 2 litres per minute, work done is more than 550 watts, and rise in heart rate is about 75–100 per cent, i.e., it increases from a basal heart rate of 80 per minute to 150 per minute or more.

Table 30.1 WHO's grading of exercise.

Grade (and level) of exercise	Heart rate (per minute)	O$_2$ consumption (l/min)	Relative load index (RLI) (% of maximum O$_2$ consumption)	Metabolic equivalent task (MET)
I (Mild)	<100	0.4–0.8	<25	<3
II (Moderate)	100–125	0.8–1.6	25–50	3.1–4.5
III (Heavy)	125–150	1.6–2.4	51–75	4.6–7
IV (Severe)	>150	>2.4	>75	>7

Types of Exercises

Exercise may be isotonic or isometric. Differences between isotonic and isometric exercises are presented in Table 30.2.

Table 30.2   Differences between isometric and isotonic exercises.

	Isotonic exercise	Isometric exercise
Length of muscle	Shortening occurs	Remains same
Muscle tension	No change	Tension increases
External work	Work is done	No work done
Blood pressure	SBP increases moderately Change in DBP varies according to severity of exercise	SBP and DBP rise sharply
Cardiac parameters	CO increases significantly due to proportionate increase in both HR and SV	Change in SV is relatively less
Blood flow to exercising muscle	Blood flow to exercising muscle increases substantially	Blood flow to exercising muscle decreases due to compression of blood vessels by contracting muscle
Examples	Walking, jogging, running, cycling, swimming, dancing	Weightlifting (before lifting), pushing against wall

SBP = systolic blood pressure; DBP = diastolic blood pressure; CO= cardiac output; SV = stroke volume

Isotonic exercise

In isotonic exercise, there is a **change in muscle length,** and the exercise is **phasic in nature.** Common examples are walking, jogging, and running.

Cardiovascular changes in isotonic exercise

1. **Heart rate increases** proportionately with the severity of exercise.
2. **Cardiac output increases** markedly due to the increase in heart rate and stroke volume.
3. **Systolic pressure increases**.
4. **Diastolic pressure** increases in mild exercise, usually does not change or increases or decreases slightly in moderate exercise, and could decrease in severe exercise or may remain the same or slightly increase.
5. **Blood flow** to the exercising muscle **increases**.

Isometric exercise

Isometric exercise is any exercise in which there is **no change in the length** of the muscles. The exercising muscle remains contracted throughout the maneuver (e.g., pushing against the wall). Therefore, this type of exercise is tonic in nature.

Cardiovascular changes in isometric exercise

1. **Heart rate rises** at the beginning of exercise. This is mainly due to **decreased vagal tone**. Increased discharge of cardiac sympathetic fibres may also contribute to this.
2. Stroke volume changes relatively little.
3. Systolic and diastolic pressures rise sharply.
4. **Blood flow** to the exercising muscles **decreases**.

The cardiovascular responses to isometric exercise are different because the exercising muscles are tonically contracted during exercise. **Peripheral resistance increases**, which **increases diastolic pressure** significantly in isometric exercise.

METHODS TO STUDY THE EFFECTS OF ACUTE ISOTONIC EXERCISE ON PULSE RATE AND BP

Principle

Cardiovascular functions alter during exercise. Pulse rate and blood pressure are recorded before and immediately after exercise. The results are compared to study the effect of exercise on these parameters.

Requirements

1. Stethoscope
2. Sphygmomanometer

Procedure

1. Record the blood pressure (using a sphygmomanometer) and the pulse rate of the given subject after 5 minutes of rest.
2. Ask the subject to perform **spot-jogging for a period of 5 minutes**.
3. Record the pulse rate and blood pressure immediately, 2, 4, 6, 8, and 10 minutes after the exercise.
4. Calculate the pulse pressure, mean pressure, and rate pressure product and compare the pre- and post-exercise values.

Note: Rate pressure product =
Systolic pressure × Heart rate × 10^{-2}.
RPP is a good index of myocardial function.

5. Record your observations in a tabular form.

Observation and Results

1. Record your observations as shown in Table 30.3.
2. Calculate the degree of exercise from HR calculation as depicted in the table.

3. Plot graphs for changes in each parameter over time.
4. Note that heart rate and systolic pressure rise significantly immediately after exercise.
5. Since five-minute spot jogging is a mild exercise, diastolic pressure usually rises (or may not change). Pulse pressure changes accordingly.
6. Also note that blood pressure returns to normal within 5–7 minutes of the termination of exercise, whereas the heart rate takes longer to return to normal.

Table 30.3 Observations of changes with exercise.

	PR	SBP	DBP	PP	MAP	RPP
Basal (before exercise)						
Immediately after exercise						
Two minutes after exercise						
Four minutes after exercise						
Six minutes after exercise						
Eight minutes after exercise						
Ten minutes after exercise						

PR = pulse rate; SBP = systolic blood pressure; DBP = diastolic blood pressure; PP = pulse pressure; MAP = mean arterial pressure; RPP = rate pressure product

Precautions

1. The pre- and post-exercise heart rate and blood pressure should be **recorded in the same position**.

> **Note:** To eliminate the effect of posture on BP, it should be recorded in the standing position both before and after exercise. If BP is recorded in the supine or sitting posture before exercise, then post-exercise BP should also be recorded in the same position. Since exercise is performed in the erect posture, it is better to record BP in the standing posture.

2. The subject should be encouraged to **exercise properly for five minutes**.
3. For the first recording following exercise (immediately after exercise), blood pressure and pulse rate should be recorded as quickly as possible.

DISCUSSION

Effects of Acute Isotonic Exercise

Cardiovascular changes

Heart rate: Heart rate increases with exercise. The degree of increase *depends on the severity of the exercise*. The maximum heart rate achieved during exercise decreases with age. In children, the heart rate can rise up to 200 beats per minute or more; in adults, it seldom rises above this and in elderly subjects, it rarely goes beyond 150.

Cardiac output: There occurs a *marked increase in cardiac output*. Cardiac output may increase even up to 25 litres per minute or more. Increase in cardiac output is due to increase in heart rate and stroke volume. Tachycardia and increased stroke volume occur due to *increased activity in the noradrenergic sympathetic nerves* to the heart. Sympathetic activity increases by psychic stimuli and stimulation of receptors in the muscles, joints, and tendons. The *inhibition of vagal tone* also contributes to tachycardia.

1. **Stroke volume increases** due to increased myocardial contractility by sympathetic stimulation and due to increased venous return.
2. **Venous return increases** due to sympathetic venoconstriction and increased skeletal muscle pump activity.
3. **Increased thoracic pump** and mobilization of blood from the splanchnic and cutaneous beds also contribute to increased venous return.

Systolic blood pressure: Systolic pressure **rises markedly**. This occurs due to increased cardiac output.

Diastolic blood pressure: Diastolic pressure **increases in mild exercise** due to sympathetic vasoconstriction. In **moderate exercise**, diastolic pressure increases, remains stable, or falls. In **severe exercise, *diastolic pressure usually falls*** or remains the same or exhibits a mild increase.

1. The fall in diastolic pressure occurs due to the *vasodilation in the exercising muscle*. The blood vessels in the skeletal vascular bed receive sympathetic vasodilator fibres. Therefore, vasodilation occurs in the skeletal bed.
2. In addition, the *systemic blood vessels also dilate* in severe exercise due to: i) rise in body temperature (**thermal vasodilation**) and ii) deposition of metabolites like lactic acid, K^+, and CO_2 in the active tissues (**metabolic vasodilation**).

Total peripheral resistance decreases due to vasodilation. Therefore, despite increased sympathetic activity, diastolic pressure may fall during severe exercise/may not change/may display mild increase.

Muscle blood flow: Blood flow to the skeletal muscle **increases due to vasodilation** in the skeletal bed. There is vasoconstriction in the cutaneous and splanchnic circulation. As a result, blood is diverted from the cutaneous and visceral circulation to the skeletal vascular bed. The **initial increase** in blood flow is due to *neural mechanisms,* and **continued blood flow** is due to **local mechanisms**.

1. **Neural mechanism** refers to the *activation of the sympathetic vasodilator system* and a decrease in tonic vasoconstrictor discharge.
2. **Local mechanisms** are *accumulation of metabolites* and rise in temperature in the active muscles. Vasodilation opens up many closed capillaries.

Respiratory changes

1. There is **hyperventilation** and an increased oxygen supply to the tissues. Hyperventilation also removes excess CO_2 and heat produced by the active tissues.
2. Respiratory minute volume increases linearly with work rate.
3. Pulmonary blood flow increases, which increases perfusion of the alveoli.

Other changes

1. The body's metabolic rate increases.
2. The body temperature increases.
3. Catecholamine secretion from the adrenal medulla and glucocorticoid secretion from the adrenal cortex increase.
4. Glycogenolysis is stimulated in the liver and skeletal muscles.
5. Lipolysis occurs in prolonged aerobic exercise.

Effect of Regular Exercise (Training) on Health

On the cardiovascular system

There is profound improvement in cardiovascular function. The **basal heart rate decreases** due to **increased vagal tone**. Stroke volume increases due to increased myocardial muscle mass. A **trained subject** achieves the required cardiac output during exercise mainly by increasing his stroke volume rather than his heart rate, whereas an **untrained individual** achieves the same cardiac output mainly by increasing his heart rate. The blood pressure is usually maintained within the normal range. Hypertension usually does not occur, unless it is associated with some secondary pathology.

Regular exercise decreases cholesterol, TG, and LDL, and **increases HDL**. This decrease in bad lipids slows down the process of atherosclerosis and **decreases cardiovascular risks** in diabetes, hypertension, stroke, and other lifestyle disorders.

On the respiratory system

There is an **increase in breathing capacity and VO_{2max}**. VO_{2max} is the product of maximal cardiac output and maximal oxygen extraction by the tissues. Both these parameters increase with training.

On the skeletal muscles

The size of the muscles and work capability increase. The number of mitochondria and the enzymes involved in oxidative metabolism increases. The number of capillaries increases, which results in increased extraction of oxygen.

On the mind

Exercise **improves memory** and intellectual mental functions.

Clinical Significance

Exercise therapy: Exercise is becoming popular nowadays because of its visible **therapeutic benefits** in lifestyle disorders. It is regularly prescribed as part of treatment for patients who have cardiovascular diseases, especially ***hypertension and myocardial infarction***. It has been seen that isotonic exercise (mild to moderate) performed regularly, decreases blood pressure significantly in otherwise resistant cases of hypertension. Exercise also improves cardiac performance in patients who have myocardial infarction and prevents infarction in subjects at risk. Exercise also improves joint functions and is therefore prescribed for patients with chronic arthritis and degenerative joint diseases.

VIVA

1. *What are the various types of exercise?*
   (**Ans.** Exercises are classified as isotonic and isometric and aerobic and anaerobic exercises.

   Isotonic and isometric exercise: Isotonic exercises involve active body movements. The two types of isotonic contractions are **concentric isotonic**—where a muscle shortens and produces movement (e.g., flexion of the elbow), and **eccentric isotonic**—where a muscle gradually lengthens while continuing to contract (e.g., slowly lowering a weight during weightlifting). In **isometric exercises**, muscle tension is generated without shortening of the muscle.

   Aerobic and anaerobic exercise: Aerobics exercises are sustained activities that use oxygen to meet the energy demands of the muscles. These exercises are beneficial to the cardiovascular and respiratory systems. Examples include jogging, cycling, spot running, swimming, skipping rope, etc. **Anaerobic exercises** are short-duration, high-intensity activities where oxygen is not the primary energy source. These exercises rely on stored energy in the muscles and include activities like sprinting. Due to their intensity, anaerobic exercises can only be maintained for a brief period.

2. *How do you determine the severity of exercise?* (**Ans.** Refer to page 203, Table 30.1.)

3. *What are the differences between isotonic and isometric exercise?* (Ans. Refer to page 204, Table 30.2.)
4. *What are the cardiovascular responses to acute exercise?* (Ans. Refer to page 205, under the heading 'Effects of Acute Exercise'.)
5. *What are the causes of increased cardiac output in exercise?* (Ans. Refer to page 205, under the heading 'Cardiovascular changes'.)
6. *What is the cause of systolic rise in blood pressure in exercise?* (Ans. Refer to page 205, under the heading 'Physiological basis of CV changes'.)
7. *Why does diastolic pressure not change or decrease in moderate to severe exercise?* (Ans. Refer to page 205, under the heading 'Cardiovascular changes'.)
8. *Why does heart rate take more time than blood pressure to return to normal level following exercise?*
   (Ans. Heart rate increases in exercise due to increased sympathetic activity. Sympathetic activity takes time to return to normal, therefore the heart normalizes slowly. BP returns to normal in 5–7 minutes due to muscle relaxation with stoppage of exercise, which produces vasodilation.)
9. *What are the effects of exercise on the respiratory system?* (Ans. Refer to page 206, under the heading 'On Respiratory System'.)
10. *What are the benefits of performing regular exercise?* (Ans. Refer to page 206, under the heading 'Exercise Therapy'.)
11. *What are the differences in CV responses to exercise among trained and untrained individuals?* (Ans. Refer to Chapter 32, Page 212.)
12. *What are sympathetic vasodilator fibres?*
    (Ans. Sympathetic vasodilator fibres are: i. sympathetic fibres supplying the blood vessels of skeletal muscles, and ii) sympathetic fibres supplying the blood vessels of sweat glands in the skin.)
13. *What are the CV changes in isometric exercise?* (Ans. Refer to page 206, under the heading 'Isometric Exercise', read CV changes in isometric exercise.)

31 Cardiac Efficiency Tests (Exercise Stress Testing): Treadmill and Master's Step Test

Learning Objectives

After completing this practical, you will be able to (MUST KNOW):

1. Explain exercise stress testing and its physiological basis.
2. List the indications and contraindications of cardiac efficiency tests.
3. Define target heart rate and explain its importance.
4. List the various cardiac efficiency tests for the upper and lower limbs.
5. List the pre-test procedures for treadmill testing.
6. Name the commonly used GXT protocols for treadmill testing.
7. List the cardiovascular changes and normal ECG responses to graded exercise.
8. List the exercise-test termination criteria.
9. Explain the basic principle and procedure of bicycle ergometry.
10. Understand the basic principle and procedure of Master's step test or Harvard step test.
11. Name the tests for upper extremity exercise testing and mention their principles.

You may also be able to (DESIRABLE TO KNOW):

1. Describe and explain the cardiovascular effects of graded treadmill.
2. Describe data collection and interpretation of treadmill testing with reference to MET.
3. Calculate cardiac efficiency index in the Harvard step test.
4. Calculate the energy cost of work using bicycle ergometry.
5. Explain the physiological principle and basic methods of treadmill exercise and Master's step test.
6. Describe the principle of arm ergometry.
7. Explain the exercise test response.

PY3.15: Demonstrate the effects of mild, moderate, and severe exercise and record changes in cardiorespiratory parameters.

PY5.12: Record blood pressure and pulse rate at rest and in different grades of exercise and posture in a volunteer or in a simulated environment.

INTRODUCTION

Exercise Stress Testing

Assessments of cardiovascular functions during rest are poor predictors of cardiac performance as there is substantial cardiovascular reserve capacity. Exercise is currently the most convenient way of stimulating the myocardium to demand maximal blood flow so that even a mild impairment of coronary blood flow capacity becomes detectable.

Physiological Basis

Cardiac efficiency tests (**exercise tolerance tests** or **exercise stress testing**) are performed to assess the response of the cardiovascular system to a standardized exercise schedule. These tests are highly efficient at assessing the efficiency of the heart functions.

As described in the preceding chapter, during exercise, there is a progressive increase in the heart rate and blood pressure; after the exercise, these parameters return to the pre-exercise levels in a few minutes. Thus, the **ability to attain a peak rise, the magnitude of rise, the ability to recover, and the speed of recovery** determine the cardiac efficiency of the individual. Therefore, these tests are called cardiac efficiency tests.

The response to physical exercise depends on the cardiac reserve (i.e., efficiency of the myocardial performance), skeletal muscle power, level of training, state of motivation, and the status of nutrition. Hence, cardiac efficiency tests are often used to assess physical fitness in an individual during recruitments into the army, police force, jobs that require the use of firearms, etc.

Indications for exercise testing

1. Assessment of cardio-respiratory fitness during recruitments into the army, police, etc.
2. Evaluation of patients with chest pain.
3. Evaluation of the functional capacity of the heart of a cardiac patient.
4. Evaluation of patients after myocardial infarction.

5. Evaluation of patients after coronary artery bypass surgery.
6. Screening for latent coronary artery disease.
7. Evaluation of patients with valvular heart disease.
8. Evaluation of arrhythmias.

Contraindications to stress test

1. Impending or acute myocardial infarction
2. Unstable angina
3. Severe hypertension
4. Congestive heart failure
5. Severe aortic stenosis
6. Uncontrolled arrhythmias

METHODS OF PERFORMING EXERCISE STRESS TESTING

Principle

The patient is made to exercise up to 90% of his estimated maximal heart rate, which is calculated based on the subject's age, sex, and physical training. Cardiac efficiency is tested by analyzing the patient's ability to achieve the **target heart rate**.

There are *two broad categories* of exercise stress testing: dynamic lower extremity testing and dynamic upper extremity testing. The **lower extremity tests** include treadmill, bicycle ergometry, and Master's step test and **upper extremity testing** consists of arm ergometry.

Dynamic Lower Extremity Testing

1. **Treadmill**: Treadmill testing is the most widely used method for exercise testing. It involves taking simultaneous recordings from multiple leads of ECG on a computerized treadmill. The subject exercises **until he achieves his target heart rate** or is unable to continue because of chest pain, dyspnea, and intolerable fatigue. Several standardised protocols are used, including the **Bruce, Naughton, and Balke-Ware protocols**. In different protocols, the analyses of the heart rate achievement is different.
2. **Bicycle ergometry:** This is used when a patient is unable to perform treadmill exercise. It is the method of choice during radionuclide ventriculography and for dynamic testing during cardiac catheterization. However, bicycle ergometry is the usual method of assessing cardiac–respiratory fitness in normal health and diseased conditions. The details of bicycle ergometry are **described in Chapter 25** (in the third section of the chapter, '**Energy Cost of Work**').
3. Master's Step Test/Harvard Step Test: Described below.

Computerised Treadmill Testing

Requirements

1. Heavy-duty treadmill (e.g., GE T2100)
2. Computer system with requisite software (Cardiosoft)
3. Exercise ECG monitoring system (CAM32)
4. Exercise blood pressure monitoring system (Suntech Tango)
5. Emergency resuscitation cart and trolley
6. Couch for pre- and post-exercise recordings, sphygmomanometer, and stethoscope (Fig. 31.1)
7. Room temperature to be maintained at 20–22°C; consent forms and data sheets should be filled for recording all physiological parameters
8. **Personnel requirements:** Exercise physiologist, general physician (at least with MBBS degree), multi-purpose lab technician

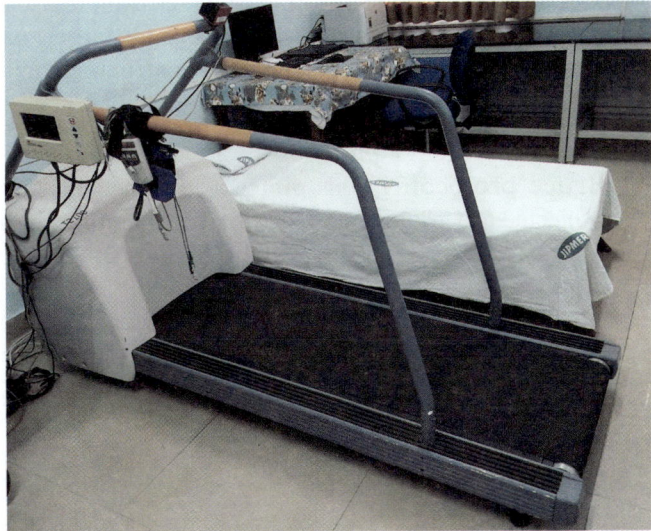

Fig. 31.1   The treadmill machine with all accessories. (*Courtesy:* CV Research Lab, JIPMER, Puducherry, India.)

Procedure

Pre-test procedure

1. Instruct the participants to refrain from ingesting food, alcohol, caffeine, or tobacco within 3 hours of testing and to avoid significant exertion or exercise on the day of the assessment.
2. Obtain **written and informed consent** from the participant after explaining the entire procedure.
3. Obtain a thorough medical history, general physical examination, and laboratory tests, if required (blood glucose, lipid profile).
4. Record anthropometric parameters (height, weight, BMI).
5. Resting supine heart rate and blood pressure measurements, resting ECG recording, **heart rate and blood pressure recording after five minutes of assuming standing posture**.

Exercise testing and protocols

Computerized treadmill exercise stress ECG testing of healthy individuals is used to assess their cardio-respiratory fitness (CRF) by estimating their **maximal oxygen consumption (VO$_{2max}$)**. This is based on the principle that the **heart rate response** of a healthy person subjected to a graded exercise of incremental work output shows a linear relationship with his VO$_{2max}$. A graded exercise of incremental work output is devised into a treadmill by sequentially increasing the **treadmill speed and inclination**.

The primary aim of **graded exercise testing (GXT)** is to determine the subject's heart rate response to the given workload and use the total test duration result in **validated prediction equations** to predict VO$_{2max}$. Both maximal and sub-maximal intensity of GXT using a treadmill can be performed to assess the CRF, however, maximal GXT provides a better estimate of VO$_{2max}$. The decision to use a maximal or sub-maximal exercise test depends largely on the reasons for the test, risk level of the client/patient, and the availability of appropriate equipment and personnel.

Commonly used GXT protocols

1. **Bruce protocol**: In this protocol, the participant is subjected to a **graded exercise with incremental stages** (of treadmill speed and inclination), **each lasting three minutes** or until a steady state is achieved.
2. **Modified Bruce protocol**: This protocol is similar to the Bruce protocol, except for two additional stages of lesser workload at the beginning. This protocol is **suitable for older individuals**.
3. **Bruce ramp protocol**: In this protocol, the incremental **graded stages are of twenty seconds'** duration, thereby, providing no room for achieving steady-state conditions.

Treadmill testing provides a familiar form of exercise and, if the correct protocol is chosen, can accommodate the least physically fit to the fittest individuals across the continuum of walking to running speeds. Nevertheless, a practice session might be necessary in some cases to permit habituation and reduce anxiety. Treadmills **must be calibrated** to ensure the accuracy of the test. Additionally, to ensure accuracy of metabolic work output, the subject should be discouraged from holding on to the support rails, particularly when VO$_{2max}$ is estimated instead of being directly measured. Extensive use of the handrails often leads to significant overestimation of VO$_{2max}$.

Expected cardiovascular changes during graded exercise

1. There is an increase in heart rate, stroke volume, cardiac output, systolic blood pressure, mean arterial pressure, and rate pressure product (RPP).
2. Diastolic blood pressure usually shows an unequivocal response.
3. Decrease in total peripheral resistance.

Normal ECG response to exercise

1. Minor and insignificant changes in P wave morphology
2. Superimposition of the P and T waves of successive beats
3. Increases in septal Q wave amplitude
4. Slight decreases in R wave amplitude
5. Increases in T wave amplitude (although wide variability exists among clients/patients)
6. Minimal shortening of the QRS duration
7. Depression of the J point
8. Rate-related shortening of the QT interval

Exercise test termination criteria (ACSM criteria)

1. **Onset of angina** or angina-like symptoms
2. **Drop in SBP** of ≥ 10 mmHg with an increase in work rate or if SBP decreases below the value obtained in
3. the same position prior to testing
4. **Excessive rise in BP**—systolic pressure > 250 mmHg and/or diastolic pressure > 115 mmHg
5. **Shortness of breath**, wheezing, leg cramps, or claudication
6. **Signs of poor perfusion**—light-headedness, confusion, ataxia, pallor, cyanosis, nausea, or cold and clammy skin
7. **Failure of HR to increase** with increased exercise intensity
8. Noticeable **change in heart rhythm** by palpation or auscultation
9. Subject requests to stop
10. Physical or verbal manifestations of severe fatigue
11. Failure of the testing equipment

Post-test procedure

Post-exercise monitoring should continue in the supine position for **at least 6 minutes after exercise** or until ECG changes return to baseline and significant signs and symptoms resolve.

1. **ST-segment changes** that occur only during the post-exercise period are currently recognized to be an **important diagnostic part of the test**.
2. HR and BP should also return to near baseline levels before discontinuation of monitoring.

Data collection and interpretation

At the end of the procedure, we arrive at the following data: **i)** pre-exercise heart rate and blood pressure after five minutes of supine rest, **ii)** pre-exercise heart rate and blood pressure after five minutes of assuming the standing posture, **iii)** maximal heart rate, **iv)** maximal RPP, **v)** total treadmill exercise test time, **vi)** derived VO$_{2max}$, **vii)** cumulative METs (metabolic equivalents of tasks), **viii)** cumulative work output achieved, and **ix)** recovery heart rate and blood pressure.

VO_2 is calculated using the following formula:

$$VO_2 = HC + VC + RMR$$

Where HC (horizontal component) = speed of the treadmill × 0.1

VC (vertical component) = speed of the treadmill × 1.8 x grade

RMR (resting metabolic rate) = 3.5 ml/kg/min

METs is calculated by the following formula:

$$METs = VO_2 / 3.5$$

Cumulative METs is the METs calculated for each stage and successively added to the calculated METs value of the subsequent stage. This is continued until the end of the test.

Work output of exercise: Work output of exercise is calculated using the formula:

Work output = body weight (kg) × vertical displacement (m) × total time (min)

Where vertical displacement = percentage grade × speed of the treadmill m/min)

The work output is **calculated for each stage** and successively added to the calculated work output of the subsequent stage. This is continued until the end of the test.

Master's Step Test/Harvard Step Test

This method of exercise testing is routinely practiced in clinical physiology labs for cardiovascular fitness (physical fitness) assessment, which **measures aerobic capacity and recovery rate**.

▪ Principle

In this test, the subject walks up and down over a device (Master's step device/Harvard step device) at a specific pace for a set duration, after which his pulse recovery rate is measured.

▪ Requirements

Master's step device: This device has a total of **three steps**, two of which are 9 inches above the floor, and the top step is 18 inches high (Fig. 31.2). The exercise is carried out for a **prescribed number of ascents**. The workload achieved in this test is usually too low to be of any significant clinical use. Therefore, after the advent of the treadmill and bicycle ergometer, this method of exercise testing has lost its popularity and is seldom used in clinical set-ups these days. Alternatively, the **Harvard step device** is used.

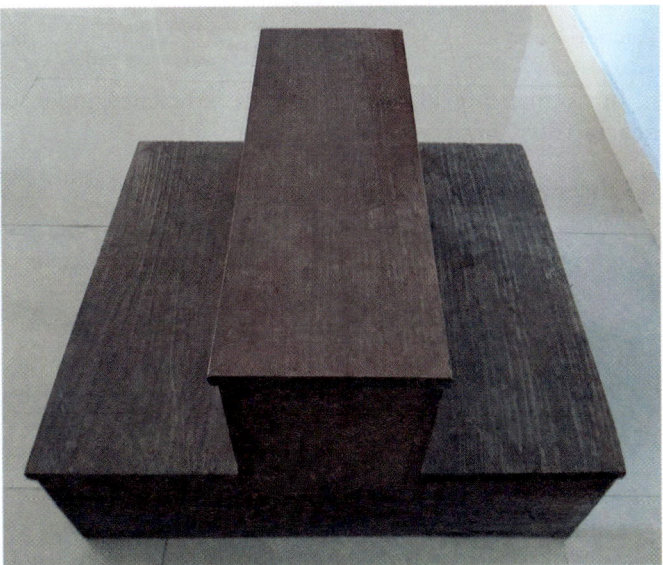

Fig. 31.2 Wooden device with having three steps for performing the Master's step test. Note that the two side steps are 9 inches high and the central step is 18 inches high (20 inches high for men and 16 inches high for women).

▪ Procedure

The test is conducted in **three major steps**: warm up, stepping, and rest/recovery.

1. Record the subject's basal pulse rate.
2. Ask the subject to warm up by performing some stretching or light exercise for a minute.
3. Instruct the subject to alternately hop on each foot while alternatively climbing on to the two steps. The subject should step on and off the steps **30 times per minute** (one step every two seconds) for five minutes or until he has exerted himself fully. Then, note the pulse rate.
4. Ask the subject to rest on a chair. During rest, note the pulse rate for 30 seconds at the end of every minute (at 1 – 1.5, 2 – 2.5, and 3 – 3.5 minutes). Add the pulse rate of the 3 recordings of 30 seconds' duration each.
5. Repeat the test if needed, depending on the physical ability of the subject.

Note: If the heart is healthy, there should be little disturbance in breathing. The pulse rate should not increase more than 10–20 beats per minute and should return to pre-exercise level in 1–5 minutes.

6. Calculate the cardiac efficiency (physical fitness) index.

▪ Cardiac efficiency (physical fitness) index

Cardiac efficiency index is calculated by following formula.

$$\text{Cardiac efficiency index} = \frac{\text{Duration of exercise in seconds}}{2 \times \text{Sum of heart rate in the recovery period}} \times 100$$

In normal individuals, the cardiac efficiency index **is nearly 100%** but is more in sportspersons.

■ Observation and results

1. In a tabular format, record the pre-exercise and rest pulse rate and the sum of the pulse rate during recovery.
2. Calculate and note the **efficiency or fitness index**.

For example, if the individual completes the test in 5 min (300 seconds) and the total heartbeat in the recovery period (of 30 seconds each of three recordings) add up to 150.

$$300 \times 100 \,/\, 2 \times 150 = 300,00/300 = 100$$

Thus, the fitness index of the subject is 100%.

3. Report your results about the fitness of the individual, as per the fitness index rating given below.

Efficiency (fitness) index interpretation

Over 90%: Excellent
81–90%: Good
55–80%: Average
Below 55%: Poor

■ Clinical application

The Harvard step test is a cardiovascular fitness assessment that measures **aerobic capacity and recovery rate**. Though it is not usually practiced in medicine or on cardiology patients for cardiac fitness assessments, it is routinely used in physiology and sports science for physical fitness measurements. A person with a test **value >90%** is considered to be healthy and fit. Standardization of **step height and step rate and the accurate measurement of recovery pulse rate** are key to precision of the result of the test. **BMI prior training and the endurance capacity** of the individual contribute to results.

Dynamic Upper Extremity Testing

Arm ergometry

This is sometimes used in patients with peripheral vascular disease affecting the lower limbs or orthopedic abnormalities. Arm ergometry is less sensitive than leg ergometry for eliciting exercise-induced ischemia.

Arm ergometry is performed using **Mosso's ergograph** or a **hand dynamometer** (details in Chapter 34).

DISCUSSION

Exercise Test Response

Exercise responses are mainly assessed by **ECG changes**. When the **heart rate increases** with exercise, a number of **predictable changes occur in the normal ECG**: i) the PR interval shortens, ii) the P wave becomes taller, iii) the atrial repolarization rate becomes prominent, causing depression of the PQ segment, which results in— iv) J point (junction between S wave and ST segment) depression, which is usually of a short duration, and v) the ST segment becomes upsloping and slightly convex and returns to baseline within 0.04 second after the J point.

The abnormal changes in ECG are analyzed with recordings obtained before, during, and after the termination of the test and interpreted accordingly.

Differences Between Trained and Untrained Individuals

During exercise, trained individuals exhibit several physiological advantages as compared to untrained individuals. These include higher VO_{2max} (maximum oxygen uptake), increased capillary density in muscles, greater glycogen storage capacity, and a more efficient ability to utilize fat as fuel. Furthermore, trained individuals often have lower resting heart rates, faster heart rate recovery after exercise, and a lower increase in blood pressure during exercise.

Cardio-respiratory adaptations

VO_{2max}: Trained individuals have significantly higher VO_{2max}, meaning they can utilize more oxygen during exercise, leading to increased aerobic capacity.

Heart rate: Trained individuals tend to have lower resting heart rates and a faster recovery rate after exercise, indicating a more efficient cardiovascular system.

Blood pressure: Trained individuals experience a smaller increase in blood pressure during exercise compared to untrained individuals, likely due to improved cardiovascular efficiency.

Muscle adaptations

Capillary density: Trained muscles have a higher density of capillaries, facilitating greater blood flow and nutrient delivery to muscle tissues.

Glycogen storage: Trained muscles have an increased capacity and quicker means to store glycogen, providing a readily available energy source during exercise.

Metabolic efficiency: Trained muscles become more efficient at utilizing fat for energy, sparing glycogen stores and allowing for longer durations of exercise.

Hormonal and metabolic adaptations

Hormonal response: Trained individuals may exhibit a different hormonal response to exercise compared to untrained individuals, with po)tential differences in stress hormones, endorphins, growth hormone (GH) levels during and after exercise. Trained individuals have more GH and endorphins and less stress hormones.

Metabolic efficiency: Trained individuals may have a higher metabolic efficiency, meaning they need less oxygen to produce the same amount of power during exercise. They also have a better blood glucose regulation mechanism.

VIVA

1. *What do you mean by exercise stress testing? What is its physiological basis?* (Ans. Refer to page 208, under the heading 'Introduction', read Exercise Stress Testing, Physiological Basis.)

2. *What are the indications and contraindications of cardiac efficiency tests?* (Ans. Refer to page 208-209, under the 'Indications' and 'Contraindications'.)

3. *What is target heart rate? What is its importance?* (Ans. Refer to page 209, under the heading 'Methods.' ... 'Principle'.)

4. *Name the various cardiac efficiency tests for lower and upper limbs.* (Ans. Refer to page 209, under the heading 'Basic Principle', read 'Types of Exercise Stress Testing'.)

5. *What are the pre-test procedures for treadmill testing?* (Ans. Refer to page 209, under the heading 'Procedure of...', read 'Pre-test Procedure'.)

6. *What are the commonly used GXT protocols for treadmill testing?* (Ans. Refer to page 210, under the heading 'Exercise Testing and Protocols', read 'Commonly used GXT protocols'.)

7. *What are the normal ECG responses to graded exercise?* (Ans. Refer to page 210, under the heading 'Normal ECG Responses...'.)

8. *What are criteria for the termination of the exercise-test?* (Ans. Refer to page 210, under the heading 'Exercise Test Termination Criteria')

9. *What is the basic principle and procedure of bicycle ergometry?* (Ans. Refer to heading 'Bicycle Ergometry'; Chapter 25, under the heading 'Energy Cost of Work'.)

10. *What are the basic principles and the procedure of Master's step test or Harvard step test?* (Ans. Refer to page 211, under the heading 'Master's step test or Harvard step test')

11. *What are the tests for upper extremity exercise testing and mention their principles?* (Ans. Refer to page 212, see 'Dynamic Upper Extremity Testing')

12. *What are the cardiovascular effects of graded treadmill exercise?* (Ans. Refer to page 210, under the heading 'Expected Cardiovascular Changes...'.)

13. *How do you interpret treadmill testing with reference to MET?* (Ans. Refer to page 210, under the heading 'Data Collection and Interpretation'.)

14. *How do you calculate cardiac efficiency index in Harvard step test?* (Ans. Refer to page 211, under the heading 'Harvard Step Test' and the subheading 'Procedure' and 'Cardiac efficiency index'.)

15. *How the energy cost of work calculated using bicycle ergometry?* (Ans. Refer to Chapter 25, under the heading 'Bicycle Ergometry' and the subheading 'Energy cost of work'.)

16. *What is the physiological principle of Master's step test?* (Ans. Refer to page 211, under the heading 'Master's step test' and the subheading 'Principle'.)

17. *What are the major steps of Master's step test?* (Ans. Refer to page 211, under the heading 'Master's step test' and the subheading 'Procedure'.)

18. *How is fitness index calculated in Master's step test? How is the result interpreted?* (Ans. Refer to page 211, under the heading 'Master's step test' and the subheading 'Observation and results'.)

19. *What are exercise test responses?* (Ans. Refer to page 212, under the heading 'Discussion' and the subheading 'Exercise test responses'.)

20. *What are the differences in cardiovascular and other physiological responses between trained and untrained individuals?* (Ans. Refer to page 212, under the heading 'Discussion' and the subheading 'Differences Between Trained...'.)

32 | Nerve Conduction Study and Demonstration of H reflex

Learning Objectives

After completing this practical, you will be able to (MUST KNOW):

1. Explain the importance of the study of nerve conduction in clinical physiology.
2. Classify nerve fibres.
3. Explain the difference in nerve conduction in myelinated and unmyelinated fibres.
4. List the factors that affect nerve conduction.
5. State the principle of nerve conduction study.
6. Explain the basic process of nerve conduction.

7. List the precautions taken during the recording of nerve conduction.
8. Understand the principle of H reflex recording and its importance.

You may also be able to (DESIRABLE TO KNOW):

1. Correlate the findings of nerve conduction with the clinical abnormality.
2. List the causes and effects of some of the common neuropathies.
3. Draw a schematic diagram of H reflex arc.

INTRODUCTION

Nerve conduction study (NCS) is part of the **electrodiagnostic procedures** that help in *establishing the type and degree of abnormalities of the nerves*. NCS establishes diagnosis very early and more accurately than other electrodiagnostic techniques. This is because of its *sensitivity in detecting conduction slowing* (or block), which is an *early indicator of nerve entrapment* or peripheral neuropathy, the problems most frequently encountered in neurology clinics.

Electrodiagnostic Testing

Electrodiagnostic or **electro-neurodiagnostic** testing actually involves **two different tests**: i) the **nerve conduction study** (NCS) and ii) the **electromyography (EMG) testing**. These tests are usually conducted when a patient has experienced muscle pain or cramping or sensations of weakness, numbness, or tingling. Conditions that can be diagnosed and/or monitored with the aid of electrodiagnostic testing include amyotrophic lateral sclerosis (ALS), brachial plexus injuries, carpal tunnel syndrome, cubital tunnel syndrome (ulnar nerve entrapment), herniated disc ('slipped disc'), Parsonage–Turner syndrome, radiculopathy, thoracic outlet syndrome, myopathies, other neuropathies, and neuromuscular diseases.

To interpret the results of nerve conduction studies, one should know the anatomical course of the nerve, the muscle supplied by the nerve, the normal conduction velocity of the nerve, the physiological basis of the conduction of impulse in the nerves, the pathophysiologic responses of the nerve and muscle to dysfunction, and the biological electrical signals.

Anatomical and Physiological Aspects

The conduction velocity of the nerve depends on **the fibre diameter, degree of myelination, and the internodal distance**.

Fibre diameter: The diameter of nerve axons varies between 0.2 and 20 μm. As the axon increases in size, the myelin sheath becomes thicker, and the internodal distance becomes longer. The conduction therefore becomes faster.

Myelination: Nerve fibres are classified as *myelinated and unmyelinated*. The myelinated axons are surrounded by Schwann cells; there is no Schwann sheath in unmyelinated fibres.

Internodal distance: Internodal distance, which is the distance between the two nodes of Ranvier, depends on the spacing of Schwann cells at the time of myelination during development. Proliferation of Schwann cells does not occur afterwards, but the internodal distance increases during the growth of the nerve. Thus, *the fibres myelinated early have a longer internodal distance, larger diameter, and wider spacing* at the nodes of Ranvier.

Classification of Nerve Fibres

Nerve fibres are classified (**Erlanger-Gasser classification**) into **groups A, B, and C** depending on the fibre diameter (Table 32.1).

1. **Group A fibres** contain both afferent and efferent myelinated somatic fibres of small, medium, and large diameters (1–20 μm). They are subclassified into α, β, γ and δ in the order of descending diameter and conduction velocity.

2. **Group B fibres** consist only of small preganglionic myelinated axons of the autonomous nervous system (1–3 μm).

3. **Group C fibres** consist of small unmyelinated fibres, which are present in visceral afferents, pain and temperature afferents and preganglionic autonomic efferents (2–2.2 μm).

Table 32.1 Classification of nerve fibres

Fibre types	Fibre diameter (μm)	Conduction velocity (m/s)	Function
Aα	12–20	70–120	Somatic motor and proprioception
Aβ	5–12	30–70	Touch—pressure
Aγ	3–6	15–30	Motor to muscle spindle
Aδ	2–5	12–30	Pain, cold, and touch
B	<3	3–15	Autonomic preganglionic fibres
C-dorsal root fibre	0.4–1.2	0.5–2	Somatic sensations
C-sympathetic fibre	0.3–1.3	0.7–2.3	Postganglionic sympathetic fibres

Impulse Conduction

The action potential originating in the axons is propagated in either direction from its site of origin. This conduction is continuous in unmyelinated and saltatory in myelinated fibres.

Myelinated fibres: Conduction is much faster in myelinated fibres than in unmyelinated fibres. Myelin thickness is inversely related to internodal capacitance and conductance. Therefore, conduction velocity increases with increasing myelin in the axon.

As the myelin sheath becomes thinner, the internodal conductance and capacitance increase in conditions of *segmental demyelination or during remyelination*. This causes a greater loss of local current before reaching the next node of Ranvier, which results in a failure to activate the nodes of Ranvier. This results in a *conduction block*. The segmental demyelination of smaller fibres may result in continuous conduction instead of saltatory conduction.

Unmyelinated fibres: Impulse conduction in unmyelinated fibres is *much slower* than in myelinated fibres. The conduction velocity is slow due to the continuous nature of conduction. The conduction velocity further slows down in conditions of focal compression, which may occur due to demyelination or decrease in the diameter of the fibres.

Factors That Affect Nerve Conduction

A number of **physiological and technical factors** can influence the result of nerve conduction studies.

Physiological factors

1. **Temperature:** Nerve temperature is the single most important factor that affects conduction velocity. The nerve conduction velocity is **directly related to intraneuronal temperature,** which in turn depends on internal body temperature. *Five per cent increase in conduction velocity occurs per degree Celsius rise of body temperature*, from 30°C to 40°C. Conversely, low temperature decreases the conduction velocity. For each degree Celsius fall in temperature, the latency increases by 0.3 ms and velocity decreases by 2.4 m/s. The change in conduction velocity due to alteration in body temperature is attributed to the **effect of temperature on sodium channels** in the nerves. Therefore, the laboratory temperature should ideally be maintained between 20°C and 25°C.

2. **Age:** Age significantly affects nerve conduction. Conduction velocity of nerves is **low in infants and children**. In neonates, it is nearly half of the adult values. It **attains the adult value by 3–5 years of age**, then remains relatively stable until sixty years of age, after which it starts declining at a rate of 1.5 per cent per decade. This is related to the gradual loss of larger neurons with ageing.

3. **Height:** An *inverse relationship* exists between the height of an individual and the velocity of nerve conduction. This is because shorter nerves conduct faster than longer nerves of the same age group. **In tall subjects**, distal conduction slowing occurs due to *greater axonal tapering and lesser myelination*. Tall individuals are also subjected to more loss of large-sized axons with ageing because of higher metabolic stress related to supplying the more distal axon.

4. **Limbs:** In the upper limbs, conduction velocity is higher; this too is attributed to the length of the nerves. The **factors that contribute** to the differences in the conduction velocity of the nerves in the upper and lower limbs are as follows:

   - Abrupt distal axonal tapering in the lower limbs
   - Shorter internodal distance in the lower limbs

- Progressive reduction in axonal diameter in the lower limbs
- Lower temperature of the feet compared to hands

5. **Gender:** Gender is known to affect nerve conduction. In general, nerve conduction is more in males.

Technical factors

Technical factors that affect nerve conduction may be due to a defect in the stimulating system or due to a defect in the recording system.

Stimulating system: Failure of the stimulating system may result in small responses or no response.

1. **Faulty location of stimulator:** The stimulator may be placed wrongly on the skin surface, or the nerve may be stimulated submaximally. In such cases, the stimulator should be relocated close to the nerve and pressed firmly.
2. **Fat or edema between stimulator and nerve:** In some conditions such as obesity or edema, needle electrodes may be used, as the impulse may not reach the target properly otherwise.
3. **Bridge formation between anode and cathode:** An important source of failure of the stimulating systems is the shunting of current between the anode and cathode either by sweat or the formation of a bridge by conducting jelly.

Recording system: Results may be erroneous if the recording system is defective, especially if the connection is faulty.

1. **Damage in the electrode wire**: The intactness of the recording system is tested by asking the subject to contract the muscle with the electrode in position. If the cable is damaged, the stimulus-induced muscle twitches cause movement-related potential.
2. **Incorrect position of active or reference electrode:** An initial positivity preceding the peak of compound muscle action potential suggests incorrect positioning of the active electrode. The recorded potential is also distorted if the reference electrode is located in an active rather than a remote region in relation to muscle action potential.
3. **Wrongly connected preamplifier/wrong settings of gain, sweep, or filter**: Amplifier filters can change all the components (amplitude, latency and duration) of the recorded response.

METHODS OF NERVE CONDUCTION STUDY

Principle

Nerve conduction study requires an external stimulation that initiates depolarization simultaneously in all the axons of the nerve to produce a recordable response. The response is recorded by stimulating the nerve at two different points. Conduction velocity is determined by studying the difference in latencies of the responses compared with the distance between the two points. Nerve conduction study involves the study of motor and sensory conduction.

Principles of motor nerve conduction

Measurement of motor nerve conduction includes studying the onset of latency, its duration, and the amplitude of **compound muscle action potential (CMAP)** and nerve conduction velocity. The onset of latency is the time in ms from the stimulus artefact to the first negative deflection of CMAP (Fig. 32.1). This is achieved by stimulating the nerve at least at two points along its course. The motor nerve conduction velocity is calculated by measuring the **distance between two points of stimulation in mm and dividing it by the latency difference in ms** (Fig. 32.2). The nerve conduction velocity is expressed as m/s.

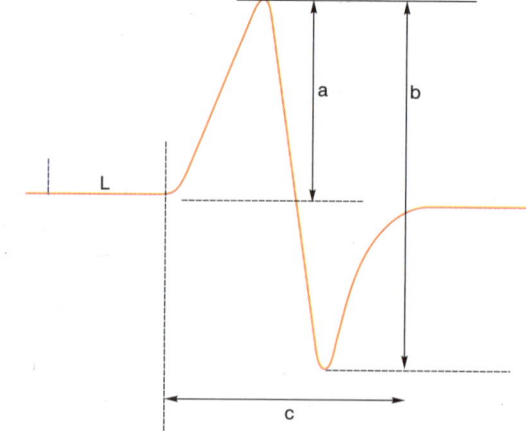

Fig. 32.1   Compound muscle action potential (CMAP) (L: latency; a: base-to-peak amplitude; b: peak-to-peak amplitude; c: duration of CMAP).

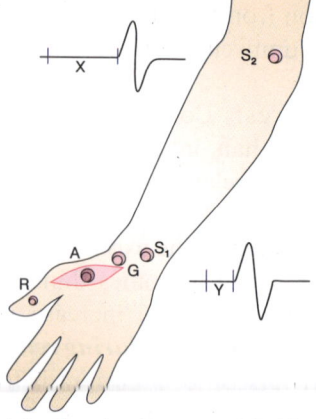

Fig. 32.2   2 Principle of motor neuron conduction. The conduction velocity is calculated by dividing the distance between the proximal (S2) and distal (S1) stimulating electrodes by the difference in the proximal (X) and distal latency (Y) (R: reference electrodes; G: ground electrode; A: active recording electrode).

Principles of sensory nerve conduction

Like motor nerve conduction study, sensory nerve conduction measurement includes the study of onset latency, amplitude, duration of **sensory nerve action potential (SNAP),** and nerve conduction velocity. Sensory nerve conduction can be measured orthodromically or antidromically. **In orthodromic conduction,** *a distal portion of the nerve (e.g., the digital nerve) is stimulated*, and SNAP is recorded at a proximal point along the nerve. **In antidromic sensory nerve conduction,** the nerve is stimulated at a proximal point, and the nerve action potential is recorded distally. The latency of orthodromic potential is measured from the stimulus artefact to the initial positive or subsequent negative peak. The *initial positive peak in SNAP having a triphasic appearance* is a feature of orthodromic potential. In antidromic potential, the initial positivity in SNAP is absent. The sensory conduction velocity is calculated by *dividing the distance (mm) between the stimulating and the recording site by the latency (ms)*. The **amplitude of SNAP** suggests the density of nerve fibres, whereas the **duration** suggests the number of slow-conducting fibres.

Requirements

1. Stimulator
2. Stimulating and recording electrodes
3. Preamplifier and oscilloscope of nerve conduction machine (Fig. 32.3).
4. Electrode jelly
5. Spirit

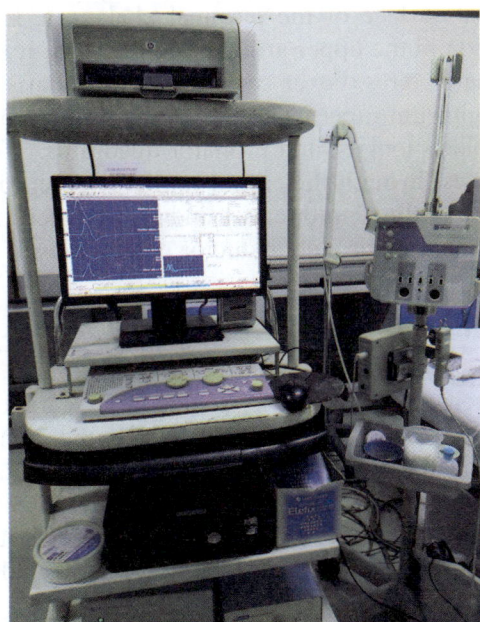

Fig. 32.3 Nerve conduction machine (preamplifier and oscilloscope). (Courtesy: EP-EMG Lab, Physiology Department, JIPMER, Puducherry, India.)

Procedure

1. Clean the area and the skin overlying the nerve with spirit at the proximal and the distal ends.
2. Fix the cup electrode on the skin overlying the muscle supplied by the nerve.
3. Connect the electrodes to the oscilloscope through the preamplifier.
4. Keep the sweep at 5 ms/cm.
5. With the help of stimulating electrodes, **stimulate the nerve, first at the distal end** (Fig. 32.4A), and observe the action potential on the oscilloscope.

Note: The stimulus artifact, which is due to current leak, appears at the beginning of the sweep. This is useful for noting the point of stimulus. The latent period is the interval between the beginning of the stimulus artifact and the first deflection of the muscle potential.

6. Then, **stimulate the nerve at the proximal end** and record the action potential (Fig. 32.4B). Note the latent period.
7. Record NCS for the upper limb nerves (ulnar, median, radial) and for lower limb nerves (femoral, sciatic, common peroneal, tibial, etc.)

A)
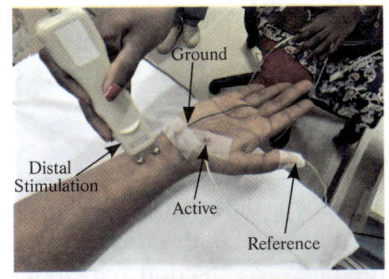

B)
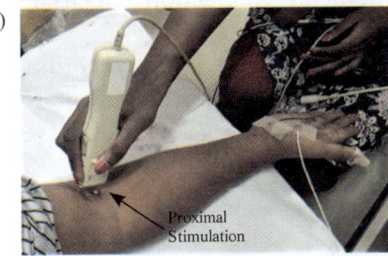

Fig. 32.4 Procedure of nerve conduction study: (A) Median nerve, stimulation of the distal end and (B) median nerve, proximal stimulation.

Note: The difference between the two latent periods gives the time taken by the impulse to travel from the proximal point to the distal point.

8. Measure the distance between the points of stimulation.
9. Measure the latent period of both distal and proximal action potentials (Fig. 32.5).
10. Calculate the conduction velocity in m/s by the following formula:

$$\text{Conduction velocity} = \frac{\text{Distance}}{\text{Difference in latent periods}}$$

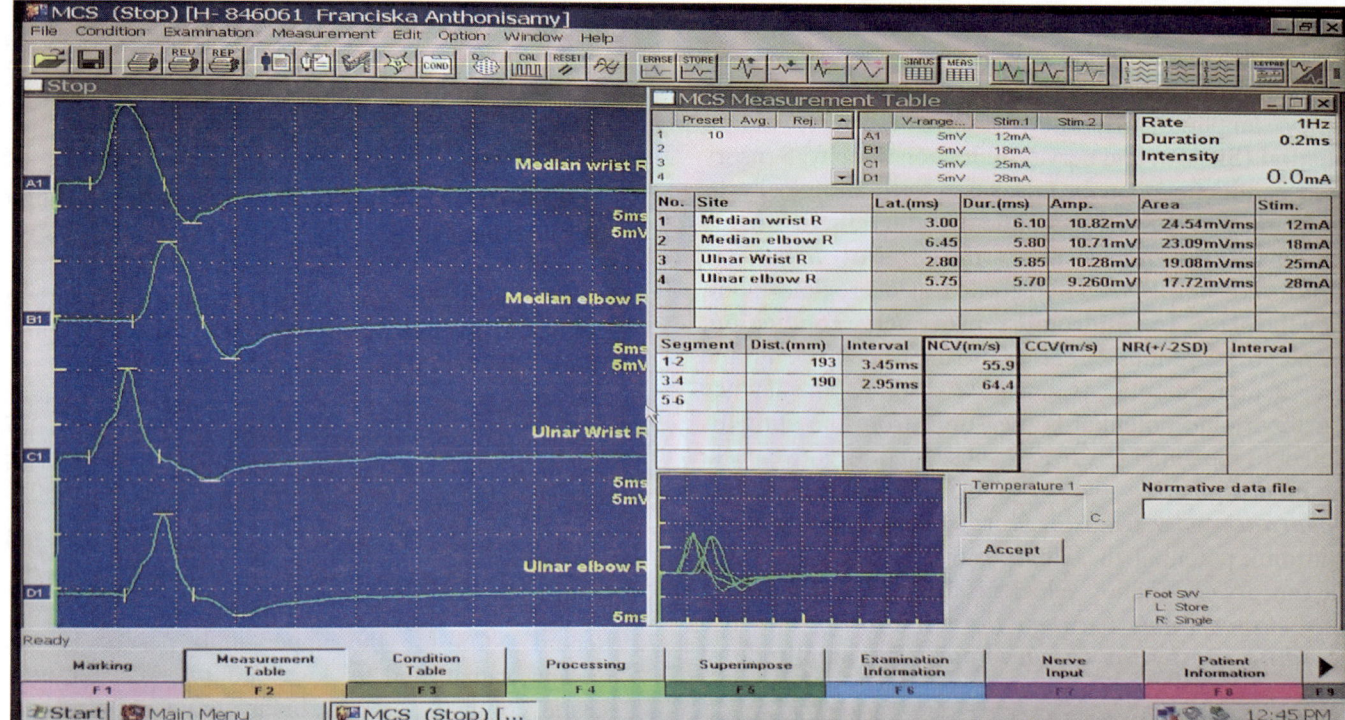

Fig. 32.5   Recording of CMAP of median nerve at distal end (A1 tracing); CMAP of median nerve at proximal end (B1 tracing); CMAP of ulnar nerve at distal end (C1 tracing); CMAP of ulnar nerve at proximal end (D1 tracing). Note the details of the values for latency, duration, amplitude, and conduction velocity for each nerve on the right side of the recording display (CMAP: Compound muscle [nerve] action potential).

Observation and Results

1. Enter the latency, duration, and amplitude of each nerve of both limbs of both sides in a tabular format.
2. Express the nerve conduction velocity in meters per second (m/s) for each nerve.
3. Report your findings. In the recording shown in Fig. 32.5, the conduction velocity of the median nerve is 55.9 m/s. This is a normal nerve conduction report.

Precautions

1. The subject should be properly instructed and motivated to provide full cooperation.
2. The subject should be fully relaxed.
3. The room should be quiet and comfortable.
4. The subject should be grounded properly.

DISCUSSION

Recording of nerve conduction study is ordered in neurological practice to assess the velocity of conduction of impulses in the nerve. The important nerves tested are the median, ulnar, and radial nerves and the brachial plexus in the upper limbs, and sciatic, femoral, common peroneal, tibial, and sural nerves in the lower limbs.

Median Nerve

The median nerve (**C5–T1**) is a mixed nerve. It supplies the flexors of the forearm and the thenar muscles of the hand. It is sensory to the lateral aspect of the palm and the dorsal surface of the terminal phalanges. It has no innervation in the upper arm. **In the forearm, it supplies** the pronator teres, flexor carpi radialis, palmaris longus, flexor digitorum superficialis, flexor digitorum profundus, flexor pollicis longus, and pronator quadratus. The nerve then **passes through the carpal tunnel** to enter the hand, where **it supplies** lumbricals I and II, opponens pollicis, flexor pollicis brevis, and abductor pollicis brevis.

Median Entrapment Neuropathy

The entrapment (compression) neuropathy of the median nerve often occurs during its course in the carpal tunnel. In fact, the **carpal tunnel syndrome** is the commonest entrapment neuropathy seen in a neurology clinic. **Pronator teres syndrome** of the median nerve (entrapment of the nerve between the heads of the pronator teres, through which the nerve descends into the forearm from the arm) occurs occasionally.

In these syndromes, the conduction of the median nerve decreases. The nerve conduction decreases distal to the site of compression.

Causes of carpal tunnel syndrome: The common causes of carpal tunnel syndrome are:

1. Rheumatoid arthritis
2. Overuse of wrist (too much computer work)
3. Hypothyroidism
4. Acromegaly

Ulnar Nerve

The ulnar nerve arises from **C7–T1** through the medial cord of the brachial plexus. It does not supply any muscle in the upper arm. It passes through the condylar groove in the elbow, to enter the forearm, where it passes through the cubital tunnel. Here, it supplies the flexor carpi ulnaris. Then, it supplies the flexor digitorum profundus III and IV. At the wrist, it **passes through Guyon's canal,** where it bifurcates to form a **superficial sensory and a deep motor branch.** The **motor branch** supplies hypothenar muscles and the abductor pollicis, the medial half of the flexor pollicis, the interosseous and the third and fourth lumbricals.

Ulnar neuropathy

Ulnar nerve neuropathy can occur at the elbow, the distal forearm, and the wrist.

Ulnar nerve lesion at the elbow: There are two vulnerable sites for lesions of the ulnar nerve in the elbow: the condylar groove and the cubital tunnel.

1. *At condylar groove*: Repeated pressure, fracture of ulna, leprosy
2. *At cubital tunnel*: Arthritis, ganglion

Ulnar nerve lesion in the distal forearm: The ulnar nerve in the distal forearm can be damaged by trauma or chronic repetitive ergonomic stress. It is usually associated with median and radial nerve involvement. The ulnar nerve may be compressed in the middle of the upper arm by the head while sleeping.

Ulnar nerve lesion at the wrist:

1. **Lesion proximal to the branch to hypothenar muscles:** This produces profound weakness of the interossei and lumbricals, which is associated with mild hypothenar weakness. The sensations remain normal.
2. **Lesion distal to the branch to hypothenar muscles:** This causes weakness of the interossei and lumbricals, but not of the hypothenar muscles. The sensation remains normal.
3. **Lesion before the division of the superficial and deep branches:** A lesion at this site causes weakness of the intrinsic muscles of the hand supplied by the ulnar nerve and impairment of sensation in the area of distribution of the superficial branch.

4. **Lesion of the superficial branch of the ulnar nerve:** There is impairment of sensations in the areas supplied by the superficial branch. The motor conduction remains normal.

Radial Nerve

The posterior cord of the brachial plexus extends as the radial nerve. It has the **root value of C5–T1**. It supplies the triceps and then descends into the spiral groove of the humerus. It supplies the brachioradialis and extensor carpi radialis and longus. In the proximal part of the forearm, it divides into the posterior interosseous and superficial radial nerves. The **posterior interosseous nerve** supplies the supinator, abductor pollicis longus, extensor carpi ulnaris, extensor digitorum, extensor digiti minimi, extensor pollicis longus, and extensor indices. The **superficial cutaneous nerve** supplies the dorsum of the hand.

Radial neuropathy

A lesion of the radial nerve causes *wrist drop*. The radial nerve may be affected in the axilla, behind the humerus (retrohumeral), in the proximal forearm or distal forearm.

In the axilla: Lesion of radial nerve in the axilla usually occurs due to *compression during sleep*. There is weakness in all the muscles supplied by the radial nerve, including the triceps. The motor and sensory nerve conduction of the radial nerve reveals abnormality.

Retrohumeral lesion: This is the *commonest form* of radial nerve palsies. It occurs due to compression as in **Saturday night paralysis** or following general anesthesia.

In proximal forearm: The posterior interosseous nerve is involved in the lesion of the radial nerve in the proximal forearm. The posterior interosseous nerve is a *pure motor nerve*. There is weakness in the extensors of the wrist and metacarpophalangeal joints. Motor conduction study reveals reduced CMAP. The radial sensory conduction remains normal.

In distal forearm: This affects the superficial sensory nerve. Therefore, it results in pure sensory loss in the distribution of the radial nerve. Motor conduction remains normal.

Brachial Plexus

The brachial plexus (**C5–T1**) carries the fibres that provide motor and sensory supply of the shoulder girdle, upper trunk, and upper limb. It has **two trunks** (suprascapular and subclavian) and **three cords** (medial, posterior and lateral). The *medial cord* gives rise to the medial pectoral, the medial cutaneous nerve of the arm, and the medial cutaneous nerve of the forearm. The *posterior cord* gives rise to the superior subscapular, thoracodorsal, and inferior subscapular nerves. The *lateral cord* forms the lateral pectoral nerve. The *terminal branches* of the brachial plexus form the musculocutaneous, axillary, radial, median, and ulnar nerves.

Nerve conduction in the brachial plexus can be measured by *stimulating at Erb's point*. The **F waves** have been used in assessing conduction in the proximal portion of the nerves, plexus, or roots. The brachial plexus is involved in brachial neuritis, thoracic outlet compression syndrome, radiation-induced plexopathy, and obstetric and congenital brachial plexus palsy in newborns.

Femoral Nerve

The femoral nerve has the **root value of L2–4**. It innervates the extensors of the knee. It carries sensations from the anteromedial thigh, medial leg, and foot. In its intra-abdominal course, it supplies the iliopsoas muscle. It emerges from the pelvis under the inguinal ligament and divides into the anterior and posterior branches. The *anterior division* supplies the anterior and medial thigh, and the *posterior division* supplies the knee and hip joint and quadriceps muscle and terminates as the saphenous nerve.

Femoral neuropathy
■ Causes
Femoral neuropathy is caused by the following:
1. Diabetes mellitus
2. Vertebral tumours
3. Compression of the inguinal ligament during prolonged surgery in the lithotomy position

In femoral neuropathy, the motor conduction abnormalities include decreased conduction velocity and low CMAP amplitude. Compression at the level of the inguinal ligament results in conduction block, which can be detected by stimulating the femoral nerve above and below the inguinal ligament and comparing the CMAP.

Saphenous Nerve

This is a **purely sensory nerve**. It is the **largest and longest branch** of the femoral nerve. Any lesion of the saphenous nerve, which occurs in laceration injuries or during surgery for varicose veins, results in sensory impairment in the medial aspect of the knee, leg, and foot. There is no defect in motor conduction.

Sciatic Nerve

The sciatic nerve is the **largest nerve of the body**. It has medial and lateral trunks. The *medial trunk* below

the popliteal fossa continues as the tibial nerve, and the *lateral trunk* continues as the common peroneal nerve. Sciatic neuropathy commonly results from fracture dislocation of the hip joint, hip replacement surgery, prolonged compression during anesthesia or sitting in an awkward position, or sometimes due to gluteal injection. Electrophysiological evaluation involves motor conduction studies of the peroneal and posterior tibial, and sensory conduction of the sural and superficial peroneal nerve.

Common Peroneal Nerve

The common peroneal nerve winds around the neck of the fibula and descends to divide into the superficial and deep peroneal nerves. The **superficial peroneal nerve** innervates the peroneus longus and peroneus brevis and then supplies the lateral and dorsal portions of the lower leg and dorsum of the foot. The **deep peroneal nerve** supplies the muscles of the anterior compartment.
Causes of common peroneal nerve lesion: Neuropathy usually occurs due to compression of the common peroneal nerve as it winds around the fibula. The following are some of the causes of common peroneal nerve lesions:
1. Plaster cast
2. Tight bandage
3. Fracture neck of fibula
4. Habitual crossing of the legs
Nerve conduction studies reveal defects in both motor and sensory conduction.

Tibial Nerve

This is the continuation of the medial trunk of the sciatic nerve below the popliteal fossa. It supplies both heads of the gastrocnemius, soleus and tibialis posterior muscle. It descends and passes through the tarsal tunnel and supplies the intrinsic foot muscles.
Tibial neuropathy: The tibial nerve is frequently affected in cases of leprosy. Lesion of the tibial nerve results in the weakness of the plantar flexors, invertors, and intrinsic foot muscles. The nerve is also involved in tarsal tunnel syndrome.

Nerve conduction reveals impairment in both motor and sensory conduction. The tarsal tunnel syndrome is diagnosed by demonstrating a conduction block and latency prolongation across the tarsal tunnel.

Sural Nerve

The sural nerve is the **root value of S1 and S2**. It is derived from both the tibial and peroneal nerves. It is a **purely sensory nerve**. It innervates the posterolateral part of the distal leg and the lateral aspect of the foot. In sural neuropathy, there are abnormalities in sensory conduction.

Demonstration of H Reflex

The H reflex (or **Hoffmann's reflex**) is a reflectory reaction of muscles to electrical stimulation of sensory fibres (Ia afferents stemming from muscle spindles) in their innervating nerves. H reflex is a **monosynaptic spinal reflex**, used in nerve conduction velocity (NCV) studies to assess the integrity of the monosynaptic reflex arc and spinal cord excitability.

Principle

The H-reflex test is performed with an electric stimulator, which usually gives a square-wave current of short duration and small amplitude (higher stimulations might involve alpha fibres, causing an F-wave, which compromises the results), and an EMG set to record the muscle response. It is elicited by electrically **stimulating Ia afferent fibres**, which are large-diameter sensory fibres.

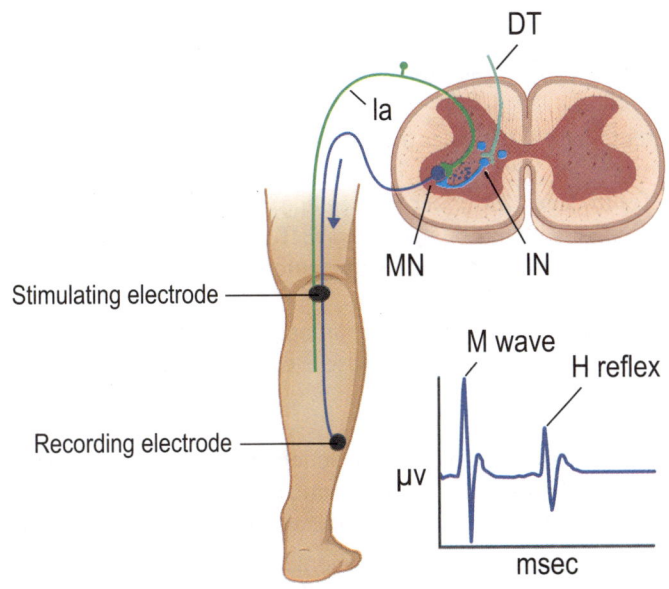

Fig. 32.6   The schematic diagram of H reflex recording. Note that H reflex wave (H wave) appears after the M wave in the recording. M wave is the early motor response that precedes the H reflex (Ia: Ia afferent fibres; MN: motor neuron, IN: interneuron, DT: descending tract).

Procedure

Electrical stimulation: A *low-intensity electrical stimulus* is applied to a mixed nerve, such as the tibial nerve, to **activate Ia afferent fibres**.

Sensory input: Ia fibres transmit the signal to the spinal cord, where they **synapse with alpha motor neurons**.

Motor response: The alpha motor neurons then generate a **reflex response** in the target muscle, typically the soleus, causing a measurable contraction. The response is usually a clearly distinguished wave, called the **H wave**, 28–35 ms after the stimulus (Fig. 32.6), not to be confused with an F wave.

> **Note:** H reflex is analogous to the mechanically-induced spinal stretch reflex (e.g., the kneejerk reflex). The primary difference between the H reflex and the spinal stretch reflex is that the H reflex bypasses the muscle spindle, and, therefore, is a **valuable tool** for assessing the *modulation of monosynaptic reflex activity* in the spinal cord.

Clinical applications of the H reflex

The H reflex provides valuable information about peripheral nerve function and can help differentiate between various neuropathies and radiculopathies, particularly those involving the S1 nerve root.

Assessing peripheral nerve function: The H reflex can help in evaluating the function of the peripheral nerves, especially in cases of neuropathy and radiculopathy.

Differentiating S1 and L5 radiculopathies: It is particularly useful in distinguishing between S1 and L5 radiculopathies, which can have similar EMG recordings.

Evaluating spinal cord excitability: The H reflex can provide insights into the excitability of the spinal cord and the integrity of the monosynaptic reflex arc.

Monitoring neuromuscular conditions: Changes in the H reflex can indicate changes in peripheral and central nerve conditions, making it a sensitive measure for evaluating neuromuscular conditions.

Distinguishing H reflex from other reflexes

F wave: The F wave is a later response elicited by stimulating the motor nerve, while the H reflex is elicited by stimulating sensory nerves.

M wave: The M wave is the early motor response that precedes the H reflex.

B reflex: The B reflex is another late response that can be recorded in addition to the H reflex.

VIVA

1. *What is the importance of nerve conduction study in clinical medicine?* (**Ans.** Refer to page 214, under the heading 'Introduction'.)
2. *How does myelination affect the conduction velocity of the nerves?* (**Ans.** Refer to page 214, under the heading 'Anatomical and Physiological Aspects'.)
3. *How are nerve fibres classified?* (**Ans.** Refer to page 214–215 see Table 32.1.)

4. *What are the factors that affect nerve conduction?* (Ans. Refer to page 215, under the heading 'Factors Affecting Nerve Conduction'.)

5. *What is the principle of nerve conduction?* (Ans. Refer to page 216, under the heading 'Methods. . .' and the subheading 'Principle'.)

6. *What is the course and innervation of the median nerve?* (Ans. Refer to page 216, under the heading 'Methods' and the subheading 'Principle'.)

7. *What are the waves of compound muscle action potential (CMAP)?* (Ans. Refer to page 216, under the heading 'Principle of motor nerve conduction'.)

8. *What are the waves of sensory nerve action potential (SNAP)?* (Ans. Refer to page 217, under the heading 'Principle of sensory nerve conduction'.)

9. *How is the conduction velocity in a nerve calculated?* (Ans. Refer to page 217, under the heading 'Procedure', point no. 9.)

10. *What are the common sites and causes of median neuropathy?* (Ans. Refer to page 218, under the heading 'Median Nerve'.)

11. *What are the effects of median neuropathy at different sites?* (Ans. Refer to page 218, under the heading 'Median entrapment neuropathy'.)

12. *What is the course and innervation of the ulnar nerve?* (Ans. Refer to page 219, under the heading 'Ulnar Nerve'.)

13. *What are the common sites and effects of ulnar neuropathy?* (Ans. Refer to page 219, under the heading 'Ulnar neuropathy'.)

14. *What are the effects of ulnar neuropathy at different sites?* (Ans. Refer to page 219, under the heading 'Ulnar Nerve Lesions'.)

15. *What is the course and innervation of the radial nerve?* (Ans. Refer to page 219, under the heading 'Radial Nerve'.)

16. *What are the common sites and causes of radial neuropathy?* (Ans. Refer to page 219, under the heading 'Radial neuropathy'.)

17. *What are the effects of radial neuropathy at different sites?* (Ans. Refer to page 219, under the heading 'Radial neuropathy'.)

18. *What is the course and innervation of the femoral nerve?* (Ans. Refer to page 220, under the heading 'Femoral Nerve'.)

19. *What is the common site of lesion on the femoral nerve?* (Ans. Refer to page 220, under the heading 'Femoral neuropathy'.)

20. *What are the causes and effects of femoral neuropathy?* (Ans. Refer to page 220, under the heading 'Femoral neuropathy'.)

21. *What is the course and innervation of the common peroneal nerve?* (Ans. Refer to page 220, under the heading 'Common peroneal nerve'.)

22. *What are the common sites and causes of common peroneal neuropathy?* (Ans. Refer to page 220, under the heading 'Common causes of peroneal nerve lesion'.)

23. *What are the effects of common peroneal neuropathy?* (Ans. Refer to page 220, under the heading 'Common peroneal nerve lesion'.)

24. *What is the course and innervation of the tibial nerve?* (Ans. Refer to page 220, under the heading 'Tibial nerve'.)

25. *What are the common sites and causes of lesion of the tibial nerve?* (Ans. Refer to page 220, see 'Tibial nerve'.)

26. *What are the effects of tibial neuropathy?* (Ans. Refer to page 220, under the heading 'Tibial neuropathy'.)

27. *What is the F wave? What is its significance?*
(Ans. The F wave is recorded from the muscle. When a supramaximal stimulus is applied, an action potential travels up the motor nerve and ventral root to the motor neuron, and is reflected back down to the muscle, causing a delayed muscle contraction.)

28. *What is H reflex and what is its significance?*
(Ans. An H reflex is usually recorded in the soleus muscle using a submaximal stimulus. The action potential travels in the proprioceptive Ia sensory fibre within the nerve, and through the dorsal root and a monosynaptic reflex arc, it reaches the motor neuron, resulting in a late muscle contraction. It is a sensitive test for detecting S1 radiculopathy.)

29. *How is the H reflex differentiated from the F wave, M wave, and B reflex?* (Ans. Refer to page 221, under the heading 'H reflex' and the subheading 'Distinguishing H reflex from...'.)

30. *What are the clinical utilities of H reflex?* (Ans. Refer to page 221, under the heading 'H reflex' and the subheading 'Clinical application...'.)

31. *What are the other clinical phenomena associated with the name Hoffman?*
(Ans. There are two more clinical entities associated with the name Hoffman.

i). **Hoffmann sign:** This test is used to detect upper motor neuron lesions, particularly involving the cervical spinal cord. It is performed by flicking the nail of the middle finger. A positive response—characterized by involuntary flexion of the thumb and/or index finger—suggests corticospinal tract dysfunction. It is often referred to as the 'Babinski sign of the upper limb'.

ii). **Hoffman sign of tetany:** Electrical or mechanical stimulation of the sensory nerve produces muscle spasm. It is usually performed on the ulnar nerve in cases of tetany caused by hypoparathyroidism.

33 | Electromyography

Learning Objectives

After completing this practical, you will be able to (MUST KNOW):
1. Explain the importance of performing EMG in clinical physiology.
2. List the uses of EMG.
3. Describe the types and features of motor unit potentials.
4. List factors that affect motor unit potentials.
5. Describe the principle of EMG and the precautions to be taken while recording it.

You may also be able to (DESIRABLE TO KNOW):
1. Explain insertional activity.
2. List the different types and common causes of spontaneous activity.

INTRODUCTION

Electromyography (EMG) refers to the **recording of action potentials of muscle fibres** firing singly or in groups near the needle electrode in a muscle. The muscle action potential, when recorded by a needle, usually has **three phases**. The rise time and fall of muscle action potential depends on the distance of the recording electrode from the muscle fibres.

Each muscle is composed of thousands of muscle fibres, each of which is a complex multinucleated cell of variable length and diameter. Each muscle fibre receives a nerve twig from a motor neuron in the anterior horn of the spinal cord. A single motor neuron and the group of muscle fibres innervated by it are together known as a **motor unit** (Fig. 33.1). The rate and pattern of firing of muscle fibres of a motor unit depend on the stimuli that travel through the nerve. A **denervated muscle** exhibits unstable membrane potential and fires spontaneously, without stimulation.

Motor Unit Potential (MUP)

The motor unit potential is the **sum of the action potentials produced in the muscle supplied by an anterior horn cell**. The muscle fibres discharge synchronously near the needle electrode. Therefore, the MUP has higher amplitude and longer duration than the action potential produced by a single muscle fibre. The MUPs can be characterised by their **firing pattern and appearance**. With mild contraction, the firing rates of MUPs are normally 5–15 Hz. With additional firing during muscle contraction, there is recruitment of MUPs. The recruitment of MUPs depends on the size principle. According to the **size principle**, motor neurons are recruited in the order of size from small to large.

Features

The MUP is characterised by its duration, number of phases, amplitude, and the rate of rise of the first component (Fig. 33.2).

Duration: The duration is measured from the **initial take-off to the point of return to the baseline**. It varies from 5–15 ms. It is shorter in children and longer in elderly subjects.

The duration of MUP is a measure of:
- Conduction velocity
- Length of the muscle fibre
- Membrane excitability
- Synchrony of different muscle fibres of a motor unit

Note: Motor unit potentials (MUPs) of brief duration are a common finding in myopathies, myasthenia gravis, and the initial phase of nerve regeneration. In contrast, LMN lesions and some types of myositis are associated with MUPs exhibiting extended duration.

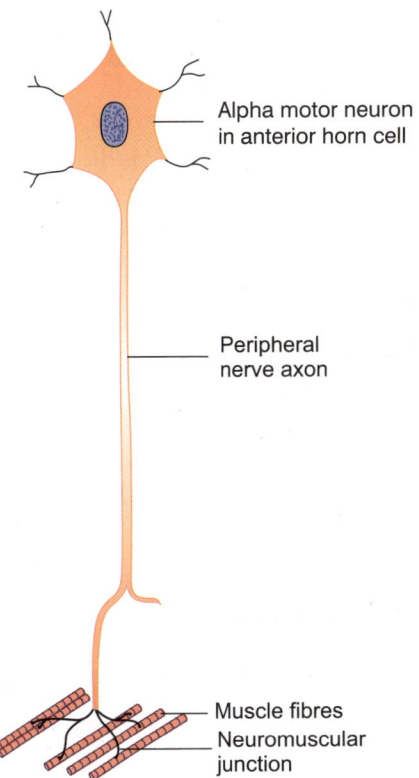

Alpha motor neuron in anterior horn cell

Peripheral nerve axon

Muscle fibres
Neuromuscular junction

Fig. 33.1 Schematic representation of a typical motor unit.

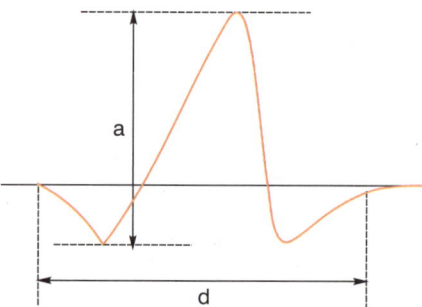

Fig. 33.2 Normal motor unit potential (a: amplitude; d: duration; note the first positive wave (1st downward wave from the baseline), the negative wave (upward wave from baseline), and the second positive wave (2nd downward wave from the baseline). **Rise time** is the duration from the initial positive wave to the peak of the negative wave.

Phases: Usually, **MUP is triphasic**—positive, negative, and positive. **Phase** is defined as the portion of the MUP between the departure and the return to the baseline. An MUP with more than four phases is called a *polyphasic MUP*. Normally, the polyphasic potentials do not exceed 5–15 per cent of the total MUP population. The presence of more polyphasic potentials indicates desynchronization or dropout of muscles.

Amplitude: Amplitude is measured from the maximum peak of the negative phase to the maximum peak of the positive phase. It depends on the following:

- Size of the muscle fibres
- Density of the muscle fibres
- Synchrony of firing
- Proximity of the needle to the muscle fibre
- Types of muscles examined
- Muscle temperature
- Age of the subject

Rise time: The rise time of MUP is the duration from the initial positive to the subsequent negative peak. The usual rise time is less than 500 μs. If it is more than 500 μs, the increased resistance and capacitance of the intervening tissue could be responsible.

Factors that affect MUP

Technical factors

1. Types of needle electrode
2. Characteristics of the recording surface
3. Electrical characteristics of the cable
4. Preamplifier and amplifier
5. Method of recording

Physiological factors

1. Age of the patient (older individuals tend to have higher MUPs)
2. Muscle examined
3. Temperature

METHOD OF PERFORMING ELECTROMYOGRAPHY

Principle

A resting muscle does not show recordable electrical potential. If allowed to contract, it does. With increased force of contraction, the amplitude of the potential increases.

Requirements

1. Cathode ray oscilloscope (CRO)
2. Preamplifier and amplifier (Fig. 33.3)
3. Recording electrodes
4. Electrode paste
5. Spirit

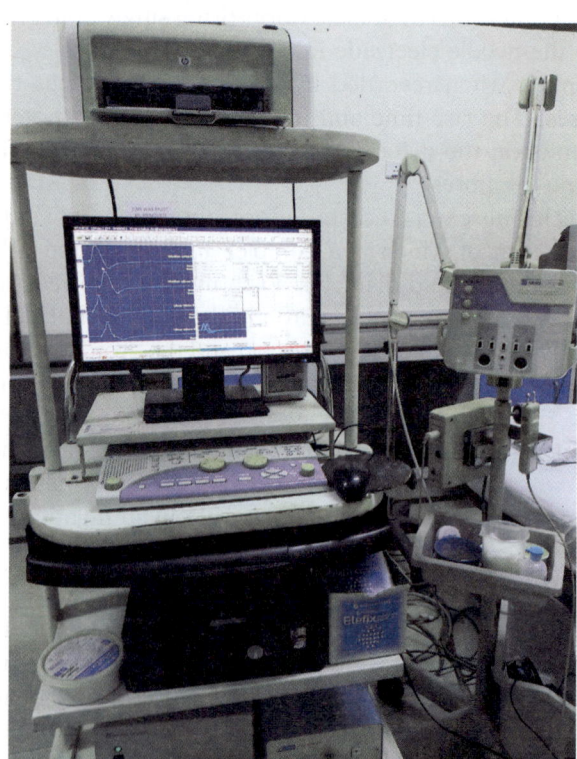

Fig. 33.3 Nerve conduction machine (preamplifier and oscilloscope). (*Courtesy:* EP-EMG Lab, Physiology Department, JIPMER, Puducherry, India.)

Recording electrodes: There are different types of recording electrodes are broadly divided into **needle electrodes and surface** electrodes. The different types of needle electrodes are:

1. Concentric needle electrodes
2. Monopolar needle electrodes
3. Single-fibre needle electrodes
4. Macro-needle electrodes

The concentric needle electrodes are the most commonly used electrodes in clinical practice. A **concentric needle electrode** consists of a 24–26-gauge needle with a fine wire in its lumen. The recording area of the tip of the needle is $125 \times 580 \ \mu m^2$. In this electrode, the *shaft of the needle is considered as the active electrode*, thus, reducing the surrounding muscle noise. The **monopolar needle electrode** is a solid, 22–30-gauge teflon-coated needle with a bare tip. The MUP recorded by a monopolar electrode is slightly higher in amplitude and longer in duration.

Procedure for Surface EMG

1. Clean the skin overlying the muscle with spirit.
2. Fix a set of three electrodes on the skin over the muscle (one for ground, and the other two for recording EMG) with a small amount of electrode paste. The electrode paste minimises the skin–electrode resistance.
3. Connect the electrodes through the preamplifier to the oscilloscopes.
4. Observe the resting potentials in the oscilloscope.
5. Ask the subject to contract the muscle and observe the potentials.

Procedure for Needle EMG

1. Clean the skin overlying the muscle with spirit. Fix the ground electrode.
2. Insert the concentric needle electrode into the muscle to be tested.
3. Observe the potentials in the oscilloscope during insertion.
4. Ask the subject to contract the muscle and observe the potentials.
5. Move the needle in different directions in the muscle and record the potential.

Observation and Results

The following activities are observed during recording EMG:
1. Insertional activity
2. Spontaneous activity
3. Voluntary activity
4. Write down your final opinion on EMG based on the three above-mentioned activities and state whether they are normal or abnormal (details of abnormal patterns are given in 'Discussion' below).

Precautions

1. The subject should be properly instructed and motivated to cooperate fully during the procedure.
2. The subject should be fully relaxed.
3. The room should be calming and comfortable.
4. The subject should be grounded properly.

DISCUSSION

While EMG is a valuable tool for identifying motor neuron diseases and neuromuscular transmission deficits, it can also help differentiate these conditions from particular muscle disorders like muscular dystrophy, myopathies, and neuropathies. A typical muscle fibre maintains a resting membrane potential (RMP) and produces an action potential (AP) when stimulated to contract. However, following denervation, a muscle fibre undergoes certain changes, leading to an unstable membrane potential and the occurrence of spontaneous twitching.

Motor Unit Potentials (Fig. 33.4A)

Types
1. Short-duration MUP
2. Long-duration MUP
3. Polyphasic MUP
4. Mixed pattern MUP
5. Doublets MUP

1. **Short-duration MUPs:** These are usually low-amplitude MUPs (Fig. 33.4C). They have rapid recruitment with minimal effort. These are found in diseases associated with the loss of muscle fibres.

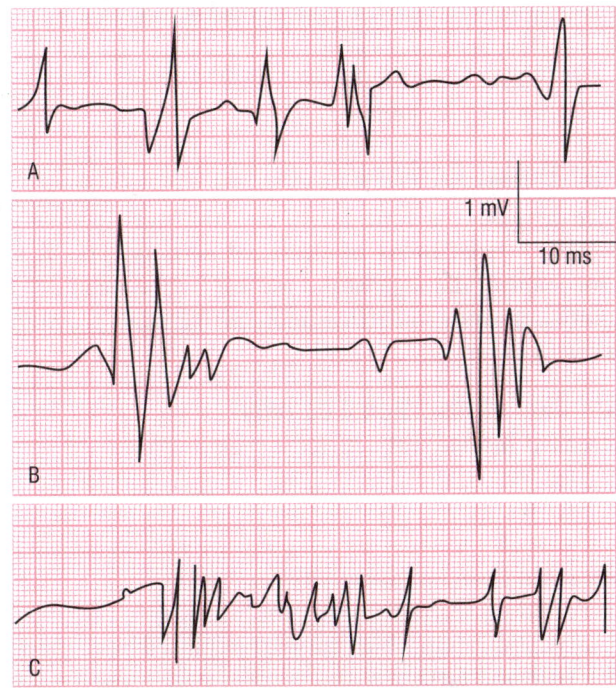

Fig. 33.4 Motor unit potentials: **(A)** Normal; **(B)** neurogenic (MUPs are larger, prolonged, and polyphasic); and **(C)** myopathic (MUPs have low amplitude).

Short-duration MUPs are commonly seen in:

i. Myopathies (endocrine and metabolic)
ii. Neuromuscular junction disorder
iii. The early stages of reinnervation after nerve damage

2. **Long-duration MUPs:** These are generally associated with high amplitude and poor recruitment (Fig. 33.4B). Long-duration MUPs are commonly seen in:
   i. Motor neuron disease
   ii. Neuropathies
   iii. Chronic myositis

3. **Polyphasic MUPs:** When there are more than four phases in MUP, they are called polyphasic. They are commonly seen in:
   i. Myopathies, where there is regeneration of fibres and increased fibre density
   ii. Neurogenic diseases, where there is regeneration of axons

4. **Mixed pattern of MUPs:** In a mixed pattern of MUPs, short-duration MUPs, long-duration MUPs, and polyphasic MUPs are all seen. This pattern is seen in both myopathies and neuropathies.

5. **Doublets, triplets, or multiplets:** Normally, MUPs are discharged as a single potential in a semi-rhythmic fashion. In some diseased conditions, the rhythm of MUPs is disturbed. It then occurs in bursts of two or more at an interval of 10–30 ms. These are called *doublets, triplets, or multiplets* depending on the number of bursts. This is commonly seen in:
   i. Hyperventilation
   ii. Motor neuron disease
   iii. Muscle ischemia

Insertional Activity

When a needle is introduced into the muscle, there is normally a **brief burst of electrical activity**. This is due to mechanical damage of the muscle by the needle. This activity appears as *positive or negative high-frequency spikes in clusters*.

Alteration of insertional activity

Increased insertional activity is seen in:
1. Denervated muscles
2. Myotonia
3. Familial

Decreased insertional activity is seen in:
1. Periodic paralysis (during the attack)
2. Myopathies (in which muscle is replaced by connective tissue and fat)

3. Insertional activity is lower in calf muscles

Spontaneous Activity

Normally, there is **no spontaneous electrical activity** (after the decay of insertional activity). However, a type of spontaneous activity is recorded in the end plate zone, which appears as monophasic negative waves of less than 100 µV and durations of 1–3 ms. The end plate potentials are known as **end plate noise**. The end plate spikes occur due to the mechanical activation of nerve terminals by the needle.

The various types of **abnormal spontaneous activities** are as follows:
1. Fibrillations
2. Fasciculations
3. Complex repetitive discharges (CRD)
4. Cramp potentials

Fibrillations

Fibrillations are **spontaneously occurring action potentials from a single muscle fibre**. They *fire regularly* at a rate of 1–15 Hz with amplitudes of 20–200 µV and durations of 1–5 ms when recorded by a concentric needle. Fibrillations are biphasic or triphasic waves **with *initial positivity*** (this differentiates them from end plate spikes).

▌Causes

1. **Neurogenic diseases:** Anterior horn cell disease and axonal neuropathy
2. **Diseases of neuromuscular junction:** Myasthenia gravis and botulism
3. **Myogenic diseases:** Myositis and muscle trauma

Fasciculations

Fasciculation potentials are **spontaneous activities generated by a number of muscle fibres** belonging to whole or a part of a motor unit. They occur *randomly and irregularly* at variable rates of 1–500 per minute. Their size and shape depend on the motor units from which they arise and the distance of the recording electrode from the motor unit.

▌Causes

1. **Physiological:** Benign fasciculations, muscle cramps
2. **Neurological:** Root compression, amyotrophic lateral sclerosis, syringomyelia

Complex repetitive discharge

This refers to the **repetitive and synchronous firing of a group of muscle fibres**. They have amplitudes of 50 μV–1 mV, durations of 50–100 ms, and frequency of 5–100 Hz.

▋ Causes

1. Polymyositis
2. Poliomyelitis
3. Spinal muscular atrophy
4. Chronic neuropathies

Cramp potentials

During a muscle cramp, the spontaneous discharges of potential occur at 40–60 Hz, usually with abrupt onset and cessation.

▋ Causes

1. Salt depletion
2. Chronic neurogenic atrophy
3. Pregnancy
4. Also seen in healthy persons

VIVA

1. *What are the clinical uses of electromyography?* (Ans. Refer to page 223, under the heading 'Introduction'.)
2. *What is the motor unit potential (MUP)?* (Ans. Refer to page 223, under the heading 'Motor Unit Potential'.)
3. *What are the features of MUPs?* (Ans. Refer to page 223, under the heading 'Motor Unit Potential' and the subheading 'Features'.)
4. *What are the factors that affect MUPs?* (Ans. Refer to page 224, under the heading 'Factor that Affect MUP'.)
5. *What is the principle of EMG?* (Ans. Refer to page 224, under the heading 'Methods' and the subheading 'Principle'.)
6. *What are the types of needles used in EMG recording?* (Ans. Refer to page 224, under the heading 'Methods' and the subheading 'Requirements – Recording Electrodes'.)
7. *What are the precautions taken for EMG recordings?* (Ans. Refer to page 225, under the heading 'Precautions'.)
8. *What are the different types of activities recorded in an EMG?*
   (Ans. In EMG recordings, two types of activities are seen: insertional activity and spontaneous activity. Details on page 226.)
9. *What are the different types of MUPs?*
   (Ans. Abnormal MUPs are broadly classified as neurogenic and myopathic MUPs. Details in Fig. 33.4, page 225.)
10. *What are the features of short-duration MUPs? In what conditions are they seen?* (Ans. Refer to page 226, under the heading 'Motor Unit Potentials' and the subheading 'Short-duration MUPs'.)
11. *What are the features of long-duration MUPs? In what conditions are they seen?* (Ans. Refer to page 226, under the heading 'Motor Unit Potentials' and the subheading 'Long-duration MUPs'.)
12. *What are the features of polyphasic MUPs? In what conditions are they seen?* (Ans. Refer to page 226, under the heading 'Motor Unit Potentials' and the subheading 'Polyphasic MUPs'.)
13. *What are the features of mixed pattern MUPs? In what conditions are they seen?* (Ans. Refer to page 226, under the heading 'Motor Unit Potentials' and the subheading 'Mixed pattern of MUPs'.)
14. *What is doublet or multiplet MUPs? In what condition is it seen?* (Ans. Refer to page 226, the heading 'Motor Unit Potentials' and the subheading 'Doublet or multiplet MUPs'.)
15. *What is insertional activity? What are the conditions in which insertional activities increase and decrease?* (Ans. Refer to page 226, under the heading 'Insertional Activity'.)
16. *What is spontaneous activity? What are the different types of spontaneous activity?* (Ans. Refer to page 226, under the heading 'Spontaneous Activity'.)
17. *What are the features and causes of fibrillation?* (Ans. Refer to page 226, under the heading 'Fibrillation'.)
18. *What are the features and causes of fasciculation?* (Ans. Refer to page 226, under the heading 'Fasciculation'.)
19. *What are the features and causes of complex repetitive discharge?* (Ans. Refer to page 227, under the heading 'Complex Repetitive Discharge'.)
20. *What is cramp potential? In what conditions is it seen?* (Ans. Refer to page 227, under the heading 'Cramp Potentials'.)

34 Mosso's Ergography, Study of Fatigue, and Use of Handgrip Dynamometer

Learning Objectives

After completing this practical, you will be able to (MUST KNOW):
1. State the importance of performing this practical in human physiology.
2. Define ergography.
3. Perform Mosso's ergography and use the handgrip dynamometer to study the hand–muscle performance and the phenomenon of fatigue.
4. List the precautions of performing ergography.
5. Calculate the work done.

6. List the factors that affect fatigue and work done.
7. Name the sites of fatigue in human beings.
8. Calculate mechanical efficiency

You may also be able to (DESIRABLE TO KNOW):
1. Explain the factors that affect the performance.
2. Explain the effect of venous and arterial occlusion and motivation on work done.
3. Explain the sites of fatigue in humans.

PY3.14: Perform ergography.

MOSSO'S ERGOGRAPHY AND STUDY OF FATIGUE

INTRODUCTION

Ergography is the recording of an ergogram. It was first described by **Angelo Mosso** in 1890; therefore, it is also called Mosso's ergography. An **ergogram** is a recording of the voluntary contractions of the skeletal muscles of a human being on a moving kymograph. **Erg** is a unit of energy equal to 10^{-7} joules, derived from '*ergon*', a Greek word meaning 'work'. **Ergograph** is the machine used for recording voluntary muscle contractions.

Mosso's ergography is performed to assess the performance (the ability to work) of the flexors of the fingers of the hand. It is also used to study the phenomenon of fatigue in human skeletal muscles.

Muscle fatigue is defined as the process in which muscle function diminishes with use to the point that it can no longer perform its expected function with the same level or intensity as when rested (exhaustion).

Factors That Affect Performance

1. **Age:** Young adults can perform better than children and elderly individuals.
2. **Gender:** Men can perform voluntary contractions better than women.

3. **Height:** Taller people usually perform better than those who are short.
4. **Physical build:** Persons with sound physical build can perform better than the obese or very thin.
5. **Training:** A physically trained individual can always perform better than untrained people.
6. **Race:** Europeans and Caucasians perform better than Asians.
7. **Motivation:** Encouragement and motivation stimulate the reward system in the brain and improve performance.
8. **Environmental factors:** Environmental temperature and humidity greatly influence performance.

Factors That Affect Fatigue

1. The degree of work
2. The duration of work

In Mosso's ergography, fatigue is affected by:
1. **The weight to be lifted:** When the weight to be lifted increases, fatigue occurs early.
2. **The frequency of contractions:** Fatigue occurs early when the frequency of contractions increases.
3. **Motivation:** Encouragement delays fatigue.
4. **Blood supply to the exercising muscle:** Venous and arterial occlusion accelerate fatigue.

The following **factors cause muscle fatigue**:
- Depletion of nutrients (oxygen, creatine phosphate, ATP)
- Depletion of neurotransmitters
- Accumulation of metabolites

METHOD OF ERGOGRAPHY

Principle

Using Mosso's ergogram, the subject contracts the flexors of his fingers against resistance until the fingers are fatigued. The work done is calculated to study the effect of various factors on the performance.

Requirements

1. **Mosso's ergograph** (Fig. 34.1): This is the apparatus (in the laboratory setting) used to record an ergogram. In Mosso's ergograph, the fingers and forearm can be fixed in the appropriate holders. A cord passing over a pulley and carrying a load of 3 kg at one end is attached to a sliding plate. This sliding plate is connected through a sling to the finger, the flexors of which are being studied. The metal plates also carry a writing lever which makes markings on a slow-moving drum. When the middle finger is flexed, the load is lifted, the distance through which the load is lifted is marked by the writing lever on the drum.
2. **Metronome**: This instrument (Fig. 34.2) is used in experiments requiring an interrupter adjusted from 40 to 200 contacts/min. The frequency of interruption is adjusted by sliding the clip on a sideways-movable metal plate in front of a graduated scale. The position of the clip on the scale gives the frequency at which the sound is delivered.
3. Electrical kymograph
4. Sphygmomanometer
5. A set of 500 g weights

Procedure

1. Provide proper instructions to the subject.
2. Insert the subject's index and ring fingers into the fixed-tube holders, leaving the middle finger to pull the load (Fig. 34.3A and B).
3. Set the metronome to oscillate once in two seconds.
4. Connect the sling to the middle finger.
5. Ask the subject to lift the load using maximal contractions of the flexors of the middle finger and to repeat the movement every two seconds, in sync with the metronome oscillations.
6. Ask the subject to continue (lifting the load) until they can no longer do so.

Note: The record of the contractions obtained in the drum is called an ergogram.

7. Allow the subject to rest for 15 minutes.
8. After rest, ask her to repeat the procedure until the load can no longer be lifted.
9. When the subject can no longer lift the weight, encourage her (to study the effect of encouragement) to keep trying, and record the ergogram.
10. Allow the subject to rest for 15 minutes. Then, obtain the ergogram after venous occlusion.

Note: Venous occlusion is obtained by tying a BP cuff around the subject's arm and raising and maintaining the pressure at 40 mmHg. This occludes the veins in the arms.

11. Allow the subject to rest for 15 minutes. Then, obtain the ergogram after arterial occlusion.

Note: Arterial occlusion is obtained by raising the pressure to 200 mmHg and keeping the BP cuff inflated till the experiment is over. This occludes veins as well as arteries.

12. Study the ergogram of each condition and calculate the work done (as described below) for each.

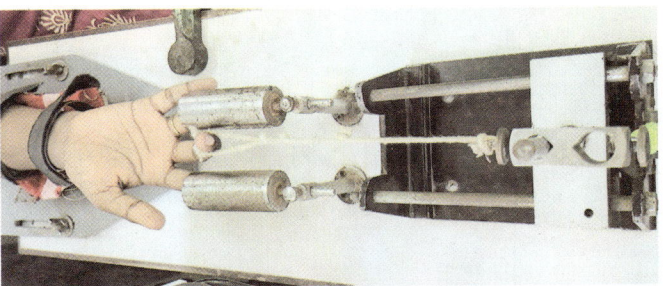

Fig. 34.1 Mosso's ergograph. Note the arrangement of the arm fixing clamp and finger-holder.

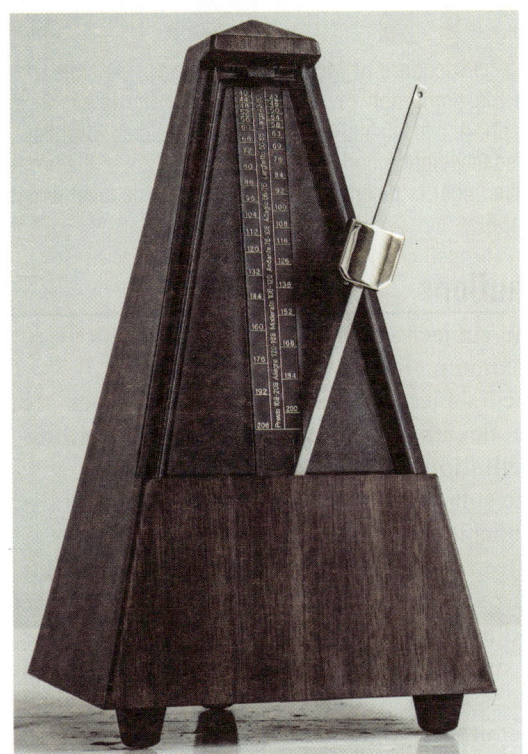

Fig. 34.2 Color photograph of a vintage metronome against a gray background. (*Courtesy*: Shutterstock/Konstantin Kolosov.)

A)

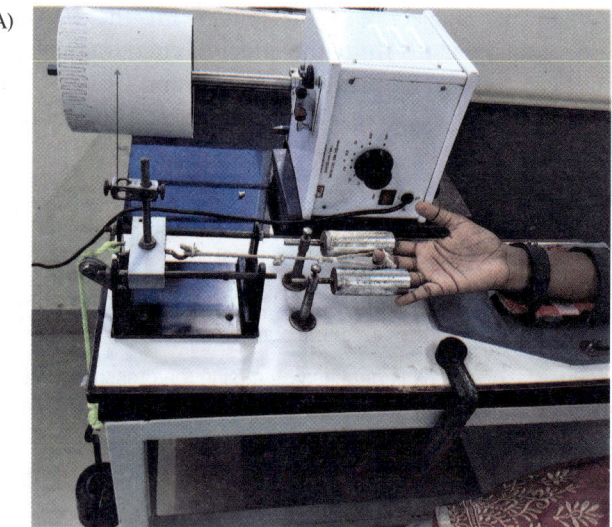

B)

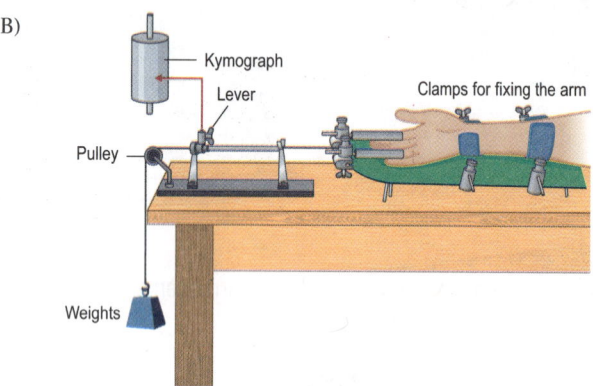

Kymograph

Lever

Clamps for fixing the arm

Pulley

Weights

Fig. 34.3   Procedure of Mosso's ergography. (A) Note the various parts of the ergograph (1. Writing point of the lever; 2. drum; 3. kymograph; 4. arm-fixing clamp; 5. finger holder; 6. pulley; 7. cord connected to weights) and (B) schematic diagram of the procedure—the middle finger is pulling the weights, while the level writes on the kymograph.

Precautions

1. The subject should be instructed properly to put in maximum effort.
2. The subject should move the finger (contract the flexors of the middle finger) according to the **oscillations of the metronome**.
3. The subject should continue to do the work until she is unable to lift the load.
4. Fifteen minutes of rest should be provided between all the procedures (**encouragement, venous occlusion, and arterial occlusion**).
5. To study the **effect of encouragement and motivation**, the subject should be properly and adequately encouraged to do her best.
6. To **obtain venous occlusion**, the BP cuff pressure should be *raised to 40 mmHg* and maintained at the same pressure till the subject is fatigued.

7. To **obtain arterial occlusion**, the BP cuff pressure should be *raised to 200 mmHg* and maintained at the same pressure till the subject is fatigued.

Calculation

Calculate the work done for each ergogram using the following formula:

$$W = F \times S.$$

Where W is the work done (in kg–m), F is the load (in kg), and S is the total distance (in metres) through which the load is lifted. S is the sum of all the vertical amplitudes in each ergogram, i.e., the total length of all vertical lines.

Observation and Results

Study the **amplitude of contractions** and the **time of onset of fatigue**.

1. Calculate the work done for all the four settings (normal, encouragement, venous occlusion, arterial occlusion).
2. Note that the work done improves with encouragement and decreases with venous and arterial occlusion (Fig. 34.4).
3. Motivation and encouragement increase the amplitude of contractions and delay the onset of fatigue.
4. Venous occlusion decreases the amplitude of contractions and shortens the onset of fatigue.
5. Arterial occlusion further decreases the amplitude of contractions and brings on early onset of fatigue.

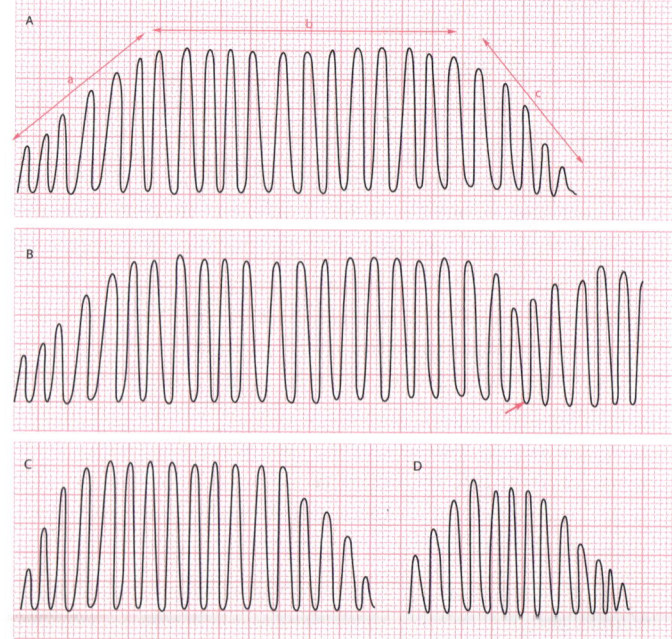

Fig. 34.4   (A) Normal ergogram (**a.** rising phase; **b.** plateau phase; c. falling phase); **(B)** effect of encouragement (arrows indicate the starting of encouragement prior to which is the normal recording); **(C)** effect of venous occlusion; and **(D)** effect of arterial occlusion.

DISCUSSION

Mosso's ergography is performed to study the work done by the flexors of the fingers and to study the phenomenon of fatigue in human skeletal muscles.

Encouragement

Encouragement and motivation improve the subject's performance. The exact mechanism of motivation increasing the performance is not known. The **prefrontal cortex** is part of the reward system in the brain, which on stimulation, increases bar pressing among experimental animals. It is possible that, in human beings too, encouragement stimulates the **frontal lobe** of the cortex, which increases the activity in the motor cortex. This, in turn, stimulates the flexor muscles by increasing the activity in the corresponding motor neurons.

Venous Occlusion

Venous occlusion decreases the work done due to the **accumulation of metabolites** in the muscle. Metabolites like lactic acid are removed from the tissue by the veins. Accumulation of metabolites decreases muscle performance.

Arterial Occlusion

Arterial occlusion decreases the work done maximally because it **prevents the supply of nutrients** to the muscle. Nutrients, especially oxygen, are essential for metabolic oxidation in the tissues to provide energy (ATP). Therefore, intact blood supply to the muscle is a minimum requirement for its functioning. The sphygmomanometer pressure that occludes the artery also occludes the veins. Therefore, arterial occlusion is accompanied by venous occlusion and consequently, the work done decreases maximally.

Sites of Fatigue in Human Beings

In human beings, **fatigue is mostly a central phenomenon** as it is observed in the present study that encouragement enhances performance and prolongs onset of complete fatigue. Though motivation prolongs or delays fatigue, the **site of fatigue could be the muscle** followed by **neuromuscular junction**, as rest helps in recovery and continuation of the work. The nerve is theoretically unfatiguable.

Merton's experiment: The original experiments performed by **P A Merton** (1954) on in-situ human muscle showed an important underlying cause of **decline in force (fatigue) is indeed within the muscle**, namely the **accumulation of metabolic products** of activity.

USE OF HANDGRIP DYNAMOMETER

INTRODUCTION

The handgrip dynamometer is used for exercising the upper limb muscles, especially of the hand and forearm.

METHOD OF USING THE HANDGRIP DYNAMOMETER

Requirement

Handgrip dynamometer: This device uses a spring to measure the maximum isometric contractions of hand and forearm muscles. It has a handle and a graduated pressure scale on a circular metal plate (Fig. 34.5). The results are read manually from the scale.

Procedure

1. Explain the procedure and the use of the instrument to the subject. Ask the subject to sit comfortably with his arms at his sides and elbows slightly bent.

> **Note:** The dominant hand should be used for the exercise to get the best grip of the device.

2. Ask the subject to squeeze the spring and note the tension developed (Fig. 34.6).
3. Instruct the subject to make two more attempts with an interval of about a minute between the trials to avoid fatigue. Calculate the average of these readings. This is called T_{max} (**maximal isometric tension**).

> **Note:** The scale needs to be reset to zero after each test.

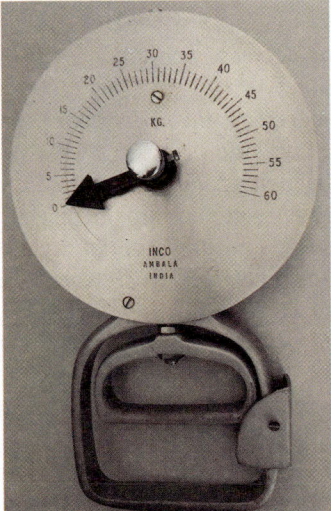 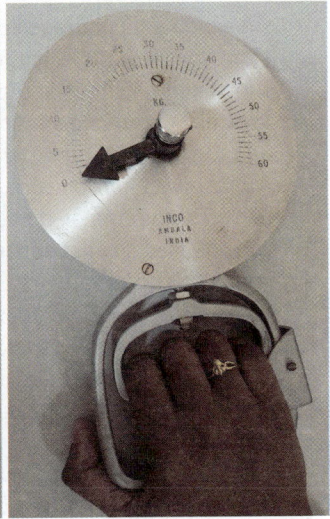

Fig. 34.5 Handgrip dynamometer (spring type).

Fig. 34.6 Procedure of testing muscle strength (work done) using a handgrip dynamometer.

4. **Determine the endurance time** for 60–80% of T_{max}. This is the time of the onset of fatigue after starting the exercise on the dynamometer.

5. After resting for 2–3 minutes, measure the endurance time for 60–80% of T_{max}, first after **occlusion of the veins** and then **after occlusion of the arteries** with a BP cuff on the upper arm.

Observation and results

Note the T_{max} values for each maneuver. The T_{max} varies widely between 30 and 50 kg. It depends on many factors such as sex, age, muscle strength, hand dominance, and level of training.

DISCUSSION

Factors Affecting T_{max}

T_{max} depends on age, gender, muscle strength, hand dominance, time of the day, nutrition, and sensitivity to fatigue and pain. There may be a slight difference in values between the two hands.

Venous and Arterial Occlusion

Venous occlusion reduces the performance due to accumulation of metabolites and arterial occlusion considerably decreases work done and facilitates early onset of fatigue due to decreased nutrition supply to muscle.

Encouragement

Encouragement and motivation enhance the performance.

Calculation of Work Done and of Mechanical Efficiency

Calculation of work done and calculation of mechanical efficiency have been described in Chapter 25, under the headings 'Energy Cost of Work' and 'Bicycle Ergometry'.

VIVA

1. *What is the use of Mosso's ergography in physiology? Who invented this procedure and in what year?* (Ans. Refer to page 228, under the heading 'Introduction'.)

2. *What do you mean by erg, ergon, ergogram and ergography?* (Ans. Refer to page 228, under the heading 'Introduction'.)

3. *What are the precautions taken for Mosso's ergography?* (Ans. Refer to page 229, under the heading 'Precautions'.)

4. *What are the factors that affect performance (the work done)?* (Ans. Refer to page 228, under the heading 'Factors that Affect Performance'.)

5. *Define muscle fatigue.* (Ans. Refer to page 228, under the heading 'Introduction' and subheading 'Fatigue'.)

6. *What are the factors that affect fatigue?* (Ans. Refer to page 228, under the heading 'Factors that Affect Fatigue'.)

7. *What are the factors that delay and facilitate fatigue?* (Ans. Refer to page 228, under the heading 'Factors that Affect Fatigue'.)

8. *How does encouragement improve physical performance?* (Ans. Refer to page 231, under the heading 'Discussion' and the subheading 'Encouragement'.)

9. *Why does venous occlusion decrease performance?* (Ans. Refer to page 231, under the heading 'Discussion' and the subheading 'Venous occlusion'.)

10. *Why does arterial occlusion decrease the performance maximally?* (Ans. Refer to page 231, under the heading 'Discussion' and the subheading 'Arterial occlusion'.)

11. *Name one condition each in human beings where venous or arterial occlusion can impair muscular performance.*
(Ans. Thrombosis of the leg veins due to **thrombophlebitis** is an example of venous occlusion, wherein the venous return is decreased so that fatigue sets in early. Arterial occlusion occurs in **Buerger's disease**, which is usually seen in chronic smokers; these patients experience pain while walking because the narrowed vessels cannot keep pace with increased demands of muscles for oxygen.)

12. *What is the primary site of fatigue in human beings?* (Ans. Refer to page 231, under the heading 'Discussion' and the subheading 'Site of fatigue'.)

13. *How can you determine the primary site of fatigue in an intact muscle?* (Ans. Refer to page 231, under the subheading 'Site of fatigue' and the write-up on 'Merton's experiment'.)

14. *How does fatigue in this experiment compare with fatigue in frog's nerve-muscle preparation?*
(Ans. In frog's nerve-muscle preparation, there is no blood supply. Therefore, fatigue sets in early. The seat of the fatigue is the neuromuscular junction. In Mosso's ergography, the seat of fatigue appears to be a central phenomenon, though muscle could also be the site of fatigue.)

15. *What are the neurotransmitters that delay fatigue and promote fatigue?*
(Ans. Several neurotransmitters play a role in either delaying or promoting fatigue, primarily by influencing alertness, motivation, and endurance. Neurotransmitters that delay fatigue are mainly **dopamine and norepinephrine**. Neurotransmitters that promote fatigue are mainly **adenosine, serotonin, and low serotonin to dopamine ratio**.)

35 | Visual and Auditory Reaction Times

Learning Objectives

After completing this practical, you will be able to (MUST KNOW):

1. Define reaction time, visual reaction time, and auditory reaction time.
2. Determine the reaction time to visual and auditory stimuli.
3. List the factors affecting visual reaction time and auditory reaction time.
4. Understand the physiological importance of learning visual reaction time and auditory reaction time.

INTRODUCTION

Reaction time (RT) is a measure of the **quickness with which an individual responds to a stimulus**. RT plays an important role in our daily lives as it has several practical implications.

Definition and Concept

RT is defined as the **interval of time between the presentation of the stimulus and appearance of appropriate voluntary response** in the subject. A T Welford described **three types of RT**:

1. **Simple RT**: There is one stimulus and one response.
2. **Recognition RT:** In this type of RT, there are multiple stimuli. The subject should respond to some stimuli and not respond to others.
3. **Choice RT:** There are multiple stimuli and multiple responses.

Human RT is determined by a complex nervous system that **recognises various stimuli**. Neurons relay the *message of sensory stimulation to the brain;* this message travels *from the brain to the spinal cord* and then reaches the person's hands and fingers. The motor neurons then instruct the hands and fingers to react in a particular way. The accepted values for mean simple RTs in healthy adults are about 190 ms for light stimuli (**visual RT**) and about 160 ms for sound stimuli (**auditory RT**).

Factors Affecting RT

RT in response to a situation can significantly influence our lives due its practical implications. Fast RTs can produce rewards (e.g., in sports), whereas slow RT can produce grave consequences (e.g., driving and road safety issues).

Factors that can affect RT include age, gender, hand dominance (left or right), vision (central vs. peripheral), level of practice, fatigue, fasting, breathing cycle, personality type, exercise, and intelligence.

METHODS OF DETERMINING REACTION TIMES

Manual Method

Principle

Reaction time is the time interval between the application of an adequate stimulus and the voluntary motor response to it. It varies with the complexity of the reflex and interrelated sensory pathways associated with the course of the impulse as it travels to the centre.

Requirements

1. Two tapping keys (K1, K2)
2. Signal marker
3. Short-circuiting key
4. Bulb
5. Low-voltage current (6V DC mains)
6. Kymograph with drum

Procedure

▌**Visual reaction time (VRT)**

1. Set up a **circuit with two tapping keys** (termed as K1 and K2), an **electromagnetic signal maker,** and **a bulb** connected in series to the **6V DC mains current source**.
2. Connect the kymograph to record the movement of the signal marker.
3. Instruct the subject to press the tapping key K1.

Note: The subject should be given some training to be alert and to release the key the moment the bulb is lit up.

4. Without making a sound, gently **press the K2 key to light up the bulb**.

> **Note:** This event is marked on the drum with the signal marker as **Event 1 (E1)**. The **subject, as instructed, releases K2**, which is marked on the drum as **Event 2**.

5. Record a time tracing below the event recordings by using a tuning fork of 100 Hz and **calculate VRT from the time interval between E1 and E2**.

Auditory reaction time (ART)

1. Remove the bulb from the circuit.
2. Instruct the subject to press the tapping key K1.
3. Press the **tapping key K2 to produce the sound**—this is marked as **Event 1 (E1)**.
4. Instruct the subject to release the K2 key as soon as he hears the sound—this is marked on the drum as **Event 2 (E2)**.

> **Note:** The subject should be alert and release the key the moment he hears the tapping sound.

5. Calculate ART from the **time interval between E1 and E2**.

Precautions

1. The subject should not face the examiner.

> **Note:** The subject should respond to the visual and auditory stimuli and not to the movement of the examiner's hand.

2. The subject should remain alert throughout the procedure.
3. The examiner's key should be released without making any noise for VRT.

Normal values

Visual reaction time: 200–400 ms
Auditory reaction time: 100–200 ms

> **Note:** Normally, **VRT is more than ART** because visual responses involve chemical mechanisms for information processing, chiefly for the conversion from a photon to a bioelectric stimulus, which takes a lot longer than the conversion from a pressure wave to bioelectric stimuli.

Determination of RT Using Software

Reaction time testing is also done using Inquisit 4.0 software released in 2013 by Millisecond Software in Seattle, Washington.

During the **visual RT (VRT) task**, in the centre of a white screen, the participant is presented with a black fixation cross that is followed after variable time intervals by a target stimulus—a red circle.

• The subject is asked to concentrate on the fixation cross and press the 'space bar' key as quickly as possible once the red circle (target stimulus) appears on the screen.

In a simple **auditory RT (ART) task**, after variable time intervals, the sound is played for the participant for 30 seconds through speakers.

• The task is to press the space bar as soon as the sound is presented.
• The subject is thoroughly acquainted with the procedure, and practice trials need to be given before taking the test.

By default, the time intervals are randomly chosen from 2000 ms, 3000 ms, 4000 ms, 5000 ms, 6000 ms, 7000 ms, and 8000 ms. For each stimulus, five readings are taken, and the respective *fastest RT for each stimulus is recorded*. The readings are taken during a fixed time and in a quiet, secluded room.

Using A Digital Audio-Visual Reaction Timer

Requirements

A–V reaction timer: In this system, there are *two sides*, one is the *operator's side* and the other is the *trainer's side*.

There are **three switches and three lights on both sides**. The switches on the operator's side are responsible for lighting up the lights, while the switches on the trainer's side turn off the lights (Fig. 35.1).

The **main features** of the reaction timer are: i) modes of operation for both light and sound, ii) functions for light and sound, iii) LCD display for recording the reaction time, iv) soft-touch switches, iv) different colours and larger LED screen, and v) audible beeps for the sound operation.

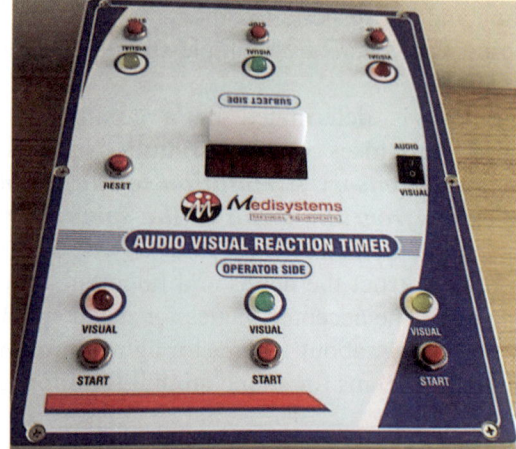

Fig. 35.1 Audio-visual reaction timer. Note the arrangements on the operator's side and the trainer's side.

Procedure

1. **Switch on any light quite suddenly** and ask the trainer to react to the action by **turning off the light immediately** from his side. The time taken by the

trainer is called *reaction time* and is noted on the timer.

2. Similarly, in the second mode, there are **three different melodies/tones**. The operator plays one of these sounds, and the trainer is asked to turn it off immediately and as soon as he can.

3. Thus, the operator can operate anyfunction—light or sound—and the trainer is to react very fast to turn the same off.

4. Note the reaction time displayed on the LED screen.

Observation and results

1. The minimum time taken by the trainer to react is said to be the **reaction time.**

2. Note the reaction time for visual stimuli

3. Note the reaction time for auditory stimuli.

DISCUSSION

Physiological Significance

Since reaction time is defined as the interval of time between the presentation of the stimulus and the appearance of the appropriate voluntary response in a subject, a number of **external environmental stimuli** of different modalities influence it. There are various sensory modalities, and the human body responds to various stimuli at different speeds. This plays an important role in routine activities as well as in an emergency. For example, while driving a vehicle, it is necessary to apply the brakes as quickly as possible when required. Reaction time becomes an important component of information processing, as it indexes speed of stimulus processing and response programming.

Components of RT

Reaction time mainly has **two components:**

1. **Mental processing time:** It is the time required by the responder to *perceive, identify, and analyse* a stimulus, and *decide* the proper motor response.

2. **Movement time:** It is the time required to *perform a movement* after deciding how to respond.

In simple reaction time, there is one stimulus and one response. **In recognition reaction time**, there are some stimuli that should be responded to and others that should not get a response. **In choice reaction time**, there are multiple stimuli and multiple responses.

1. In **simple reaction time**, the stimulus and the response are one. Therefore, to complete a task, only the identification of the stimulus and its proper response are required.

2. In **choice reaction time**, there are multiple stimuli and appropriate responses; after the identification of the stimulus among the many stimuli, one response out of the many responses has to be verified.

   • In choice reaction time, the task involves more mental processes, requiring more time.

   • The **choice auditory reaction, the time taken is more** than that the simple auditory reaction time.

Note: Choice reaction time is generally longer than simple reaction time due to the increased mental workload. Thus, the **choice auditory reaction time would be more** than simple auditory reaction time.

Alterations in RT

The reaction time can be **decreased with practice and training**. It can also be decreased by increasing **alertness and concentration**. The reaction time becomes **prolonged** with advancing age, fatigue, distractions, and muscular weakness.

VIVA

1. *Define reaction time, visual reaction time, and auditory reaction time.* (Ans. Refer to page 233, under the heading 'Introduction'.)

2. *What are the types of RT?* (Ans. Refer to page 233, under the heading 'Definition and Concept'.)

3. *What are the normal values of visual reaction time and auditory reaction time?* (Ans. Refer to page 234, under the heading 'Normal Values'.)

4. *Explain why ART is less than VRT.* (Ans. Refer to page 235, under the heading 'Discussion'.)

5. *What are the components of RT?* (Ans. Refer to page 235, under the heading 'Discussion' and the subheading 'Components of RT'.)

6. *List the factors affecting visual reaction time and auditory reaction time.* (Ans. Refer to page 233, under the heading 'Factors Affecting RT'.)

7. *Explain the application of visual reaction time and auditory reaction time in daily life.* (Ans. Refer to page 235, under the heading 'Discussion'.)

8. *In which conditions RT is decreased or prolonged?* (Ans. Refer to page 235, under the heading 'Discussion' and the subheading 'Alteration in RT'.)

36 | Electroencephalogram

Learning Objectives

After completing this practical, you will be able to (MUST KNOW):
1. Define EEG.
2. Name EEG waves and rhythms.
3. Understand the basic principle of EEG recordings.
4. List the uses of EEG.
5. Appreciate the clinical applications of EEG in common epilepsies and other neurological disorders.
6. Define brain death.
7. List the criteria for the diagnosis of brain death.

PY10.12: Identify normal EEG forms.

INTRODUCTION

Electroencephalogram (EEG) is a *record of the spontaneous electrical activities generated in the cerebral cortex,* which are picked up from the brain's surface through electrodes placed on designated sites on the scalp. These electrical activities reflect the electrical currents that flow in the extracellular spaces in the brain. The electrical currents also reflect the **summated effects of innumerable excitatory and inhibitory synaptic potentials** upon the cortical neurons. These spontaneous activities of cortical neurons are greatly influenced by the afferent inputs arising from the thalamus and brainstem reticular formation. These afferent impulses entrain the cortical neurons to produce most of the characteristic rhythmic EEG waves.

Electroencephalography is the procedure of recording EEG using a sensitive device called an **electroencephalograph**. EEG is the best diagnostic tool available for assessing the abnormalities of electrical activities of the brain. Therefore, it is very helpful in diagnosing epilepsies and for studying sleep and sleep disorders.

Specialities in EEG Recording

In 1929, **Hans Berger**, a German psychiatrist, demonstrated for the first time that the electrical activities of the human brain could be recorded using external electrodes placed on the scalp. He called this recording an electroencephalogram. As the EEG waves are of very low voltage, they require amplification before recording.
1. **EEG leads** may be bipolar (comparing the potentials between two active leads) or unipolar (measuring the potential changes at a single lead against a reference lead placed on the ear, nose, or chin).
2. EEG electrodes are solder or silver-silver chloride discs of 0.5 cm diameter.
3. The recording is done with the subject preferably in the recumbent position, with his head and neck supported to ensure that the posterior electrodes are secure.
4. Usually, four leads are attached to the scalp by means of adhesive material on standard skull locations on either side.
5. A **multi-channel pen recorder** is used to record the activities from the **eight or more leads simultaneously**.
6. The EEG waves are analysed manually or using a computer.

EEG Waves

EEG waves are described in terms of their frequency, which usually ranges from 1 to 30 Hz, and amplitude, which ranges from **20 to 100 μV**. The characteristics of EEG waves vary according to the state of consciousness.
1. When the **individual is fully alert** (sensory inputs are maximum), the waves are generally of **high frequency and low amplitude** with as many units **asynchronized**.
2. When the person is **minimally alert**, as in deep sleep (least sensory input), the waves are of **low frequency and high amplitude** and **synchronized**.
3. Absence of EEG waves indicates brain death.

EEG Wave Patterns and Rhythms

EEG **wave patterns** are classified into **four types**: α, β, θ, and δ according to their frequency. The characteristic features of the various EEG rhythms are presented below.

Alpha rhythm

This is also called the **Berger rhythm**. Frequency ranges from **8–13 Hz** and amplitude from **50–100 μV** (Fig. 36.1).
1. This is the most prominent EEG rhythm seen in a **normal adult at rest** (awake but relaxed) with his eyes closed.
2. It is found in the posterior half of the brain, especially in **the parieto-occipital regions**.
3. A normal alpha rhythm is **synchronized** (synchronous and symmetric) over the cerebral hemispheres, which is seen during quiet alertness with eyes closed.

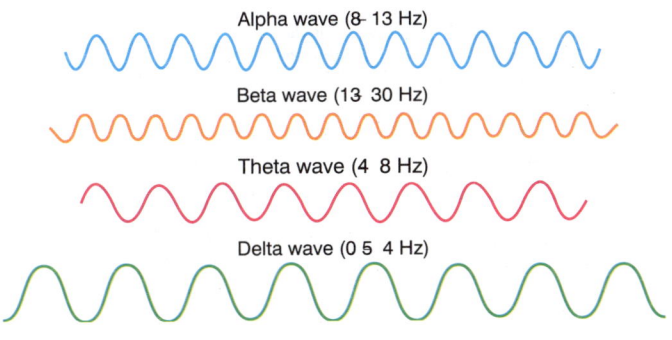

Alpha wave (8–13 Hz)

Beta wave (13–30 Hz)

Theta wave (4–8 Hz)

Delta wave (0.5–4 Hz)

Fig. 36.1 EEG waves.

Alpha block

The alpha rhythm **disappears once the subject opens his eyes** and engages in mental effort such as mental arithmetic. The regular alpha rhythm is replaced by irregular low-voltage activity. This phenomenon is known as alpha block or **desynchronization**. It is also called arousal or **alerting response**.

Factors affecting α wave frequency

The frequency of alpha rhythm is **decreased** by hypoglycemia, hypothermia, high arterial pressure, and low levels of glucocorticoids. High blood glucose, increased body temperature, low arterial pressure, and high levels of glucocorticoids increase the frequency of alpha rhythm.

Beta rhythm

The normal frequency of beta waves ranges from **13 to 30 Hz** with low amplitude, ranging from **5–10 μV**.
1. This type of rhythm is seen in adults when their **eyes are open**.
2. These waves appear in the **posterior regions of the brain**. However, beta rhythms are sometimes seen in the frontal regions regardless of whether the eyes are closed or open.

Theta rhythm

The normal frequency of theta waves ranges from **4 to 8 Hz** with high amplitude.
1. Theta rhythm is usually **seen in normal children**.
2. It also occurs **during moderate sleep**.
3. It may sometimes appear in adults when they are severely disappointed or depressed.

Delta rhythm

The frequency of delta waves ranges from **0.5 to 4 Hz** and amplitude from **20 to 200 μV**.
1. Delta rhythm occurs normally **during deep sleep**.
2. Its appearance in an alert state in an adult suggests serious organic brain damage.

EEG Rhythms in Infants and Children

The EEG recordings in children show a wide range of patterns.
1. In awake infants, the EEG typically shows a fast **beta rhythm**.
2. The rhythm speeds up during childhood, and a **theta rhythm** appears.
3. As the child matures, the **theta rhythm** is replaced by the **faster alpha rhythms**.
4. The **alpha rhythm of adults** gradually appears **during adolescence**.
5. The theta rhythm is prominent in the temporal or parietal region, while alpha rhythms are in the occipital region.

METHOD TO RECORD AN EEG

Principle

EEG reflects spontaneous brain electrical activities recorded from the surface of the scalp. It measures changes in electric potential caused by a large number of electric dipoles generated in the neural network—**either excitatory (EPSP) or inhibitory (IPSP) potentials**. When these potentials get summed up spatially or temporally, they become strong enough to be picked up by the electrodes placed on the surface (of the scalp) by the principle of volume conduction. The signals picked up by special bioelectric sensors are of very low amplitude; they have to be amplified and then converted into a set of numeric values (analog to digital conversion), which accurately represent the original bioelectric signal. The converted signal can then be displayed in the form of traces, stored on magnetic disks, printed, or processed in several ways.

Requirements

A **computerised EEG System with video monitoring** is ideal for quality EEG recording and analysis. The Galileo video-assisted EEG system (Fig. 36.2) is one such system. The hardware used is BE Light (EB Neuro) and the **software** used for acquisition is Galileo Suite (EB Neuro). A schematic diagram of the hardware is presented in Fig. 36.3.

Procedure

Preparation of the subject

The electrodes (gold/silver) are applied to the scalp surface with the help of **conductive paste** (Ten20 paste), and are held in place by adhesives, suction, or pressure from caps or headbands. To maintain a constant relationship between the location of the electrode and the underlying cerebral structures, a **system of electrode placement** is necessary. Although other systems like Gibbsian, Michigan, and Houston have been used successfully, the majority of EEG labs throughout the world utilise the **10–20 International System of Electrode Placement**.

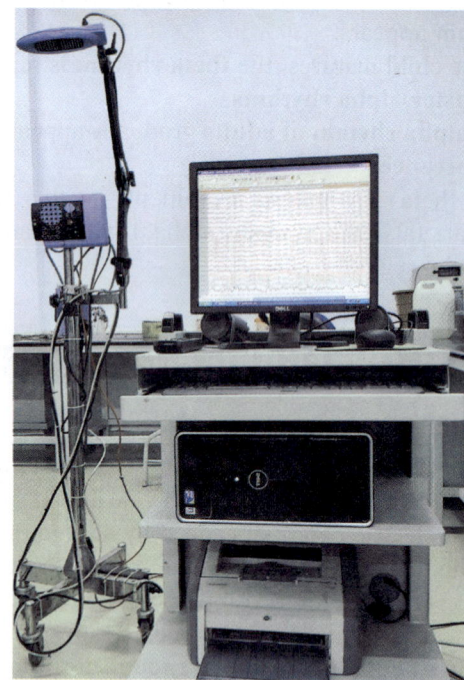

Fig. 36.2 EEG machine with all its accessories. (*Courtesy*: Neurophysiology Lab, Physiology Department, JIPMER, Puducherry, India.)

Standard electrode placement uses **21 electrodes** as prescribed by the 10–20 International Federation of Societies for EEG and Clinical Neurophysiology in 1958. This system is based on percentages of the total head size; the anatomical landmarks for measurement are the nasion, the inion, **the left and right pre-auricular points** (tragus).

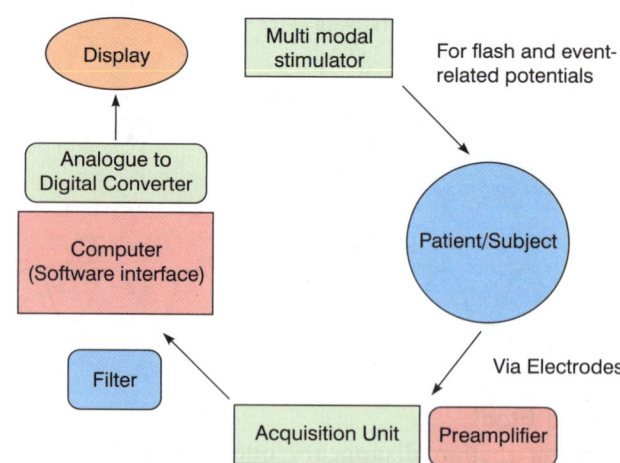

Fig. 36.3   Schematic diagram of an EEG hardware unit.

Position of the electrodes

Electrodes are placed based on anatomical landmarks of the scalp:

1. The electrode placement should be symmetrical in the sagittal plane and more strictly on the landmarks.
2. Electrodes should be spaced equally along the anteroposterior and transverse axes of the head.
3. The designation of the position of electrodes should be in terms of brain area, e.g., frontal, parietal, temporal, occipital, etc.

Electrode nomenclature

F – Electrode over frontal lobe
T – Electrode over temporal lobe
C – Electrode over central area
Fp – Electrode over frontopolar
O – Electrode over the occipital lobe
P – Electrode over the parietal lobe
Z – Midline electrodes

Odd numbers refer to electrodes over the left hemisphere, while even numbers refer to electrodes over the right hemisphere (Fig. 36.4).

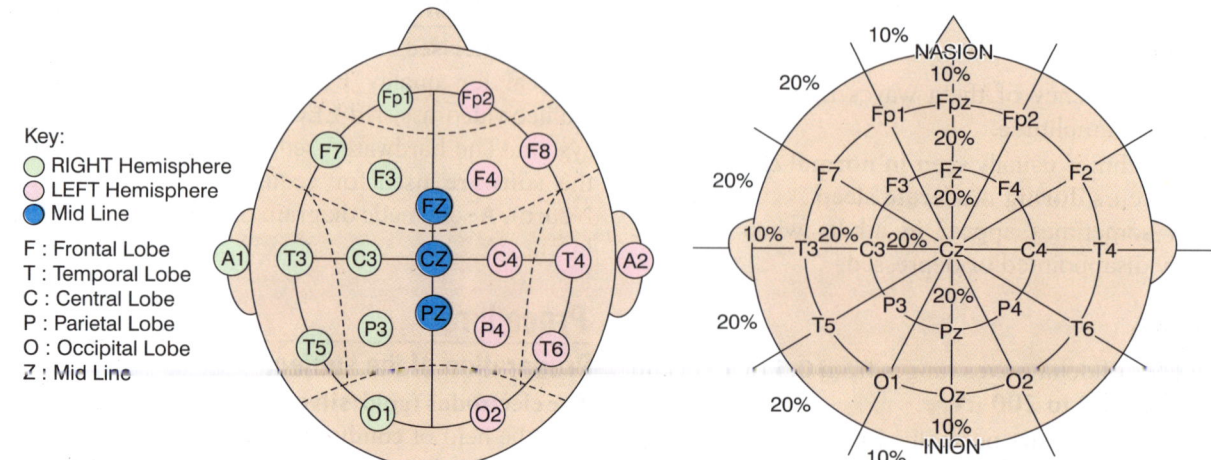

Fig. 36.4   International 10–20 system of electrode placement.

International 10–20 system of measurement

1. Measure the distance from the nasion to inion on the sagittal line. Mark 50% (of the nasion–inion distance) perpendicular to the tape: **Cz**.
2. Measure and mark 10% up from the nasion on the sagittal line: **Fpz**; 10% up from inion: **Oz**.
3. Measure and mark 20% from Fpz towards **Cz** on the sagittal line: **Fz**; 20% anteriorly on the sagittal line from **Oz** towards **Cz** on the sagittal line: **Pz**.
4. Measure the distance from the left and right pre-auricular points (tragus) on the coronal line: (A1 and A2).
5. Measure and mark 50% (of the inter-tragal line) perpendicular to the tape: **Cz**.
6. Measure and mark 10% up from the pre-auricular point: **T3** on the left and **T4** on the right.
7. Measure the head circumference connecting the 4 points: **Fpz** anteriorly, **T4** on the right, **Oz** posteriorly, and **T3** on the left).
8. Measure 5% of the head circumference on either side of **Fpz**: **Fp1** on the left and **Fp2** on the right.
9. Measure 5% of the head circumference on either side of **Oz**: **O1** on the left and **O2** on the right.
10. Measure 10% of the head circumference on either side of **T3**: **F7** anteriorly and **T5** posteriorly on the left side.
11. Measure 10% of the head circumference on either side of **T4**: **F8** anteriorly and **T6** posteriorly on the right side.
12. On the coronal line between **T3** and **Cz** (20% of the inter-tragal line): **C3** on the left side and **C4** in between **Cz** and **T4** on the right side.

EEG software

The acquisition unit transmits data to the software—Galileo NT in this case. The acquired data are sampled and displayed as a digital polygraph in the window of the system, which can be customised according to the investigator's requirements.

Important terminology in EEG recording

Sensitivity: It is defined as the *ratio of input voltage to pen deflection*. It is expressed in microvolts per millimetre (μV/mm). A commonly used sensitivity is **7 μV/mm**, which, for a calibration signal of 50 μV, results in a deflection of 7.1 mm. Sensitivity of the EEG equipment for routine recording should be set in the **range of 5–10 μV/mm** of pen deflection.

Filters: These selectively restrict the frequency domain of a signal.

1. **High-pass filters** allow a high-frequency input to pass through while eliminating the rapidly changing low frequencies (low-frequency filters) and are set at 0.5 Hz.
2. **Low-pass filters** allow low frequencies to pass through while eliminating the rapidly changing high frequencies (high-frequency filters) and are set at 70 Hz.

Filtering can be done electronically by resistors, capacitors, and amplifiers and digitally by mathematical algorithms.

Notch filter: The 50 Hz (notch) filter can prevent the distortion or attenuation of signals by electrical line noise; it should therefore only be used when other measures against 50 Hz interference fail.

Epoch: A digital display of 10 seconds/page should be utilised for routine recordings.

Montage: The representation of the EEG channels is referred to as a montage (Fig. 36.5).

1. **Bipolar montage:** Each channel represents the difference between two adjacent electrodes. The entire montage consists of a series of these channels.
2. **Referential montage:** Each channel represents the difference between a certain electrode and a designated reference electrode (normally the ear/vertex reference electrode; A1 on the left side and A2 on the right side).
3. **Average reference montage:** The outputs of all the amplifiers are summed and averaged, and this averaged signal is used as the common reference for each channel.
4. **Laplacian montage:** Each channel represents the difference between an electrode and a weighted average of the surrounding electrodes.

Instructions to Subject (or Patient)

1. Ask the subject to come to the test after a hair wash with an oil-free scalp (to avoid a sticky scalp).
2. For activating procedures, give proper instruction; for example, sleep deprivation at night (only 3–4 hours of sleep are advisable).
3. Advise the subject to avoid caffeinated drinks before the procedure.
4. Discuss with the clinician about withholding drugs before the procedure, especially sedatives, antidepressants, antipsychotics, and antiepileptics. Instruct the subject accordingly.

Procedure

1. Instruct the subject to lie down comfortably on the couch and relax. It is advisable to have the head end of the bed elevated to have proper access to the scalp for electrode placement (Fig. 36.6).
2. Apply the reference electrodes on the earlobes and the ground electrode above the bridge of the nose. Place the sensitive electrodes on the scalp as per the 10–20

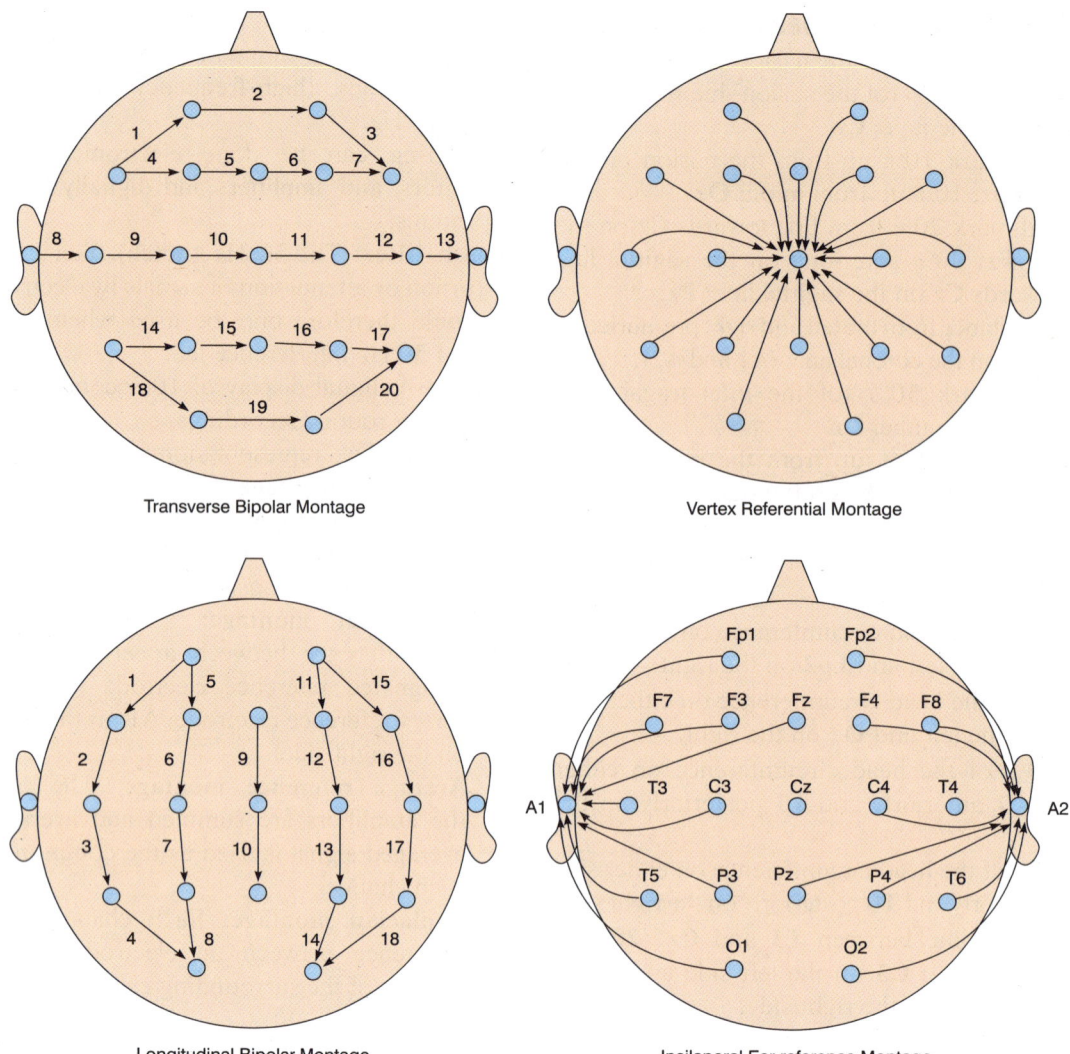

Transverse Bipolar Montage

Vertex Referential Montage

Longitudinal Bipolar Montage

Ipsilaperal Ear reference Montage

Fig. 36.5 Recording montages.

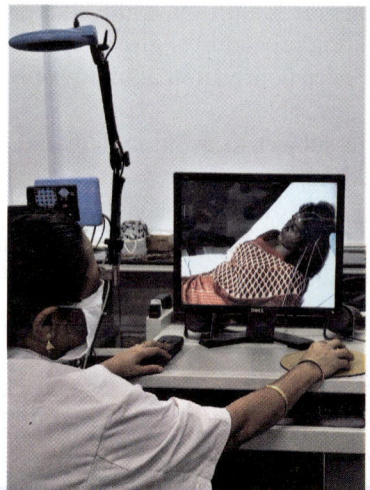

Fig. 36.6 Position of the patient while placing the electrodes on the scalp. The picture of the subject is shown on the computer screen, which is transmitted from the video clip of the system. (*Courtesy*: Ms. Bharathi Balakumar, Senior Technical Officer, Physiology Dept., JIPMER, Puducherry, India.)

system described above. Connect them to the electrode board and ensure that there are no loose connections.

3. ***Sensitivity calibration***—calibrate the machine to ensure that an input of 50 μV gives a pen deflection of 7 mm.

4. Ask the subject to close his eyes and make a test recording.

Note: Normally, the alpha rhythm is recorded. Records are taken simultaneously from multiple analogous areas of the scalp over at least a 20-minute period.

5. ***Effect of opening the eyes***—ask the subject to open his eyes and note the effect.

Note: The alpha rhythm is immediately replaced by desynchronization, i.e., fast, irregular activity. When the subject is asked to close his eyes, the alpha rhythm reappears.

6. ***Photic stimulation***—as the record is running, deliver light flashes at the rate of 25/sec for 5 seconds, first with the eyes closed, then with the eyes open.

Note: Normally, there may be no change, but in diseases like epilepsy, the delta rhythm may appear. In some cases, an epileptic attack may be precipitated.

7. Note the images on the video in case of an epileptic attack. Correlate the EEG waves with the flickering on the television to ensure the result in an attack of epilepsy.

8. *Effect of hyperventilation*—ask the subject to take deep breaths for 3 minutes.

Note: Normally, the frequency of alpha waves decreases due to low PCO_2, and the record may show a theta or delta rhythm. An epileptic attack may be precipitated along with abnormal patterns of waves, which may be correlated with the video recording of the seizure movements.

Precautions

1. Avoid kinking of the wires to prevent physical damage to these sensitive wires.
2. Clean the electrodes properly after use; this prevents corrosion.
3. Prepare the skin properly before placing the electrodes; this decreases the impedance.
4. Apply conducting (Ten20) paste judiciously; it should be adequate for conduction of the signal but not in excess, because an excess of the paste would result in salt-bridge artefacts, which should be avoided.

Observation and Results

Carefully note, read, and analyse the EEG waves of all the tracings as recorded for each electrode (Fig. 36.7).

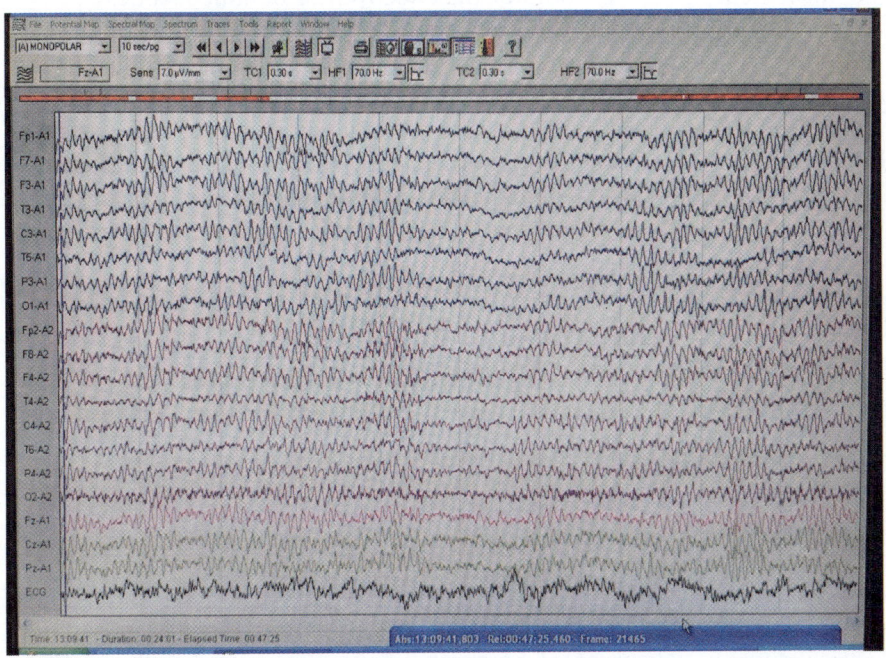

Fig. 36.7 EEG waves as originally recorded on the computer screen. Note the waves against each electrode, demarcated on the extreme left side against each tracing.

EEG analysis

The following should be looked for and interpreted in an EEG montage:

1. **Frequency of the waves:** Based on their frequency, the waves can be classified as: gamma (>30 Hz), beta (13–30 Hz), alpha (8–12 Hz), theta (4–7 Hz), and delta (<4 Hz).

2. **Epileptiform waves:**
   - *Spike:* Sharply contoured waveform with a duration of <70 ms.
   - *Sharp wave:* Sharply contoured waveform with a duration of 70–200 ms.

3. **Complex waves:** Two wave patterns together, e.g., spike followed by a 'slow wave spike'—'slow wave' complex.

4. **Amplitude of waves:** Amplitude is the size of the waveforms (µV), often measured peak to peak. Amplitude can be reported as a numerical range (20 to 40 µV) or in descriptive terms as low (0 to 25 µV), moderate (25 to 75 µV), or high (>75 µV) amplitude. Some pathological conditions are associated with enormous amplitudes of hundreds of microvolts, such as hypoarrhythmia, a chaotic pattern seen in severe infantile epilepsy. The degree to which the original waveform signal is amplified in the computer is called **gain**.

5. **Polarity:** Electrical signals approaching an electrode are sensed as positive deflections, and those spreading away from it are sensed as negative deflections. Polarity reversal helps in localising the focus of epileptiform discharge.

6. **Phase:** Refers to that part of the waveform that begins in one direction (up or down) and then changes its direction in the next turn. Depending upon the turns, waves can be classified as monophasic, biphasic, and triphasic.

7. **Rhythmicity:** Refers to the appearance of uninterrupted monomorphic waveforms. Based on rhythmicity, they can be classified as rhythmic, irregular, and semi-rhythmic patterns.

8. **Reactivity:** The degree of changes that occur in an EEG in response to exogenous or endogenous stimulation is called reactivity. The test for reactivity is routine in EEG recording. The usual stimuli are opening and closing of eyes, arithmetic calculations, and orientation questions.

9. **Activation:** It is the appearance of a particular pattern in response to an activating procedure. Activation procedures are carried out to induce epileptiform waves during the interictal phase to aid in the diagnosis of the condition. The commonly used activation procedures are sleep deprivation, hyperventilation, and photic stimulation.

10. **Synchrony:** Simultaneous occurrence of *similar waveforms over each hemisphere* is called synchrony of waveforms. Normal EEG activity is usually synchronous over the left and right hemispheres, both for relatively continuous background activities and more sporadic waveforms (e.g., 'K complexes', the high-amplitude biphasic slow waves seen in stage 2 sleep, should have simultaneous onset over both hemispheres). **Loss of synchrony** is observed in *damage to the corpus callosum* and severe *disorders of cortical function*. Lack of synchrony can also indicate that the location where the waveform appears first may be closer to the origin of that activity; this helps with the *localisation of abnormal or epileptiform activity*.

11. **Symmetry:** This is a comparison of waveform patterns based on their spatial distribution in the left and right hemispheres.

EEG artefacts

Biological artefacts: These include ECG artefacts, eye movement artefacts (blinking, side-to-side movements, eyelid flutter, and slow, roving eye movement in a drowsy state), muscle artefacts, pulse artefacts, respiratory movement artefacts, glossokinetic (tongue movement-induced) artefacts, tremor-induced head movements, sweat artefact, and induced artefacts.

Technical artefacts: These include artefacts caused due to electrical interference (50 Hz electrical line artefact), excess paste use (salt-bridge artefact), and electrode pop-out from the scalp.

Instrumental artefacts: These include errors due to portable air pumps, monitoring devices in the ICU, respirator, lights and lamps, fans, air conditioner, pneumatic boots, heating and cooling blankets, electric beds, intravenous infusion pumps, feeding delivery systems, elevators, computers, telephones, diathermy, dialysis machine, and X-ray equipment.

Quantitative EEG

The numerical data analyses of EEG to provide supportive diagnosis for the clinical condition form the basis of quantitative EEG. The waves can be analysed by using Fast Fourier Transform analysis (FFT), power spectral analysis, or wavelet analysis. Increased abnormal electrical activity (as in an epileptic focus) or decreased conductance (as in brain injury) can be picked by alterations in the power spectrum confined to a topographic area.

DISCUSSION

The electroencephalogram (EEG) represents the electrical activity inside the brain as recorded by electrodes placed on the scalp. EEG is an important tool used by neurophysiologists, neurologists, and neurosurgeons. It is a non-invasive technique, and in conjunction with imaging techniques like CT scan and MRI, it is effective in **diagnosing abnormal electrical activities** in the brain, causing seizure disorders. EEG is also effectively used in diagnosing **sleep disorders** as it forms an essential component of **polysomnography**. Other uses in the clinical setting include the diagnosis of **encephalopathy** and monitoring of comatose patients in the ICU for confirming **brain death**.

Clinical Applications of EEG

1. To confirm seizure activity
2. To study sleep physiology and diagnose sleep disorders—polysomnography
3. In encephalopathies—generalised slowing, burst suppression
4. To confirm brain death in comatose patients—absent electrical activity (electrically silent/near silent)
5. To monitor the depth of anesthesia—used to decide the optimal dose of anesthesia
6. To monitor prognosis in seizure disorders
7. To monitor the effectiveness of antiepileptics
8. For EEG biofeedback

In current practice, EEG is widely used as one of the tools to **intra-operatively monitor** the depth of anesthesia, to assess burst suppression and extent of cortical excision in epileptic surgery. EEG signals are also used as **neurofeedback/biofeedback** inputs, suggesting the effectiveness of specific brainwave entrainment procedures.

Limitations of EEG Studies

1. Preparing the subject is a tedious process
2. Technical expertise is needed for signal acquisition
3. Poor signal-to-noise ratio
4. Poor spatial resolution compared to imaging techniques
5. Does not use signals from deeper layers of the brain

Diagnosis of Epilepsies and Other Problems

Epilepsy (seizure or fit) is defined as the intermittent disorder of cerebral function associated with a sudden uncontrolled discharge of cerebral neurons, which may or may not be accompanied by loss of consciousness. The epileptogenic focus in the cerebral cortex discharges irregular slow waves, or sometimes, high-voltage waves that can be recorded in the EEG.

There are **two groups** of epilepsy:

I. **Generalised seizures** with loss of consciousness associated with generalised synchronous EEG discharge from both hemispheres. Examples include:

1. **Grand mal epilepsy** is characterised by immediate loss of consciousness followed by sustained contraction of limb muscles (*tonic phase*) and then jerky movements due to rhythmic contraction–relaxation of limb muscles (*clonic phase*). In EEG, **fast activities** are recorded in the tonic phase, and slow activities in the clonic phase.

2. **Petit mal epilepsy (absence seizure)** manifests in the form of a short-lived loss of consciousness with mild or no motor activity. EEG recording shows **doublets consisting of a spike and a dome**. Three such doublets occur typically per second.

II. **Focal epilepsy**, the manifestations of which depend on the site of the cortex from which the discharge occurs, e.g., temporal lobe epilepsy and Jacksonian (motor cortex) epilepsy.

Though EEG confirms the type of epilepsy recordings between the attacks may be normal.

Intracranial Space-occupying Lesion

Cerebral tumours do not directly produce abnormal electrical activity. They compress adjoining neurons and suppress their normal rhythms, which manifests as **irregular or slow waves**. This helps in localising cerebral tumours. Fluid collection, as occurs in subdural hematoma, can suppress neurons and produce local abnormal EEG waves.

Diagnosis of Sleep Disturbances

Analysis of sleep and the diagnosis of sleep disorders are accomplished with the help of EEG.

Brain Death

EEG can confirm brain death when it shows no electrical activity more than 2 microvolts, at a sensitivity of 2 microvolts/mm for at least 30 seconds. Also, it should show no reactivity to intense somatosensory stimuli.

Definition and meaning

According to the American Academy of Neurology's guidelines, brain death is clinically equivalent to the **irreversible loss of all brain stem functions**, which refers to the impossibility of recovery, regardless of any medical intervention. However, patients with brain death could be maintained physiologically for prolonged periods in the intensive care units.

Criteria for the diagnosis of brain death

Brain death **can be assessed** by performing physical examination, apnea test, and ancillary tests.

I. **Physical examination**: This includes checking for response to pain and assessment of brain stem reflexes. Loss of eye response and motor reflexes in response to deep pain stimuli are features of brain death. Brain death can be confirmed if **brain stem reflexes are lost**, including:

1. **CN II:** Loss of light reflex, pupils should be mid-dilated, 4–9 mm, and not reactive to light.
2. **CN III, IV, VI:** Eye motion is lost in reaction to head movement (Doll's eyes).
3. **CN V, VII:** Loss of corneal reflex.
4. **CN VIII:** Loss of oculovestibular reflex (caloric test)—upon irrigating the ear with 60 ml of ice water, the corresponding eye will not move towards the irrigated ear.
5. **CN IX:** Loss of gag reflex.
6. **CN X:** Loss of cough reflex

II. **Apnea test:** This test is used to assess the brain's ability to drive pulmonary function in response to the rise of CO_2. During the test, oxygen should be supplemented using a cannula connected to the endotracheal tube at 6 l/min. In the case of loss of respiratory drive, CO_2 is expected to rise by 5 mmHg every minute in the first 2 minutes, then by 2 mmHg every minute. A rise of CO_2 more than 20 mmHg above the baseline is consistent with brain death.

III. **Ancillary tests:** Two types of ancillary tests are considered if there is uncertainty of diagnosis or if the apnea test cannot be performed.

1. For the detection of cessation of cerebral blood flow:

   - **Cerebral angiography:** Four-vessel angiography is considered the gold standard.
   - **Transcranial ultrasound:** This is used to assess pulsations in the middle cerebral arteries and vertebral and basilar arteries bilaterally.
   - **Computed tomogram (CT) brain angiography and MR angiography:** These tests show cessation of cerebral blood flow.
   - **Radionuclide brain imaging:** This is done using a ^{99m}Tc-isotope tracer and then imaging by SPECT brain scintigraphy. The absence of a

tracer in the brain circulation (the hollow skull phenomenon) is consistent with brain death.

2. For the detection of loss of bioelectrical activity of the brain:

- **Electroencephalogram (EEG):** This test confirms brain death when it shows no electrical activity of more than 2 microvolts at a sensitivity of 2 microvolts/mm for at least 30 seconds.

- **Somatosensory evoked potentials:** Patients with brain death show no SEP in response to bilateral median nerve stimulation and no BAEP in response to auditory stimuli.

Implications

It is crucial to **differentiate brain death from other forms of severe brain damage**, which can cause vegetative states when some of the brain functions are maintained. Recovery can occur even after prolonged periods, especially in patients with traumatic brain injuries. Another essential topic that evolved in parallel with brain death is the need to **obtain organs for transplantation**. According to the **'dead donor rule'**, organ procurement can occur only after death. So, for patients who are brain dead, the procurement of viable organs is allowed, even if they still have some circulatory and pulmonary functions.

VIVA

1. *Define EEG.* (**Ans.** Refer to page 236, under the heading 'Introduction'.)
2. *What are EEG waves? What do they represent?* (**Ans.** Refer to page 236, under the heading 'EEG Waves'.)
3. *What are EEG wave patterns and rhythms?* (**Ans.** Refer to page 236, under the heading 'EEG Wave Patterns and Rhythms'.)
4. *What is alpha block? What is its physiological significance?* (**Ans.** Refer to page 237, under the heading 'EEG Wave Patterns and Rhythms' and the subheading 'Alpha block'.)
5. *What are EEG rhythms in infants and children?* (**Ans.** Refer to page 237, under the heading 'EEG Rhythms in Infants and Children'.)
6. *What is the basic principle of EEG recording?* (**Ans.** Refer to page 237, under the heading 'Methods' and the subheading 'Principle'.)
7. *How do you prepare a subject for EEG recording?* (**Ans.** Refer to page 237-238, under the heading 'Procedure' and the subheading 'Preparation of the subject'.)
8. *How are EEG electrodes positioned on the head?* (**Ans.** Refer to page 238, under the heading 'Procedure' and the subheading 'Position of electrodes'; also refer to Fig. 36.4.)
9. *What do you mean by sensitivity, filters, and montage? What is their significance?* (**Ans.** Refer to page 239, under the heading 'Important Terminologies in EEG Recording'.)
10. *What are the special instructions given to the subject before taking an EEG recording?* (**Ans.** Refer to page 239, under the heading 'Instructions to Subject'.)
11. *List the precautions observed while taking an EEG recording.* (**Ans.** Refer to page 241, under the heading 'Precautions'.)
12. *What are the special features of EEG analysis?* (**Ans.** Refer to page 241, under the heading 'EEG Analysis'.)
13. *What are the possible artefacts in an EEG? How are they avoided?* (**Ans.** Refer to page 242, under the heading 'EEG Artefacts'.)
14. *What is quantitative EEG?* (**Ans.** Refer to page 242, under the heading 'Quantitative EEG'.)
15. *List the uses and applications of EEG.* (**Ans.** Refer to page 242, under the heading 'Clinical applications of EEG'.)
16. *What are the limitations of EEG investigation?* (**Ans.** Refer to page 242, under the heading 'Limitations of EEG Studies'.)
17. *What are the major types of epilepsy? What are the major EEG findings in these disorders?* (**Ans.** Refer to page 242-243, under the heading 'Diagnosis of Epilepsies'.)
18. *What is the definition of brain death? What are the criteria to detect brain death?* (**Ans.** Refer to page 243, under the heading 'Brain Death'.)
19. *What are the clinical implications of determining brain death?* (**Ans.** Refer to page 244, under the heading 'Implications'.)

37 | Autonomic Function Tests

Learning Objectives

After completing this practical, you will be able to (MUST KNOW):
1. Describe the importance of performing autonomic function tests (AFTs) in clinical physiology.
2. List the functions of ANS.
3. Enumerate the major differences between the sympathetic and parasympathetic systems.
4. List the various autonomic function tests.
5. Perform various non-invasive AFTs.
6. Explain the principle of AFTs.

7. List the precautions taken while performing AFTs.
8. State the normal values of AFTs.
9. Name the conditions in which there are alterations in AFTs.

You may also be able to (DESIRABLE TO KNOW):
1. Explain the differences between the parasympathetic and sympathetic functions.
2. Explain the physiological basis of AFTs.
3. Explain the mechanism of alteration in AFTs.

INTRODUCTION

The autonomic nervous system (ANS) has two major divisions: **sympathetic and parasympathetic**. The ANS regulates all visceral functions, metabolism, and the functions of almost all the body systems. Autonomic functions can be evaluated by a number of invasive and non-invasive tests. The non-invasive tests can be readily performed and used to confirm the diagnosis of autonomic neuropathy, whereas invasive tests require complex procedures and are used chiefly for localisation of the site of lesion.

Anatomical and Physiological Considerations

Functional Anatomy

1. The ANS is divided into the **sympathetic and parasympathetic** systems.
2. Both the divisions of the ANS have preganglionic and postganglionic neurons.
3. **Preganglionic neurons** are myelinated and cholinergic. The **postganglionic neurons** are unmyelinated and *cholinergic in the parasympathetic* division, and *adrenergic in the sympathetic division,* **except** the fibres that innervate the sweat glands and blood vessels in the skeletal muscles (**sympathetic vasodilator system**).
4. Cell bodies of the sympathetic preganglionic neurons lie in the *intermediolateral grey horns* of twelve thoracic and the first three lumbar segments of the spinal cord (Fig. 37.1A). The cell bodies of the parasympathetic preganglionic neurons lie in *four cranial nerve nuclei* (III, VII, IX, and X) in the brainstem and lateral grey horns of the 2nd–4th sacral segments of the spinal cord (Fig. 37.1B).

5. **Sympathetic preganglionic neurons** synapse with postganglionic neurons in the *paravertebral sympathetic chain* of the ganglia. The **parasympathetic preganglionic neurons** synapse with the postganglionic neurons, which are present very close to the viscera and sometimes, in the viscera.
6. The gastrointestinal system is richly innervated by the ANS. This innervation is regarded as the **enteric nervous system**, the *third division* of the ANS.

Physiological Considerations

Most organs of the body receive dual innervation from the ANS. Usually, one division causes facilitation and the other causes inhibition of functions of the organs.
1. Cholinergic neurons release acetylcholine as a neurotransmitter, whereas adrenergic neurons release norepinephrine or epinephrine.
2. The effect of parasympathetic stimulation is usually short-lived because acetylcholine is degraded rapidly. On the other hand, the effect of sympathetic stimulation lasts long and has widespread effects.
3. Cholinergic receptors are divided into muscarinic and nicotinic types, whereas adrenergic receptors are broadly categorised into α and β.
4. The parasympathetic division regulates activities that conserve and restore body energy. The sympathetic division prepares the body for emergencies (fight or flight response) and causes a loss of energy from the body.
5. The autonomic reflexes adjust the activities of smooth muscles, cardiac muscles, and glands.
6. The autonomic reflexes consist of receptors, sensory neurons, centre of integration, autonomic motor neurons, and visceral effectors.

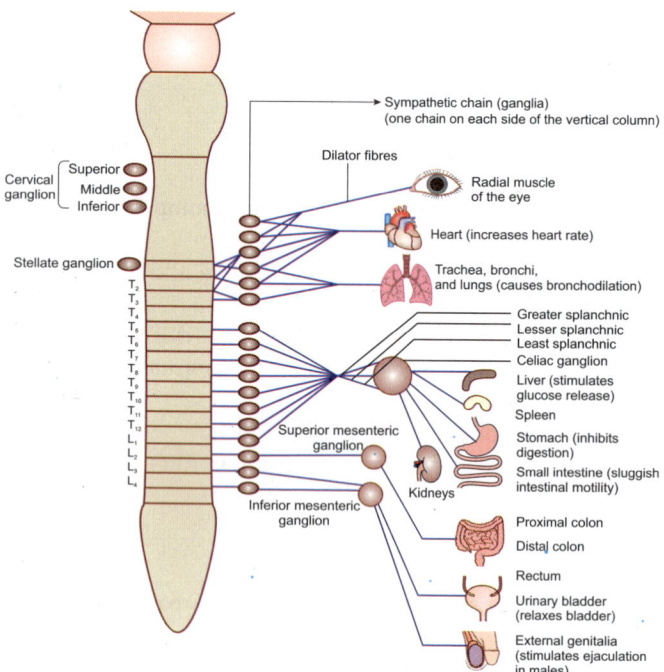

Fig. 37.1A The autonomic nervous system: The sympathetic system (*Courtesy:* Prasad J. 2019. *Textbook of Pharmacology*, 2nd edition. Hyderabad: Universities Press.)

7. The hypothalamus controls and integrates the functions of both the divisions of the ANS. The control of the cortex, especially by the limbic cortex, largely occurs during emotional states.

Autonomic Function Tests (AFTs)

AFTs have usually been described as cardiovascular AFTs and other AFTs.

Cardiovascular autonomic function tests (CAFTs)

1. Heart rate and blood pressure (BP) response to standing
2. Heart rate and BP response to passive tilting
3. Heart rate response to deep breathing
4. Valsalva ratio
5. BP response to isometric handgrip
6. Cold pressor test

Sweat tests

1. Sympathetic skin response
2. Quantitative sudomotor axon reflex test (QSART)

Vasomotor tests

1. Laser Doppler velocimetry for skin blood flow measurement with inspiratory gasp
2. Valsalva maneuver
3. Cold pressor test

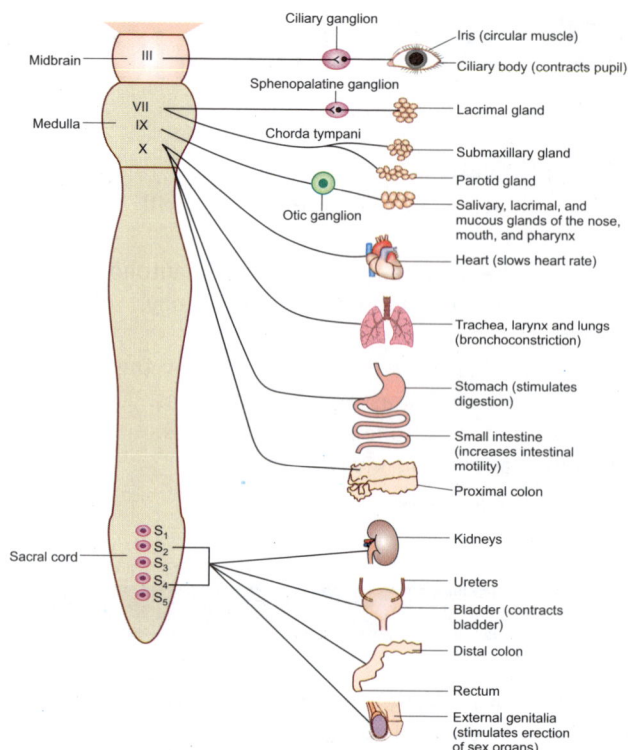

Fig. 37.1B The autonomic nervous system: The parasy mpathetic system. Note that preganglionic fibres are short in the sympathetic system and long in the parasympathetic system. The postganglionic fibres are long in the sympathetic system, close to the organs or in the organs in the parasympathetic. (*Courtesy:* Prasad J. 2019. *Textbook of Pharmacology*, 2nd edition. Hyderabad: Universities Press.)

Cardiovascular AFTs are described as the **conventional or classical autonomic function tests (CAFTs)** because they are the standard tests that can easily be performed and reproduced.

Functional classification of AFTs

▉ AFTs for assessment of sympathetic functions

1. BP response to standing/tilt
2. Cold pressor test
3. Isometric handgrip
4. Galvanic/sympathetic skin response
5. Thermoregulatory sweat test
6. Valsalva ratio
7. NE spillage test
8. QT/QS2 ratio
9. LF, LFnu, and LF-HF ratio of HRV

▉ AFTs for assessment of parasympathetic functions

1. **Resting heart rate:** Basal heart rate is a good index of parasympathetic functions since heart rate in resting conditions is a measure of vagal tone. ***Resting HR***

more than 75 indicates poor vagal tone and is considered an indicator of CV risk.

2. 30:15 ratio
3. E:I ratio
4. Valsalva ratio
5. Tachycardia ratio
6. Baroreceptor reflex sensitivity
7. Standing to lying ratio
8. HF and HFnu of HRV

METHODS OF MEASURING AUTONOMIC FUNCTIONS

Heart Rate and BP Response to Standing

Principle

On standing up from a supine position, the blood pressure immediately falls by about 20 mmHg, and the heart rate usually increases from 10 to 20 beats. These changes occur within 5–15 seconds.

Requirements

1. A multichannel polygraph with provisions to record beat-to-beat variation in heart rate
2. NIBP monitor or a servoplethysmo-manometer (Finapres)

Note: Though a polygraph and NIBP should be used ideally, this test can also be performed with a sphygmomanometer and an ECG machine, which are routinely used clinically.

Procedure

1. Ask the subject to lie down in the supine position.
2. Connect the ECG electrodes from the subject to the polygraph, and connect the pulse cap of the NIBP to one of the subject's fingers or tie the cuff of the NIBP around the subject's arm.
3. Ask the subject to relax completely for a minimum of 10 minutes.
4. Record the basal heart rate and blood pressure from the polygraph and NIBP.
5. Ask the subject to stand up and immediately note the change in heart rate and blood pressure from the monitoring screen of the polygraph and NIBP.
6. Record blood pressure and heart rate serially for 1–3 minutes after standing.
7. Determine the **30:15 R–R ratio** from the ECG recording of the polygraph.

Note: The longest R–R interval (slowest heart rate) occurring about 30 beats after standing divided by the shortest R–R interval (fastest heart rate), which occurs at about 15 beats after standing, gives the 30:15 R–R ratio. 30:15 ratio (**cardiovagal effect**) is a measure of **parasympathetic function**.

Observation and results

1. Note the HR response to standing and calculate the 30:15 ratio.
2. Note the systolic and diastolic BP responses to standing.
3. Write down your opinion on the results.

Note: The normal value of 30:15 ratio is 1.04. A ratio less than **1.04** is considered autonomic deficiency. A fall in SBP of more than 20 mmHg and DBP more than 10 mmHg upon standing is indicative of orthostatic hypotension.

Precautions

1. The subject should relax completely in the supine position for 10–20 minutes before recording the basal blood pressure and heart rate.
2. When the subject stands up, he should lean (passive standing) against a wall to avoid the effect of muscular effort of active standing on heart rate and blood pressure.
3. Changes in heart rate and blood pressure should be observed within 15 seconds of standing.

Heart Rate and BP Response to Passive Tilting

Principle

The cardiovascular response to changes in position is tested by **tilting (passively) the subject using a tilt table**. The early responses are similar but not identical to those of standing. The early response to tilting, which occurs in 30–60 seconds, reflects the autonomic cardiovascular reflexes; changes that occur after 30–60 seconds reflect neurocardiogenic reflex.

Requirements

1. Tilt table
2. ECG electrodes
3. NIBP
4. Multichannel polygraph

Procedure

1. Ask the subject to lie down on the tilt table.
2. Connect ECG electrodes to the polygraph and connect the NIBP.
3. Ask the subject to relax for 10 minutes.
4. Record the baseline heart rate and blood pressure.
5. Position the head side of the tilt table to an inclination of 80° (80° head-up tilt) from the horizontal.

Note: Heart rate and blood pressure response to passive tilt with the head down (head-down tilt) can also be recorded.

6. Immediately record the heart rate and blood pressure, and then record these at one-minute intervals for three minutes.

Observation and results

Note the HR and BP responses to passive tilting are similar to those of active standing (described above).

Precautions

1. The subject should be instructed properly about the procedure.
2. The subject should be completely relaxed for a minimum of 10 minutes before recording basal heart rate and ECG.
3. Changes in heart rate and blood pressure to tilt should be recorded accurately.

Valsalva Ratio

Principle

The Valsalva ratio is a measure of the changes in the heart rate that take place during a brief period of forced expiration against a closed glottis or mouthpiece (Valsalva maneuver). During and after the Valsalva maneuver, there will be changes in cardiac vagal efferent and sympathetic vasomotor activity, resulting from the stimulation of the carotid sinus, aortic arch baroreceptors, and other intrathoracic stretch receptors.

Requirements

1. A mercury manometer
2. Nose clip
3. Mouthpiece
4. Electrocardiograph

Procedure

1. Provide proper instructions to the subject on how to exhale forcefully into the manometer and maintain the pressure at 40 mmHg.

> Note: The subject may be allowed to practice the procedure till he is capable of performing it properly.

2. Ask the subject to lie down in a semi-recumbent or sitting position.
3. Close the subject's nostrils with the help of the nose clip.
4. Place a mouthpiece into the subject's mouth and connect the mercury manometer to it.
5. Switch on the ECG machine for continuous recording.
6. Ask the subject to breathe forcefully into the mercury manometer and then ask him to **maintain the expiratory pressure at 40 mmHg** for 10–15 seconds.
7. Record ECG changes throughout the procedure, and 30 seconds before and after the procedure.
8. **Repeat the procedure three times** with a gap of five minutes between the maneuvers.
9. Calculate the Valsalva ratio and **take the largest ratio of the three** (which represents the best performance) for consideration.

> Note: The Valsalva ratio is calculated by dividing the longest inter-beat interval after the maneuver by the shortest inter-beat interval during the maneuver.

Observation and results

1. **Calculate the Valsalva ratio** (VR):

   VR is the ratio of the longest R–R interval during phase IV to the shortest R–R interval during phase II.

   $$VR = \frac{\text{Longest R} - \text{R interval during phase IV}}{\text{Shortest R} - \text{R interval during phase II}}$$

2. Report your findings as normal or abnormal. A VR above **1.45 is normal**, and a value below 1.2 is abnormal.

Precautions

1. The subject should be instructed properly.
2. The subject should be allowed to practice the maneuver before the actual test.
3. The subject should maintain the pressure in the manometer constantly at 40 mmHg throughout the maneuver (10–15 seconds).
4. The procedure should be repeated three times, and the best of the three values should be considered.

Heart Rate Response to Deep Breathing

Principle

Heart rate increases during inspiration due to decreased cardiac vagal activity and decreases during expiration due to increased vagal activity. This is detected by recording the heart rate while the subject is breathing deeply.

Requirements

1. ECG apparatus with electrodes
2. ECG jelly

Procedure

There are two methods used for determining heart rate variation with breathing. One method monitors a single deep breath, and the other method monitors deep breathing at a rate of six breaths per minute. Usually, the method using six breaths per minute is used to determine heart rate variation with respiration.

1. Provide proper instructions to the subject.
2. Ask the subject to lie down comfortably in the supine position with the head elevated to 30°.
3. Connect ECG electrodes to record the lead II ECG.
4. Ask the subject to breathe deeply at a rate of six breaths per minute (allowing 5 seconds each for inspiration and expiration).
5. Record the maximum and minimum heart rate with each respiratory cycle.
6. Determine the expiration to inspiration ratio (**E:I ratio**).

Note: The E:I ratio is the ratio of the mean of maximum R–R intervals during deep expiration (slow HR) to the mean of minimum R–R intervals during deep inspiration (fast HR). The E:I ratio can also be calculated following a single deep breath.

Observation and results

1. Note the deep breathing difference (DBD) in HR during the respiratory cycle, i.e., the difference between the maximum (in inspiration) and the minimum (in expiration). Note that DBD is >18 beats/min in adults up to the age of 40 years.
2. Note the E/I ratio. The **normal E/I ratio range is 1.23–1.08** between the ages of 16 to 60 years.
3. Report the results with your comments.

Precautions

1. The subject should be instructed properly to take six breaths per minute.
2. The subject should be relaxed and comfortable before performing the test.

BP Response to Isometric Handgrip

Principle

Sustained handgrip against resistance causes an increase in heart rate and blood pressure. These responses are detected using ECG and blood pressure monitors.

Requirements

1. ECG electrodes and ECG machine
2. NIBP monitor/sphygmomanometer
3. Handgrip spring dynamometer

Procedure

1. Provide proper instructions to the subject about the test.
2. Ask the subject to lie down in a semi-recumbent position.
3. Connect the ECG electrodes for lead II recording and NIBP monitor/sphygmomanometer for blood pressure measurement. Tie the **BP cuff in the arm of the subject's non-dominant** hand, leaving the dominant hand free to perform the handgrip exercise.
4. Record the basal heart rate and blood pressure for at least 3 minutes.
5. Ask the subject to hold the dynamometer **in his dominant hand with a firm grip**.
6. Ask the subject to exert maximum force and note the maximum tension developed. Note the maximum isometric tension (T_{max}).
7. Ask the subject to maintain a pressure of **30 per cent of the T_{max}** for about 5 minutes.

8. Record the heart rate and **change in diastolic pressure** just before the release of the hand grip.

Note: Change in diastolic pressure is defined as the difference between the last value recorded before the release of handgrip pressure and the mean resting value calculated by averaging the last 3 minutes of recording before commencing isometric exercise.

Observation and results

1. Note the DBP just before the subject releases the handgrip pressure.
2. Note the resting DBP by averaging the pressure of the last three minutes of recording before commencing the isometric exercise.
3. Estimate the difference between the resting DBP and the isometric handgrip DBP. Also, note the difference in heart rate.
4. State your opinion on the value.

Note: The normal response to isometric handgrip is a rise in diastolic pressure of **more than 15 mmHg** and a rise in HR of about 30%.

Precautions

1. The subject should be instructed properly.
2. BP should be recorded from one arm, while the other arm is used for the handgrip exercise.
3. The basal diastolic blood pressure should be recorded.
4. The subject should maintain a pressure of 30 per cent of the maximum activity for about 5 minutes.
5. The diastolic blood pressure before the release of the grip should be recorded.

Cold Pressor Test

Principle

Submerging the hand in cold water results in a rise in systolic and diastolic pressure, which is detected by a blood pressure monitor or sphygmomanometer.

Requirements

1. NIBP monitor/sphygmomanometer
2. Ice-cold water (just below 4°C)

Procedure

1. Provide proper instructions to the subject regarding the test.
2. Tie the BP cuff around the subject's arm and record the basal blood pressure (the other arm will be submerged in cold water).
3. Take very cold water (at or below 4°C) in a container.
4. Ask the subject to submerge his other upper limbs (at least up to the wrist) in the cold water for 60 seconds.
5. Record blood pressure 30 and 60 seconds after submersion of the limb.

Observation and results

1. Note the difference in resting BP and the BP at 60 seconds of submersion.
2. Record your opinion.

> **Note:** Submerging the hand in ice-cold water increases systolic pressure by 20 mmHg and diastolic pressure by 10 mmHg. Rise of BP less than these values indicates sympathetic deficiency.

Precautions

1. The subject should be instructed to be mentally prepared to submerge his limb for one minute in the cold water.
2. The temperature of the cold water should be 4°C or less.
3. The subject should keep his limb submerged in ice-cold water for one minute (not less than 30 seconds).
4. BP should be recorded in the opposite limb.

Sympathetic Skin Response

Principle

Sympathetic skin response (SSR) or **galvanic skin response (GSR)** assesses the integrity of peripheral sympathetic cholinergic (sudomotor) function by evaluating the changes in the resistance of the skin to electrical conduction.

Requirements

1. EMG equipment/polygraph with provision to record EMG
2. Electrodes

Procedure

1. Provide proper instructions to the subject about the test.
2. Connect the electrodes from the subject's hand or foot to the EMG machine or the polygraph.

> **Note:** Connect the active electrode on the palm of the hand or sole of the foot, and the reference electrode over the dorsum of the respective body part. Disc electrodes are used with electrode gel.

3. Set the low-frequency filter at 0.1 or 0.5 Hz and the high-frequency filter at 500–1000 Hz.
4. Set the apparatus to obtain the gain to record a potential of 0.5–3 mV and set the sweep to record 5 seconds after the stimulus.
5. Provide a stimulus in the form of a startling sound and record the response.
6. Record the SSR potentials and their amplitude and latency.

Observation and results

Note the latency and amplitude of SSR. The amplitude of SSR in the hands is 1.6 mV, and in the feet is 2.1 mV.

DISCUSSION

Autonomic dysfunctions are associated with many diseases such as diabetes, hypertension, obesity, heart diseases, arthritis, asthma, psychiatric disorders, and various metabolic diseases. Abnormalities of autonomic function lead to different clinical entities like orthostatic hypotension, sexual dysfunction, diarrhea, incontinence, dryness of mouth, and so on. Autonomic function tests are performed to confirm the clinical diagnosis of autonomic neuropathies and to assess the intactness of the sympathetic and parasympathetic pathways.

Heart Rate and BP Response to Standing

HR response: On changing the posture from supine to standing, the heart rate increases immediately, usually by 10–20 beats per minute. On standing, the heart rate increases until it reaches a **maximum at about the 15th beat**, after which it slows down to a **stable rate at about the 30th beat**. The ratio of R–R intervals corresponding to the 30th and 15th heartbeats is called the **30:15 ratio**.

- The 30:15 ratio is a measure of **parasympathetic function**.
- This ratio decreases with age. In young individuals, a **ratio less than 1.04 is considered abnormal**.

BP response: The blood pressure changes on standing are studied to assess the integrity of the **sympathetic system**. Immediately on standing, the blood pressure falls, but this activates the baroreceptor reflex, and blood pressure returns to normal within 15 seconds. When **systolic pressure falls by 20 mmHg** or more or **diastolic pressure falls by 10 mmHg** or more on standing, **orthostatic hypotension** is said to be present.

Heart Rate and BP Response to Tilting

Heart rate response to **head-up tilt** is especially useful in the diagnosis of **multisystem atrophy** and patients suffering from **recurrent unexplained syncope**. On changing from the recumbent to the upright position on a tilt table, there is pooling of about 30 per cent venous blood in the peripheral compartment. This decreases cardiac filling pressure and **stroke volume by 40 per cent**.

The heart rate rises immediately **due to the withdrawal of parasympathetic activity** and afterwards **due to increased sympathetic activity**.

Heart Rate Response to Deep Breathing

The variation in heart rate with respiration is known as **sinus arrhythmia**. Inspiration increases and expiration decreases the heart rate. This is primarily mediated by the parasympathetic innervation of the heart. The pulmonary stretch receptor, cardiac mechanoreceptors, and baroreceptors contribute to sinus arrhythmia.

Deep breath difference (DBD): The difference between the maximum and minimum heart rate during deep breathing is called DBD. The normal DBD is *more than 15 beats per minute* in normal individuals. It is a measure of **parasympathetic activity**. DBD decreases with age.

Table 37.1 presents the normal values of DBD, and Table 37.2 presents the normal values of E:I ratios with age.

Table 37.1   Normal values of DBD

10–40 years	>18 beats per minute
41–50 years	>16 beats per minute
51–60 years	>12 beats per minute
61–70 years	>8 beats per minute

Table 37.2   Normal values of E:I ratio

16–20 years	>1.23
21–25 years	>1.20
26–30 years	>1.18
31–35 years	>1.16
36–40 years	>1.14
41–45 years	>1.12
46–50 years	>1.11
51–55 years	>1.09
56–60 years	>1.08
61–65 years	>1.07
66–70 years	>1.06

Abnormalities in DBD/E:I ratio

Abnormalities in the DBD/E:I ratio occur in the following conditions:
1. Multisystem atrophy
2. Progressive autonomic failure
3. Diabetes
4. Autonomic neuropathy
5. Uremic patients
6. CNS depression
7. Hyperventilation
8. Pulmonary diseases

Sinus arrhythmia is **abolished by parasympathetic block** but not by sympathetic block. This indicates that HR response to deep breathing is **purely a vagal function**. In fact, HR response to deep breathing is a **classical parasympathetic function test**.

Valsalva Ratio

The Valsalva ratio is a measure of both *parasympathetic and sympathetic function*. For the response to occur in the Valsalva maneuver, the parasympathetic system acts as the afferent and efferent and the sympathetic system acts as part of the efferent pathway. Therefore, the Valsalva ratio assesses more of parasympathetic (cardiovagal) function.

Valsalva maneuver

The Valsalva maneuver has **four phases** (Fig. 37.2).
1. **Phase I**: This phase consists of the **onset of strain**. There occurs a *transient increase in blood pressure*, which lasts for a few seconds. This is due to increased intrathoracic pressure and mechanical compression of the great vessels. However, the *heart rate does not change much*.
2. **Phase II**: This is the **phase of straining**. In the **early part** of this phase, venous return decreases, which decreases cardiac output and blood pressure. This change persists for 4 seconds. In the **later part** of this phase, blood pressure returns towards normal due to increased peripheral resistance as a result of sympathetic vasoconstriction. However, the *heart rate increases steadily* throughout this phase *due to vagal withdrawal* (in the early phase) and *sympathetic activation* (in the later phase).
3. **Phase III**: This phase occurs following the **release of strain**, whereby there occurs a *transient decrease in blood pressure* lasting for a few seconds. This is caused by mechanical displacement of blood to the pulmonary vascular bed, which was under increased intrathoracic pressure. There is *little change in heart rate*.
4. **Phase IV**: This occurs with **further release of strain**. The *blood pressure slowly increases,* and the *heart rate proportionately decreases*. It occurs 15–20 seconds after the release of strain and lasts for about a minute or more. Cardiovascular changes occur due to an increase in venous return, stroke volume, and cardiac output.

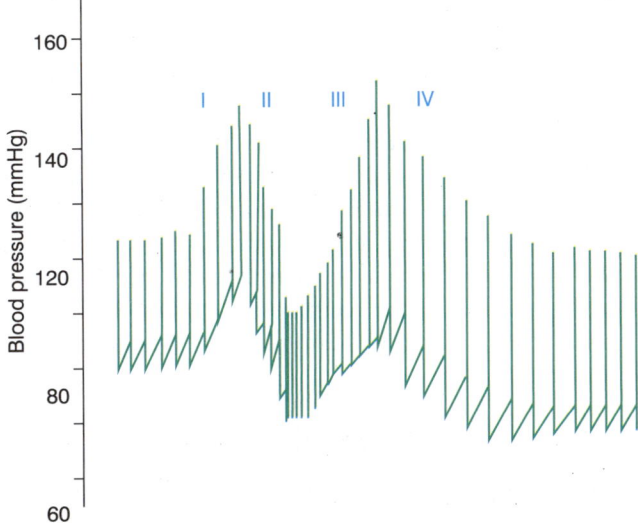

Fig. 37.2   Blood pressure changes during different phases (I, II, III, IV) of the Valsalva maneuver.

Calculation of Valsalva ratio (VR): VR is the ratio of the longest R–R interval during phase IV to the shortest R–R interval during phase II.

$$VR = \frac{\text{Longest R} - \text{R interval during phase IV}}{\text{Shortest R} - \text{R interval during phase II}}$$

Normal value of VR (Table 37.3): Valsalva ratio of *more than 1.45 is considered to be normal*. When it is 1.2–1.45, it is borderline, and if it is less than 1.2, it is regarded as abnormal.

Table 37.3   Valsalva ratios in different age groups

10–40 years	>1.5
41–50 years	>1.45
51–60 years	>1.40
61–70 years	>1.35

Tachycardia ratio: This is the ratio of the shortest RR interval during Valsalva maneuver to the longest RR interval before the effort. This is considered to be an index of *parasympathetic activity*.

Factors that affect Valsalva ratio

1. Age
2. Expiratory pressure
3. Sex
4. Duration of strain
5. Position of patient
6. Practice of yogic techniques

Clinical applications

1. Changes in the Valsalva maneuver occur due to **changes in cardiac vagal efferent** and sympathetic vasomotor activity, which are stimulated by the carotid sinus and aortic arch baroreceptors and other intrathoracic stretch receptors.
2. **Failure of heart rate to increase** during strain *suggests a sympathetic dysfunction;* **failure of heart rate to slow down** after the strain *suggests parasympathetic dysfunction*.
3. If the cardiovascular response to the Valsalva maneuver is abnormal but that to the cold pressure test is normal, the lesion is thought to be present in the baroreceptors or their afferent nerves. Such abnormalities occur commonly in diabetes, other neuropathies, multisystem atrophy, and autonomic failure.

BP Response to Isometric Handgrip

In the isometric handgrip (IHG) test, there is a rise in heart rate and blood pressure. These cardiovascular responses to isometric exercise are mediated chiefly by the influence of cardiovascular centres and partly by metabolic or mechanical changes or both in response to the contraction of the muscles that activate the small fibres in the afferent limb of the reflex arch. The normal response is a **rise in diastolic pressure of more than 15 mmHg** and a *rise in the heart rate by about 30 per cent*.

1. The rise in blood pressure is due to increased sympathetic activity, and the increase in the heart rate is due to decreased parasympathetic activity and increased sympathetic activity. This response is not influenced by age.
2. The **BP response to IHG is a pure sympathetic response** and is considered the **gold-standard** of sympathetic function tests.

Cold Pressor Test

Submerging the hand in ice-cold water **increases systolic pressure by about 20 mmHg** and *diastolic pressure by 10 mmHg*. The afferent limb of the reflex pathway consists of somatic fibres, whereas the efferent pathway consists of the sympathetic fibres. Though this test is a **classical sympathetic function test**, it requires standardisation for age and gender as the rise in BP is not equal in all subjects, and there are variations.

OTHER TESTS

Standing to Lying Ratio (SLR)

Heart rate (RR interval) response to lying down from the standing posture is assessed by a continuous recording of ECG.

1. Lying down from the standing position results in an **increase in venous return** and produces **reflex bradycardia**.
2. The ratio of the **longest RR interval while standing to the shortest RR interval while lying down** is the SLR.
3. Any value of SLR **below 1** is considered abnormal.
4. SLR is a **parasympathetic test**.

Tests for Sudomotor Functions

Sympathetic skin response

Sympathetic skin response (SSR) helps in studying the functions of **peripheral sympathetic cholinergic (sudomotor) fibres** by evaluating the changes in the resistance of the skin in response to electrical stimuli.

1. SSR is age-dependent and is present in both the hands and feet till the age of 60.

2. The composition of surface electrodes, stimulus frequency, skin temperature, and the mental state of the subject affect the parameters of SSR.
3. The latency and amplitude of SSR are measured.
4. The **amplitude of SSR in the hand is 1.6 mV** and that **in the feet is 2.1 mV.**
5. SSR is helpful in diagnosing multisystem atrophy, progressive autonomic failure, diabetes, uremia, and alcoholic neuropathy.

Thermoregulatory Sweat Test (TST)

Assessment of **sweating response to heat** also assesses sudomotor functions.
1. The subject's body temperature is raised by 1°C by exposing it to heat from an electric heater.
2. The sweating response is studied by demarcating the area of sweating with the help of either iodide starch or quinizarin powder, which change the colour of moist skin.
3. Absence of sweating in TST indicates **sympathetic pre- and post-ganglionic lesions**.

Quantitative Sudomotor Axon Reflex Test

Quantitative sudomotor axon reflex test (**QSART**) is a measure of regional autonomic function by acetylcholine (Ach)-induced sweating.
1. In this test, Ach is injected intradermally, and the sweat production rate is assessed.
2. The absence of or reduced sweating indicates a post-ganglionic lesion of sudomotor fibres (sympathetic fibres concerned with sweating).

Tests for Pupillary Functions

Pupillary function tests assess the function of the sympathetic nerve supplying the iris. Two tests are usually performed: the cocaine test and the adrenaline test.

Cocaine test

Dilation of the pupil is observed following the instillation of 4% cocaine in both eyes. Cocaine prevents the reuptake of norepinephrine at the adrenergic nerve endings. Therefore, the pupils dilate in response to cocaine. Horner's pupils, however, do not dilute.

Adrenaline test

Instillation of 1:100 or 1% noradrenaline in the eyes dilates the Horner's pupil more than the normal pupil. This is due to the mechanism of denervation hypersensitivity of the Horner's pupil.

Tests for Bladder Function

Cystometrogram (CMG) is performed to detect autonomic dysfunctions of the urinary bladder.
1. CMG reveals decreased ability of the bladder to accommodate urine.
2. The absence of accommodation to filling indicates autonomic dysfunction.
3. Also, contraction of the bladder muscle is poor in response to the act of micturition (evacuation).

Spectral Analysis of HRV and BRS

Recently, spectral analysis of **heart rate variability** (HRV) and **baroreflex sensitivity** (BRS) has evolved as a sensitive tool for assessing the integrity of sympathetic and parasympathetic functions, determining the **sympathovagal balance, and assessing CV risks** (details are given in the next two chapters).

Concept of Reactivity and Activity Tests and CAFTs

Reactivity tests

Tests that are based on stimuli or disturbances such as changes in position (standing/lying down), dipping the finger in cold water, handgrip against resistance, Valsalva maneuver, etc., are called **reactivity tests**. Accordingly, they are grouped as *sympathetic and parasympathetic reactivity tests.*

Activity tests

Tests that are performed without disturbing the subject (subject at rest—usually lying on a couch in a comfortable room for 15 to 20 minutes) are called **activity tests**.
1. Recording of resting HR and BP and HRV analysis are examples.
2. Accordingly, they are grouped as **sympathetic and parasympathetic activity tests**.
3. **Resting heart rate is a parasympathetic test,** and **resting BP is a sympathetic test.**

Conventional autonomic function tests (CAFTs)

HR and BP response to standing, HR response to deep breathing, isometric handgrip, cold pressor test, and Valsalva maneuver are routinely considered as CAFTs.

QT-QS$_2$ Ratio

This test was used in the past as part of the determination of **systolic time interval** (STI). It is an **index of the sympathetic function** of the heart.

Procedure

1. Ask the subject to lie down on the couch and relax. Attach the ECG leads and place the contact microphone on the carotid artery to record heart sounds (phonocardiogram).
2. Record lead II of the ECG and PCG simultaneously at a paper speed of 50 mm/sec.
3. Measure QT interval from the beginning of the QRS complex to the end of the T wave.
4. Measure QS$_2$ from the beginning of QRS to the first major vibration of the aortic component of the 2nd heart sound in PCG.
5. Determine the QT/QS$_2$ ratio.

Interpretation

QS$_2$ is the total **electromechanical systolic interval**. A high value indicates a greater sympathetic tone, while a low value represents low sympathetic tone.

VIVA

1. *What are the divisions of ANS? What are their general functions?* (Ans. Refer to page 246, under the heading 'Introduction'.)
2. *What are the organisations of preganglionic and postganglionic fibres in the sympathetic and parasympathetic systems?* (Ans. Refer to page 246, under the heading 'Functional Anatomy'.)
3. *What are the functions of the sympathetic and parasympathetic divisions of the ANS?* (Ans. Refer to page 246, under the heading 'Physiological considerations'.)
4. *List the classical or conventional autonomic function tests (CAFT).* (Ans. Refer to page 246, under the heading 'Autonomic Function Tests'.)
5. *Name the sympathetic and parasympathetic function tests.* (Ans. Refer to page 246, under the heading 'Classification of AFTs'.)
6. *How do you assess cardiovascular response to standing? Why is the 30:15 ratio significant?* (Ans. Refer to page 247, under the heading 'HR and BP Response to Standing'.)
7. *What is the significance of the cardiovascular response to standing?* (Ans. Refer to page 250, under the heading 'HR and BP Response to Standing'.)
8. *What are the precautions taken for testing cardiovascular response to standing?* (Ans. Refer to page 247, under the heading 'HR and BP Response to Standing' and the subheading 'Precautions'.)
9. *How do you assess cardiovascular response to passive tilting?* (Ans. Refer to page 247, under the heading 'HR and BP Response to Passive Tilting'.)
10. *What is the difference between cardiovascular response to standing and cardiovascular response to passive tilting?* (Ans. Refer to page 247, under the heading 'HR and BP Response to Passive Tilting'.)
11. *What is the Valsalva ratio? What is its significance?* (Ans. Refer to page 248, under the heading 'Valsalva Ratio'.)
12. *How is the Valsalva ratio calculated? What is the normal value of the Valsalva ratio in different age groups?* (Ans. Refer to page 248, under the heading 'Valsalva Ratio' and the subheading 'Calculation...Normal Values'.)
13. *What are the clinical applications of Valsalva ratio?* (Ans. Refer to page 248, under the heading 'Valsalva Ratio' and the subheading 'Clinical Application'.)
14. *What is the principle and procedure for the Valsalva maneuver?* (Ans. Refer to page 248, under the heading 'Valsalva Ratio' and the subheadings 'Principle' and 'Procedure'.)
15. *What are the precautions taken while performing the Valsalva maneuver?* (Ans. Refer to page 248, under the heading 'Valsalva Ratio' and the subheading 'Precautions'.)
16. *How do you assess heart rate variations with deep breathing? What is the principle of this test?* (Ans. Refer to page 251, under the heading 'Valsalva Ratio' and the subheading 'Clinical Application'.)
17. *What is the normal value of deep breathing difference (DBD) and E:I ratio in different age groups?* (Ans. Refer to page 251, under the heading 'Heart Rate Response to Deep Breathing', Tables 37.1 and 37.2.)
18. *What is sinus arrhythmia?* (Ans. Refer to page 248, under the heading 'Heart Rate Response to Deep Breathing'.)
19. *What are the conditions that alter DBD?* (Ans. Refer to page 250, under the heading 'Clinical Conditions with abnormalities of DBD'.)
20. *What is the isometric handgrip test? Explain its principle and procedure.* (Ans. Refer to page 249, under the heading 'BP response to Isometric Handgrip'.)
21. *How are the results of the isometric handgrip test interpreted?* (Ans. Refer to page 252, under the heading 'BP response to Isometric Handgrip'.)

22. *What is the cold pressure test? What is its significance?* (Ans. Refer to pages 249 and 252, under the heading 'Cold Pressor Test'.)
23. *What is sympathetic skin response (SSR)? What is its significance?* (Ans. Refer to pages 250 and 252, under the heading 'Sympathetic Skin Response'.)
24. *Name the tests for sudomotor functions.* (Ans. Refer to page 253, under the heading 'Tests for Sudomotor Functions')
25. *What is QSART? What is its significance?* (Ans. Refer to page 253, under the heading 'Quantitative Sudomotor Axon Reflex Test'.)
26. *What are the tests for pupillary functions?* (Ans. Refer to page 253, under the heading 'Tests for Pupillary Functions'.)
27. *What are the reactivity and activity tests of CAFT?* (Ans. Refer to page 253, under the heading 'Concept of Reactivity and Activity'.)
28. *What is QT/QS2 ratio? What is its physiological significance?* (Ans. Refer to page 254, under the heading 'QT/QS2 ratio'.)
29. *What is the most sensitive AFT?*
    (Ans. Spectral analysis of heart rate variability (HRV) is the most sensitive AFT. LF–HF ratio of HRV indicates sympathovagal balance. However, HRV is not an accurate test, especially for the diagnosis of autonomic dysfunctions. HRV helps in the prediction of future cardiovascular (CV) problems and is used for CV risk stratification.)
30. *What are the best sympathetic AFTs?*
    (Ans. BP response to IGH, SSR, and QSART are the best sympathetic function tests. However, BP response to IHG is considered to be the best among these due to its consistency, ease of recording, and reproducibility.)
31. *What is the best parasympathetic AFT?*
    (Ans. HR response to deep breathing is the best parasympathetic function test. Resting heart is a good index of vagal tone.)

38 | Spectral Analysis of Heart Rate Variability

Learning Objectives

After completing this practical, you will be able to (MUST KNOW):

1. Define and explain heart rate variability (HRV).
2. List the different indices (time domain and frequency domain) of HRV.
3. State the physiological importance of each HRV index.
4. Explain the principle of HRV recording.
5. Explain the concept of sympathovagal balance.
6. Explain the importance of HRV in health and disease.

You may also be able to (DESIRABLE TO KNOW):

1. Describe the different methods of HRV measurement.
2. Explain the time domain and frequency domain indices of HRV.
3. State the importance of HRV recording in assessing sympathovagal balance.
4. Explain the significance of HRV recording from other autonomic function tests.
5. Explain the clinical utility of HRV analysis.

INTRODUCTION

Heart rate variability (HRV) is the cardiac beat-to-beat variation (variation in cardiac cycle length), a physiological phenomenon that primarily occurs due to variations in cardiac activity during the respiratory cycle (**respiratory sinus arrhythmia**) at rest, though the circadian rhythm, environmental factors, and exercise also contribute to it. Variation in cardiac cycle length (the physiological basis of HRV) will be appreciated from the presentation of 2.5 seconds of heartbeat recordings, as depicted in Fig. 38.1.

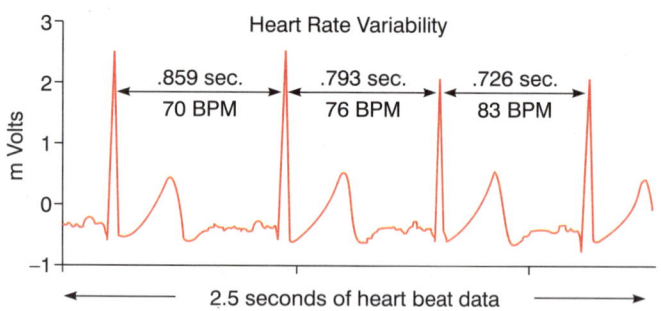

Fig. 38.1 Variation in cardiac cycle length during heartbeats, as presented in three consecutive beats here.

Resting heart rates can vary—it is 100 beats/min for some and only 60 beats/min for others for no obvious reason. The rate of the heart and its beat-to-beat variations are dependent on the *rate of discharge of the primary pacemaker, the SA node*, which is influenced by autonomic activities that are controlled in a complex way by a variety of reflexes, central irradiations, and cortical factors. As SA nodal discharge is largely controlled by parasympathetic (vagal) influence and sinus arrhythmia is primarily due to alterations in vagal tone in inspiration and expiration, **HRV is mainly influenced by vagal activity**, though both the divisions of ANS influence it. Recently, HRV has been proposed as the most sensitive indicator of autonomic function, especially for the assessment of sympathovagal balance, the balance between the sympathetic and parasympathetic activity at any given time. The state of **sympathovagal balance** is used to predict several cardiovascular (CV) dysfunctions and other dysfunctions affecting cardiovascular function; its foremost application is in *CV risk stratification*. However, the use of HRV analysis is limited in the diagnosis and management of CV and other diseases.

Technical Aspects

HRV can be **quantified in two domains: the time and frequency domains**. The time domain measures include the usual tools of assessment of variation, as is performed in statistics. Though the time domain is easier to assess, the finer aspects of variations cannot be appreciated. In a short period, the overall magnitude of HRV is assessed well, but the individual contributions of various factors are not elucidated.

On the other hand, variations in instantaneous heart rate can be **assessed spectrally**. That is, **an R–R tachogram** is plotted using the R–R intervals in the five-minute lead II ECG. The R–R tachogram is considered as a non-periodic signal which is transformed to its frequency spectrum using the **Fast Fourier Transform (FFT) algorithm or autoregressive (AR) modelling**. The biggest advantage of this complex mathematical transformation is that the distribution of the magnitude of variation in different frequency bands corresponds to the activity of different physiological systems. The entire frequency spectrum, 0.0 – 0.4 Hz, is divided as follows.

HRV components

The power spectrum of HRV in mammals usually reveals **three spectral components** (Fig. 38.2):

1. A high-frequency band (HF): 0.15–0.4 Hz
2. A low-frequency band (LF): 0.04–0.15 Hz
3. A very low-frequency band (VLF): 0.0–0.04 Hz

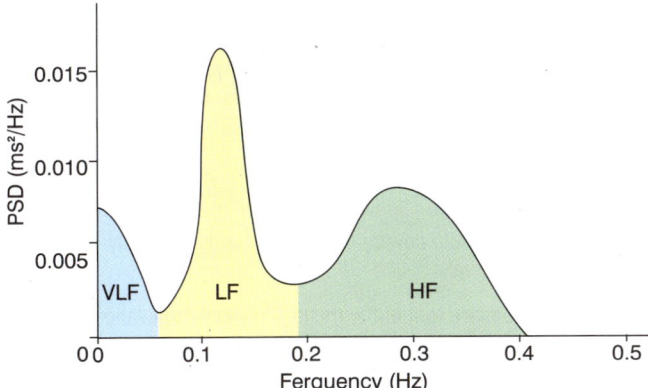

Fig. 38.2 Distribution of VLF, LF, and HF in the HRV power spectrum. Note that in this picture, the TP was 920 ms^2, of which VLF was 70 ms^2, LF was 400 ms^2, and HF was 450 ms^2.

The **HF component** is caused by *vagal activity during the respiratory cycle*. The inspiratory inhibition of vagal activity is evoked centrally in the cardiovascular centre. This explains why the heart rate fluctuates with respiratory frequency. In addition, peripheral reflexes arising from thoracic stretch receptors contribute to this so-called respiratory sinus arrhythmia (RSA). RSA is clearly abolished by atropine or vagotomy, and the power of the HF component is used as an index of **vagal modulation of cardiac function**.

The **LF component** of HRV is characterised by an oscillatory pattern with a duration of 10 seconds. This rhythm originates from self-oscillation in the vasomotor part (*sympathetic component*) of the baroreflex loop because of negative feedback and is commonly associated with synchronous fluctuations in blood pressure, the so-called **Mayer waves**. Though LF component mainly represents cardiac *sympathetic drive*, it has some parasympathetic contribution.

The **VLF component** accounts for all other heart rate changes, including those associated with *thermoregulation and humoral* (especially, the renin–angiotensin mechanism) and local factors.

Power Spectrum Analysis of HRV

The power spectrum of HRV is analysed by **two methods**: FFT and AR modelling.

Fast Fourier Transform

Any non-periodic electrophysiological signal can be described as the **sum of sine waves**. This decomposition

is called the **Fast Fourier Transform (FFT)**. The FFT is an efficient algorithm, which, with some improvements and modifications, is still in use in many applications, such as voice analysis, vibration studies, and analysis of short-term HRV (SHRV). FFT algorithms impose some constraints on the signal to be analysed because an evenly sampled, infinite, stationary time series is required.

Autoregressive modelling

An alternative method to the FFT is the autoregressive (AR) identification algorithm combined with power spectral estimation for the assessment of SHRV. This method fits the data to a previously defined model and estimates the parameters of the model. The power spectrum implied by the model is then computed.

FFT and AR modelling share a common goal—the estimation of the power spectrum of a signal. FFT-based methods are also called non-parametric methods because the time domain prior to spectral analysis is greatly simplified.

The **FFT and AR algorithms** are the most commonly used tools to study the SHRV. The final step in SHRV analysis is the application of power spectrum estimation methods to *characterise the frequency components* associated with vagal and/or sympathetic outflow. AR methods are parametric because they require prior information of the system under study. Thus, it was suggested that **FFT-based methods are still the best choice** for the assessment of SHRV in comparative studies, where no previous knowledge of the system is available. In addition, FFT algorithms are readily available in many languages, even in commercial statistical packages. Once the basic spectral content of the system is known and an initial model of the signal can be formulated, AR algorithms should be a better choice because they provide better frequency resolution and avoid the problems of spectral leakage.

The **electrocardiogram** (ECG) is the **most appropriate** signal to study SHRV because it offers the most accurate representation of electrical cardiac events. In particular, the QRS complex of the ECG *sharply defines the onset of ventricular electrical depolarization* and is the closest approach used to time the occurrence of pacemaker potentials, which in turn are modulated by the autonomic outflow.

HRV Indices

HRV analysis has two components: time domain and frequency domain. The HRV assessed by calculating indices is based on statistical operations on R–R intervals (**time domain analysis**) or by spectral analysis of an array of R–R intervals (**frequency domain analysis**). Both methods require accurate timing of R waves. The analysis can be performed on short ECG segments (lasting 0.5–5 minutes) or on 24-hour ECG recordings. The analysis of five to ten minutes of an ECG recording is called short-term HRV and of the 24-hour ECG recording is called long-term HRV.

Time domain analysis

Two types of HRV indices are distinguished in time domain analysis. Beat-to-beat or **short-term variability (STV)** indices represent fast changes in heart rate. **Long-term variability (LTV)** indices are slower fluctuations (fewer than 6 per minute). Both types of indices are calculated from the R–R intervals occurring in a chosen time window (usually between 0.5 and 5 minutes). An example of a simple STV index is the standard deviation (SD) of beat-to-beat R–R interval differences within the time window. Examples of LTV indices are the SD of all the R–R intervals, or the difference between the maximum and minimum R–R interval length within the window.

With calculated heart rate variability indices, *respiratory sinus arrhythmia contributes to STV*. In addition, the *baroreflex- and thermoregulation-related heart rate variability contributes to LTV*.

Frequency domain analysis

Since spectral analysis was introduced as a method to study heart rate variability, an increasing number of investigators have preferred this method over time domain analysis for calculating heart rate variability indices. The main **advantage of the spectral analysis** of signals is that one can study the **signal's frequency-specific oscillations**. Thus, both the amount of variability and the oscillation frequency (number of heart rate fluctuations per second) can be obtained. Spectral analysis involves decomposing the series of sequential R–R intervals into a **sum of sinusoidal functions of different amplitudes and frequencies** by the FFT algorithm. The result can be displayed (power spectrum) with the magnitude of variability as a function of frequency. Thus, the **power spectrum reflects** the amplitude of the heart rate fluctuations present at **different oscillation frequencies**.

Measurement of HRV

Time domain methods

The variation in heart rate may be evaluated by a number of methods. Perhaps the simplest assessments to perform are the time domain measures. In these methods, either the **heart rate** at any point in time or the **intervals between successive normal complexes** are determined. In a continuous ECG record, each QRS complex is detected, and the so-called normal-to-normal **(N–N) intervals** (all intervals between adjacent QRS complexes resulting from sinus node depolarization or in the instantaneous heart

rate) are determined. Simple **time domain variables** that can be calculated include: i) the mean N–N interval, ii) mean heart rate, iii) difference between the longest and shortest N–N interval, iv) the difference between night and day heart rates and so on. Selected time domain measures of HRV are listed in Table 38.1.

Table 38.1 Selected time domain measures of HRV.

Variable	Description	Physiological significance
SDNN (ms)	Standard deviation of all normal-to-normal (NN) intervals.	Overall vagal modulation of cardiac functions from beat to beat
SDRR (ms)	Standard deviation of RR intervals	Same as SDNN
RMSSD (ms)	Square root of the mean of the sum of the squares of the differences between adjacent NN intervals	Vagal modulation of cardiac functions on short-term basis
SDNN index (ms)	Mean of the standard deviations of all NN intervals for all 5-minute segments of the entire recording	Same as SDNN
NN50 count	Number of pairs of adjacent NN intervals differing by more than 50 ms in the entire recording	Short-term variability of vagal modulation
HR max – HR min (bpm)	Average difference between the highest and lowest heart rates during each respiratory cycle	Cardiac vagal modulation
pNN50 (%)	NN50 count divided by the total number of all NN intervals	Short-term variability of vagal modulation
TINN (ms)	Baseline width of the RR interval histogram	Vagal modulation of cardiac function

Statistical methods

From a series of instantaneous heart rates or cycle intervals, particularly those recorded over longer periods, traditionally 24 hours, more complex statistical time domain measures can be calculated. These may be divided into two classes: i) Those *derived from direct measurements of the N–N intervals* or instantaneous heart rate and ii) those *derived from the differences between N–N intervals*. These variables may be derived from the analysis of the total ECG recording or may be calculated using smaller segments of the recording period.

The **most commonly used measures** derived from interval differences include: i) **SDNN**, the standard deviation of all N-N intervals; ii) **RMSSD**, the square root of the mean squared differences of successive N–N intervals; iii) **NN50**, the number of interval differences of successive N–N intervals greater than 50 ms; and iv) **pNN50**, the proportion derived by dividing NN50 by the total number of N–N intervals (Table 38.1). All these measurements of short-term variation estimate high-frequency variations in heart rate and are thus highly correlated.

Geometrical methods

A series of **N–N intervals** can also be converted into a geometric pattern, such as the sample density distribution of N–N interval durations, the sample density distribution of the difference between adjacent N–N intervals, Lorenz plot of N–N or R–R intervals, and so on. A simple formula that judges the variability based on the geometric and/or graphic properties of the resulting pattern is used.

HRV triangular index measurement is the integral of the density distribution (that is, the number of all N–N intervals) divided by the maximum of the density distribution. The **main advantage** of the geometric methods lies in *their relative insensitivity to the analytical quality of the series of N–N intervals*. The **main disadvantage** of this method is the need for a *reasonable number of N–N intervals to construct* the geometric pattern.

The methods expressing overall HRV and its long- and short-term components cannot replace each other. The selection of the method used should correspond to the aim of each particular study.

Frequency domain methods

Various spectral methods for the analysis of the tachogram have been applied since the late 1960s. **Power spectral density (PSD) analysis** provides the basic information about how *power (variance) is distributed as a function of frequency*. Independent of the method used, only an estimate of the true PSD of the signal can be obtained by proper mathematical algorithms.

Methods to calculate PSD may be generally classified as **non-parametric and parametric**. In most instances, both methods provide comparable results.

The advantages of the non-parametric methods are: i) the simplicity of the algorithm used (FFT in most cases and ii) the high processing speed.

The advantages of parametric methods are: i) smoother spectral components that can be distinguished independently of pre-selected frequency bands, ii) easy post-processing of the spectrum with automatic calculation of low- and high-frequency power components and easy identification of the central frequency of each component, and iii) an accurate estimation of PSD even on a small number of samples on which the signal is supposed to remain stationary.

The **basic disadvantage** of parametric methods is the need for verification of the suitability of the chosen model and of its complexity (that is, the order of the model).

Selected frequency domain measures of HRV are listed in Table 38.2.

Table 38.2   Selected frequency domain measures of HRV.

Variable	Frequency range	Description analysis of short-term recordings (5 minutes)	Physiological significance
TP (ms^2)	Approximately <0.4 Hz	The variance of NN intervals over the temporal segment	Overall vagal potency of cardiac modulation, i.e., the heart rate variability
ULF power (ms^2)	≤0.003 Hz	Absolute power of the ultra-low-frequency band	Circadian rhythms may be the primary driver of this rhythm Core body temperature, metabolism, and RAS may also contribute
VLF (ms^2)	0–0.04 Hz	Power in very low-frequency range	Integrity of the renin–angiotensin system
LF (ms^2)	0.04–0.15 Hz	Power in low-frequency range	Primarily, the cardiac sympathetic drive
LF-normalised (LFnu)		LF power in normalised units LF/ (Total power – VLF) x 100	Cardiac sympathetic modulation independent of other powers of modulation
HF (ms^2)	0.15–0.4 Hz	Power in high-frequency range	Cardiac parasympathetic drive
HF-normalised (HFnu)		HF power in normalised units HF/ (Total Power – VLF) x 100	Cardiac parasympathetic modulation, independent of other powers of HRV
LF/HF		Ratio LF [ms^2] / HF [ms^2]	Sympathovagal balance

TP: total power; nu: normalised unit.

Spectral Components of Frequency Domain

Short-term recordings

Three main spectral components are distinguished in a spectrum calculated from short-term recordings of 5 to 10 minutes: **VLF, LF, and HF**. The distribution of the power and the central frequency of LF and HF are not fixed but may vary in relation to changes in autonomic modulations of the heart period. The physiological explanation of the **VLF component** is less clearly defined, and the existence of a specific process attributable to these heart period changes might even be questioned. The non-harmonic component, which does not have coherent properties and is affected by algorithms of baseline or trend removal, is commonly accepted as a major constituent of VLF. Thus, VLF assessed from short-term recordings (≤5 minutes) is a *dubious measure and should be avoided* when the PSD of short-term ECGs is interpreted.

The measurement of VLF, LF, and HF power components is usually made in **absolute values of power** (milliseconds squared). LF and HF may also be *measured in normalised units*, which represent the relative value of each power component in proportion to the total power minus the VLF component (Table 38.2). The representation of LF and HF in normalised units (**LFnu and HFnu**) emphasises the controlled and balanced behaviour of the two branches of the autonomic nervous system. Moreover, the normalisation tends to *minimise the effect of the changes in total power* on the values of LF and HF components. Nevertheless, *normalised units should always be quoted with absolute values* of LF and HF power in order to describe completely *the distribution of power* in spectral components. The **LF–HF ratio** provides a *better indicator of spectral powers*. Frequency domain measures are summarised in Table 38.2.

Long-term recordings

Spectral analysis may also be used to analyse the sequence of N–N intervals of the entire *24-hour period*, recorded by **Holter monitoring**. The result then includes an *ultra-low frequency (ULF) component*, in addition to the VLF, LF, and HF components. The slope of the 24-hour spectrum can also be assessed on a log–log scale by linear fitting the spectral values. The 24-hour long-term HRV analysis is a **robust method of detecting** autonomic dysfunctions, existing and impending CV risks and cardiac problems related to sympathovagal imbalance.

METHODS TO DETERMINE SPECTRAL INDICES OF HRV

Principle

Beat-to-beat variation in SA nodal discharge as recorded by ECG is computed and analysed by the software to determine the spectral indices of HRV

Requirements

1. All the equipment required for ECG recording
2. Computer with software for HRV analysis

Procedure

There are two **types of HRV recordings**: the short-term 5-minute HRV recording and the 24-hour (day–night) long-term HRV recording. As the **short-term HRV recording** is usually practised for research and clinical investigations, we shall describe its procedure as given in the Task Force Report on HRV.

1. Ask the subject to lie down comfortably in the supine position in the laboratory (5 minutes of rest).
2. Place the ECG electrodes on the subject's limbs and connect the leads to the machine for lead II ECG recording (Fig. 38.3).

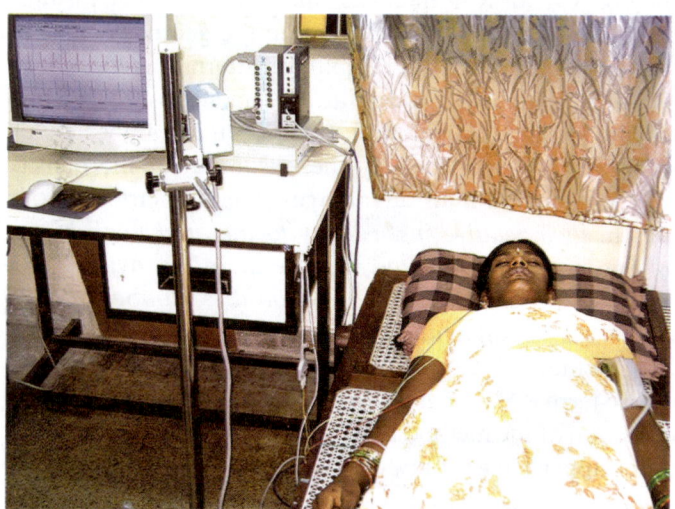

Fig. 38.3   System of short-term HRV recording. Note that the Lead II ECG signals are recorded at a rate of 1000 samples/second during supine rest using a data acquisition system (BIOPAC MP 100).

3. Acquire the ECG signals at a rate of 1000 samples/second during supine rest using a data acquisition system such as BIOPAC MP 100 (BIOPAC Inc., USA; minimum 250 Hz sampling rate).

Note: The raw ECG signal and the R–R intervals are acquired on a moving time base.

4. Transfer the data from BIOPAC to a Windows-based PC loaded with software for HRV analysis, such as Acknowledge 3.8.2 software.
5. Remove ectopic beats and artefacts from the recorded ECG.
6. Extract the R–R tachogram from the edited 256-second ECG using the R-wave detector in the AcqKnowledge software and save it in the ASCII format, which can later be used offline for short-term HRV analysis (the R–R tachogram should have a minimum of 288 R–R intervals; Fig. 38.4).
7. Perform HRV analysis using the HRV analysis software version 1.1 (Biosignal Analysis group, Finland).

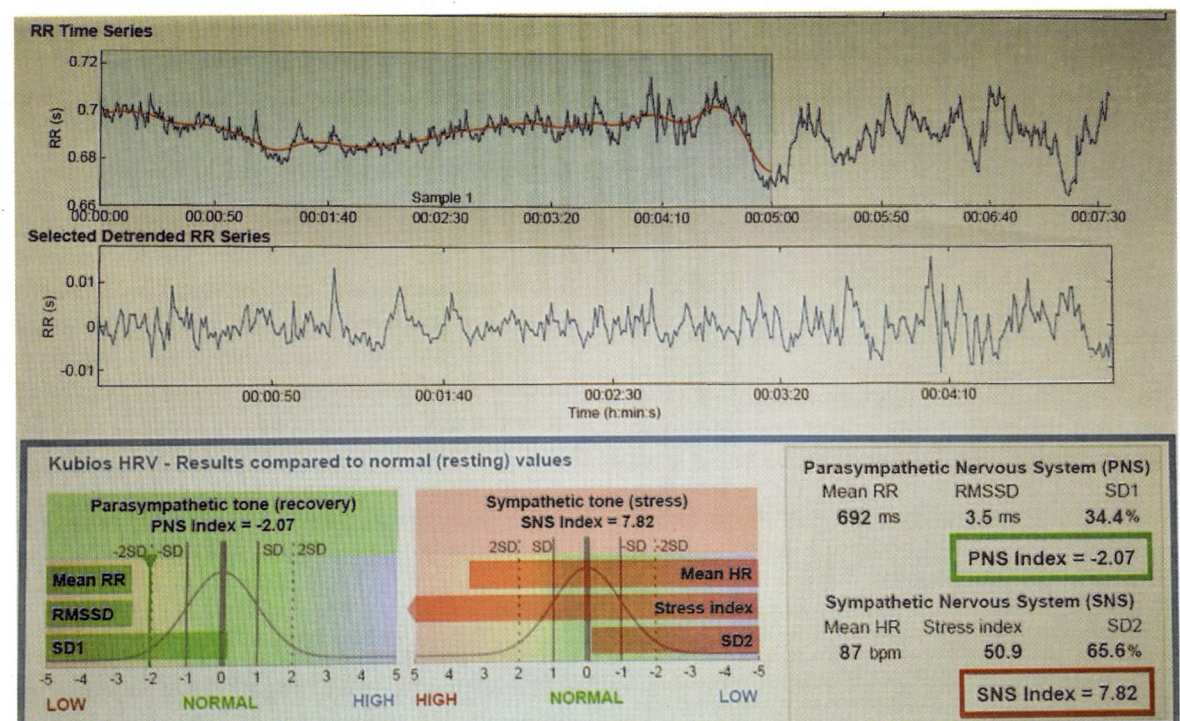

Fig. 38.4   R–R tachogram obtained from continuous ECG recordings for HRV analysis. Note that 300 R–R intervals (30 to 330) were selected from R–R interval time series (upper R–R tracing). Lower RR tracing represents selected R–R intervals. Also note the PNS index and SNS index of the parasympathetic and sympathetic drive respectively.

Note: Mean R–R is measured in second(s). Variance, defined as power in a portion of the total spectrum of frequencies, is measured in milliseconds squared (ms^2). Mean R–R is measured in seconds (s).

Different spectral indices (TP, LF, HF, LFnu, HFnu, and LF/HF ratio) and the time domain indices (mean R–R, SDNN and RMSSD) are calculated as described below.

Calculation of Time Domain Indices (TDI)

In a continuous ECG record, each QRS complex is detected, and the so-called normal-to-normal (N−N) intervals (that is, all intervals between adjacent QRS complexes resulting from sinus node depolarization) or instantaneous heart rate is determined. Simple time domain variables that are calculated include the **mean R–R**, standard deviation of normal-to-normal interval (**SDNN**), and square root of the mean squared differences of successive normal-to-normal intervals (**RMSSD**) of HRV.

Calculation of Frequency Domain Indices (FDI)

Frequency domain variables that are usually calculated include **total power (TP)**, low-frequency (**LF**) component, LF component expressed as normalised unit (**LFnu**), high-frequency (**HF**) component, HF component expressed as normalised unit (**HFnu**), and **LF/HF ratio**.

Normalising spectral powers are calculated by the following formulae:

1. $LFnu = LF/(TP - VLF) \times 100$
2. $HFnu = HF/(TP - VLF) \times 100$
3. LF/HF ratio = Ratio of LF to HF spectral powers

Precautions

1. The subject should eat a light breakfast if the recording is to be performed in the morning. The stomach should not be full and heavy.
2. The room temperature should be comfortable and constant for all recordings.
3. The subject should not have ingested coffee, tea, or soft drinks at least one hour prior to recording.
4. The subject should not have smoked or consumed alcohol two hours prior to recording.
5. The subject should not be disturbed throughout the recording.
6. All ectopics should be removed from the ECG tachogram.
7. Take all the precautions taken for ECG recording (refer to Chapter 26).

Observations, Analysis, Results, and Reporting

Meticulously study and analyse the entire recording of the HRV graph. Note the time domain and frequency domain results and assess the Poincaré plots (Fig. 38.5).

1. Assess the TP, which is the primary indicator of the overall spectral power of HRV.

2. Among TDI, note specifically the SDNN and RMSSD.
3. Among FDI, mainly note the absolute powers of LF (mainly sympathetic drive) and HF (vagal drive).
4. Note the LF/HF ratio (sympathovagal balance).
5. Assess the overall HRV indices and analyse whether the HRV indices are within the normal limit or if there is sympathetic or parasympathetic dominance.

> **Note:** As such, HRV data are highly variable in terms of age, gender, environment, region, religion, country, race, social and cultural factors, personality, stress level, training level, food habits and so on. Further, there are no normative data of HRV indices for reference. Therefore, always compare the recorded HRV data of the subject with the previous data of your own lab or with similar patients/population data, if it is available. Be careful about commenting on sympathetic and parasympathetic abnormalities just from your recordings. Always correlate them with the clinical findings of the subject and have a discussion with the clinician about the HRV report you have finalised.

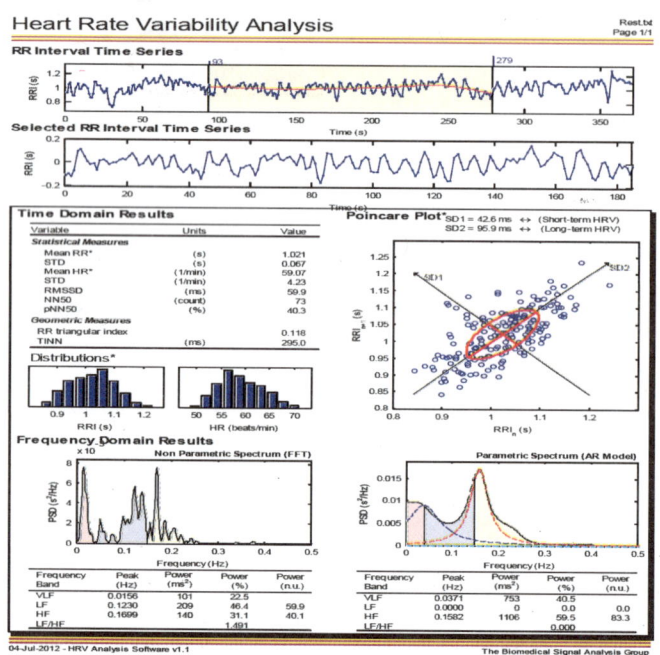

Fig. 38.5   Graph of the entire recording of HRV. Note the time domain and frequency domain results (parametric and non-parametric) and observe the Poincaré plots.

DISCUSSION

Physiological Significance

HRV analysis is used to precisely assess the efficiency of an individual's vagal control, as it reflects the heart rate variability that occurs mainly due to sinus arrhythmia. Due to inspiratory inhibition of the vagal tone, the heart rate shows fluctuations with a frequency similar to the respiratory rate. The inspiratory inhibition is evoked primarily by central irradiation of impulses from the medullary respiratory to the cardiovascular centre. Respiratory sinus arrhythmia can be abolished by atropine or vagotomy, as it is parasympathetically mediated.

HRV Analysis for the Assessment of Autonomic Functions

HRV, i.e., the degree of heart rate fluctuations around the mean heart rate, can be used as a mirror of the cardiorespiratory control system. It is a **valuable tool to investigate the sympathetic and parasympathetic functions** of the autonomic nervous system. SA nodal activity at any particular time is determined by the balance between vagal activity, which slows it, and sympathetic activity, which accelerates it.

Generally, if the *rate is lower than the intrinsic rate* of the pacemaker, it implies **predominant vagal activity**, while high heart rates are achieved by *increased sympathetic drive*.

Parasympathetic drive: The **HF component of HRV** indicates the **cardiac vagal drive of the individual**. Increased HF power (or more specifically, increased HFnu) represents increased vagal drive and **decreased HF power (decreased HFnu) represents decreased vagal drive to the heart**.

Sympathetic drive: The **LF component of HRV** mainly indicates **cardiac sympathetic drive of the individual**. **Increased LF power (or more specifically, increased LFnu) represents increased sympathetic drive,** while decreased LF power (decreased LFnu) represents decreased sympathetic drive.

Sympathovagal balance: The sympathovagal balance is assessed by the **LF–HF ratio**. Increased **LF–HF ratio reflects increased sympathetic activity**, while decreased LF–HF ratio indicates increased parasympathetic and decreased sympathetic activity.

- The relationship between **vagal stimulation** frequency and the resulting change in heart rate is hyperbolic. Changes in frequency at low heart rates have a much greater effect, which does not directly control the heart rate, but regulates the interval between successive beats. The *effect of vagal stimulation is rapid*. Vagal stimulation releases the neurotransmitter acetylcholine, which inhibits the pacemaker potentials.
- **Sympathetic responses** differ from vagal effects in that they develop *much more slowly*. Hence, *responses with longer latency* are likely to be mainly sympathetic.

HRV indirectly reflects sympathetic vascular function: Peripheral vascular resistance exhibits intrinsic oscillations with a low frequency. These oscillations can be influenced by thermal skin stimulation and are thought to arise from thermoregulatory peripheral blood flow adjustments. The **fluctuations in peripheral vascular resistance** are accompanied by *fluctuations with the same frequency in blood pressure and heart rate* and are mediated by the sympathetic nervous system. Hence, analysis of HRV also tacitly indicates the **tone of sympathetic outflow to blood vessels** and therefore implicitly reflects the individual's state of sympathetic function and susceptibility to sympathetic dysfunction.

Importance of LF–HF Ratio and Sympathovagal Balance

The HF component of HRV, which indicates the cardiac vagal drive to the heart, represents parasympathetic activity. The LF component of HRV, which mainly indicates the cardiac sympathetic drive, represents sympathetic activity.

- In healthy individuals, **HF constitutes about 60%** and LF constitutes about 40% of the total power **(TP) of HRV.** Therefore, **LF–HF ratio less than 1 indicates good cardiovascular health**.
- **The normal value of LF–HF ratio** in the general population varies from **0.5 to 1.2.** Lower LF–HF ratio (<0.5) is observed in those who *regularly practice yoga and exercise*.
- LF–HF ratio depicts the status of sympathovagal balance or imbalance.

Higher LF–HF ratio: Increased LF–HF ratio reflects *increased sympathetic activity* and decreased vagal activity (Fig. 38.6), which is invariably associated with **decreased TP**.

Lower LF–HF ratio: Decreased LF–HF ratio indicates *increased parasympathetic activity* and decreased sympathetic activity, which is invariably associated with **increased TP** (Fig. 38.7).

Clinical Applications

Though there are considerable discussions and debates regarding the physiology of HRV, it is well-correlated and studied in many clinical and pathological conditions:

1. **Association of adverse CV events:** Among HRV indices, the **total power (TP) of HRV** indicates the magnitude of heart rate variability. **Decreased TP** (decreased overall cardiac vagal modulation) has been implicated with associated *adverse cardiovascular (CV) morbidities* and mortalities in many cardiac and non-cardiac diseases.
2. **Prognostic value:** Decreased HRV (decreased total power of HRV) is observed in many cardiovascular disease conditions and generally indicates a *poor prognosis* in these conditions.
3. **Prediction of CV health:** Much before the onset of clinical symptoms of cardiovascular disease, alterations are observed in HRV, indicating that HRV could be used as a *sensitive tool in the prediction of CV health*. However, more research is required to establish the predictive value of HRV in CV dysfunctions.
4. **Post-MI prognosis:** Presently, HRV is used as a prognostic tool in conditions like post-myocardial infarction and cardiac transplantation.
5. **Surveillance in DM and MI:** The most important application of HRV analysis is the surveillance of post-infarction heart failure and diabetic patients.
6. **HRV for autonomic function assessment in many diseases:** As HRV analysis is used to assess the state of sympathovagal balance of the individual, it could be used to assess autonomic dysfunctions that happen in many diseased conditions like prehypertension, hypertension, gestational hypertension, gestational diabetes, thyroid dysfunctions, anxiety disorders, psychiatry illness, and so on.
7. **HRV for risk stratification:** Decreased HRV is well correlated with the risk of developing CV morbidities and mortality in various diseases and the risk of sudden cardiac death in patients with heart diseases.
8. **HRV analysis as a research tool:** HRV provides information about the sympathetic–parasympathetic autonomic balance and is used as a tool for the assessment of autonomic dysfunctions in clinical research.
9. **Prediction for future development of diseases**: As HRV analysis is used to assess the subtle changes in the individual's sympathovagal balance long before the clinical manifestations of the disease appear, it could be used to determine an individual's vulnerability/susceptibility to later develop a disease in which autonomic dysfunction is the primary pathophysiology of the disease, such as pregnancy-induced hypertension, prehypertension, and hypertension.
10. **Promotive and preventive health:** Improvements in HRV and CV health are observed as a result of interventions like exercise, yoga, and relaxation exercises. This can be used in future research on holistic improvement of health.
11. **HRV biofeedback therapy:** In recent years, **heart rate variability biofeedback (HRVB)** has been widely used to improve cardiovascular health and well-being. Based on the principle of HRV, the HRVB is established on breathing at an individual's resonance frequency,

Frequency domain results

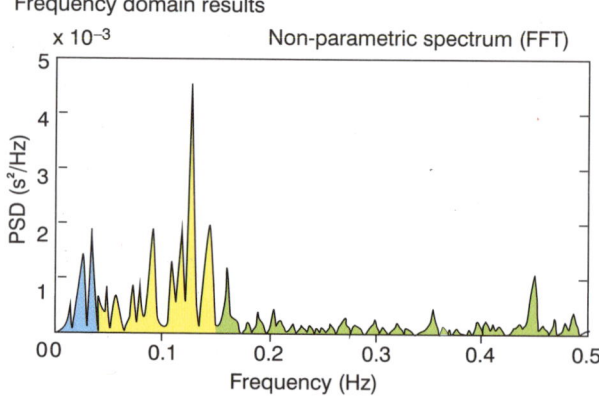

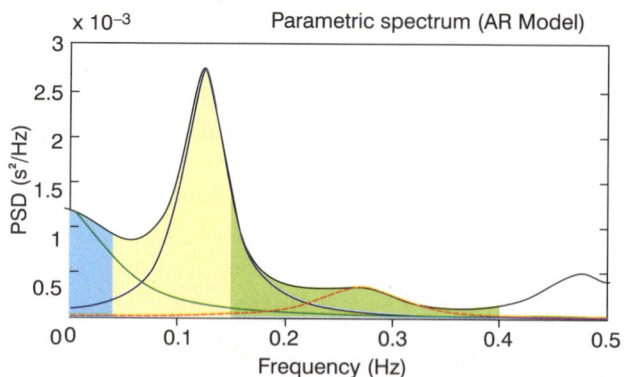

Frequency band	Peak (Hz)	Power (ms²)	Power (%)	Power (n.u.)
VLF	0.0332	22	15.4	
LF	0.1250	89	62.7	74.0
HF	0.1602	31	22.0	26.0
LF/HF			2.852	

Frequency band	Peak (Hz)	Power (ms²)	Power (%)	Power (n.u.)
VLF	0.0000	61	21.1	
LF	0.1270	189	65.9	64.6
HF	0.2734	37	13.0	12.7
LF/HF			5.077	

Fig. 38.6 Frequency domain indices of the HRV analysis of a subject having increased sympathetic activity. Refer Fig. 37.2 for PSD of VLF, LF, and HF of HRV. Note that as depicted in the parametric spectrum, the LF power (ms²) is significantly increased (189 ms²) compared to the HF power, which is grossly reduced (37 ms²), and the LF–HF ratio is increased to 5.077. Also, the total power is only 287 (VLF 61 + LF 189 + HF 37).

Frequency domain results

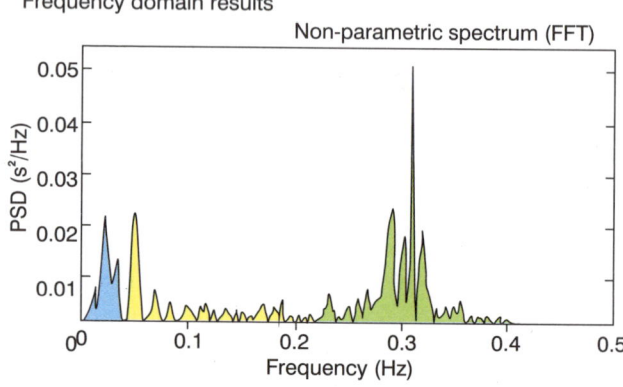

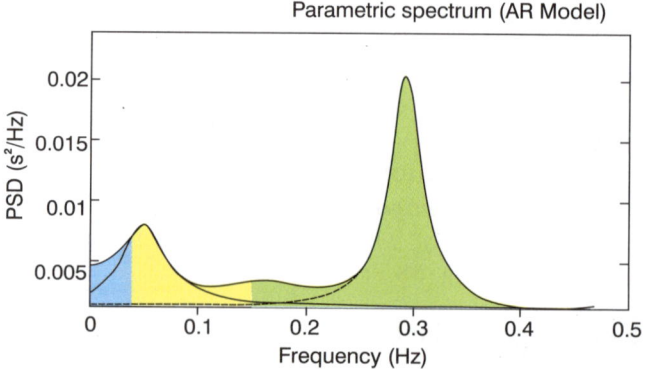

Frequency band	Peak (Hz)	Power (ms²)	Power (%)	Power (n.u.)
VLF	0.0254	247	15.2	
LF	0.0527	312	19.2	22.7
HF	0.3145	1063	65.5	77.3
LF/HF			0.293	

Frequency band	Peak (Hz)	Power (ms²)	Power (%)	Power (n.u.)
VLF	0.0000	0	0.0	
LF	0.0508	557	30.0	28.4
HF	0.3105	1301	70.0	66.3
LF/HF			0.428	

Fig. 38.7 Frequency domain indices of HRV analysis of a subject with high parasympathetic activity. Refer to Fig. 37.2 for PSD of VLF, LF, and HF of HRV. Note that as depicted in the parametric spectrum, HF power (ms²) is significantly increased (1301 ms²) as compared to the LF power, which is much less (557 ms²) and the LF–HF ratio is decreased to 0.428. Also, the total power is 1858 (VLF 0 + LF 557 + HF 1305), which is quite high and reflects increased HRV, an indicator of good CV health.

which stimulates respiratory sinus arrhythmia (RSA) and the baroreflex. HRVB is found to be useful in the management of in stress, anxiety disorders, depression, sleep disorders, cognitive deficiency, and chronic pain, and in improving CV health, memory, and emotional balance.

The clinical applicability is still limited due to the lack of established normative data of HRV for different age, gender, and ethnic groups because of its demanding technical and mathematical comprehensibility. However, with increasing use of automation and computers in medicine, the clinical applicability of HRV is bound to increase rapidly.

Limitations of HRV Analysis

1. HRV data **do not provide a concrete direction for the diagnosis** of a disease. They are mainly used as adjunctive investigations for quality of autonomic dysfunctions. HRV analysis must be done along with conventional autonomic tests (CAFTS) to know the quantitative deficiency in autonomic function.

2. **LF and LFnu are not pure sympathetic tests.** Other sympathetic markers such as increased LF-HF ratio should be analysed and correlated with CAFT sympathetic test results (e.g., handgrip test).

3. The report of HRV data **should be correlated clinically** and discussed with the clinician to confirm the nature and quantum of autonomic deficiencies.

4. HRV data are **highly variable** because they are influenced by age, gender, adiposity, environment, race, social and cultural factors, personality, stress level, training level, food habits, sleep habits, etc. Therefore, if HRV is a parameter in a research study, the **sample size of the group should be very large**, ideally 500 or above. The control group should be well-matched, especially for age and gender, with the study group.

5. Since numerous **HRV datasets are non-parametric** and non-linear due to 'SD values' often being more than 'Means', appropriate statistical tests should be employed for data analysis.

6. HRV data are **mainly used for prognostic and predictive purposes.** Interpretation of data for diagnostic means should be done very carefully.

7. As there are **no standard normative data** for HRV indices, the data of a patient's investigation should be corroborated with other data of the same lab.

8. Data of **short-term HRV should not be used for predictive purposes** because ECG recording for 5 minutes in supine rest virtually does not reveal much information of the cardiovascular oscillations and variations, especially to routine stressors. Long-term HRV recording (at least for 12 hours) by Holter monitoring is a better indicator for the prediction of CV risks.

VIVA

1. *What do you mean by HRV? What is its physiological importance?* (**Ans.** Refer to page 256, under the heading 'Introduction'.)
2. *What is sinus arrhythmia? What is its contribution to HRV?* (**Ans.** Refer to page 256, under the heading 'Introduction'.)
3. *What are the frequency distribution curves in HRV as recorded in a parametric spectrum (AR model)?* (**Ans.** Refer to page 257, under the heading 'Autoregressive Modelling'.)
4. *What are the time domain and frequency domain indices of HRV?* (**Ans.** Refer to page 258; see Tables 38.1 and 38.2.)
5. What do the time domain and frequency domain indices of HRV represent? (**Ans.** Refer to page 259, see Tables 38.1 and 38.2.)
6. *What are the methods of HRV measurement?* (**Ans.** Refer to page 260, under the heading 'Measurements of HRV'.)
7. *What is the basic principle and procedure of HRV recording?* (**Ans.** Refer to page 260, under the heading 'Methods'.)
8. *What are the pre-recording instructions given to the subject before performing HRV investigations?* (**Ans.** Refer to page 261, under the heading 'Precaution'.)
9. *What is the importance of HFnu?* (**Ans.** Refer to page 259-260, under the heading 'Short-term recordings'.)
10. *How is the normalisation done for LF and HF?* (**Ans.** Refer to page 261, under the heading 'Calculation of frequency domain indices'.)
11. *What is the importance of LFnu?* (**Ans.** Refer to page 260, under the heading 'Short-term recordings'.)
12. *What are the advantages of parametric methods of frequency domain studies?* (**Ans.** Refer to page 259, under the heading 'Frequency Domain Methods' and the subheading 'Advantages of parametric methods'.)
13. *What is the LF–HF ratio? What is its importance?* (**Ans.** Refer to page 263, under the heading 'Importance of LF–HF ratio'.)
14. *What is sympathovagal balance? What is its importance in health and disease?* (**Ans.** Refer to page 263, under the heading 'Importance of LF–HF ratio and Sympathovagal Balance'.)
15. *What is the importance of TP of HRV? How does it predict the CV health of the individual?* (**Ans.** Refer to page 263, under the heading 'Clinical Application', No. 1 and 2.)
16. *What is the application of HRV analysis in clinical medicine?* (**Ans.** Refer to page 263, under the heading 'Clinical Application'.)
17. *What are the limitations of HRV analysis?* (**Ans.** Refer to page 264, under the heading 'Limitations of HRV Analysis'.)

39 | Blood Pressure Variability and Baroreflex Sensitivity

Learning Objectives

After completing this practical, you will be able to (MUST KNOW):
1. Understand the concept of blood pressure variability (BPV).
2. Learn the principle of measurement of BPV.
3. Apprehend the applications of BPV in health and disease.
4. Define baroreflex sensitivity (BRS) and state the normal values.

5. Explain the basic principle and method of BRS measurement.
6. Outline the role of BRS in assessing the CV health of an individual.

You may also be able to (DESIRABLE TO KNOW):
1. Describe the principle and application of BPV and BRS.
2. Appreciate the applications of BRS in clinical physiology and research.

BLOOD PRESSURE VARIABILITY

INTRODUCTION

Serial blood pressure variability (BPV) recorded by continuous pulse pressure tracing of arterial pressure waves provides non-stop evaluation of hemodynamic conditions and beat-to-beat variation in blood pressure (BP). Among non-invasive methods, **finger cuff technology** is considered to be the best because it provides continuous and non-invasive monitoring of BP and other hemodynamics parameters. The finger cuff method using Finapres is superior to others because it detects changes in cardiac preload, cardiac hemodynamics, cardiac output, and peripheral circulation in addition to beat-to-beat heart rate variability.

Physiological Aspects

Since spectral indices of BPV are useful in determining the **type, degree, and quality of disturbances** in various CV diseases, **Finapres recordings** have been established as the ***gold-standard in detecting hemodynamic turbulence*** in hypertension and circulatory disorders. The important CV parameters recorded in the latest version of Finapres are:
1. Heart rate and heart rate variability
2. Systolic blood pressure and its variability
3. Diastolic blood pressure and its variability
4. Mean arterial pressure and its variability
5. Mid-cardiac cycle pressure
6. Delta-systolic pressure
7. Rate pressure product
8. Stroke volume
9. Left-ventricular ejection time
10. Maximum slope of ejection
11. Cardiac output
12. Pulse interval (inter-beat interval)
13. Mid-interval and delta-interval
14. Total peripheral resistance
15. Baroreceptor-reflex sensitivity

Except for vessel diameter and wall thickness, ventricular wall thickness, and sizes of the cardiac chambers and orifices, Finapres records almost **all the hemodynamics parameters** required for studying functional abnormalities of the cardiovascular system. Among all the BPV parameters, **baroreceptor reflex sensitivity** (BRS) is considered the most vital one in the assessment of CV function and dysfunction and CV risks in health and various clinical disorders.

METHODS OF RECORDING BPV WITH FINAPRES

Developed in the early 1980s, Finapres (**FIN**ger Arterial **PRES**sure) records arterial pressure waveforms using a finger cuff. It measures arterial pressure waveform at the level of the finger using a finger cuff.
1. Since it provided a reliable, non-invasive measurement of the beat-to-beat blood pressure variation, it was widely appreciated.
2. The first-generation Finapres™ device was developed by Wesseling et al. based on the principle of the **volume-clamp method** developed by the Czech physiologist Jan Penaz.

Principle

Finapres measurement is based on the principle of 'development of the **dynamic or pulsatile unloading of the arterial walls of the finger** using an inflatable finger cuff with built-in **photoelectric plethysmograph**. The dynamic unloading is ensured by a **fast pneumatic servo system** and a **dynamic servo setpoint adjuster** that assure arterial unloading at zero transmural pressure and consequent full transmission of arterial blood pressure to cuff air pressure. Pressure pulse waveforms obtained from the arteries of the finger provide the derivation of parameters such as heart beats, pulse rate, cardiac output, systolic, diastolic and mean pressure from beat-to beat of cardiac pumping.

Procedure

1. Explain the procedure in detail and get the subject's consent. Take the subject's anthropometric measurements—height and weight. Ask the subject to lie down on a couch and rest for 10 minutes.
2. Connect the blood pressure cuff (arrow of the cuff over the brachial artery) and tie the front-end box over the wrist of the same arm (Fig. 39.1).
   - Use the cuff size guide to choose an appropriate finger cuff.
   - The appropriate cuff should be attached to the middle phalanx of any of the middle three fingers, preferably the middle finger.
   - If the cuff does not fit any of the middle three fingers, the thumb can be used.
3. First, connect the metal plug to the front-end box so that the red dot on the plug faces upwards; then, connect the air plug.
4. **Using the finometer:** Either Finapres or a finometer is used for BPV recording.
   - Switch on the finometer and the desktop. Select finometer research and press the 'Mark' button.
   - Click on 'Enter' to fill in the subject details/describe the subject using the buttons provided on the finometer. Enter the gender, age, height, and weight of the subject.
   - Click on 'Configure' and wait for the barometric pressure to buffer to around 800 mmHg.
   - Then choose height correction so that both brachial and finger height sensors are maintained at 0 cm when placed together; then press 'Mark' (either 0 or within +/−2).
5. Attach the brachial and finger sensors to the BP cuff and finger cuff respectively.
6. Go back to the finometer to 'Describe subject' and confirm.
7. **Using the software:** The most commonly used software is Beat-scope Easy.
   - Open the programme and press 'Start'. Enter the subject's id in the window and press 'Start'.
   - Click on/select the 'Physical & RTF cal' menu in the finometer and press 'Down' to come to step.
   - Wait for 2 minutes for the physiological calibration to run. After 2 minutes, press the same

button, following which, 'Return to Flow (RTF)' caliberation will be done.
   - Come back to the desktop and switch off the Physiocal and wait for a minute for it to switch on again; then, switch it off.
8. Start the timer and take recordings for a minimum of 10 minutes. After 10 minutes, press 'Stop' and wait for 30 seconds for the measurement to get stored.
   - Click File > Save to > Other location > choose a specific folder to save the measurements in.
   - Again click File > Export > BRS > Save to the same folder (label as BRS).
9. Disconnect the brachial and finger height sensors.
   - While disconnecting the finger cuff, first disconnect the air tube and then the metal tube.
   - Remove the finger cuff with care. Remove the front-end box and the BP cuff in that order.
   - Switch off the finometer by pressing down on both the arrow buttons simultaneously.
10. **Analysis:** Open the saved text document and copy the values onto an Excel sheet after removing the semicolons.
    - After Physiocal, the values of all the parameters are obtained by averaging all the values obtained. Similarly, perform the BRS analysis on another Excel sheet.

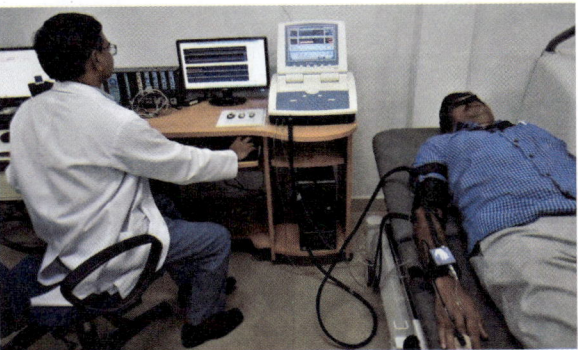

Fig. 39.1 Recording of blood pressure variability using Finapres with the subject in supine posture with the brachial cuff and finger cuff tied at the appropriate position. (*Courtesy:* Cardiovascular Research Lab, Physiology Dept., JIPMER, Puducherry, India.)

BAROREFLEX SENSITIVITY

INTRODUCTION

The integrity of the baroreceptor reflex or baroreflex sensitivity (BRS) reflects the status of sympathovagal balance or imbalance.

1. BRS assesses reciprocal increase of sympathetic activity and reduction of parasympathetic (vagal) activity, which is a precursor to the development of many CV diseases. Measurement of BRS is a **reliable tool for CV disease risk stratification**.

2. Assessment of BRS is also an ideal measure of the determination of **autonomic tone of CV functions** and circulatory homeostasis.

3. Therefore, BRS evaluation provides valuable information in clinical management, especially prognostic evaluation, risk stratification, and assessment of the treatment of various cardiac diseases.

BRS Definition and Calculation

BRS is defined as the **change in the inter-beat interval (IBI) in milliseconds per unit change in BP**. For example, when the BP rises by 10 mmHg and IBI increases by 100 ms, the BRS would be 100/100 = 10 ms/mmHg.

From this definition, it appears that there is no direct relation of BRS to the BP buffering capacity of the baroreflex; rather, it focuses more on the reflex effect on the sinus node. However, BRS accurately reflects the alteration in IBI that is the result of the influence of the parasympathetic and sympathetic tones or a combination thereof.

Physiological Basis and Importance of BRS

The baroreceptor reflex system plays a critical role in the short-term regulation of BP. Arterial baroreceptors, distributed in the walls of the carotid sinus and aortic arch, continuously provide information on alterations in blood pressure to the central nervous system.

Vago-sympathetic assessment

Baroreflex responses mediated by **vagal and sympathetic efferents** exhibit significant differences in the onset time and the delay in the execution of their effects.

- Following an immediate and considerable rise in arterial pressure, **parasympathetic activation occurs faster**. This produces an immediate response, usually between 200 and 600 ms. On the other hand, **cardiac and vasomotor sympathetic stimulation occur after a gap of 2–3 seconds**, and the peak effect of responses reaches more slowly.

- Also, *sympathetic-mediated alteration in venous return takes still longer* (more sluggish response) in fulfilling the baroreflex control of BP.

- Therefore, the potency of the baroreflex to control heart rate and BP on a beat-to-beat basis is mediated **principally through vagal activity** rather than through sympathetic activity.

- Further, baroreflex modulation of the heart rate is **greatly influenced by respiration**; the process is known as sinus arrhythmia.

- Inspiration decreases baroreceptor stimulation of vagal efferents (motoneurons) and expiration increases vagal activity (activates baroreceptor stimulation of vagal motoneurons). This is called **the respiratory gate of vagal** activity.

- Within the physiological limit of BP, baroreceptors constantly exert inhibitory effects on sympathetic efferent activity. Many neural, humoral, behavioural, and environmental factors influence the functioning of the baroreceptor reflex.

METHODS OF ASSESSING BRS

Principle

In the BPV method, the brachial artery pressure measured is the reconstructed pressure from finger pressure using generalised waveform inverse modelling and generalised level correction. Baroreceptor reflex sensitivity (BRS) and other cardiovascular parameters are measured continuously using the BPV method using Finapres, which employs the **volume-clamp technique developed by Penáz** and the **Physiocal criteria described by Wesseling**.

Procedure (in Brief)

If BRS is recorded by Finapres, the procedure of measurement is the same as that for blood pressure variability, as described above.

1. The subject is instructed to lie down on a couch for 15 minutes. Then, the brachial cuff of the Finapres is tied around at mid-arm level, 2 cm above the cubital fossa (Fig. 39.1).

   - A finger cuff of appropriate size (small, medium, or large) is tied around the middle phalanx of the middle finger, depending on the finger width. For **height correction**, two sensors are placed—one at the heart level and another at the finger level.

   - The BPV recording is obtained once the cables of the cuffs are connected to the Finometer, after a minimum of ten minutes of supine rest.

2. The '**return to flow calibration and the Physiocal**' is done for the level correction between the brachial and finger pressure during the initial 5 minutes of the recordings.

3. Following this, continuous BP recording is performed for a period of 10 minutes (Fig. 39.2).

4. The BRS is recorded as small, star-like, shining dots on the pressure-pulse wave tachogram.

Observation and Results

The important parameters obtained from the reconstructed brachial pressure tachogram include heart rate (HR), systolic BP, diastolic BP, mean arterial pressure (MAP), rate–pressure product (RPP), inter-beat interval, left ventricular ejection time (LVET), stroke volume, cardiac output, total peripheral resistance (TPR), baroreflex sensitivity (BRS), and many other cardiac parameters except data about the chamber wall thickness and valvular orifices.

1. Note the values of all the above-mentioned parameters.
2. Compare the BPV parameters (except BRS) with the values of standard normative data.
3. Compare BRS with normative values from your laboratory (as general normative data for BRS is not widely available).

4. Report the findings, particularly the BRS, as **normal** or **reduced**.

Normal values of BRS: Studies by G K Pal et al. and others from the Cardiovascular Lab, Department of Physiology, JIPMER, Puducherry, India, published from 2012–2024 and conducted on more than 2,500 subjects, have demonstrated that **BRS in the normal healthy** Indian population varies from **20–40 ms/mmHg** (Fig. 39.2). Values of **BRS between 14 and 19** are seen in pre-hypertension and prediabetes, as noted in the recording below (Fig. 39.3). **Values of 13 or less** are observed in diseased conditions and indicate a significant CV risk.

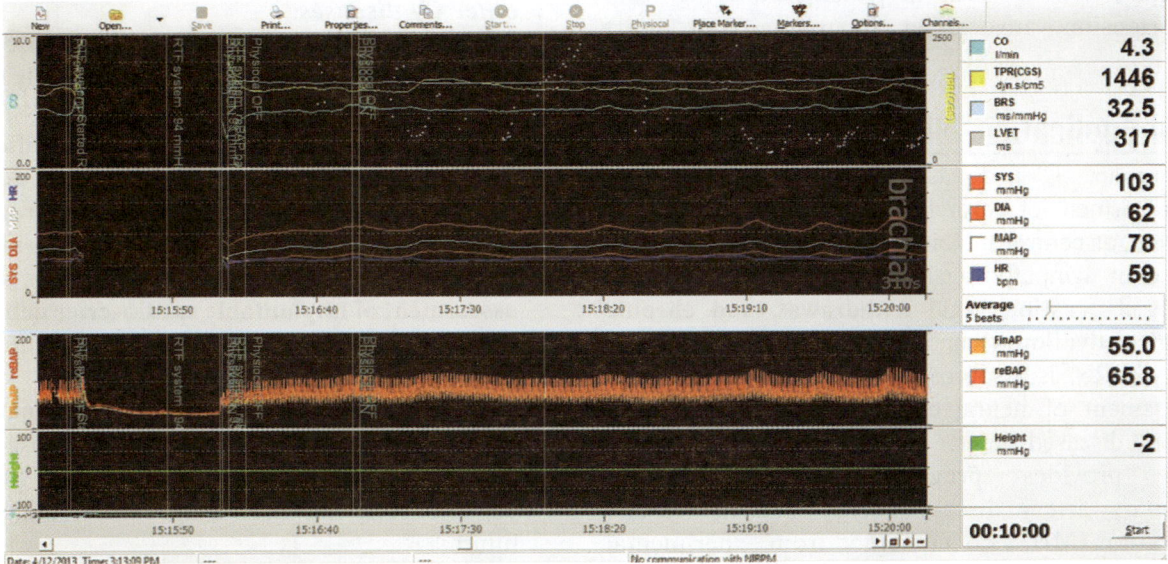

Fig. 39.2   BP variability recording by Finapres in a normal healthy (control) subject. Note that the SBP was 103 mmHg, DBP was 62 mmHg, and BRS was 32.5 ms/mmHg. BRS is recorded as small, star-like, shining dots on the pressure-pulse wave tachogram.

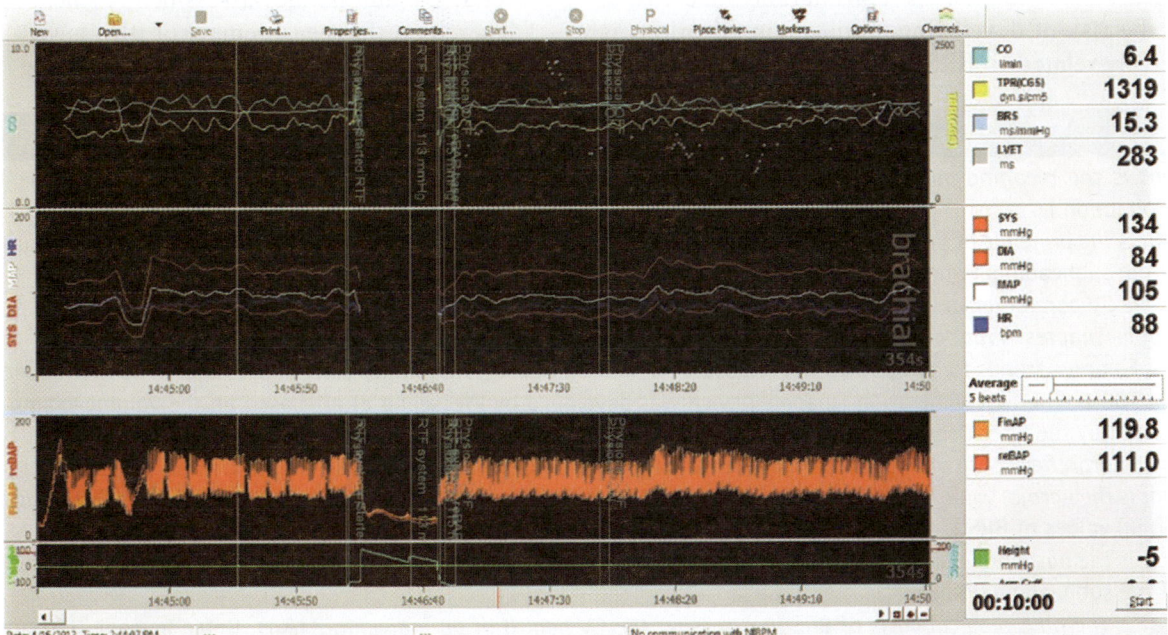

Fig. 39.3   BP variability recording by Finapres in a prehypertensive subject. Note that the SBP was 134 mmHg, DBP was 84 mmHg (pre-hypertension range), and the BRS was 15.3 ms/mmHg. The BRS was decreased due to BP in pre-hypertension range.

DISCUSSION

Physiological Applications of BRS

CV diseases are usually associated with the impairment of baroreflex activity and imbalance in sympathovagal outflow from the CNS to the heart and blood vessels, resulting in persistent sympathetic activation.

1. Chronic baroreflex-mediated sympathetic activation contributes to the progression of the underlying disease process and promotes end-organ damage.
2. **Blunted baroreflex gain** is reported to be *predictive of increased CV risk* in patients suffering from hypertension, myocardial infarction, and heart failure.

Clinical Applications of BRS

Cardiovascular (CV) diseases are often accompanied by an impairment of baroreflex mechanisms, often with a reduction of central inhibitory activity, resulting in an imbalance in sympathovagal outflow to the heart and blood vessels, **lasting vagal withdrawal, and chronic adrenergic activation**. Quantification of arterial baroreflex sensitivity (BRS) is a source of valuable information for the assessment of neural cardiovascular regulation in normal and diseased states.

1. BRS provides **prognostic information** in coronary artery disease (CAD) and myocardial infarction (MI), as documented from experimental observations and confirmed in human studies. The major observations are that baroreflex regulation of heart rate and BP is considerably decreased, and the risk of developing cardiac complications is inversely related to BRS.

2. The first human study emphasising the clinical implication of BRS was the ATRAMI study (Autonomic Tone and Reflexes After Myocardial Infarction), which analysed the utility of BRS in risk stratification of myocardial infarction patients.
   - In this study, **decreased BRS (<3 ms/mmHg)** was established as a *significant predictor of cardiac death* with a relative risk of 2.8 (95% CI 1.40–6.16), independent (statistically adjusted) of other established risk factors.
3. The importance of **reduced BRS as a CV risk** has been observed in *heart failure, hypertension, and other CV diseases*.
4. BRS has recently been reported to be reduced in **pre-hypertension, prediabetes, and in the early stages of various metabolic disorders**.
5. BRS is an important tool in **CV risk stratification** in a number of cardiovascular and metabolic disorders.
6. BRS has recently been used to **assess the prognosis of cardiac diseases** and therapeutic responses in diseases that have direct or indirect CV dysfunctions and in the **assessment of implantable cardioverter defibrillator (ICD) implantation and cardiac resynchronisation therapy (CRT)**.
7. BRS is an important **marker of sympathovagal balance**. Hence, alteration in BRS is used in the assessment of autonomic dysfunctions in clinical conditions. It has promising clinical utility in the future.
8. BRS is reported to be a better marker of autonomic balance or imbalance compared to other non-invasive tests of autonomic assessments, including HRV. Therefore, the measurement of BRS is very **useful in clinical research**.

VIVA

1. *What is the meaning and concept of blood pressure variability (BPV)?* (Ans. Refer to page 266, under the heading 'Introduction'.)
2. *What is the principle of the measurement of BPV?* (Ans. Refer to page 266, under the heading 'Methods of Measuring BPV' and the subheading 'Principle'.)
3. *List the CV parameters recorded in BPV measurement.* (Ans. Refer to page 266, under the heading 'Physiological Aspects'.)
4. *What is Finapres? What principle does it use, and who invented it?*
   (Ans. Finapres stands for **FINger Arterial PRESsure**—a method of recording finger arterial pressure. It was introduced in the early 1980s. The first-generation Finapres device was developed by **Wesseling et al.**, based on the **volume-clamp method** invented by the Czech physiologist **Jan Peňáz**.)
5. *Define baroreflex sensitivity (BRS)?* (Ans. Refer to page 267, under the heading 'BRS Definition and Calculation'.)
6. *What is the normal value of BRS?* (Ans. Refer to page 269, under the heading 'Observation and Results' and the subheading 'Normal values of BRS'.)
7. *What is the basic principle of BRS measurement?* (Ans. Refer to page 268, under the heading 'Method of Measuring BRS' and the subheading 'Principle'.)
8. *What is the physiological basis of BRS in assessing the CV health of an individual?* (Ans. Refer to page 270, under the heading 'Discussion' and the subheading 'Physiological Applications of BRS'.)

9. *What are the clinical uses of BRS?* (Ans. Refer to page 270, under the heading 'Discussion' and the subheading 'Clinical Applications of BRS'.)

10. *How is BRS measurement superior to HRV measurement?*

(Ans. BRS is considered superior to HRV due to the following reasons:

i. The measurement and analysis of BRS are more standardised, as compared to HRV.

ii. BRS is a better marker of sympathovagal balance since it assesses both limbs of baroreflex pathways, including sympathetic and parasympathetic components.

iii. BRS records all the parameters of hemodynamics, including peripheral resistance in circulation along with various cardiac functions, which are not captured by HRV.

iv. Unlike HRV, the data of BRS is not highly variable in the general population.

v. Reduced BRS is a robust marker of CV risks. S

40 Brainstem Auditory Evoked Potential

Learning Objectives

After completing this practical, you will be able to (MUST KNOW):
1. Define brainstem auditory evoked potentials (BAEPs).
2. State the physiological basis of the generation of BAEP waveforms.
3. List the physiological factors that affect BAEP waveforms.
4. Trace the auditory pathway.
5. List the normal characteristics of different BAEP waveforms.
6. Correlate the changes in waveforms with common diseases that affect the auditory pathway.

INTRODUCTION

Brainstem auditory evoked potentials (BAEPs) constitute an objective hearing test. These are the potentials recorded from the ear and the scalp in response to a brief auditory stimulation. The evoked potentials that appear following the **transduction of the acoustic stimulus** by the ear cells create an **electrical signal** that is carried through the **auditory pathway to the brainstem,** and from there to the cerebral cortex. When the signal travels, it **generates an action potential** in all the fibres. These action potentials can be **recorded at several points along the auditory pathway** and even from the surface of the body.

BAEPs assess the conduction of impulses through the auditory pathway up to the midbrain. BAEP is **primarily performed to assess** hearing in uncooperative patients and in very young children, to detect the degree of hearing loss in infants, and to assess the functions of the midpart of the brainstem.

Anatomical and Physiological Considerations

Auditory pathway

The axons of the spiral ganglion, which innervate the hair cells of the ear, form the cochlear nerve. The **first order of neurons** terminates in the *cochlear nuclei* in the medulla, from where the **second order of neurons** arises and ends in the *superior olivary nucleus*. The **third order of neurons** originates from the **superior olivary nucleus** and ascends the lateral lemniscus to project onto the *inferior colliculus*, which is the centre for auditory reflexes. From the inferior colliculi, fibres project to the *medial geniculate body* in the thalamus, and from there to the *primary auditory cortex* (area 41) (Fig. 40.1; and refer to Fig. 47.1, Chapter 47).

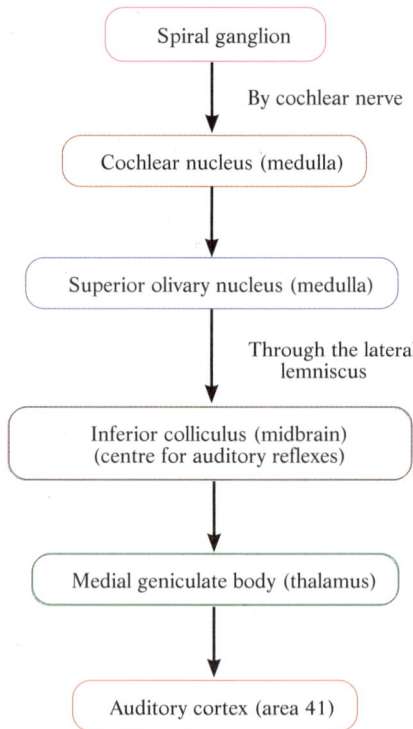

Fig. 40.1 Auditory pathway

Physiological basis of BAEPs

BAEPs are recorded within 10 ms after an **acoustic stimulus** is given. A *series of potentials* is generated corresponding to the sequential activation of different parts of the auditory pathway—peripheral, pontomedullary, pontine, and midbrain portions of the pathway.

Waves of BAEP

Five or more distinct waveforms are **recorded within 10 ms** of the auditory stimulus. These waveforms are named **I, II, III, IV, and V** (Fig. 40.2). If the recording continues, a few more positive and negative waves are recorded. These peaks are considered to originate from the following anatomical sites:

1. Waves I and II: **Cochlear nerves**
2. Wave III: **Cochlear nucleus**
3. Wave IV: **Superior olivary complex**
4. Wave V: **Nuclei of lateral lemniscus**
5. Waves VI and VII: **Inferior colliculus**

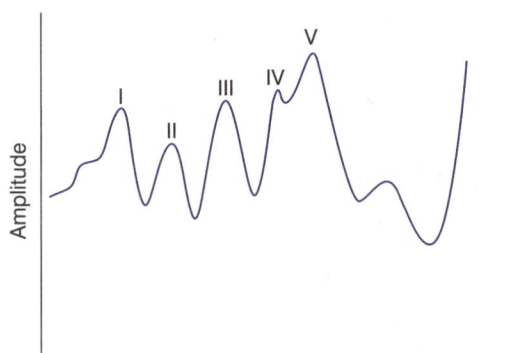

Fig. 40.2 Brainstem auditory evoked potential recorded in a normal individual.

Factors That Affect BAEP

1. **Age**: The latency of BAEP is affected by age, especially in *early childhood*. Latency is age-dependent up to two years. The effect of age is more pronounced in premature infants. *Older adults* have slightly longer I to IV interpeak latency compared to younger individuals.
2. **Sex**: Women have shorter latency and higher amplitude of BAEPs.
3. **Height**: The height of the subject has no direct correlation with the latency or amplitude of BAEPs.
4. **Temperature**: Increased body temperature decreases the latency, and decreased temperature increases the latency of BAEP.
5. **Drugs**: *Barbiturates and alcohol* prolong the latency of wave V. These drugs affect latency by decreasing the body temperature instead of directly acting on the auditory pathway.
6. **Hearing loss**: Hearing deficits affect BAEPs. Therefore, hearing tests, especially ones to detect conductive deafness and examination of the ear to diagnose ear block by cerumen, should be performed before recording BAEPs.

METHODS OF RECORDING BAEPs

Principle

A brief auditory stimulation generates action potentials in the auditory pathway. These potentials are recorded from the ear and vertex as BAEPs.

Requirements

1. Recording electrodes
2. Amplifier and average (EP-EMG machine; Fig. 40.3)
3. Electrode paste
4. Earphone

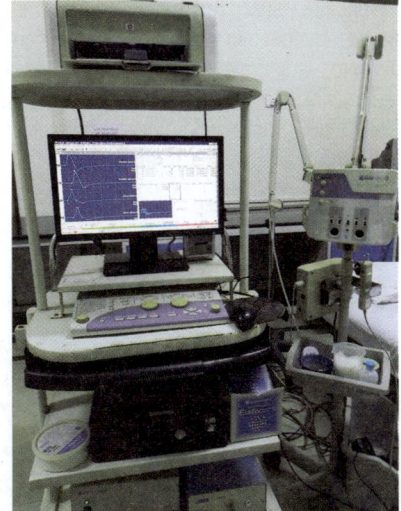

Fig. 40.3 Evoked potential-electromyogram (EP-EMG) machine with all its accessories. (Courtesy: Physiology EP-EMG Lab, JIPMER, Puducherry, India).

Procedure

1. Place the **recording electrodes** on both the ear lobes or on the mastoid process (Fig. 40.4).
2. Place the **reference electrode** on a point slightly in front of the vertex.
3. Place the **ground electrode** on a point in front of the reference electrode.
4. Connect the recording electrodes to the amplifier.
5. Use amplifications of 2,00,000–5,00,000.
6. Set the low filter at 100 Hz and the high filter at 3000 Hz.
7. Give a **brief click stimulus** that lasts for 0.1 ms.

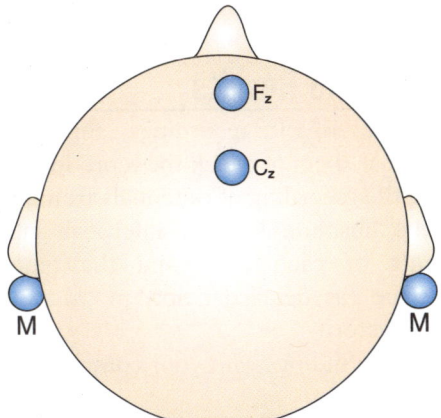

Fig. 40.4 Sites of placing electrodes for recording BAEP (M [mastoid process] for active electrode, Cz for reference and Fz for ground electrode).

Note: The stimulus applied is usually a square wave pulse. The pulse can move towards or away from the ear. The movement of the earphone towards the ear is called **condensation phase stimulus** and the movement away from the ear is called **rarefaction phase stimulus**. The amplitude of the waveforms is affected by the type of stimulus; for example, wave I amplitude is greater with rarefaction stimulus. The clicks are usually presented 10–70 times per second. Waveforms are poorly defined at faster rates. Therefore, slower or intermediate rates are preferred. A click rate of 11–31 Hz is commonly used in clinical practice. The stimulus intensity is usually kept within 40–70 dB. Some laboratories maintain the stimulus intensity at 60 dB above the hearing threshold.

8. Observe the recording of potentials from both ears (Fig. 40.5).
9. Repeat 2–3 times and see that recordings are superimposed, to check their reproducibility.

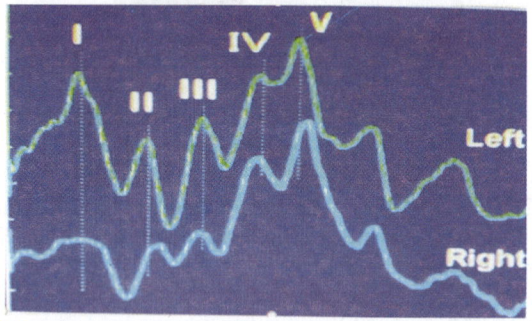

Fig. 40.5 Brainstem auditory evoked potentials recorded from both right and left sides.

Note: The BAEP repetition should be superimposed almost exactly.

Precautions

1. The subject should be properly instructed and motivated to cooperate fully.
2. The subject should be fully relaxed; hypnotics can be used to achieve maximum relaxation.
3. The room should be quiet and comfortable.
4. The skin of the scalp and mastoid should be grease-free.

Observation and Results

1. Repeat the BAEP recordings three times and superimpose them to check the reproducibility.
2. Observe the recording of potentials from both ears.
3. Note the absolute latency, interpeak latency, and amplitude of each wave and the time of their appearance (as detailed below in 'Measurement of BAEP Waveforms').
4. Report your findings with your comments.

Measurement of BAEP Waveforms

The following parameters are measured for analysing the waveforms of BAEPs:

1. Absolute latency and amplitude
2. Interpeak latencies
3. Amplitude ratio of V/I
4. Inter-ear–interpeak difference

Absolute latency and amplitude

The **absolute amplitude** is measured as the height of the wave (expressed in μv), measured from the peak of a wave to the trough of that wave. The **absolute latency** is measured as the distance (expressed in ms) from the beginning of the first wave to the peak of that wave.

Inter-peak latencies

The interpeak latencies (IPLs) that are usually measured are **I–V, I–III, and III–V**. These are measured as the distances between the peaks of the two waves (expressed in ms).

I–V interpeak latency: The normal value is 4.5 ms.

1. It represents conduction from the proximal part of the eighth nerve, through the pons, to the midbrain.
2. It is slightly less in females and more in elderly men.
3. It is **prolonged** in:
   • Demyelination
   • Degenerative diseases
   • Hypoxic brain damage

I–III interpeak latency: The normal value is about 2.5 ms.

1. It measures conduction from the eighth nerve across the subarachnoid space into the core of the lower pons.
2. It is **prolonged** in:
   • Inflammation or tumour of the eighth nerve
   • Diseases at the pontomedullary junction
   • Guillain–Barré syndrome

III–V interpeak latency: The normal value is about 2.4 ms.

1. It measures conduction from the lower pons to the midbrain.
2. It is **prolonged in** the prolongation of I–V IPL. The isolated prolongation of III–V IPL is not considered significant.

Amplitude Ratio of V/I

Wave I is generated outside, whereas wave V is generated inside the CNS. Therefore, the V/I ratio compares the relationship of the signal amplitude.

Normal value: The ratio is normally between 50 per cent and 300 per cent.

Clinical implication: If the ratio is less than 50 per cent, it suggests small amplitude of wave V, which indicates a central impairment of hearing. If the ratio is more than 300 per cent, it suggests small amplitude of wave I, which indicates peripheral hearing impairment.

DISCUSSION

Normal BAEP Waveforms

Wave I

Characteristics:

1. This is the **first prominent upgoing peak** in the ipsilateral ear recording channel. It is *reduced or absent from the contralateral ear* recording channel.
2. It appears **1.4 ms after the stimulus**.
3. The **amplitude of this wave can be increased** by using a horizontal montage, an external canal needle electrode, or a nasopharyngeal electrode, as well as by increasing stimulus intensity or decreasing the stimulus rate.

Clinical application: As it originates from the eighth nerve, this wave is *preserved in patients who have only central problems*. Those who have **peripheral hearing impairment** have reduced or absent wave I (wave II to V remain relatively normal).

Wave II

Characteristics:

1. This is a **poorly defined wave**.
2. It appears as a **small peak** following wave I. It may appear in the downward slope of wave I or in the upward slope of wave III.
3. It is more prominent in the contralateral channel recording, where it has a slightly prolonged latency compared to the ipsilateral recording.

Clinical application: It is **absent** in the *lesions of the eighth nerve*.

Wave III

Characteristics:

1. This is a **prominent upgoing** peak.
2. It is smaller and appears earlier in the contralateral channel.
3. It may sometimes appear as a bifid wave (with two peaks).

Clinical application: It is *reduced or absent* in **lesions of the cochlear nucleus**.

Wave IV

Characteristics:

1. This is a **very small wave**, which usually appears in the upward slope of wave V.
2. Sometimes, it may be absent or may appear as a very small wave at the peak of wave V, giving it a bifid appearance.

Clinical application: It *is absent* in lesions of the *superior olivary nucleus*.

Wave V

Characteristics:

1. This is the **most prominent** peak in BAEP.
2. It appears **5.5 ms after** the stimulus.
3. It usually starts above the baseline immediately following wave IV.

Clinical application: It *disappears in diseases* affecting the **lateral lemniscus and inferior colliculi**.

Clinical Applications

Changes in brainstem auditory evoked potentials (BAEPs) have been correlated with diseases affecting **different levels of the auditory pathway**. BAEP is particularly useful in **localising lesions in the brainstem** and is helpful in the **diagnosis of conditions** such as cerebellopontine angle tumour, intrinsic brainstem tumour, multiple sclerosis, coma, brain death, and strokes involving the brainstem (e.g., thrombosis of the vertebrobasilar system). It is also useful in **pediatrics for assessing auditory function in children** whose hearing cannot be tested behaviorally.

Uses of BAEP

BAEPs are used to assess the *integrity and function of the auditory pathways* from the cochlea to the brainstem. They are especially useful in diagnosing hearing loss in individuals who are unable to cooperate with traditional hearing tests, such as children and comatose patients. BAEPs are also used for **intraoperative monitoring** during surgeries involving the auditory pathway.

1. **Diagnostic tool for hearing loss:** BAEPs can help: i) identify the *type and severity of hearing loss*, especially in cases where standard audiometry is not feasible (e.g., in infants or comatose patients); ii) *differentiate between cochlear and retrocochlear hearing loss* (damage to the auditory nerve or brainstem); and iii) *estimate hearing thresholds* in individuals who cannot participate in behavioural audiometry.
2. **Neurological assessment:** BAEPs can help: i) detect *lesions in the auditory pathway,* such as tumours, demyelination, or stroke affecting the brainstem; ii) evaluate the *function of the auditory pathway* in conditions like multiple sclerosis; and iii) assess brainstem function and prognosis in comatose patients.
3. **Intraoperative monitoring:** During surgery, particularly surgery in the **posterior fossa** or near the *cerebellopontine angle*, BAEPs can be used to monitor the *integrity of the auditory pathway* and help prevent hearing loss. This is especially important

when structures like the cochlea, auditory nerve, or brainstem nuclei are at risk.

4. **Newborn hearing screening:** BAEPs are a key component of newborn hearing screening programmes, helping *identify hearing loss early in life*.

5. **Other clinical applications:** BAEPs can be used to evaluate the *effects of ototoxic drugs* on hearing.

6. **Use in research:** BAEP is used extensively in auditory research to study the functions and effects of various conditions on the auditory pathway.

VIVA

1. *What are the different waveforms seen in the recording of BAEP, and how are they generated?* (**Ans.** Refer to page 273-274, under the heading 'Waves of BAEP'.)
2. *Trace the auditory pathway.* (**Ans.** Refer to page 272, under the heading 'Auditory Pathway'.)
3. *What are the physiological factors that affect BAEP?* (**Ans.** Refer to page 273, under the heading 'Factors that affect BAEP')
4. *What are the precautions observed while taking a recording of BAEP?* (**Ans.** Refer to page 277, under the heading 'Precautions'.)
5. *What should be the stimulus intensity and duration for recording BAEP?* (**Ans.** Refer to page 273, under the heading 'Procedure', point no.7.)
6. *How can the amplitude of wave I of BAEP be improved?* (**Ans.** Refer to page 274, under the subheading 'Wave I', characteristic no. 3.)
7. *In what conditions is wave I reduced or absent?* (**Ans.** Refer to page 274, under the subheading 'Wave I', read 'Clinical application'.)
8. *What is the cause of wave II in BAEP? In what diseases is it absent?* (**Ans.** Refer to page 275, under the subheading 'Wave II'.)
9. *In which conditions is wave III absent?* (**Ans.** Refer to page 278, under the subheading 'Wave III', read 'Clinical application'.)
10. *What is the significance of wave V? In what conditions is it altered?* (**Ans.** Refer to page 275, under the subheading 'Wave V'.)
11. *What does I–V interpeak latency represent? In what conditions is it prolonged?* (**Ans.** Refer to page 274, see 'I–V interpeak latency'.)
12. *What does I–III interpeak latency represent? In what conditions is it prolonged?* (**Ans.** Refer to Page 274, see 'I-III interpeak latency'.)
13. *What does III–V interpeak latency represent? In what conditions is it prolonged?* (**Ans.** Refer to Page 274, see 'III-V interpeak latency'.)
14. *What is the significance of the V/I ratio?* (**Ans.** Refer to Page 275, under the heading 'Amplitude Ratio of V/I'.)
15. *What is the clinical utility of recording BAEP in children?* (**Ans.** Refer to page 275, under the heading 'Clinical Application'.)
16. *What are the uses of BAEP?* (**Ans.** Refer to page 275, under the heading 'Clinical Application'.)

41 | Visual Evoked Potential

Learning Objectives

After completing this practical, you will be able to (MUST KNOW):

1. Describe the significance of performing this practical in clinical physiology.
2. Define visual evoked potentials (VEPs).
3. State the physiological basis of VEPs.
4. List the factors that influence VEP.
5. List the pre-test instructions given to the subject prior to recording the VEP.
6. State the principle of recording VEP.
7. List the precautions taken during the recording of VEP.

You may also be able to (DESIRABLE TO KNOW):

1. Describe the normal waveforms of VEP.
2. List the abnormalities of VEP waveforms.
3. Name the diseases associated with different abnormalities.

INTRODUCTION

Visual evoked potentials (VEPs) are electrical potential differences recorded from the vertex in response to visual stimuli. VEPs represent the mass response of the cortical and possibly subcortical areas. Normal VEPs indicate the intactness of the entire visual system.

Anatomical and Physiological Considerations

Layers of the retina

The retina has ten layers. The outermost layer is the **pigment epithelium**. The **rods and cones** lie next to the pigment layer. They synapse with the **inner nuclear** or bipolar cells, which in turn project onto the **ganglion cell layer**. The axons of the ganglion cells form the **optic nerve**. The rods and cones are receptors that are stimulated by light impulses. The information received by them is conveyed through the bipolar and ganglion cells to the visual pathway.

Visual pathway

Fibres in the **optic nerves** terminate in the **lateral geniculate body** via the optic chiasma, which in turn project onto the **visual cortex through optic radiation** (for details, refer to Fig. 44.1, Chapter 44).

Physiological basis of VEPs

The **P_{100} waveform** of VEP is generated in the occipital cortex by the **activation of the primary visual cortex** and the activation of **areas surrounding the visual cortex** by thalamocortical fibres. The **retinal ganglion cells** are of three types: **X, Y, and W.**

1. **X cells** are small ganglion cells that mediate the **function of the cone system** (colour vision). They have small-diameter axons and small receptive fields. They are concentrated in the central portion of the visual field (central retina) and exhibit lateral inhibition. X cells provide the **substrate for pattern VEPs via the geniculate pathway.**

2. **Y cells** are large ganglion cells that mediate the **functions of the rod system**. Their axons have large diameters and large receptive fields. They are concentrated in the peripheral visual field (peripheral retinal location) and **provide the substrate for flash VEPs** via the extrageniculate pathway.

The VEPs primarily represent the **activity originating in the central visual field**, which is connected to the surface of the occipital cortex.

1. Activities originating from the **peripheral retina** are directed to the deeper regions of the visual cortex, which **attenuates the VEPs** (on peripheral retinal stimulation only).

2. The **central part of the retina** (fovea centralis) has greater cortical representation in the visual cortex, and **activities in the central visual field magnify the VEPs**.

Waveforms of VEPs

The VEPs consist of a **series of waveforms** of opposite polarities. The negative waves are denoted by N and positive waves by P, followed by their approximate latency in ms. The commonly seen waveforms are N_{75}, P_{100}, and N_{145} (Fig. 41.1). The **peak latency and peak-to-peak amplitudes** of these waves are measured. Generally, the peak latency, duration, and amplitude of P_{100} are measured.

The **normal values** of the parameters of P_{100} are as follows:

Latency (ms): 100
Amplitude (μv): 11
Duration (ms): 60

N_{75} mainly results from foveal stimulation and originates in area 17. P_{100} originates in area 19. N_{145} reflects the activity of area 18.

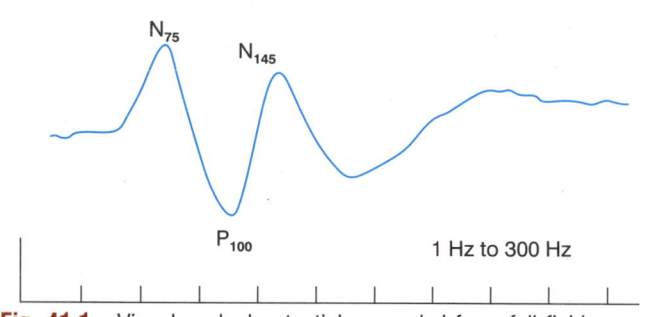

Fig. 41.1 Visual evoked potentials recorded from full-field mono-ocular stimulation.

Factors That Influence VEP

1. **Age:** The amplitude of P_{100} is high in infants and children—almost double the adult value. The adult value is reached in 5–7 years. After 50 years, the amplitude decreases.
2. **Gender:** P_{100} latency is longer in men, possibly because of the larger head size in men. However, the P_{100} amplitude is greater in women, possibly due to hormonal influences.
3. **Drugs:** Drugs that cause miosis (pupillary constriction), such as pilocarpine, increase P_{100} latency due to the decreased area of retinal illumination. In contrast, mydriatic agents decrease P_{100} latency.
4. **Eye dominance:** The duration and amplitude of P_{100} are shorter when they are recorded by stimulating the dominant eye compared to the non-dominant eye. This is attributed to neuroanatomic asymmetries in the human visual cortex.
5. **Eye movement:** The amplitude of P_{100} is decreased by eye movement, but its latency remains unaffected.
6. **Visual acuity:** With decreased visual acuity, the amplitude of P_{100} decreases, whereas its latency remains normal.

METHODS OF RECORDING VEP

Principle

The stimulation of the visual pathway generates activities in the visual cortex. A visual stimulus is presented to the subject a selected number of times, and the cerebral responses are amplified, averaged by a computer, and displayed on the oscilloscope screen or printed out on paper.

There are different methods of measuring VEP:
1. Pattern reversal VEP
2. Flash VEP
3. Goggle VEP

The **pattern reversal VEP** is most commonly used for adult patients who can follow the light. The **flash** VEP is used for infants, individuals with very poor visual acuity, or those in a coma. The **goggle VEP** is used for children.

Requirements

1. Standard disc EEG electrodes
2. Preamplifier and amplifier (Fig. 40.3)
3. Oscilloscope
4. Electrode paste

Procedure

For best results, proper instructions should be given to the subject, and a thorough eye examination should be conducted.

Pre-test instructions

1. The procedure should be explained in detail to the subject to ensure full cooperation.
2. The subject should avoid applying hair spray or oil after the last hair wash.
3. If the subject uses optical lenses, they should be worn during the test.
4. The subject should be instructed not to use miotics or mydriatics 12 hours before the test.
5. A full ophthalmological examination should be carried out to determine the visual acuity, the pupillary diameter, and the field of vision.
6. If any field defect is present, electrodes may be placed laterally in addition to midline electrodes, as field defects can alter the potential field distribution of P_{100}.

Steps of the test

1. Prepare the skin by abrading and degreasing.
2. Place the recording electrode at O_Z (Fig. 41.2) using conducting jelly or electrode paste.
3. Place the reference electrode at F_{PZ} or 12 cm above the nasion.
4. Place the ground electrode at the wrist.
5. Keep the electrode impedance below 5 kΩ.
6. Use amplification ranging from 20,000–1,00,000 to record pattern shift visual evoked potentials (PSVEPs).
7. Set low-cut filters at 1–3 Hz and high-cut filters at 100–300 Hz.

Note: The filter setting should be kept constant.

8. Maintain the sweep duration at 250–500 ms.
9. Stimulate visual pathways by different photic stimulation and record the responses (Fig. 41.3).
10. Compare the obtained tracing with the normal one (as shown in Fig. 41.1).

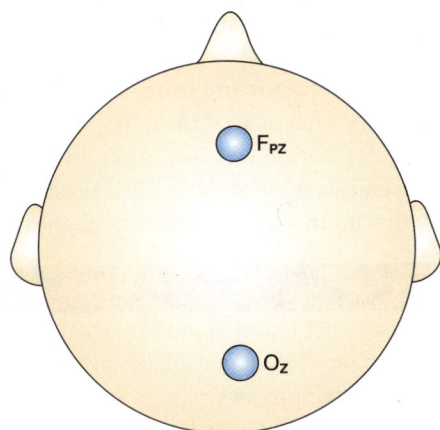

Fig. 41.2 Sites of placement of electrodes for recording VEP (reference electrode at the point F$_{PZ}$, recording electrode at O$_Z$, and the ground electrode at the wrist).

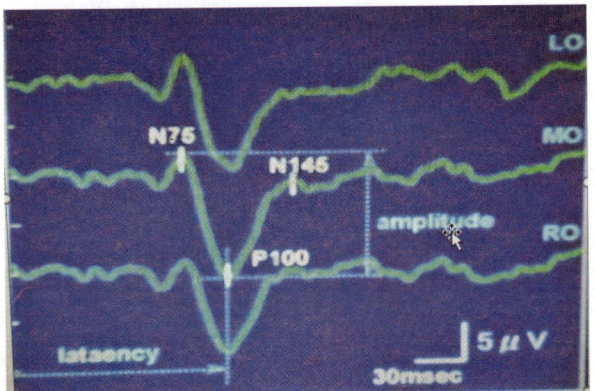

Fig. 41.3 Visual evoked potentials (LO: left occipital; MO: mid-occipital; RO: right occipital).

Precautions

1. The subject should be instructed properly.
2. The skin of the scalp should be grease-free.
3. Mydriatics and miotics should not be used for a minimum of 12 hours before the test.
4. Visual acuity, pupillary diameter, and field of vision must be checked before starting the test.
5. Additional lateral electrodes should be used if there is any visual field defect.
6. Electrode impedance should be kept below 5 kΩ.
7. The amplification range should be between 20,000 and 1,00,000 for recording pattern shift VEP.
8. The filter setting should be kept constant.
9. The subject should not sleep during the procedure.

Observation and Results

1. Measure the peak latency, duration, and amplitude of P$_{100}$.
2. Report your findings, and state whether they are normal or abnormal.
3. The **normal values** of P$_{100}$ are—latency: 100 ms; amplitude: 11 µv; and duration: 60 ms.

DISCUSSION

For recording VEPs, the **eyes are tested one at a time**. Each eye projects to the occipital cortex through the optic chiasma. Therefore, **unilateral VEP abnormality** is obtained by *full-field mono-ocular stimulation* and is likely to be due to a pre-chiasmal lesion. If the pattern shift visual evoked potential (PSVEP) is abnormal bilaterally, it becomes difficult to locate the anatomical site of the defect.

VEP Abnormalities

The common VEP abnormalities are as follows:
1. **Prolongation of latency:** The commonest cause of prolonged latency of P$_{100}$ is *demyelination of the optic pathways*. The amplitude remains normal.
2. **Amplitude reduction:** Amplitude reduction of P$_{100}$ occurs in *ischemic optic neuropathy*, which causes axonal loss. The latency remains normal. It also occurs in *refractive errors, media opacities* (e.g., lens opacity) and *retinal diseases*.
3. **Combined latency and amplitude defects:** These occur in *optic nerve compression*, which causes segmental demyelination and axonal loss.
4. **Shape abnormalities:** Usually, two types are observed:
    i. **Bifid P$_{100}$**—two peaks are observed. This is seen rarely in normal individuals. It indicates abnormality.
    ii. **W-shaped VEP**—when two peaks are separated by 10–50 ms, it forms a W-shaped P$_{100}$ waveform.

Clinical Applications

Visual evoked potential (VEP) studies provide a sensitive method for detecting **abnormalities in the visual pathways**, especially *anterior to the optic chiasma*. Although VEP abnormalities are *non-specific* and not characteristic of any particular etiology, they can support the clinical diagnosis of various conditions, including demyelinating diseases, ischemic optic neuropathy, nutritional and toxic optic neuropathies, hereditary and degenerative diseases, lesions affecting the anterior visual pathways, and cortical blindness.

Uses of VEP

VEPs are primarily used to assess the integrity of the visual pathway—**from the retina to the visual cortex**. They are valuable for *diagnosing conditions* such as multiple sclerosis and optic neuritis, and for *evaluating vision* in children or adults who cannot read eye charts.
1. **Diagnosing neurological disorders:** Multiple sclerosis, optic neuritis, other conditions (anterior ischemic optic neuropathy, compressive lesions).

2. **Assessing visual function in specific populations:**
   i. **Children and infants:** VEPs can be used to evaluate vision in individuals who cannot cooperate with traditional eye exams, like children and those with developmental delays.
   ii. **Individuals with visual impairments:** VEPs can help assess visual acuity in individuals with vision loss, even if they are unable to understand the concept of vision.

3. **Monitoring treatment and progression of conditions:** VEPs can be used to track the effectiveness of treatments for conditions like multiple sclerosis.

4. **Research and development:** VEP is used commonly in research that addresses the neural mechanisms of vision.

VIVA

1. *What is the clinical application of VEP?* (**Ans.** Refer to page 279, under the heading 'Clinical Significance'.)
2. *What is the physiological basis of VEP?* (**Ans.** Refer to page 277, under the heading 'Physiological Basis of VEPs'.)
3. *What are the waveforms of VEP?* (**Ans.** Refer to page 277, under the heading 'Waveforms of VEP'.)
4. *What are the factors that affect VEP?* (**Ans.** Refer to page 278, under the heading 'Factors that Influence VEP'.)
5. *What are the pre-test instructions given to the subject prior to recording VEP?* (**Ans.** Refer to page 278, under the heading 'Pre-test Instructions'.)
6. *What are the components of the visual pathway?* (**Ans.** Refer to page 277, under the heading 'Visual Pathway'.)
7. *What are the precautions taken while recording VEP?* (**Ans.** Refer to page 279, under the heading 'Precautions'.)
8. *What are the different VEP abnormalities?* (**Ans.** Refer to page 279, under the heading 'VEP Abnormalities'.)
9. *What are the causes of latency prolongation and amplitude reduction of VEP?* (**Ans.** Refer to page 279, under the heading 'VEP Abnormalities', points no. 1 and 2.)
10. *What are the uses of VEP study?* (**Ans.** Refer to page 279, under the heading 'Uses of VEP'.)

42 | Somatosensory Evoked Potential

Learning Objectives

After completing this practical, you will be able to (MUST KNOW):

1. Describe the clinical significance of the study of somatosensory evoked potentials (SEPs).
2. Define somatosensory evoked potentials (SEPs).
3. Trace the sensory pathway for proprioception.
4. State the basic principle of recording SEPs.

You will also be able to (DESIRABLE TO KNOW):

1. Explain the physiological basis of different latencies and amplitudes of various waveforms of SEPs.
2. List the common abnormalities of latencies and amplitudes of various waveforms of SEPs.

INTRODUCTION

Somatosensory evoked potentials (SEPs) are the potentials generated by *large-diameter fibres* (sensory fibres) in response to a sensory stimulus applied to them anywhere in their course, either in the peripheral or in the central portion of the pathway. The potentials recorded have *different latencies* and are accordingly called **short-, intermediate-, and long-latency potentials**.

1. The **short-latency SEPs** appear within 50 ms of stimulation; these are *clinically important*.
2. The **intermediate- and long-latency potentials** lie within 50–100 ms and 100–300 ms, respectively; these are *not clinically significant* because they are highly variable and inconsistent.

Due to their long course—starting from sensory receptors on the body surface, and transversing through the peripheral nerves to the spinal cord, and onward to the cerebral cortex—sensory pathways are potentially vulnerable to lesions at various sites. The SEPs assess the *intactness of the sensory pathway,* and the long course makes it easy to evaluate.

Anatomical and Physiological Considerations

Sensory pathways

SEPs assess the intactness of the pathway for proprioception (as they involve large-diameter fibres). Proprioceptors are present in and around joints (joint capsules), muscles, and tendons. The **first order of neurons** carries impulses from the receptors to the spinal cord in type A fibres and ascends the dorsal column of the spinal cord to terminate in the gracile and cuneate nuclei in the medulla of the same side. The **second order of neurons** originates from the gracile and cuneate nuclei in the medulla, crosses to the opposite side, and ascends in the medial lemniscus to reach the VPL nucleus of the thalamus. From here, the **third order of neurons** projects into the sensory cortex through the thalamocortical radiation.

Physiological basis of SEPs

The SEPs can be recorded by **stimulating any large peripheral nerve**. However, in clinical practice, SEPs are commonly recorded from the *median and posterior tibial nerves*.

Median SEPs

The stimulation of the **median nerve** generates a number of waveforms. Negative waves are designated by N, and positive waves are designated by P. Normally, the **significant negative waves** recorded are N_9, N_{11}, N_{13}, N_{18}, and N_{20}, and the **positive waves** are P_{14} and P_{25}. Clinically, P_{14} *is considered more significant*.

N_9: Generated by the brachial plexus.

N_{11}: Generated by the dorsal cervical root, ascending volley in the posterior column of C_5.

N_{13}: Generated by the rostral cervical cord.

P_{14}: Generated by the *medial lemniscus and brainstem collaterals*.

N_{18}: Generated by the rostral brainstem nuclei, the thalamus.

N_{20}: Generated by the VPL nucleus of the thalamus, the primary sensory cortex.

Tibial SEPs

Tibial SEPs are recorded from the posterior **tibial nerve**. The important waveforms are N_8, N_{22}, N_{28}, and P_{37}.

N_8: Generated by the tibial or sciatic nerve.

N_{22}: Generated by the dorsal grey matter of the lumbar spinal cord.

N_{28}: Generated by the cervical spinal cord.

P_{37}: Generated by the primary sensory cortex.

Factors That Affect SEPs

1. **Age:** In **infants and children**, N_9 and N_{15} potentials of median SEPs appear early. In **elderly individuals**, most of the latencies are longer by about 10 per cent

after the age of 55. The interpeak latencies are shorter with increasing age, which indicates slowing of conduction in the peripheral nerves in old age.

2. **Gender:** Women have a shorter central conduction time.

3. **Temperature:** Peripheral nerve conduction **decreases with decrease in limb temperature**. Changes in body temperature affect the conduction in the peripheral portion of the pathway more than the central portion. *Temperature and latency have a linear relationship*.

4. **Sleep:** The amplitude of the peak component of N_{20} is lower in sleep than in the waking state.

5. **Drugs:** SEPs are resistant to most drugs. Therefore, sedatives like diazepam can be used if needed. The patient can continue to take them if he has already been advised by the physician to take them while recording SEPs. Sedatives are used for uncooperative patients.

METHODS OF RECORDING SEPs
Principle

The stimulation of sensory nerves generates action potentials that are carried by the ascending pathways to the sensory cortex, from where these are recorded as SEPs; they are usually recorded from the large conducting fibres in the sensory pathway.

Requirements

1. Electrodes
2. Amplifier (EP-EMG machine; Fig. 40.3)
3. Averager
4. Oscilloscope
5. Electrode paste

Procedure

Pre-test instructions

1. Provide proper instructions to the subject to ensure their full cooperation.
2. Ensure that the subject is fully relaxed in the supine position with their head supported (to relax the neck muscles).
3. Use mild hypnotics, if needed, to ensure relaxation.
4. Ensure that the room is quiet and comfortable.
5. Prior to recording, obtain information about the nerve (features of nerve injury and so on).

Steps (in brief)

(SEPs recorded from the posterior tibial nerve are described here.)

Place the ground electrode about 5 cm above the medial malleolus. Stimulate the posterior tibial nerve just posterior to the medial malleolus, and the recording electrode at various points on the body as depicted in Fig. 42.1.

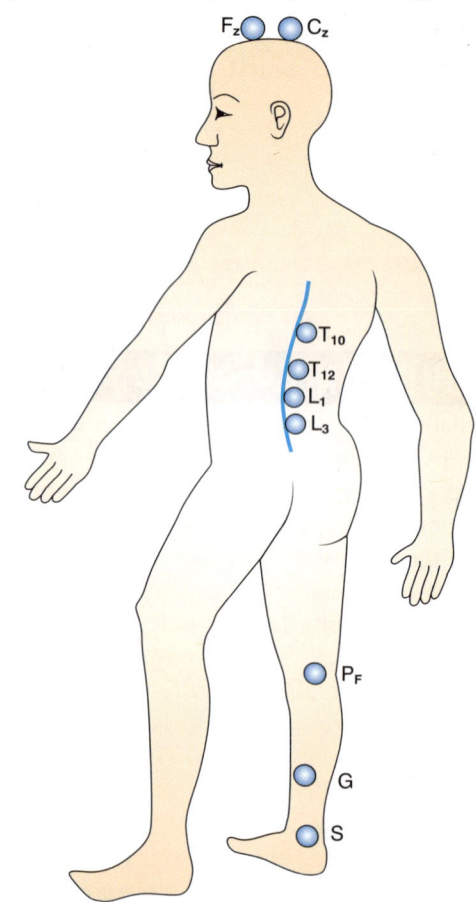

Fig. 42.1   Sites of placing electrodes for recording posttibial SEP (S: stimulating electrode; G: ground electrode; F_z, C_z, T_{10}, T_{12}, L_3, and P_F (popliteal fossa): recording electrodes).

Precautions

1. Provide proper instructions and motivation to the subject to ensure full cooperation.
2. Ensure that the subject is fully relaxed. If required, hypnotics can be used to achieve maximum relaxation.
3. Ensure that the room is quiet and comfortable.

Observation and Results

1. Study the **latency and amplitude** of N_8, N_{22}, P_{37}, and N_{45} from the recorded tracings. For example, P_{37} and N_{45} can be studied from the C_z–F_z recording (Fig. 42.2).
2. Measure the **interpeak latencies** between important waves as described below for both median and tibial SEPs.
3. Summarise your findings and report the results.

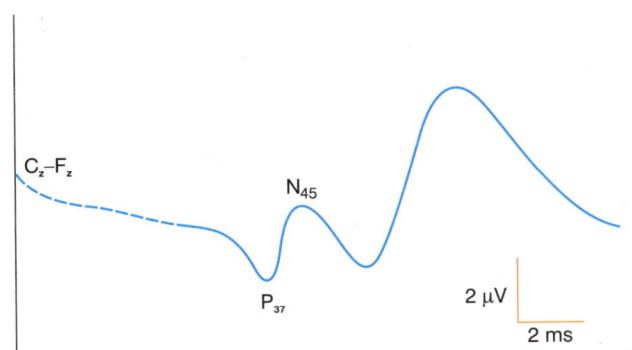

Fig. 42.2 Normal waveforms of SEP (C_z–F_z) of the posterior tibial nerve.

Median SEPs

The following parameters are measured for the analysis of median SEPs.

1. Latency
2. Amplitude
3. Interpeak latency

Amplitude and latency: The amplitude and latency of N_9, N_{11}, N_{13}, N_{18}, N_{20}, and P_{25} waveforms are measured. These latencies are prolonged, and the amplitudes are reduced in diseases at different parts of the sensory pathway that they represent.

Interpeak latency: The *two important interpeak latencies* (IPL) are clinically significant. These are N_9, N_{11}, and N_{13}–N_{20} IPL.

1. **N_9–N_{11} IPL** represents the conduction time from the brachial plexus to the spinal cord. Therefore, it is delayed by any lesion between the brachial plexus and the spinal cord.
2. **N_{13}–N_{20} IPL** represents central sensory conduction time. Therefore, it is delayed in any condition that affects the central sensory pathway, i.e., the pathway from the spinal cord to the cortex.

Tibial SEPs

Like median SEPs, the **latency and amplitude** of N_8, N_{22}, and P_{37} are measured. The *two important interpeak latencies* (IPL) are clinically significant. These are N_8–P_{37}, and N_{22}–P_{37} IPL.

1. **N_8–P_{37} IPL** is used to measure the conduction time in both peripheral and central pathways.

2. **N_{22}–P37 IPL** is used to measure the conduction time in the central pathway, that is, from the lumbar spinal cord to the sensory cortex.

DISCUSSION
Clinical Applications of SEPs

SEPs are used to assess the integrity of the somatosensory pathways, which are responsible for transmitting sensory information from the body to the brain. They have a good correlation with impairment of joint position and vibration sensation, but not with pain and touch. For an abnormality in SEP to occur, a significant degree of sensory impairment must take place.

In general: i) *latency abnormalities* are more pronounced in demyelinating diseases, ii) *amplitude abnormalities* are more common in ischemic lesions, and iii) a combination of *latency and amplitude abnormalities* is seen in compressive lesions.

Thus, SEPs are helpful in the diagnosis of the **nature and degree of sensory abnormalities** in demyelinating diseases, vascular lesions, infections of the spinal cord and brain, like acute transverse myelitis, Pott's paraplegia, degenerative diseases like cervical and lumbar spondylosis, and nutritional myopathies.

1. **Neurological disorders:** SEPs can help diagnose and monitor various neurological disorders, including multiple sclerosis, spinal cord injuries and infections, and peripheral neuropathies and myopathies.
2. **Intraoperative monitoring:** SEPs are used during surgery, especially spinal surgery, to monitor the function of the spinal cord and prevent nerve damage.
3. **Infant neurodevelopment:** SEPs can be used to assess the progress or status of the **development of sensory pathways** in infants and predict potential neurological issues.
4. **Localisation of lesions:** SEPs can help localise lesions or damage within the somatosensory pathways.

Thus, SEPs are **non-invasive neurophysiological tests that provide valuable information about the function of the somatosensory system**, aiding in the diagnosis and management of various neurological conditions.

VIVA

1. *What is somatosensory evoked potential (SEP)?* (Ans. Refer to page 281, under the heading 'Introduction'.)
2. *What is the actual sensation assessed by SEPs and why?* (Ans. Refer to page 281, under the heading 'Introduction'.)
3. *Trace the pathway of proprioception.* (Ans. Refer to page 281, under the heading 'Sensory Pathways'.)
4. *What are the different waveforms of median SEPs? How are they produced?* (Ans. Refer to page 281, under the heading 'Physiological Basis...' and the subheading 'Median SEP'.)
5. *What are the different waveforms of tibial SEPs? How are they produced?* (Ans. Refer to page 281, under the heading 'Physiological Basis...' and the subheading 'Tibial SEP'.)

6. *What are the factors that affect SEPs?* (**Ans.** Refer to page 281–282, under the heading 'Factors that affect SEP'.)
7. *What are the pre-test instructions and steps of recording SEPs?* (**Ans.** Refer to page 282, under the heading 'Procedure' and the subheadings 'Pre-test Instructions' and 'Steps (in brief)'.)
8. *What is the principle of recording SEPs?* (**Ans.** Refer to page 282, under the heading 'Methods' and the subheading 'Principle'.)
9. *What are the precautions taken for recording SEPs?* (**Ans.** Refer to page 282, under the heading 'Methods' and the subheading 'Precautions'.)
10. *What is the information obtained from the amplitude and latency of SEPs?* (**Ans.** Refer to page 282–283, under the heading 'Observation and Results' and the subheadings 'Median SEP' and 'Tibial SEP'.)
11. *Which interpeak latencies of median SEPs are clinically important? What do they represent?* (**Ans.** Refer to page 283, under the heading 'Observation and Results' and the subheadings 'Median SEP' and 'Tibial SEP'.)
12. *What is the clinical significance of the study of SEPs?* (**Ans.** Refer to page 283, under the heading 'Clinical Applications of SEPs'.)
13. *What are the uses of SEPs?* (**Ans.** Refer to page 283, under the heading 'Clinical Applications of SEPs'.)

43 | Motor Evoked Potential

Learning Objectives

After completing this practical, you will be able to (MUST KNOW):
1. Define motor-evoked potentials (MEPs).
2. Differentiate between sensory evoked potentials and MEPs.
3. Trace the pathway for the corticospinal tract.
4. Explain the principle of recording MEPs.
5. List the common abnormalities of MEP recordings.
6. List the clinical uses of MEPs.

INTRODUCTION

The sensory evoked potentials (visual, auditory, and somatosensory) are recorded from the cerebral cortex or from the sensory pathways following the application of sensory stimulation, whereas **motor evoked potentials (MEPs) are recorded from the muscles** (as EMG responses) following the **stimulation of the motor cortex or spinal cord**. MEPs can be recorded by **two types of stimulations**: electrical and magnetic. The recording of MEPs using transcranial electrical stimulation is painful. Therefore, magnetic stimulation (using a magnetic stimulator) of the cortex is performed to record MEPs. **MEPs are higher in amplitude** and easier to record in contrast to other evoked potentials.

Anatomical and Physiological Considerations

Corticospinal Tract
Refer to Chapter 58.

Physiological basis
Transcranial stimulation can be carried out by electrical or magnetic stimulation.
Electrical stimulation: This is performed with a bipolar or unipolar montage. For transcranial stimulation, **anodal stimulation is preferred** over cathodal stimulation. MEPs are restricted to the **muscles contralateral to the side of cortical stimulation**.
1. **Cortical stimulation** excites the pyramidal cells in the cortex, which in turn stimulate the corticospinal fibres.
2. The **spinal cord can be stimulated** by high-voltage electrical stimulation, either in the cervical or lumbar region. For spinal cord stimulation, **cathodal stimulation** is preferred.
   Electrical stimulation of the spinal cord stimulates the peripheral motor axons close to the spinal cord and the muscle innervated by the axon.
Magnetic stimulation: Magnetic stimulation is **more advantageous** than electrical stimulation as it is painless and can stimulate the deep structures.

METHODS OF RECORDING MEPs

Principle
Motor evoked potentials are recorded as **EMG responses from the muscles** by stimulating the motor cortex or the spinal cord.

Requirements
1. Magnetic or electrical stimulator
2. Electrodes

Procedure

Pre-test instructions
1. The subject and the operator should remove all magnetic objects like watches and keep them at a minimum distance of 50 cm from the stimulator.
2. Enquiries should be made about devices like cardiac pacemakers, cochlear devices, and so on, because electrical or magnetic stimulations are contraindicated in patients with such devices.
3. Electrical stimulation should not be performed in patients with craniotomies. However, magnetic stimulation can be carried out in such patients.
4. Elicit the history of epilepsy from the subject, as transcranial stimulation must be avoided in epileptic patients.
5. Enquire about the use of hypnotics, anticonvulsants, and anxiolytics by the patient as these drugs affect the MEPs.

Steps
1. Brief the subject about the test.
2. Place the magnetic stimulator on the vertex according to the direction of the current flow needed to stimulate the specific area of the cortex and record the MEP from the target muscle (Fig. 43.1). **Butterfly stimulators** are used for deep penetration of the pulses beneath the scalp and for recording MEPs from the upper limb and hand muscles.
3. For recording of MEPs from the target muscles, place the **surface EMG electrodes over the muscle**.

4. Use magnetic stimulation to stimulate the spinal roots and peripheral nerves and record the MEPs from the target muscle.

5. Increase the stimulator output gradually in steps of 10–20 per cent.

6. Ask the subject to slightly contract the target muscle for cortical stimulation and relax the target muscle for spinal stimulation.

7. Record the central motor conduction time (CMCT) by detecting the difference in the latencies of the cortical and spinal stimulation (Fig. 43.1A and B).

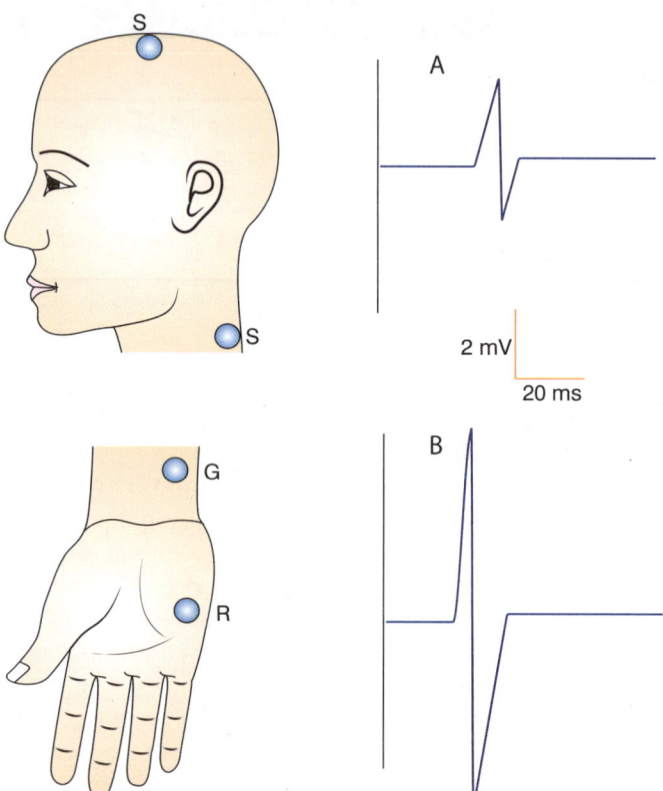

Fig. 43.1 Sites for placing electrodes for recording MEP (S: stimulating electrodes; G: grounding electrode; R: recording electrode placed on abductor digiti minimi; A: response to cortical or scalp stimulation; B: response to spinal or neck stimulation).

Observations and Results

1. **Measurement of CMCT:** Central motor conduction time (CMCT) is measured by subtracting the latency of the MEP on spinal stimulation from that on cortical stimulation. The latency difference is then compared with the distance between two stimulating electrodes.

2. Report your findings with comments.

Precautions

All the pre-test instructions can be considered as precautions for recording MEPs.

DISCUSSION

Normal Values

The normal values of latency and duration of central motor conduction time (ms) of various muscles are presented in Table 43.1.

Table 43.1 Normal values of latency and central motor conduction time (ms)

Muscle	Latency	CMCT
Deltoid	10.6 ± 1.0	4.9 ± 0.5
Biceps	11.6 ± 1.2	4.9 ± 0.5
Thenar	20.1 ± 1.8	6.4 ± 0.3
Tibialis anterior	26.7 ± 2.3	13.2 ± 0.7
Anal sphincter	22.8 ± 3.6	13.3 ± 2.3

MEP Abnormalities

Two major MEPs abnormalities are:

1. **Prolongation of CMCT:** This indicates a slowing down in the central pathways. A significant increase in CMCT is found in demyelinating conditions like multiple sclerosis.

2. **Inexcitability of motor pathways:** This occurs in the following conditions:
   i. Degeneration or damage to the corticospinal tract
   ii. Motor neuron disease

Clinical Applications

Central motor conduction studies are a valuable tool for both the diagnosis and prognosis of various neurological diseases. They are especially important in **diagnosing demyelinating diseases, stroke, degenerative conditions, hereditary ataxia, acute transverse myelitis, encephalitis, and Parkinson's disease.**

Uses of MEPs

Motor evoked potentials (MEPs) are used to assess the **integrity of motor pathways** extending from the brain to the muscles. This can be a valuable tool for monitoring spinal cord function during surgery. Stimulation for MEPs can be achieved using transcranial magnetic stimulation (TMS) or electrical stimulation.

Applications include the following:

1. **Monitoring spinal cord function during surgery:** MEPs are used to monitor the function of the motor pathways during surgical procedures, especially those involving the brain and spine.

2. **Detecting potential neurological injury:** Changes in MEP parameters, like amplitude or latency, can indicate an impending neurological injury or changes in spinal cord function, which can alert surgeons to adjust their procedures.

3. **Diagnosis of motor diseases:** MEPs play a significant role in diagnosing and evaluating the prognosis of disorders such as demyelinating diseases, stroke, degenerative conditions, hereditary ataxia, acute transverse myelitis, encephalitis, and Parkinson's disease.

4. **Assessing motor pathways:** MEPs can help assess the conduction and excitability of the corticospinal system, which is important for understanding how the brain controls movements.

5. **Use of MEPs in research:** MEPs are used now-a-days in medical research of the topics that propose to study the mechanisms of motor control and pathophysiology of various neurological disorders of the motor system.

Thus, MEPs are valuable tools for monitoring motor pathways during surgical procedures, assessing integrity of the motor system and localizing spinal cord injuries and detecting their severity. By analysing the amplitude, latency, and other parameters of the MEPs, clinicians can gain insights into the pathophysiology of motor disorders affecting central and peripheral nervous system.

VIVA

1. *What do you mean by MEPs?* (Ans. Refer to page 285, under the heading 'Introduction'.)
2. *How does MEP differ from EMG?* (Ans. Refer to page 285, under the heading 'Introduction'.)
3. *What is the physiological basis of EMG?* (Ans. Refer to page 285, under the heading 'Introduction' and the subheading 'Physiological basis'.)
4. *What are the types of stimulations used for MEP recordings? What are the differences between them?* (Ans. Refer to page 285, under the heading 'Physiological Basis' and the subheadings 'Electrical stimulation' and 'Magnetic stimulation'.)
5. *What are the important steps of MEP recording?* (Ans. Refer to page 285, under the heading 'Procedure' and the subheading 'Steps'.)
6. *What are the normal values of CMCT of various muscles?* (Ans. Refer to page 286, under the heading 'Discussion' and the subheading 'Normal values'.)
7. *What are the MEP abnormalities and the physiological basis of these abnormalities?* (Ans. Refer to page 286, under the heading 'Discussion' and the subheading 'MEP Abnormalities'.)
8. *What is the clinical significance of MEPs in clinical physiology?* (Ans. Refer to page 286-287, under the heading 'Discussion' and the subheading 'Clinical Applications of MEPs'.)
9. *What are the uses of MEP investigation?* (Ans. Refer to page 286-287, under the heading 'Clinical Applications of MEPs'.)

44 | Perimetry and Demonstration of Various Visual Phenomena

Learning Objectives

After completing this practical, you will be able to (MUST KNOW):

1. Appreciate the importance of perimetry in clinical physiology.
2. Define field of vision, visual axis, isopters, meridians, and blind spot (scotoma).
3. Read the perimeter chart.
4. State the principle of perimetry.
5. Chart the field of vision by using a perimeter.
6. List the precautions for perimetry.
7. Explain the extent of the visual field in different quadrants.
8. List the factors that affect the field of vision.
9. Trace the visual pathway.
10. Name the visual field defects with lesions at various levels of the visual pathway.
11. Demonstrate the test for physiological blind spot.
12. Explain stereoscopic vision.
13. Comprehend dominance of the eye.
14. Understand subjective visual sensations and effect of mechanical stimulation of the eye.

You may also be able to (DESIRABLE TO KNOW):

1. Name and describe different perimeters.
2. Describe a perimeter chart.
3. Explain physiological and pathological blind spots.
4. Explain the effect of lesions on the visual pathway.
5. Explain the mechanism of stereoscopic vision.

PY10.20: Demonstrate: (i) Testing of visual acuity, colour, and field of vision, (ii) Hearing, (iii) Testing for smell, and (iv) Taste sensation in a volunteer/simulated environment.

INTRODUCTION

Perimetry is the method of accurately **charting the peripheral field of vision** using a perimeter. A **perimeter** is an instrument used to determine the field of vision. Clinically, the field of **vision is roughly determined at the patient's bedside** by the **confrontation method** (described in Chapter 56), which gives a rough idea of the field of vision. Perimetry is performed to **detect the exact nature and extent of defects in the field of vision**. These defects occur due to lesions at various levels of the visual pathway.

The Visual Pathway

Visual fibres originate in the nerve cell layer in the retina (from **bipolar and ganglion cells**). The neurons travel as **optic nerves** to the optic chiasma, where *partial decussation* of the fibres takes place. The fibre coming from the temporal side of the retina (which receives information from the nasal half of the visual field) remains uncrossed, whereas the fibre emerging from the nasal hemiretina (which receives information from the temporal half of the visual field) crosses to the opposite side at the **optic chiasma**. Thus, the **optic tract** contains fibres from the temporal hemiretina of the same side and the nasal hemiretina of the opposite side. This means that the left optic tracts carry the fibres from the left halves of both retinas and the right optic tract from the right halves of both retinas. Most fibres in the optic tract terminate in the **lateral geniculate body** of the thalamus, from where the second order of neurons originates and ascends the **geniculocalcarine pathway** to reach the **visual cortex.** Some fibres from the optic tract enter the superior colliculus, from where the fibres project to the pretectal area, which through projection in *Edinger-Westphal nucleus*, mediate visual reflexes (Fig. 44.1). The fibres originating from the lateral geniculate body form a loop at their origin called the *Meyer's loop*.

Field of Vision

The portion of the external world visible to the eye when the *gaze is fixed at a particular point* is called the field of vision. The visual field mainly depends on the size and colour of the object used for mapping the field. In the temporal side of the fixation point, at about 12°–15°, a **scotoma (blind spot)** is located, in which perception of light does not occur. This is called **physiological scotoma,** and it corresponds to the **optic disc** in the retina, which does not contain rods and cones. It measures approximately **7.5° in height and 5.5° in width**. The visual fields of both eyes overlap in their medial part to form the area of **binocular vision**, in which objects are seen by both eyes. The extent of the visual field is described in the 'Discussion' section.

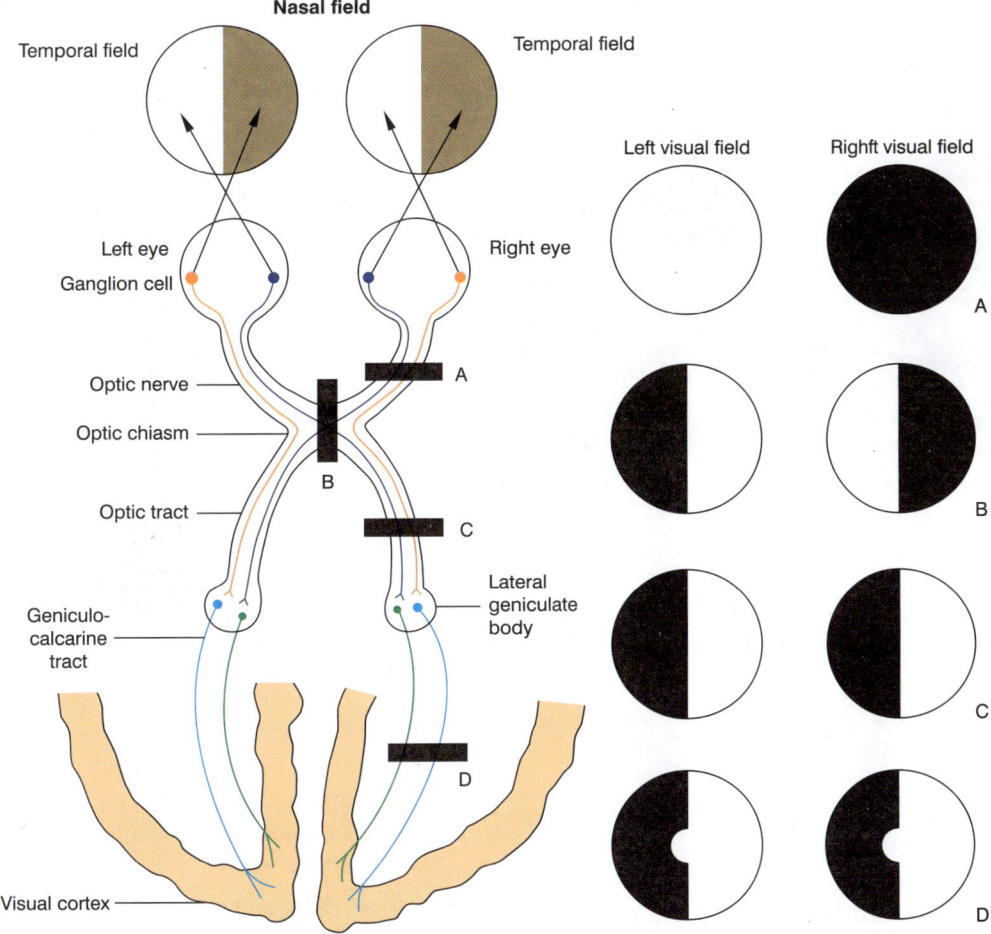

Fig. 44.1 Effects of lesions at various levels of the visual pathway: **A:** Lesion of the right optic nerve produces blindness in the right eye; **B:** Lesion of the optic chiasma produces bitemporal hemianopia; **C:** Lesion of the right optic tract produces left homonymous hemianopia; **D:** Lesion of the right geniculocalcarine tract produces left homonymous hemianopia with macular sparing.

METHOD OF PERIMETRY

Principle

The part of the external world visible to a person when he fixes his gaze on an object is called the field of vision. The method of charting the field of vision is called perimetry. The field of vision charted with one eye (the other eye closed) gives the field of vision for that eye. One eye is covered while the other is fixed on a central point. A small target is moved towards this central point along the selected meridians. Along each meridian, the location where the object first becomes visible is plotted in degrees; this process is repeated in all meridians. The determination of the visual field by the confrontation method is described in Chapter 55 (2nd cranial nerve).

Requirements

1. **Perimeter:** This is an instrument that accurately maps the field of vision. There are different types of

perimeters available. The commonly used perimeters are *Priestley–Smith's perimeter, Lister's perimeter, and the student's perimeter* (a simple hand perimeter). The most commonly used perimeter in physiology laboratories is Lister's perimeter.

Lister's perimeter: This consists of a broad, concave, metal arc that can be rotated around its centre, both clockwise and anticlockwise (Fig. 44.2). The metallic arc is graduated in degrees. There is a groove in one limb of the metallic arc into which a test object is fitted. The concavity of the arc faces the subject. The arc rotates through various angles on a pivot in any direction along with the test object. There are two metallic chin rests. At the back of the perimeter, there is an arrangement for fixing the perimeter chart.

Priestley–Smith's perimeter: This device is also used in many laboratories (Fig. 44.3).

Student perimeter: In this perimeter, the inclination of the arc is read from a plastic dial fitted behind the mirror (Fig. 44.4). When an object is moved along

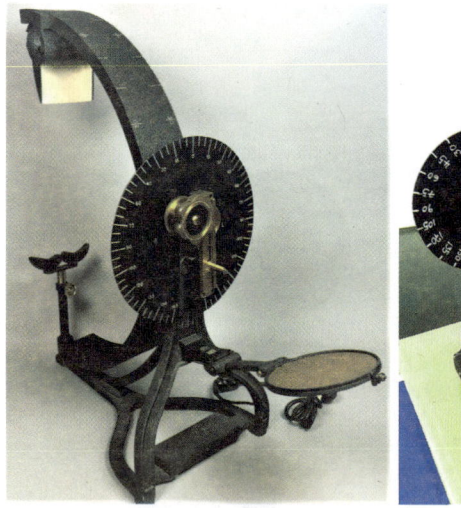

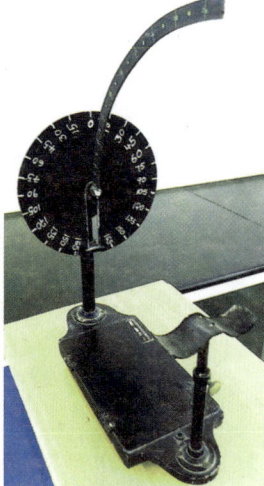

Fig. 44.2 Lister's perimeter (1: **Fig. 44.3** Priestley–metallic arc; 2: removable shield; 3: Smith's perimeter. chart plate; and 4: chin rest).

the inside of the arc, it becomes visible. The angle it subtends at the fixation point (i.e., the mirror) in a given meridian can be read from the scale engraved on the outside of the arc. The readings (the meridian and the angle) are then transferred to the corresponding points on the chart.

2. **Perimeter chart:** The centre of the chart (Fig. 44.5) corresponds to the visual axis. The concentric circles around the centre denote the point of equal visual acuity; these are called **isopters** and are **marked in degrees** (at 10° intervals) from the central fixation points. Perimeter charts contain lines through the centre of the circle denoting various meridians in degrees. These radii (meridians) are marked at 15° intervals. A black oval dot present on the horizontal meridian (15° on either side of the central fixation point) corresponds to the **normal blind spot**. For comparison with the normal field of vision, right and left visual fields are marked on the chart as dotted lines. For mapping the visual field, the chart is fixed to the back of the perimeter.

3. **Test objects:** Test objects of different colours and diameters are used. Usually, the sizes of the test objects are 3, 5, 10, 15, and 20 mm. The test object is fitted into a carrier, which moves in a groove in one limb of the metal arc. The test object moves with a knob, which causes the movement of a pin on the back of the metal arc. The most commonly used object is white and 5 mm in size.

Procedure

1. Read the perimeter chart.
2. Provide proper instructions to the subject.

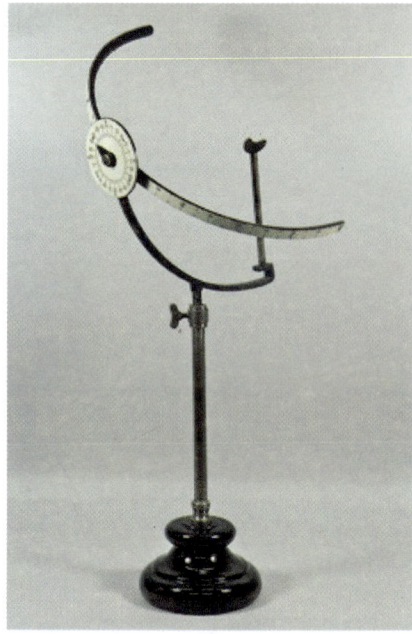

Fig. 44.4 Student perimeter.

3. Ask the subject to sit on a stool comfortably in front of the perimeter.
4. Arrange the perimeter in such a way that the concavity of the arc faces the subject.
5. Ask the subject to sit straight and rest his chin on one of the chin rests.

Note: When the field of vision of the right eye is to be tested, the subject should rest his chin on the left chin rest. This brings his right eye in line with the fixation point.

6. Focus the eye to be examined on the fixed object, which is a white object, 5 mm in size, placed at the centre of the metallic arc.

Note: It should be emphasised that the subject's gaze should be fixed on the object throughout the maneuver.

7. Fix the metallic arc in one meridian.
8. Move the test object (which is fixed to the carrier along the arc) gradually from the periphery (90°) towards the central fixation point and ask the subject to indicate when he first sees the object. Note this point.
9. Note this reading in degrees on the arc by making a marking on the chart for that meridian.
10. Repeat the procedure at 15° intervals till the field of vision is plotted in all meridians of the four quadrants.

Note: The blind spot is marked along the horizontal meridian in the temporal quadrant.

11. Mark the point of disappearance by bringing the test object towards the centre after the initial appearance in the field and the point of reappearance with further

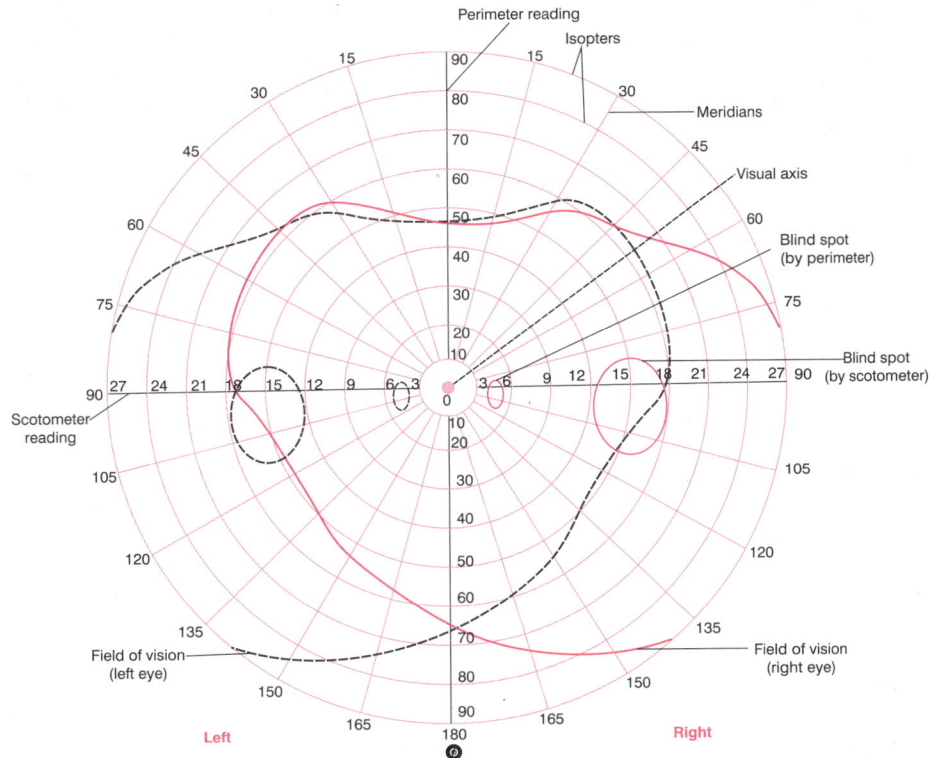

Fig. 44.5 Lister's perimeter chart.

movement of the object in the same line. This indicates the size of the blind spot.

12. Repeat the entire procedure for the other eye on the same chart.

Observation and Results

1. Observe the obtained field of vision and compare it with the normal visual field depicted in the chart.
2. Note the site and size of the blind spot.
3. Report your results with your comments.

Precautions

1. Provide proper instructions to the subject.
2. Before mapping the field of vision, study the perimetry chart thoroughly.
3. While testing one eye, ensure that the other eye is closed.
4. Fix the eye on the central fixation point.
5. Repeat the procedure at 15° intervals till the field of vision is plotted in all meridians.
6. Carry out the mapping in the clockwise direction.
7. Mark the blind spot along the horizontal meridian in the temporal quadrant.
8. Test the field of vision for both eyes separately.
9. Ensure that there is adequate illumination throughout the procedure.
10. Ask the subject to remove his glasses if he normally uses them; otherwise, the field of vision will be restricted.

DISCUSSION

The visual field of each eye is the portion of the external world visible to that eye. Theoretically, the visual field should be circular, but it is actually *restricted by the nose medially and the roof of the orbit superiorly*. Mapping of visual fields is one of the most important tests in clinical neurology to detect different diseases of the brain, especially those that affect the visual pathway.

The visual field is divided into peripheral and central fields of vision. The peripheral field of vision is mapped by perimetry, whereas the **central field of vision** is mapped with the help of a *tangent screen (Bjerrum's screen)* on which a white target is moved across a black screen.

Factors That Affect the Field of Vision

1. **Colour of the object:** Visual acuity is better for a white object than for coloured objects. Thus, the field of vision is better delineated with a white object. Roughly, the field of vision obtained by using blue and yellow objects is 10° less, and that obtained by using red and green objects is 20° less than the visual field obtained by a white object.
2. **Size of the object:** The larger the object, the better is the visual acuity. However, **a standard-sized object** is typically used during **perimetry tests** to ensure consistency.

3. **Brightness of the object:** Brightness, contrast, and illumination affect visual acuity and consequently, the field of vision.
4. **Illumination:** Poor illumination decreases the visual field.

Normal Field of Vision

The normal field of vision with a white object, 5 mm in size, is as follows:

Temporal: 100° (since there is no anatomical obstruction on the temporal side of the eyes, the extent of the field of vision in this quadrant is more)

Inferior: 75° (the maxilla of the cheek is an anatomical obstruction and reduces the extent of the field in this quadrant)

Superior: 60° (the supraorbital margin forms an anatomical obstruction and reduces the extent of the field in this quadrant)

Nasal: 60° (the nasal bridge forms an anatomical obstruction and reduces the extent of the field in this quadrant)

Visual Field Defects

A defect on the same side of both visual fields is called a **homonymous defect**; a defect in half of the visual field is called **hemianopia**. A defect in the opposite sides of the visual field is called a **heteronymous defect** (Fig. 44.1).

Complete blindness: This occurs due to lesions of the optic nerves. If the lesion is on one side, it causes blindness of that eye.

Heteronymous hemianopia: Lesions that *affect the optic chiasma*, e.g., tumours of the pituitary gland expanding the sella turcica, cause this defect. Bitemporal hemianopia is common, whereas binasal hemianopia is rare.

Homonymous hemianopia: A *lesion of the optic tract* causes this defect. A lesion of the right side of the optic tract produces left homonymous hemianopia, and a lesion of the left optic tract produces right homonymous hemianopia.

Homonymous hemianopia with macular sparing: A *lesion in the geniculocalcarine tract* causes this defect. Macular sparing (loss of peripheral vision with intact macular vision) occurs because the macular representation is separate from that of the peripheral field and is large relative to that of the peripheral fields. Therefore, the lesion in the occipital cortex must extend to large areas to affect peripheral as well as macular vision.

DEMONSTRATION OF VARIOUS VISUAL PHENOMENA

Demonstration of Physiological Blind Spot

The physiological blind spot is the naturally occurring *area in the visual field of each eye where no vision can be perceived*. It is a zone of functional blindness that all normally sighted people have in each eye due to the absence of photoreceptors where the optic nerve passes through the surface of the retina.

It is located on the nasal side (towards the nose) of the retina, where the optic nerve enters and exits the retina; there are no photoreceptor cells in the retina at this spot. The most common test to detect the physiological blind spot, also known as the **optic disc spot**, is a **visual field test using perimetry**. Simple 'blind spot' tests using an object like a finger or a card with a dot and cross can also demonstrate the blind spot.

Mariotte's experiment: French scientist **Edme Mariotte** (1620–1684) first described the blind spot in the 1660s. Edme Mariotte's experiment revealed the existence of a blind spot where *no image is perceived*. The blind spot is typically located about 15 degrees temporally (towards the outer edge of the eye) from the point of fixation. The size of the blind spot is approximately *5.5 degrees wide and 7.5 degrees in height*. Mariotte's experiment involved observing a visual field and noticing that a specific area was not perceived, thus identifying the blind spot. Mariotte explained that the blind spot is a *monocular visual field defect*, meaning that it is present when only one eye is used for viewing. Because our eyes have overlapping visual fields, the blind spot in one eye is usually not noticeable when both eyes are open.

1. Testing the blind spot by visual field tests

i. **Confrontation visual field evaluation using perimetry:** This is a basic test in which the patient covers one eye and is asked to identify an object or the number of fingers presented in the periphery.
ii. **Tangent screen:** Tests the central 30° of the visual field.
iii. **Amsler grid:** Measures the central visual field occupied by the macula.
iv. **Goldmann visual field (GVF) perimetry:** Uses a bowl-shaped perimeter with bright light targets.

These tests identify blind spots and pinpoint the location and size of the blind spot.

2. Simple 'blind spot' tests (using objects)

These tests demonstrate the location of the blind spot in a simple way. The patient covers one eye and focuses on a fixed point (like a cross on a card) with the other eye. As an object (like a dot on the card or a finger) is moved across the visual field, the patient will notice a point where the object disappears and then reappears as it's moved further across the visual field. The disappearance and reappearance denote the blind spot.

Demonstration of Stereoscopic Vision

Stereoscopic vision is the ability to perceive **three-dimensional shapes and distances** using two eyes. This is also known as **depth perception**, a fundamental aspect of binocular vision where the brain processes slight differences in the images received by each eye, creating a sense of depth and solidity. This process is called **stereopsis**, which relies on the *brain's ability to merge these two-dimensional images* from each eye into a *single, three-dimensional perception*.

Physiological significance

Depth perception: Stereoscopic vision is crucial for the *accurate perception of depth*, which is essential for tasks like judging distance, catching a ball, or navigating an environment.

Binocular vision: It relies on the coordinated functioning of both eyes and the *brain's ability to process binocular cues*.

Procedures

1. Thread a needle first with both eyes open. Then, repeat the experiment with one eye and then with the other eye. Note the time it takes in each case. The visual perception is much better with both eyes open.
2. Hold a matchbox about 25 cm in front of your eyes. Draw its appearance as seen with only the right eye, and then with the left eye. Compare the two sketches. The normal mechanism of vision fuses the two slightly different images into one to give an impression of solidity.

Factors affecting stereoscopic vision

The proper development of stereoscopic vision requires good vision in each eye and precise eye movements.

Impairment of stereoscopic vision: Stereoscopic vision can be impaired or lost in individuals with significant visual field defects, such as homonymous hemianopia, resulting from brain injury or stroke. Conditions like strabismus (misalignment of the eyes) or amblyopia (lazy eye) can affect stereoscopic vision due to disrupted binocular fusion.

Dominance of the Eye

Eye dominance, which is also known as **ocular dominance**, denotes the brain's preference for inputs from one eye over the other. While both eyes contribute to vision, the dominant eye exerts a greater influence on visual perception and spatial awareness.

Dominance is task-dependent: The dominant eye can be different for different tasks, such as sighting a target (motor dominance) or binocular rivalry (sensory dominance).

Relationship with handedness: Eye dominance often aligns with handedness; right-handed individuals are more likely to have a right-dominant eye.

Procedure

Several tests, including the **hole-in-the-card test** and **Porta test**, can help determine which eye is dominant.

Procedure: Form a circle with your thumb and index finger, and holding it at arm's length, look through it with both eyes open at a small object across the room, say, a door handle. Close one eye and then the other. The eye that sees the object within the circle is your dominant eye.

Physiological significance

The dominant eye plays a more prominent role in **depth perception**, **spatial awareness**, and **overall visual processing**. Eye dominance is a natural phenomenon where the brain favours inputs from one eye, influencing visual perception and spatial awareness.

Subjective Visual Sensations

Subjective visual sensations are visual experiences that arise from internal brain activity rather than external visual stimuli. These sensations are not based on what is physically present in the environment but are generated by the brain itself. Examples include *seeing flashes of light, spots, or other visual phenomena* without an external object or stimulus.

Causes

Subjective visual sensations can be associated with the following conditions:

1. **Medical conditions:** Migraines, glaucoma, retinal detachments, and other eye conditions can cause subjective visual sensations.
2. **Stress and anxiety:** Intense stress or anxiety can lead to visual disturbances.
3. **Medications:** Some medications can have side effects that include visual sensations. Examples include drugs like antidepressants, antiepileptic drugs, Digoxin, Sildenafil, and antihistaminics.
4. **Neurological conditions:** In some cases, subjective visual sensations can be related to neurological conditions or damage.

Procedure

Close one eye and look at the sky with the other. Try to concentrate on what you see. You will observe small, circular, semi-transparent, grey specks/or zigzag wispy filaments/or hair-like objects that drift across the field of vision. These are called **floaters**. If you try to focus on them, they drift away or sink down; if you jerk your eye up, they rise up but sink down or float away once again.

Physiological significance

1. Some individuals are more susceptible to experiencing subjective visual sensations due to higher sensitivity to light or patterns, which can lead to visual discomfort or sensory overload.
2. Distinguishing between subjective and objective visual sensations is important for accurate diagnosis and treatment of visual problems.

Mechanical Stimulation of the Eye

Mechanical compression of the eye stimulates the eye and evokes different sensations. Mechanical stimulation of the retina, in particular, can evoke visual sensations known as **phosphenes**. These sensations can manifest as various visual phenomena, such as darkening, coloured patches, or even complex light patterns.

Phosphenes: These are visual sensations perceived when the eye is not exposed to light but is still stimulated, often by pressure or mechanical means.

Mechanism

Applying pressure to the eye or surrounding area can mechanically stimulate the cells of the retina, including the photoreceptors. This supports Muller's law of specific nerve energy, which states that different types of stimuli applied to a sensory organ produce the sensation peculiar to that receptor. In this case, for the retina, the natural stimulus of light requires minimal energy to stimulate the rods and cones, while a mechanical stimulus requires many times the energy needed by the normal stimulus.

Procedure

Rubbing or pressing on the closed eyelids: Close your eyes and press on the outer corner of an eye with the index finger. This pressure produces an impression of a dark circular spot surrounded by a bright circle in the field of vision directly opposite the point of pressure. These visual sensations are called pressure phosphenes. They are caused by inadequate retinal stimulation.

Potential therapeutic applications

Mechanical stimulation of the retina is being explored as a potential treatment for photoreceptor degenerative diseases.

VIVA

1. *What is perimetry?* (Ans. Refer to page 288, under the heading 'Introduction'.)
2. *What is the clinical utility of determining the field of vision?* (Ans. Refer to page 288, under the heading 'Introduction'.)
3. *Which parts of the retina are tested in perimetry? How is acuity of vision tested?*
   (Ans. Perimetry tests most parts of the retina except the macular region, which contains the fovea centralis. The fovea contains only cones and is the region of most acute vision. The acuity of vision is tested with a Snellen chart for distant vision and a Jaeger chart for near vision.)
4. *What are the different types of perimeters?* (Ans. Refer to page 289, under the heading 'Requirements' and the subheading 'Perimeters'.)
5. *How is the perimeter chart read and interpreted?* (Ans. Refer to page 290, under the heading 'Requirements' and the subheading 'Perimeter Chart'.)
6. *What are the sizes of the test objects? Which one is usually selected for perimetry?* (Ans. Refer to page 290, under the heading 'Requirements' and the subheading 'Test objects'.)
7. *How is the blind spot mapped in perimetry?* (Ans. Refer to page 285, under the heading 'Procedure'.)
8. *What are the important precautions taken while performing perimetry?* (Ans. Refer to page 292, under the heading 'Precautions'.)
9. *Why is the visual field not circular?* (Ans. Refer to page 291, under the heading 'Discussion'.)
10. *What is the size of the normal field of vision? Detail the field of vision in its four dimensions.* (Ans. Refer to page 292, under the heading 'Normal Field of Vision', read 'Temporal, Inferior, Superior, and Nasal' extents.)
11. *What are the factors that affect the field of vision?* (Ans. Refer to page 291, under the heading 'Factors that affect the field of vision'.)
12. *Are all objects seen clearly within the field of vision?*
    (Ans. No, only objects whose images fall on the **macula** [the central part of the retina] are seen in **sharp detail**, with **bright and distinct colours**. As objects move away from the centre of focus, they become **less clear**, and colours are **harder to recognise**. For example, while reading, only about **10 mm** of text is seen in sharp focus at a time. The **peripheral retina** is not good for fine detail or colour, but it is **very sensitive to movement**, flashes of light, and motion. This is why we often notice a moving object **out of the corner of our eye** before seeing it clearly by looking straight at it.)

13. *What is the field of vision oval and restricted?*
(Ans. The visual field or field of view is the oval-cone of space. It is subdivided as follows: i. The right and left visual fields, seen by the right and left eyes respectively; ii. The binocular segment, which is seen by both eyes; and iii. The right and left monocular segments outside of the binocular segment to the right and the left.

The peripheral field of each eye extends up to about 100° on the temporal side; about 65–75° downwards, which is limited by the cheek; 55–60° on the nasal side, which is limited by the nose; and about 55–60° upwards, where it is limited by the brow. The peripheral field is widest for the white, and smaller for blue, red, and green colours in that order.

14. *Trace the visual pathway.* (Ans. Refer to page 288, under the heading 'Visual pathway'.)
15. *Name the visual field defects produced by lesions at various levels in the visual pathway.* (Ans. Refer to page 292, under the heading 'Visual Field Defects'.)
16. *Define heteronymous hemianopia and name its causes.* (Ans. Refer to page 292, under the heading 'Visual Field Defects' and the subheading 'heteronymous hemianopia'.)
17. *How is the central field of vision determined?* (Ans. Refer to page 292.)
18. *Define homonymous hemianopia and name its causes* (Ans. Refer to page 292, under the heading 'Visual Field Defects' and the subheading 'homonymous hemianopia'.)
19. *What is physiological blind spot? What is its significance?* (Ans. Refer to page 292, under the heading 'Demonstration of Physiological Blind Spot'.)
20. *Name the scientist who first demonstrated the physiological blind spot. What is Mariotte's experiment?* (Ans. Refer to page 292, under the heading 'Demonstration of Physiological Blind Spot' and the subheading 'Mariotte's experiment'.)
21. *What are the methods of determining blind spot?* (Ans. Refer to page 292, under the heading 'Demonstration of Physiological Blind Spot'.)
22. *What is scotoma?*
(Ans. A **scotoma** is a small **blind spot** in the visual field, **not including the normal physiological blind spot** we all have. It is important to **detect and map** scotomas in clinical exams, as they can be a sign of problems. Scotomas can be caused by damage to the **retina, optic nerve**, or due to **neurological conditions** like **migraine, multiple sclerosis, stroke, or head injury**.)
23. *What is dominance of the eye? How is it demonstrated?* (Ans. Refer to page 293, under the heading 'Dominance of the Eye'.)
24. *What is the physiological and clinical significance of ocular dominance?* (Ans. Refer to page 293, under the heading 'Dominance of Eye'.)
25. *What is stereoscopic vision? State its clinical importance and the method to demonstrate it.* (Ans. Refer to page 293, under the heading 'Stereoscopic vision'.)
26. *What are the subjective visual sensations? What is its clinical significance?* (Ans. Refer to page 293, under the heading 'Subjective Visual Sensations'.)
27. *What is the effect of mechanical stimulation of the eye? What is its physiological significance?* (Ans. Refer to page 294, under the heading 'Mechanical Stimulation of the Eye'.)

45 | Visual Acuity (Tests for Distant Vision and Near Vision) and Other Related Phenomena

Learning Objectives

After completing this practical, you will be able to (MUST KNOW):

1. Explain the importance of determining visual acuity in clinical medicine.
2. Define visual acuity.
3. List the factors that affect visual acuity.
4. Determine the visual acuity for distant and near vision.
5. List the precautions taken for determining visual acuity.
6. Define myopia and hypermetropia.
7. Name the type of lens used to correct the defects of visual acuity for distant and near vision.

PY10.20: Demonstrate: (i) Testing of visual acuity, colour, and field of vision, (ii) hearing, (iii) testing for smell, and (iv) taste sensation in a volunteer/ simulated environment.

INTRODUCTION

Visual acuity is defined as the **resolving power of the eyes,** i.e., the extent to which the *eye can perceive the details and contours of an object*. It can be explained in terms of *minimum separable distance*, that is, the smallest gap by which two lines can be separated and still be seen as two separate lines. Visual acuity is the **function of cones**. It is tested separately for distant vision and near vision.

Factors Affecting Visual Acuity

Visual acuity is affected by **three factors**: optical factors, retinal factors, and stimulus factors.

Optical factors

The **image-forming mechanism** is the primary factor that determines visual acuity. *Optical aberrations and defects* of the image-forming mechanism decrease visual acuity.

Retinal factors

Visual acuity is the function of the cones. *Cones are more in number at the centre* (densely packed in the fovea centralis) than in the periphery of the retina. Therefore, visual acuity is **maximal at the fovea and less in the periphery** of the retina.

Stimulus factors

The main stimulus factors are the **size and colour of the object**.

Size of the object: The size of the object and its distance from the eye affect visual acuity. Visual acuity is directly proportional to the **visual angle** (VA).

$$VA = \frac{\text{Size of the object}}{\text{Distance of the object from the eye}}$$

Colour of the object: Visual acuity is *better for white objects than for coloured objects*.

Brightness, contrast, exposure time: Visual acuity also depends on the brightness of the stimulus, the contrast between the stimulus and the background, and the length of time for which the subject is exposed to the stimulus.

METHODS TO TEST VISUAL ACUITY

Test for Distant Vision

Principle

A series of letters of varying sizes is constructed in such a way that the top letter is visible to normal eyes at 60 metres, and the subsequent lines at 36, 24, 18, 12, 9, 6, and 5 metres respectively. Visual acuity is recorded according to the formula **V = d / D**, where V is the visual acuity, d is the distance at which the letters are read, and D is the distance at which the letters should be read.

Requirements

Snellen's chart: Snellen's letters are depicted on a cardboard (Fig. 45.1) with eight rows of black letters of different fonts. The topmost line can be read by a normal subject at a distance of 60 metres and subsequent lines at 36, 24, 18, 12, 9, 6, and 5 metres, respectively.

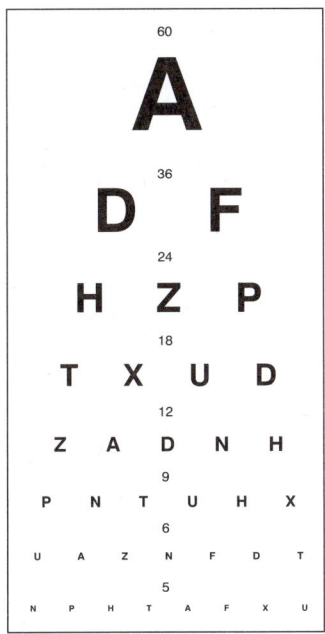

Fig. 45.1   Snellen's chart.

For uneducated or illiterate persons, the **Landolt ring chart** is used (Fig. 45.2).

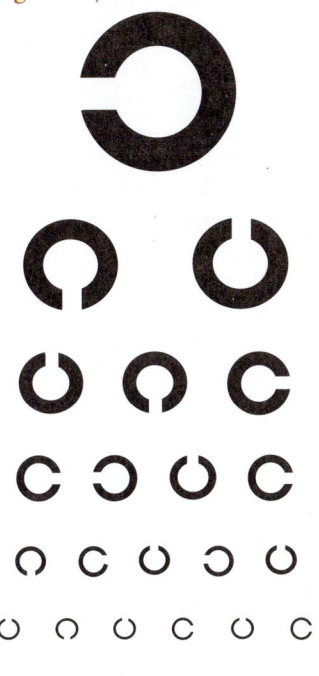

Fig. 45.2   Landolt ring chart.

Procedure

1. Provide proper instructions to the subject.
2. Ask the subject to sit at a **distance of 6 metres** from the chart (d = 6).
3. Ask him to close one of his eyes and read the chart with the other eye.
4. Note up to which line the subject is able to read comfortably.
5. Ask him to repeat the procedure with the other eye.

Precautions

1. Provide proper instructions to the subject.
2. Ascertain whether the subject knows the letters (language) written on the Snellen's chart.
3. Ensure that the Snellen's chart is well-lit.
4. Ensure that the patient sits exactly at a distance of 6 metres from the chart.
5. Test each eye separately.
6. If the subject wears glasses, test the visual acuity with and without them.

Observation

If only the top letter of the chart is visible, the visual acuity is 6/60. If the subject can read the lowest line, the visual acuity is 6/5, that is, he has better than normal vision. **Normal visual acuity is 6/6.** Accordingly, visual acuity is expressed as 6/6, 6/9, 6/12, 6/18, 6/24, and 6/36, respectively, depending on the line up to which the subject can read. If his visual acuity is less than 6/60, that is, the subject cannot read the top line from a distance of 6 metres, he should move closer until he can read the top letter. If the top letter is visible at 2 metres, the visual acuity is expressed as 2/60. If the acuity of vision is less than 1/60, the subject is asked to count fingers held up (**finger counting method**) or to perceive hand movement (**hand movement method**). If the subject cannot count the fingers or perceive hand movement, a light is focused in front of his eyes, and he is asked whether he perceives the light (**light perception method**).

Test for Near Vision

Principle

The visual acuity for near vision is tested using the Jaeger's chart at ordinary reading distance. This consists of letters of various sizes based on the principle of *Printer's point system.*

Requirement

Jaeger's chart: This chart (Fig. 45.3) consists of letters of various sizes on the Printer's point system. The smallest point is N_5, and the largest point is N_{36}.

Procedure

1. Provide proper instructions to the subject.
2. Ensure that the **room is well-lit** and that the subject is seated comfortably.
3. Hold the Jaeger's chart at a **distance of 10–12 inches** from the subject's eyes.
4. Ask the subject to read the letters of different sizes.
5. Note the smallest size of letters that the subject can read comfortably.
6. Repeat the test separately for each eye with the other eye closed.

N5

When I was ten years old, my father had a small estate near Satara where he used to take us during the holidays. It was situated in rough and uncultivated country side where wild animals were often seen. Once we heard that there was a panther in the surroundings who was killing the cattle and attacking the villagers. Father had warned me not to wander for from home in the evenings. I had made friends with a your villager called Ramu.

N6

Ramu used to drive the cattle to graze and bring them back to shelter at the end of the day. He was lean and of a short build and was barely fifteen. He used to be my companion whenever I meet him winding his way home. One afternoon, just about five o'clock, early in the month of March, chance brought us together.

N8

As there had been considerable variation in the series of Jaeger's test types produced by different printers, a new series of standard graduated test types for near vision has been recommended by the Faculty of Opthalmologist of England in which Times Roman types are used with standard spacing.

N10

The eye to be examined is anaesthetised with 1% solution in anaethine and the instrument is lightly pressed against the eye in the suspected area. If there is a solid tumour, the pupil remains dark. Then the instrument is placed on another region when the pupil is found to be read.

Fig. 45.3   Jaeger's chart.

Precautions

1. It should be ascertained that the subject knows the language in which the letters are written.
2. The room should be adequately lit.
3. The Jaeger's chart should be kept at a distance of about 25 cm from the subject's eyes.
4. The test should be performed with both eyes open. It should also be performed separately for each eye with the other eye closed.

Observation and results

1. Note the smallest size of letters that the subject can read.
2. Record the results for both eyes.
3. Record your comments on the results.

DISCUSSION

The normal visual acuity is **6/6**, i.e., the subject should be able to **read up to the seventh line**. If his visual acuity is less than 6/6, it is considered to be reduced. To correct the acuity of vision, concave lenses are prescribed after performing a thorough *postmydriatic examination* of the eye.

If the subject wears glasses, the **type of lens used** should be mentioned. The examiner can detect the type of lens by holding the lens in front of the eye and looking at an object through it. When the lens is moved from side to side, if the object appears to move in the opposite direction, the *lens is convex*; if the object moves in the same direction, the *lens is concave*. Concave lenses are used to correct **myopia**, while convex lenses are used for **hypermetropia**.

For **young children**, simple pictures printed on a chart based on *Snellen's principle* can be used. Another test used for children is the **Sheridan–Gardiner test,** in which Snellen's letters are matched with different types of objects. For people who cannot read, the 'E' test is effective.

Myopia

Myopia or **short-sightedness** is an error of refraction in which parallel rays of light coming from a distant object are focused *in front of the retina*. The person cannot see distant objects. This condition is corrected *using concave lenses*.

Hypermetropia

Hypermetropia or **long-sightedness** is an error of refraction in which parallel rays of light coming from a distant object are **focused behind the retina**. Thus, the person cannot see objects that are nearby. This defect is corrected **using convex lenses**.

OTHER RELATED VISUAL PHENOMENA

Other phenomena related to visual acuity are the **demonstration of near point, demonstration of near response and accommodation, and demonstration of Purkinje–Samson images**.

Near Point

The near point of the eye refers to the **closest distance an object can be placed and still be seen clearly and without strain**. For a normal young adult, this distance is **approximately 25 cm** (about 1 foot).

Factors affecting near point

Vision correction: People with certain eye conditions, such as myopia (near-sightedness) or presbyopia (age-related farsightedness), may have a near point that is closer or farther than 25 cm, respectively.

Age: The near point is also affected by age, with the ability to accommodate (focus on near objects) generally decreasing with age.

Procedure

1. Ask the subject to sit near a window with sufficient daylight and ask him to cover one eye with a cupped hand.
2. Hold a pencil in front of the other eye and slowly move it perfectly along a meter stick toward the eye until it can no longer be seen in sharp focus.
3. *Record the distance between the pencil and the eye.* This is the near point of that eye.
4. Measure the near point for the other eye as well.
5. If the subject wears glasses, measure the near point with and without glasses.
6. Lastly, measure the near point with both eyes open.

Demonstration of Near Response and Accommodation

The near response refers to the coordinated visual response that *allows eyes to focus on objects that are nearby*. It involves three key actions: **convergence** (eyes moving inward to focus on the nearby object), **accommodation** (the lens thickening to focus on the object), and **pupillary constriction** (pupils narrowing to reduce the amount of light entering the eye).

1. **Accommodation:** The *ciliary muscles of the eye contract*, causing the lens to *become thicker and more curved*. This change in curvature allows the eye to focus on a near object, which would otherwise be blurry.
2. **Convergence:** The eyes *move inward, towards the nose*, so that both eyes focus on the nearby object. This ensures that a single, clear image is seen rather than two images.
3. **Pupillary constriction:** The pupils narrow in size, *reducing the amount of light* entering the eye. This helps to *improve the sharpness* of the image on the retina and can *reduce glare*.

Procedure

1. Ask the subject to sit near a window and fix his eyes on a distant object.
2. Quickly bring your finger in front of his eyes and ask him to focus his eyes on it.
3. Note the convergence of the eyes and constriction of the pupil.

4. The increase in the curvature of the lens can be seen on ophthalmic examination (for details, refer to Chapter 56, *Examination of Cranial Nerves*; see 'Oculomotor Nerve').

This three-part response is called the **near response** or **accommodation reflex**.

Measurement of Range of Accommodation

The **far point** is the farthest point from the eye at which an object is seen clearly.

Procedure

1. Determine the far point of vision using a method similar to that used for measuring the near point.
2. If the subject is emmetropic (has normal vision), it will be noticeably far away. A distance of 6 meters from the eye is considered the practical far point because light rays coming from this distance are parallel.
3. If the patient wears glasses, record the near and the far points with and without glasses.
4. Calculate the range of accommodation, i.e., the distance between the far and near points for each eye, separately.

Demonstration of Purkinje–Sanson Images

Purkinje–Sanson images are reflections of objects formed within the eye, arising from the refractory surfaces of the cornea and lens. These images are named after the scientists who discovered them—**Jan Evangelista Purkinje** and **Louis Joseph Sanson**.

Typically, **four Purkinje-Sanson images are observed**, numbered I, II, III, and IV, each originating from different ocular surfaces.

Image I (P1): Reflected from the *anterior (outer) surface of the cornea*, it is the brightest and most easily visible.

Image II (P2): Reflected from the *posterior (inner) surface of the cornea*.

Image III (P3): Reflected from the *anterior surface of the lens*.

Image IV (P4): Reflected from the *posterior surface of the lens*; it is the only inverted image among the four.

Procedure

This experiment is conducted in a dark room. The subject should be seated comfortably on a chair.

1. Hold a burning candle to one side of the subject's eye and observe the images of the candle flame from the other side.
2. The **following images** are observed:
   i. On the anterior surface of the cornea, **image 1**— *bright and upright*.
   ii. On the posterior surface of the cornea, **image 2**—*upright, but not clearly visible*.

iii. On the anterior surface of the lens (near the centre of the pupil), **image 3**—*upright, somewhat larger, and not so bright*.

iv. On the posterior surface of the lens, **image 4**—*smaller and inverted*, but not so easily seen.

3. Ask the subject to look to the wall of the room. While observing the images carefully, hold a finger in front of his eye and ask him to look at it.

4. Image 3 (i.e., on the anterior surface of the lens) moves closer to Image 1 (anterior surface of the cornea), which also becomes smaller and brighter. This shows that during accommodation for near vision, the anterior surface of the lens moves forward, i.e., the anterior surface becomes more convex. This (anterior surface of the lens that becomes more convex) is better appreciated with a phakoscopic examination during accommodation reflex.

Clinical Applications

1. **Eye tracking:** Purkinje images, particularly P1 and P4, are used by eye tracking systems to monitor eye movements.

2. **Keratometry and corneal topography:** P1 is used to measure corneal curvature and shape.

3. **Accommodation and lens changes:** Changes in the position and curvature of the lens during accommodation can be assessed using Purkinje images.

4. **Cataract and aphakia diagnosis:** Purkinje images can help in diagnosing and monitoring conditions like cataracts and aphakia (absence of the natural lens).

VIVA

1. *Define visual acuity.* (**Ans.** Refer to page 296, under the heading 'Introduction'.)
2. *What are the factors that affect visual acuity?* (**Ans.** Refer to page 296, under the heading 'Factor Affecting...'.)
3. *What is visual angle? How does it affect visual acuity?* (**Ans.** Refer to page 296, under the heading 'Factor Affecting...' under the subheading 'Stimulus factor...size of object'.)
4. *How do you test visual acuity for distant vision?* (**Ans.** Refer to page 296, under the heading 'Methods'.)
5. *How is the Snellen's chart interpreted?* (**Ans.** Refer to page 296-297, under the heading 'Requirements...Snellen's Chart'.)
6. *How is the visual acuity tested for illiterate persons?* (**Ans.** Refer to page 297, under the heading 'Requirements...Landolt ring chart', Fig. 44.2'.)
7. *If a patient's acuity of vision is less than 1/60, how is the visual acuity tested?* (**Ans.** Refer to page 297, under the heading 'Observation' and the subheading 'Finger counting method'.)
8. *How do you test visual acuity for near vision?* (**Ans.** Refer to page 292, under the heading 'Test for Near Vision'.)
9. *How is Jaegar's chart read and interpreted? What is the point system for near vision testing?* (**Ans.** Refer to page 297, under the heading 'Test for Near Vision' and the subheading 'Principle' and 'Requirements'.)
10. *What are the precautions for the tests of visual acuity?* (**Ans.** Refer to page 298, under the heading 'Precautions'.)
11. *What is the Sheridan-Gardiner test? What is its significance?* (**Ans.** Refer to page 298, under the heading 'Sheridan-Gardiner test'.)
12. *What is myopia? How do you correct it?* (**Ans.** Refer to page 298, under the heading 'Myopia'.)
13. *What is hypermetropia? How do you correct it?* (**Ans.** Refer to page 298, under the heading 'Hypermetropia'.)
14. *Define near point, what factors affect it and how is it tested?* (**Ans.** Refer to page 298, under the heading 'Near Point'.)
15. *What is near response? How is it measured? How is accommodation range measured?* (**Ans.** Refer to page 299, under the heading 'Near Response'.)
16. *How are the Purkinje-Sanson images tested? What is the clinical importance of this assessment?* (**Ans.** Refer to page 299, under the heading 'Purkinje-Sanson images'.)

46 | Colour Vision

Learning Objectives

After completing this practical, you will be able to (MUST KNOW):
1. Explain the clinical importance of performing the test for colour vision.
2. Test the colour vision using the Ishihara chart.
3. Explain the functions of the cone systems.
4. Trace the pathway of the colour vision.
5. Classify and define different types of colour blindness.

You may also be able to (DESIRABLE TO KNOW):
1. Name the theories of colour vision.
2. Explain different types of colour blindness and the modes of transmission of the condition.
3. Describe other methods of detecting colour vision.

PY10.20: Demonstrate: (i) Testing of visual acuity, colour, and field of vision, (ii) hearing, (iii) testing for smell, and (iv) taste sensation in a volunteer/simulated environment.

INTRODUCTION

The human eye has the ability to respond to all wavelengths of light from 400–700 nm. This is called the visible part of the spectrum. The sense of colour is **perceived by cones**. There are **three types** of cone systems: **red, green, and blue**. There are also *three types of cone pigments*: **cyanolabe, chlorolabe, and erythrolabe**, which respond to specific parts of the spectrum. Each cone shows maximum absorption of light at a particular wavelength. Due to *differential stimulation of the three types of cones* by different wavelengths of light, the human eye perceives all the colours.

For example, a wavelength of 580 nm stimulates red cones maximally and results in the perception of the colour red. It also stimulates the green cones to some extent, resulting in the perception of the colour orange. Likewise, the wavelength of 535 nm stimulates green cones, and the wavelength 445 nm stimulates blue cones maximally, therefore, we perceive the colours green and blue.

There are **three primary colours**—*red, green, and blue*—each responding maximally to light of certain wavelengths. When colours are mixed in appropriate amounts, the object looks white. Therefore, for any colour, there is a complementary colour which, when properly mixed with it, produces white.

Pathway of Colour Vision

Neurons carrying colour vision in the optic nerve pass through the **optic tract** to reach the parvocellular part of the **lateral geniculate body** (LGB) of the thalamus. From the *parvocellular laminas* of the LGB, fibres project to the **blob regions** in layer four of the **visual cortex**. Blobs are clusters of cells arranged in a mosaic in the visual cortex and are concerned with colour vision.

Mechanism of Colour Vision

There are **two mechanisms** of colour vision: the retinal and the cortical.

Retinal mechanism

The retinal mechanism of colour vision is based on **Young and Helmholtz's theory**. According to this theory, the perception of the three primary colours is possible due to the *presence of three types of cone systems* in the retina, each containing a specific pigment which is maximally sensitive to one type of primary colour.

Cortical mechanism

The *colour-sensitive ganglion cells* project onto the cells of the **lateral geniculate body (single opponent cells)**, which in turn, project onto the cells of the **primary visual cortex (double opponent cells)**. The cortical cells in turn, project onto **area 18**. It is believed that different colours are perceived due to the activities in the primary visual cortex and the cortical association areas.

METHODS TO TEST COLOUR VISION

Ishihara's Chart Method

There are different methods of detecting colour vision. Of these, the Ishihara chart is the most routinely used.

Principle

Colour vision is tested by using Ishihara's chart, which consists of **lithographic plates** on which numbers are drawn using **coloured spots** amidst other parts of different colours and sizes. The subject reads the number and traces the pathway by appreciating the colour.

Requirements

Ishihara's chart: This consists of lithographic plates in which numerals are drawn using different colour spots (Fig. 45.1). The colour of these spots is such that they are likely to be confused with spots in the background by people with defective colour vision. These plates are so constructed that a person with colour vision defect will read a different number than a person with normal colour vision.

Procedure

1. Provide proper instructions to the subject.
2. Ask the subject to sit comfortably in a well-lit room.
3. Instruct the subject to read the numbers or trace the lines in each plate of the book.
4. Observe whether he is able to read the number or trace the pathway properly.

Observation and results

1. Note whether the subject is able to trace the lines on each plate.
2. Observe whether the subject has read the numbers on the coloured plates correctly.
3. Record your observations and report the results.

Precautions

1. The room should be adequately lit.
2. All the plates of the book should be read.

3. While reading the plates, a maximum of 5–10 seconds should be allowed per plate.

Other Methods

There are **two other methods** of testing colour vision: the Edridge–Green lantern test and Holmgren's wool-matching test.

Edridge–Green lantern test

In this test, various coloured lights are projected using a **lantern**, and the subject is asked to **identify the colours** presented. The lantern contains the following colours: pure red, red of different intensities, yellow, green, signal green, blue and purple.

- The subject sits in a dimly illuminated room, 6 meters away from the lantern.
- He names the colour of the light, focused through the glass fixed on a rotating disc in the lantern.

This test is usually employed for *railway recruitment*.

Holmgren's wool-matching test

In this test, the subject is asked to perform a series of colour-matching tasks from a **collection of wool of different colours**. There are three sets of coloured wool: test colours, matching colours, and confusing colours. The subject matches different colours of the three groups.

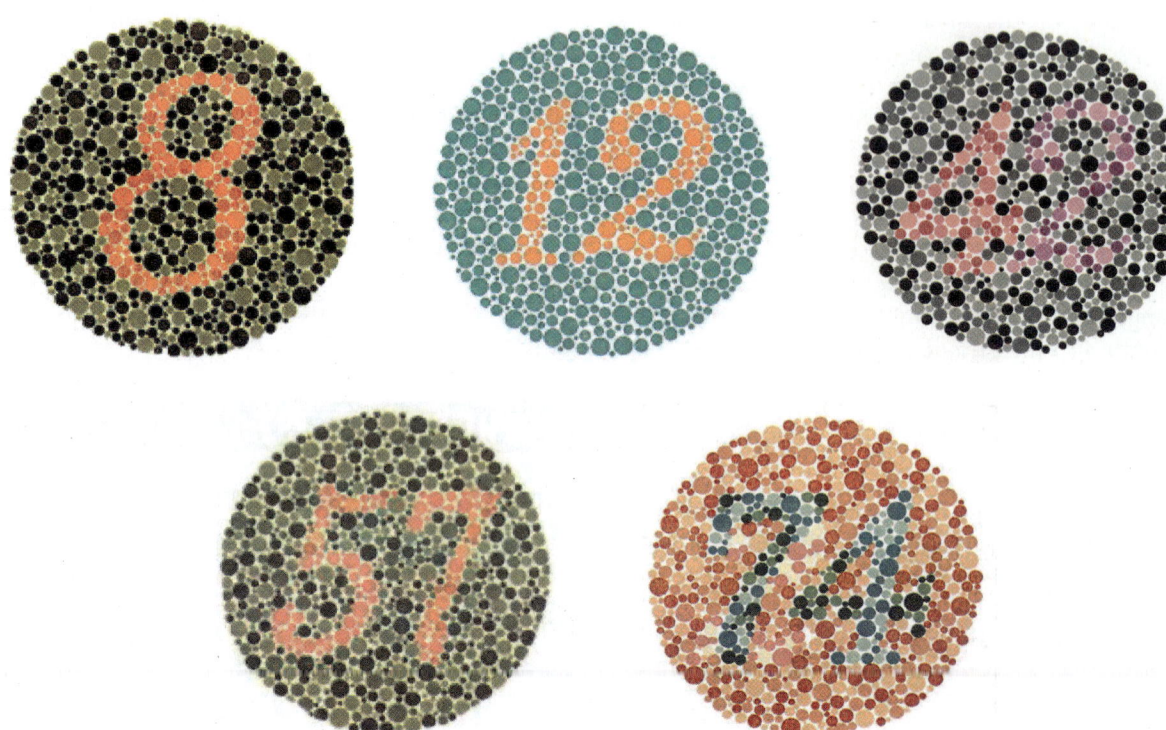

Fig. 46.1 Lithographic plates of Ishihara's chart.

DISCUSSION

Clinical Significance

The test for the intactness of colour vision is performed routinely as part of the medical screening **for recruitment** into government jobs or **admission into** professional courses. Intact colour vision is mandatory for occupations related to *driving, traffic services, railways, and the armed forces*. A defect in the perception of colour is called **colour blindness**.

Types of Colour Blindness

Colour blindness is classified into three types:

1. **Trichromats:** Trichromats are of two types: *protanomaly and deuteranomaly*. The person is less sensitive to one of the primary colours.
2. **Dichromats:** Dichromats are of **three types**: *protanopia, deuteranopia, and tritanopia*. The person perceives two primary colours.

3. **Monochromats:** The person perceives only one primary colour.

The suffix '**anomaly**' represents *colour weakness* and the suffix '**anopia**' represents *colour blindness*. The prefixes '**prot**', '**deuter**', and '**trit**' represent *red, green, and blue colour defects*, respectively. For example, protanomaly means weakness of the perception of red, and protanopia means blindness for red. A **trichromat** has all the three cone systems, but one system may be weak (*protanomaly or deuteranomaly*). A **dichromat** is an individual having only two cone systems, and one cone system absent. Depending on the absence of a cone system, a subject can be *protanopic, deuteranopic, or tritanopic*. A **monochromat** is a person having only one cone system, with two systems absent.

Colour blindness is inherited as an **X-linked recessive**. This occurs due to an abnormal gene on the X chromosome. Women are carriers but suffer from the disease only when both X chromosomes carry the defective gene.

VIVA

1. *What is the clinical significance of the test of colour vision?* (**Ans.** Refer to page 301, under the heading 'Introduction'.)
2. *What are the three primary colours? How are they perceived by different cone systems?* (**Ans.** Refer to page 301, under the heading 'Introduction'.)
3. *What is the pathway for colour vision?* (**Ans.** Refer to page 301, under the heading 'Pathway of colour vision'.)
4. *How is the Ishihara chart prepared?* (**Ans.** Refer to page 302, under the heading 'Requirements' and the subheading 'Ishihara chart'.)
5. *What chart is used for detecting colour blindness? What is its principle?* (**Ans.** Refer to page 301, under the heading 'Methods of test colour vision' and the subheading 'Principle'.)
6. *What do you mean by colour blindness? How do you classify it?* (**Ans.** Refer to page 303, under the heading 'Types of Colour Blindness'.)
7. *What is the mode of transmission of colour blindness?* (**Ans.** Refer to page 303, under the heading 'Types of Colour Blindness'.)
8. *What are the mechanisms of colour vision?* (**Ans.** Refer to page 301, under the heading 'Mechanism of Colour Vision'.)
9. *What is the principle of Young Helmhotlz's theory of colour vision?* (**Ans.** Refer to page 301, under the heading 'Retinal mechanism'.)
10. *What are the other methods of detecting colour vision? What is the principle behind each of these methods?* (**Ans.** Refer to page 302, under the heading 'Other methods'.)

47 | Hearing Tests including Audiometry, Localisation and Masking of Sounds

Learning Objectives

After completing this practical, you will be able to (MUST KNOW):

1. Elucidate the importance of performing this practical in clinical physiology.
2. Name the hearing tests.
3. State the principles of the tuning fork test.
4. Perform and interpret the tuning fork test.
5. List the precautions to be taken for the tuning fork test.
6. Differentiate conductive deafness from neural deafness.
7. Understand the principle and use of audiometry

8. Learn the concept and importance of localisation of sound.
9. Mention the meaning and benefits of masking of sound.

You may also be able to (DESIRABLE TO KNOW):

1. Trace the auditory pathway.
2. State the attributes of sounds.
3. State the principles of audiometry and BAEP.
4. Explain the abnormalities of hearing tests.
5. Know the procedure and uses of audiometry, localisation of sound, and masking of sound.

PY10.20: Demonstrate: (i) Testing of visual acuity, colour, and field of vision, (ii) hearing, (iii) testing for smell, and (iv) taste sensation in a volunteer/simulated environment.

HEARING TESTS

INTRODUCTION

Hearing tests are commonly performed by audiologists to detect the **type and degree of hearing loss** for prescribing hearing aids. Hearing tests also help neurologists to establish the extent of lesions, especially if the brainstem is involved in the pathological process.

Anatomical and Physiological Considerations

Physiological basis

■ Characteristics of sound

The perception and interpretation of sound are complex phenomena. There are **four attributes of sound**: frequency, intensity, direction, and pattern. The sound waves are **sensed by the hair cells** of the cochlea, and the impulses are transmitted to the auditory cortex by a very complex pathway. The actual **perception and interpretation** of most aspects of sound take place in the **auditory cortex**.

Frequency: The frequency (**pitch**) of the sound stimuli is **detected by the basilar membrane**. Sharpening of frequency occurs in the hair cells and auditory neurons.

- The cells in the **auditory cortex** only respond to a **narrow range of sound frequencies**. The frequency of the nerve impulses is related to the intensity of the stimulus.
- The higher the frequency, the higher is the pitch. **Pitch discrimination** is possible because different frequencies cause vibrations in different regions of the basilar membrane.
- Each segment of the basilar membrane is thus tuned for a particular pitch: high-pitched sounds near the base of the cochlea and low-pitched sounds near the apex of the cochlea.

Note: The entire audible frequency ranges from 16–20, 000 Hz (1 hertz = 1 cycle/sec). The term *infrasound* refers to frequencies below 16 Hz, whereas *ultrasound* refers to frequencies above 20,000 Hz. The **human ear is most sensitive** to frequencies between **500 and 5000 Hz**. The average **conversation voice frequency** is 120 Hz in males and 250 Hz in females. Though the human ear cannot hear (perceive) ultrasound, bats, dogs, and other animals can.

Intensity: Intensity (**loudness**) of the sound is coded as early as at the receptor level. **Outer hair cells respond to weaker stimuli** because of the lower threshold of the cilia of the outer hair cells, which are embedded in the tectorial membrane. Within the **auditory cortex**, *certain neurons are maximally sensitive* to a **specific intensity of the stimulus**, enabling fine discrimination of loudness.

Direction: The direction of sound is judged by the **difference in time and intensity** at which it arrives at the two ears. Though the direction of sound is detected by the superior olivary nucleus, the **auditory cortex is essential for the perception** of the direction of sound.

Pattern: The pattern (**timber** or quality) of sound is the *sequence in which different components of the sound appear*. This property of sound is recognised by the **auditory cortex alone**.

Mechanism of Hearing

The sound waves striking the tympanic membrane are magnified by the ossicles and set the basilar membrane to vibrate. This results in the movement of the **hair cells of the organ of Corti**. The bending of the cilia of hair cells transduces mechanical vibrations into action potentials, which are transmitted through the **auditory pathway** to the primary auditory areas of the cerebral cortex (Brodmann's areas 41, 42).

Auditory pathway (Fig. 47.1)

The axons of the spiral ganglion, which innervate the hair cells of the ear, form the **cochlear nerve** (8th cranial nerve).

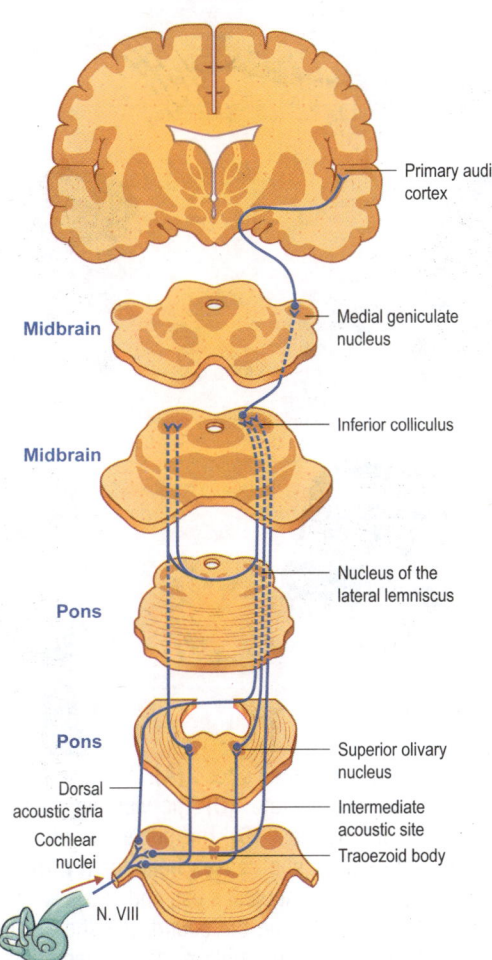

Fig. 47.1   Auditory pathway (N.VIII: Cochlear part of the 8th cranial nerve, i.e., the vestibulo-cochlear nerve).

The **first order of neurons** terminates in the **cochlear nuclei** in the medulla, from where the **second order of neurons** arises and ends in the **superior olivary nucleus**. The **third order of neurons** originates from the **superior olivary nucleus** and ascends the lateral lemniscus to project onto the **inferior colliculus**, which is the centre for auditory reflexes. From the inferior colliculi, a number of fibres project onto the **medial geniculate body** in the thalamus, and from there to the **primary auditory cortex** (area 41).

Types of Hearing Tests

A number of hearing tests have been developed to detect hearing loss:

1. Watch test
2. Tuning fork test
3. Audiometry
4. Recording of brainstem auditory evoked potentials (BAEP)

The commonly used hearing test in clinical practice is the tuning fork test.

METHODS OF ASSESSING HEARING

Watch Test

Principle

Sound is sensed by the hair cells in the ear and conducted via auditory pathways to the auditory cortex. A defect in either perception or conduction of sound can lead to hearing loss.

Requirement

1. Wristwatch

Procedure

1. Ask the subject to close his eyes.
2. Ask him to plug one ear with a finger.
3. Slowly bring a ticking wristwatch from a distance toward the uncovered ear. Ask the subject to indicate the moment they first hear the sound.
4. Note the distance at which the subject hears the sound of the wristwatch.
5. Repeat these steps for the other ear.
6. Compare the results with those of a normal subject to assess for hearing loss.

Disadvantages

1. It detects only gross hearing impairment.
2. It cannot detect the nature and degree of hearing loss.

TUNING FORK TESTS

Tuning fork tests are based on the **principle** that *sound is conducted to the ear by the air* (air conduction).

Therefore, deafness can be detected by *testing air conduction or by directly stimulating the bone* that conducts sound. There are **three types** of tuning fork tests: **Rinne's test, Weber's test, and Schwabach test.**

Requirements

Tuning fork: A tuning fork of **512 Hz** (Fig. 47.2) is commonly used for all these tests. Tuning forks of higher frequency like 512 Hz or 256 Hz produce *more sound than vibration*, whereas tuning forks with lower frequency produce more vibration than sound. Therefore, **512 Hz or 256 Hz** tuning forks are preferred for hearing tests (Fig. 47.2).

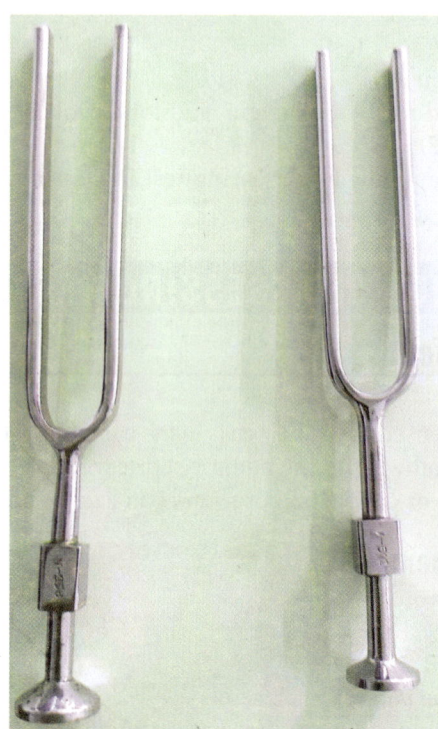

Fig. 47.2   Tuning forks for hearing tests. The longer one is 256 Hz and the shorter one is 512 Hz.

Rinne's Test

Principle

Rinne's test compares hearing ability through the mediums of bone and air; this means that there is a comparison of bone conduction with air conduction of the same ear.

Procedure

1. Provide proper instructions to the subject.

   Note: Instruct the subject to raise her finger when she stops hearing the sound of the vibrating tuning fork.

2. Hold the stem of the tuning fork between the thumb and the index finger in such a way that the fingers do not touch the blades of the tuning fork (Fig. 47.3A).

3. Make the tuning fork vibrate by suddenly striking the blades of the fork against the hypothenar eminence (Fig. 47.3B) or the thigh.

4. Immediately place the base of the vibrating tuning fork **on the mastoid process** (Fig. 47.3C) of one side and ask the subject to raise her finger when she ceases to hear the sound (Fig. 47.3D).

5. Once she stops hearing, hold the vibrating tuning fork *very close to her ear* (Fig. 47.3E) and ask her whether she hears the sound. When she stops hearing it, bring the tuning fork *close to your own ear* to confirm whether the vibrating sounds have actually stopped (Fig. 47.3F).

6. Record your observation.

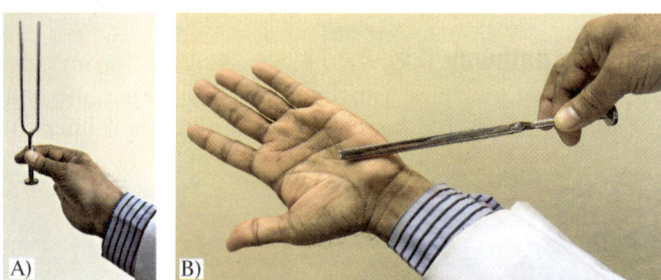

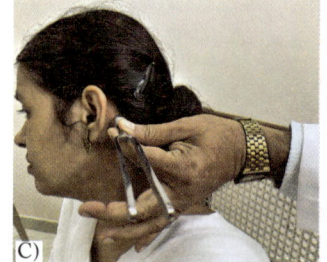 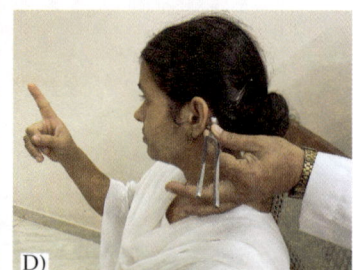

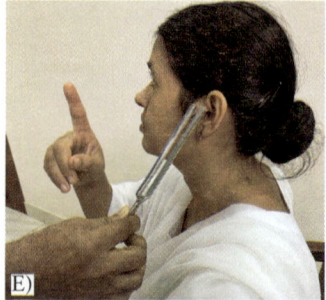 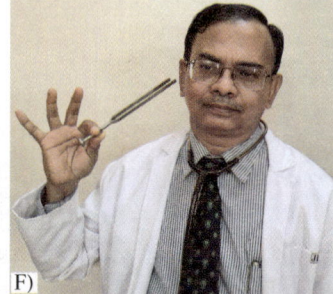

Fig. 47.3   Methodology of Rinne's test: **(A)** The tuning fork is held properly; **(B)** It is made to vibrate; **(C)** The vibrating tuning fork is placed on the mastoid process; **(D)** The subject is asked to raise her finger immediately after she ceases hearing; **(E)** The vibrating tuning fork is kept close to the subject's ear, and she is asked to raise her finger once she stops hearing the sound; **(F)** The tuning fork is brought to the examiner's ear to confirm that the vibrating sounds have actually stopped.

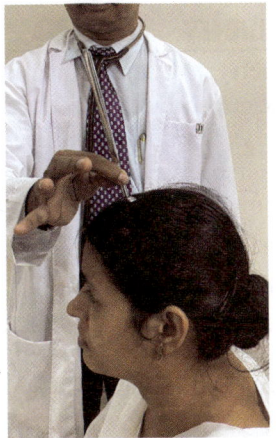

Fig. 47.4 Methodology of Weber's test: The vibrating tuning fork is placed on the centre of the vertex of the skull, and the subject is instructed to indicate whether she hears equally on both sides or if the sound is better heard in one ear.

Observation and results

Write down your observations along with your comments (for details, refer to Table 47.1):

1. If air conduction is greater than bone conduction (Rinne-positive): Normal
2. If bone conduction is greater than air conduction (Rinne-negative): Conductive deafness
3. Both air and bone conduction are absent: Complete nerve deafness
4. Air conduction is greater than bone conduction in the defective ear (Rinne-false-positive): Partial nerve deafness

Precautions

1. Proper instructions should be given to the subject.
2. The tuning fork should be held by the stem, taking care **not to touch the blades**.
3. To start the vibration in the tuning fork, the fork should be stroked against the hypothenar eminence or the thigh, not against the table or another hard surface, because the loud sound produced could disturb others and may damage the tuning fork.
4. If the subject **stops hearing the sound**, the examiner should bring the fork close to his own ear (considering the examiner has normal hearing) for comparison.

Weber's Test

Principle

Weber's test compares the bone conduction of the two ears.

Procedure

1. Provide proper instructions to the subject.
2. Make the tuning fork vibrate by striking the blades of the fork against the hypothenar eminence or the thigh.

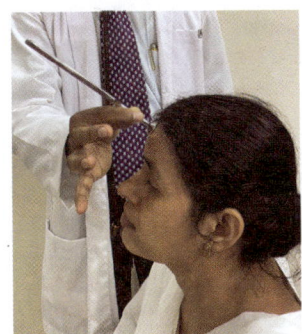

Fig. 47.5 Alternate method to perform Weber's test: The vibrating tuning fork is placed on the centre of the subject's forehead, and the subject is instructed to indicate whether she hears equally on both sides or if the sound is better heard in one ear.

3. Place the base of the vibrating tuning fork **on the vertex of the skull** (Fig. 47.4) or *on the subject's forehead* (Fig. 47.5).
4. Ask the subject to indicate whether she **hears equally on both sides** or if the sound is better heard in one ear.

Observation and results

1. Sound is heard equally in both ears: Normal
2. Sound is better heard in the defective ear (lateralised to the defective ear): Conduction deafness in a defective ear
3. Sound is better heard in the healthy ear (lateralised to the healthy ear): Partial nerve deafness in a defective ear

Precautions

1. Proper instructions should be given to the subject (the subject should understand the procedure of the test).
2. To make the tuning fork vibrate, the blades of the fork should be struck against the hypothenar eminence or the thigh.

Schwabach Test

Principle

This test compares the bone conduction of the subject with that of the examiner.

Procedure

1. Provide proper instructions to the subject.
2. Make the tuning fork vibrate.
3. Place the vibrating tuning fork over the **subject's mastoid process** (Fig. 47.6A).
4. Ask the subject to *raise her finger* when she stops hearing the sound (Fig. 47.6B).
5. Immediately bring the tuning fork towards yourself and place it *on your mastoid process* to check if you still hear the sound (Fig. 47.6C).

Observation and results

1. Bone conduction of the subject is equal to the bone conduction of the examiner: Normal

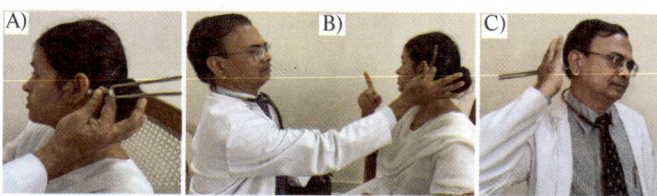

Fig. 47.6 Methodology for Schwabach test. **(A)** The vibrating tuning fork is placed on the mastoid process; **(B)** The subject is asked to raise her finger immediately after she stops hearing **(C)** The examiner places the same tuning fork on his mastoid process to check whether the sounds are still audible.

2. Bone conduction of the subject is better than the bone conduction of the examiner: Conduction deafness in the subject

3. Bone conduction of the subject is worse than the bone conduction of the examiner: Partial nerve deafness in the subject

Precautions

1. Proper instructions should be given to the subject.
2. Once the subject stops hearing the sound, a comparison should be made against the examiner by placing the tuning fork on his mastoid process.

The interpretation of the results of hearing tests is summarised in Table 47.1.

AUDIOMETRY

Audiometry is an objective and accurate method to assess the **degree of deafness and the frequency range** at which it manifests. Audiometry helps determine if someone has hearing loss, and the **nature of that loss** (e.g., conductive, sensorineural, or mixed). This is done by using an **audiometer,** which is an *electroacoustic device*.

Types of Audiometry

Pure-tone audiometry: Measures hearing sensitivity to different frequencies of sound.
Speech audiometry: Evaluates a person's ability to understand speech, in both quiet and noisy environments.
Impedance audiometry: Measures the middle ear's function.

Principle

Audiometry involves measuring **hearing sensitivity to different frequencies and intensities of sound**. It can help in *identifying the type and severity of any hearing loss*. The results are often displayed on an *audiogram*—a graph that shows a person's *hearing thresholds at different frequencies*.

Audiogram: The audiometer provides *pure tones of different frequencies* at various *levels of loudness or intensity* from an oscillator connected via an amplifier to the earphones. Generally, the audiometer provides a **minimum of 7 tones** (250, 500, 1000, 2000, 3000, 4000, and 8000 Hz). The intensity of each tonal frequency can be increased. The lowest decibel at which the patient hears the tone is called the **threshold**. A graph is plotted showing the **audiometric threshold as a function of frequency discrimination** (Fig. 47.7). This graph is called an **audiogram**.

Procedure

1. The test is conducted in a soundproof room. One ear is tested at a time with the help of an earphone.
2. A trained professional (an audiologist) presents a series of pure tones (single frequencies) to the patient through earphones or a bone conduction oscillator.

Table 47.1   Observation and inference of hearing tests.

Name of the test	Observation	Inference
Rinne's test	i) Air conduction is greater than bone conduction (Rinne-positive) ii) Bone conduction is greater than air conduction (Rinne-negative) iii) Both air and bone conduction are absent iv) Air conduction is greater than bone conduction in the defective ear (Rinne-false positive)	i) Normal ii) Conduction deafness iii) Complete nerve deafness iv) Partial nerve deafness
Weber's Test	i) Sound is heard equally in both ears ii) Sound is better heard in the defective ear (lateralised to the defective ear) iii) Sound is better heard in the healthy ear (lateralised to the healthy ear)	i) Normal ii) Conduction deafness in the defective ear iii) Partial nerve deafness in the defective ear
Schwabach Test	i) Bone conduction of the subject is equal to the bone conduction of the examiner ii) Bone conduction of the subject is better than the bone conduction of the examiner iii) Bone conduction of the subject is worse than the bone conduction of the examiner	i) Normal ii) Conduction deafness in the subject iii) Partial nerve deafness in the subject

3. The lowest intensity (measured in decibels) at which a sound is heard is recorded for each frequency, creating a graph called an audiogram.
4. The subject flashes a light when they hear the sound.
5. At each frequency, the threshold intensity is determined and plotted against a graph as a percentage of normal hearing.

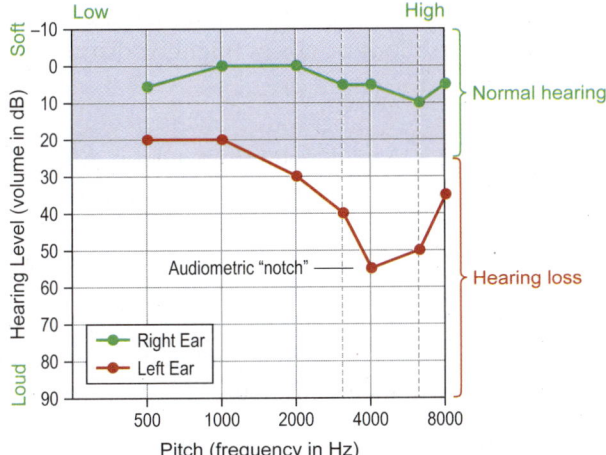

Fig. 47.7 Pure tone audiogram. Note that the audiometry reveals moderate degree of hearing loss in the left ear. The hearing in the right ear is normal.

Observation and Results

1. Note the lowest intensity (measured in decibels) at which a sound is heard for each frequency.
2. Plot a graph of threshold intensity at each frequency.

Applications

1. The audiogram provides valuable information about a person's **hearing abilities**, including the **degree and type of hearing loss**.
2. Audiometry is used for **hearing screenings**, **diagnosing hearing loss**, and evaluating the **effectiveness of hearing aids** or other **treatments**.

Brainstem Auditory Evoked Potential

Brainstem auditory evoked potential (BAEP) or **auditory brainstem response** (ABR) is an accurate method to differentiate organic deafness from functional deafness and to determine the exact site of hearing loss. BAEPs are **electrical responses** that can be recorded from the scalp in response to acoustic stimuli. Recently, BAEP has been **used for IONM** to monitor auditory pathway function. It has become essential in **diagnosing hearing loss**, acoustic tumours, and cerebellopontine angle tumours. The details of BAEP are described in Chapter 40.

LOCALISATION OF SOUNDS

Sound localisation refers to the ability to **determine the direction of a sound source**. There are two different aspects to sound localisation. This ability is crucial for navigating our environment, identifying threats, and understanding communication. It relies on the brain processing *subtle differences in the sound signals* reaching each ear, known as **binaural cues**. There are *two categories* of sound localisation.

1. **Absolute localisation or localisation acuity:** It refers to the ability to judge the absolute position of a sound source in three-dimensional space.
2. **Relative localisation:** It refers to the ability to detect a shift in the absolute position of the sound source.

Binaural Effect

The use of both ears to perceive sound is defined as *binaural hearing*. This ability makes it possible to identify the location of sound far more effectively. The ability to judge the position of the source of sound with both ears is called the *binaural effect*. *Two factors* are involved in this process:

1. The **difference in the loudness** of the sounds at the two ears.
2. The **difference in the interval** of sound at the two ears, i.e., the **phase difference** or **interval between equal phases** of sound waves entering the two ears.

Note: The human ear can gauge the direction of a sound's origin on a 0.00003 second difference in its interval at the two ears. When we want to localise a sound coming from a distance, we turn our head until the sound is equally loud in the two ears. The direction in which we are facing is the direction of the sound's origin.

Binaural cues: The brain uses *two types* of binaural cues:

1. **Interaural time difference (ITD):** The difference in *time it takes* for a sound to reach each ear.
2. **Interaural level difference (ILD):** The difference in *intensity (loudness) of the sound* reaching each ear.

Monaural cues: Some sound localisation also relies on monaural cues, which are differences in the sound signal that can be detected by a single ear, such as the filtering of sound by the head and torso.

Factors Affecting Sound Localisation

Head shape and size: These factors influence how sound waves are modified as they travel to the ears, affecting the effectiveness of monaural cues.

Environment: Reverberations and echoes can make it tougher to localise sounds.

Frequency and intensity of sound: The frequency and intensity of the sound can also influence how well it can be localised.

Method to Assess the Ability to Localise Sounds

Procedure

1. Ask the subject to sit in a quiet room and close his eyes.
2. Use a pair of forceps to produce clicking noises behind, in front of, and to each side of his head, one after the other, and ask him to locate the direction of sound in each case.

Observation and results

In your workbook, record the subject's ability to localise the sound as excellent, good, fair, or poor.

Applications of Localisation of Sound

Everyday life: Identifying the direction of approaching vehicles, recognising the source of an alarm, or understanding where someone is speaking from.

Robotics for navigation: Developing robotic systems that can navigate and interact with their environment based on sound.

Hearing aids: Helping individuals with hearing loss to better localise sounds.

MASKING OF SOUND

Sound masking or auditory masking is a method of **reducing the perception of unwanted sounds by introducing a different, generated sound** into the environment. It is the process by which the threshold of hearing for one sound is raised by the presence of another sound, i.e., when a signal—the sound that is desired to be heard—is *made inaudible by a masker*, noise or unwanted sound that is present throughout the signal. For example, if someone listens to a soft and a loud sound at the same time, they may not hear the soft sound because it is masked by the loud sound. The loud sound has a greater masking effect if the soft sound lies within the same frequency range, but masking also occurs when the soft sound is outside the frequency range of the loud sound.

Principle

Sound masking relies on the **principle of auditory masking**, where a louder sound can mask a weaker, less audible one. This technique is often used to **enhance privacy** in open office spaces and other areas where unwanted conversations or noises might be distracting.

Procedure

1. Ask the subject to read aloud from a book. After a few seconds, make a rattling noise near his ear using a tin box containing some metal objects.
2. The subject automatically increases the intensity of his voice.
3. In contrast, someone feigning deafness (malingering) may raise their voice unnaturally, revealing inconsistency in their behaviour.

Special features

Adding a background sound: Sound masking systems introduce a specific type of background sound, often described as a *'blanket' of sound*, to the environment.

Masking unwanted sounds: This background sound is designed to be disruptive to human speech, making it more difficult to understand conversations or other sounds from a distance.

Enhancing privacy and focus: By making conversations less intelligible, sound masking can improve privacy and reduce distractions, allowing individuals to focus better.

Applications and benefits

1. **Improved privacy:** Sound masking can help protect confidential conversations in areas like medical offices, law firms, and businesses.
2. **Reduced distractions:** In open office spaces, sound masking can help reduce the impact of background noises and conversations, making it easier to concentrate.
3. **Cost-effective alternative to noise control:** Sound masking is a more affordable option compared to costly structural changes or soundproofing.
4. **Flexibility and customisation:** Sound masking systems can be customised to fit specific needs, with adjustable settings to tailor the sound masking field to different zones and environments.

DISCUSSION

HEARING TESTS

Rinne's Test

This test compares bone conduction with air conduction of the same ear. If the hearing is normal, the subject will hear the sound of the vibrating fork by air conduction even after he has ceased hearing by bone conduction, because air conduction is better than bone conduction. This is called **Rinne-positive**. In *conduction deafness*, vibrations in the air are not heard after bone conduction is over, i.e., bone conduction is better than air conduction. This is **Rinne-negative**. In *total nerve deafness*, no sound is heard in either case. In partial nerve deafness, the Rinne's test becomes *false positive* (Table 47.1).

Weber's Test

Normally, sound is **heard equally in both ears**. If sound is heard better in the defective ear, the hearing loss is due to *conduction deafness*. If the sound is louder in the normal ear, the hearing loss *in the defective ear is due to nerve deafness*.

Schwabach Test

If the subject is normal, *bone conduction of the subject* is equal to *bone conduction of the examiner*. In *conduction deafness*, bone conduction is better than normal. In *nerve deafness*, bone conduction is worse than normal.

MASKING OF SOUND

Sound masking is not a form of active noise control, as it *does not physically eliminate noise*. It relies on the natural ability of the human auditory system to *prioritise louder sounds*. Sound masking can be particularly effective in situations where physical barriers or noise reduction measures are impractical or costly.

OSPE

I.   Perform Rinne's test on the given subject.
Steps
1. Give proper instructions to the subject. Instruct him to raise the finger when he stops hearing the sound of the vibrating tuning fork.
2. Hold the stem of the tuning fork between the thumb and the index finger in such a way that the fingers do not touch the blades of the tuning fork.

Make the tuning fork vibrate by stroking the blades of the fork against the hypothenar eminence.
3. Immediately place the base of the vibrating tuning fork on the mastoid process of one side of the subject and ask him to raise his finger when he ceases to hear the sound.
4. Once he stops hearing the sound, hold the vibrating tuning fork very close to his ear and ask him whether he hears the sound.
5. When he stops hearing it, bring the tuning fork close to your ear to confirm whether the sound has actually stopped.
6. Repeat on the other side (if asked to perform the test on both sides) and report your observations.

II.   Perform Weber's test on the given subject.
Steps
1. Provide proper instructions to the subject.
2. Hold the stem of the tuning fork between the thumb and the index finger in such a way that the fingers do not touch the blades of the tuning fork and make the tuning fork vibrate by stroking the blades of the fork against the hypothenar eminence.
3. Immediately place the base of the vibrating tuning fork on the vertex of the skull or on the forehead of the subject.
4. Ask the subject to indicate whether he hears equally on both sides or if the sound is better heard in one ear.
5. Note and report the findings.

III.   Perform Schwabach test on the given subject.
Steps
1. Provide proper instructions to the subject. Instruct him to raise a finger when he stops hearing the sound of the vibrating tuning fork.
2. Hold the stem of the tuning fork between the thumb and the index finger in such a way that the fingers do not touch the blades of the tuning fork. Make the tuning fork vibrate by suddenly stroking the blades of the fork against the hypothenar eminence.
3. Immediately place the base of the vibrating tuning fork on the mastoid process of one side of the subject and ask him to raise his finger when he ceases to hear the sound.
4. Once he stops hearing, immediately place the vibrating tuning fork on your mastoid process to assess if the sounds have actually stopped.
5. Repeat on the other side (if asked to perform the test on both sides) and report.

1. *What are the clinical uses of hearing tests?* (Ans. Refer to page 304, under the heading 'Introduction'.)
2. *What are the attributes of sound?* (Ans. Refer to page 304, under the heading 'Physiological Basis' and the subheading 'Characteristics of sound'.)
3. *What is the mechanism of hearing?* (Ans. Refer to page 305, under the heading 'Mechanism of Hearing'.)
4. *Trace the auditory pathway* (Ans. Refer to page 305, under the heading 'Auditory Pathway'.)
5. *What are the different hearing tests?* (Ans. Refer to page 305, under the heading 'Hearing Tests'.)
6. *What is the principle and use of the watch test?* (Ans. Refer to page 305, under the heading 'Watch test'.)
7. *What are the basic principles of hearing tests?* (Ans. Refer to page 305-306, under the heading 'Tuning Fork Tests'.)
8. *What are the tuning fork tests?* (Ans. Refer to page 305, under the heading 'Tuning Fork Tests'.)
9. *Why is a tuning fork of higher frequency used for hearing tests?* (Ans. Refer to page 306, under the heading 'Tuning Fork Tests' and the subheading 'Requirements'.)
10. *How is Rinne's test performed? What precautions are taken for this test?* (Ans. Refer to page 306, under the heading 'Rinne's test'.)
11. *What is the significance of the Rinne test? What do you mean by Rinne-positive and Rinne-negative?* (Ans. Refer to page 311, under the heading 'Discussion' and the subheading 'Rinne's test' and Table 47.1.)
12. *How is Weber's test performed? What are the precautions taken to perform this test?* (Ans. Refer to page 307, under the heading 'Weber test'.)
13. *How do you differentiate nerve deafness from conduction deafness using Weber's test?* (Ans. Refer to page 307, under the heading 'Discussion' and the subheading 'Weber test' and Table 47.1.)
14. *How is Schwabach test performed? What precautions should be taken while performing this test?* (Ans. Refer to page 307, under the heading 'Schwabach test'.)
15. *What are the clinical uses of the Schwabach test?* (Ans. Refer to page 311, under the heading 'Discussion', read 'Schwabach Test' and Table 47.1.)
16. *How are the observations and inferences made in hearing tests?* (Ans. Refer to page 308, see Table 47.1.)
17. *What are the principle and types of audiometry?* (Ans. Refer to page 308, under the heading 'Audiometry'.)
18. *How is the audiogram read and interpreted? What are the uses of audiometry?* (Ans. Refer to page 308, under the heading 'Audiometry' and the subheading 'Audiogram'.)
19. *What is BAEP? What are its uses?* (Ans. Refer to page 309, under the heading 'BAEP'.)
20. *What is localisation of sound? How is it tested?* (Ans. Refer to page 309, under the heading 'Localisation of sound'.)
21. *What are the factors that influence sound localisation? What are the applications of it?* (Ans. Refer to page 309, under the heading 'Localisation of sound'.)
22. *What is masking of sounds? What are its benefits?* (Ans. Refer to page 309, under the heading 'Masking of sound'.)

48 | Examination of Taste and Smell

Learning Objectives

After completing this practical, you will be able to (MUST KNOW):

1. Describe the importance of the examination of taste and smell in clinical physiology.
2. Name the primary tastes.
3. Explain the distribution of receptors for primary tastes in the tongue.
4. Name the cranial nerves that carry the sensations of smell and taste.
5. Examine the sensations of smell and taste.

6. List the precautions taken while performing the practical.
7. Name the conditions that alter the sensations of taste and smell.

You may also be able to (DESIRABLE TO KNOW):

1. Trace the auditory pathway.
2. Trace the pathway for taste and smell.
3. Explain the physiological bases of the abnormalities associated with taste and smell.

PY10.20: Demonstrate: (i) Testing of visual acuity, colour, and field of vision, (ii) Hearing, (iii) Testing for smell, and (iv) Taste sensation in a volunteer/simulated environment.

SENSATION OF TASTE

INTRODUCTION

Taste receptors are present in taste buds, which are distributed in the papillae of the tongue and the mucous membrane of the oral cavity. The seventh cranial nerve carries the sensation of taste from the anterior two-thirds of the tongue; the ninth cranial nerve carries the sensation of taste from the posterior third of the tongue; and the tenth cranial nerve carries the sensation from the pharyngeal region.

Basic Taste Modalities

There are **four primary tastes**: *sweet, sour, salt, and bitter*. Receptors for these tastes are different and are distributed in different parts of the tongue. A fifth taste sensation—**umami**—has been added by the Japanese to the list.

Sweet: Receptors for sweet taste are chiefly present on the tip of the tongue.

Salt: Receptors for salt taste are chiefly present in the centre of the dorsum of the tongue.

Sour: Receptors for sour taste are chiefly distributed in the lateral portions of the tongue.

Bitter: Receptors for bitter taste are chiefly distributed at the back of the tongue.

Umami: The umami taste is *produced by glutamate*, which is present in purine 5-ribonucleotides such as inositol monophosphate (IMP) and guanosine monophosphate

(GMP). *Glutamate is present as a flavour enhancer* in monosodium glutamate (MSG), a food additive used extensively in Asian cooking. Glutamate binds to and activates a cation channel that permits Na^+ and Ca^{++} entry, causing depolarisation of the receptor cell.

Taste Pathway

The *first order of neurons* carries the sensation of taste from the receptors in the **seventh, ninth, and tenth cranial nerves** to the nucleus tractus solitarius (NTS) in the medulla. The *second order of neurons* arises from the NTS and ascend the **medial lemniscus** to the **thalamus**. The *third order of neurons* arises from the thalamus and projects into the lower part of the postcentral gyrus (Fig. 48.1).

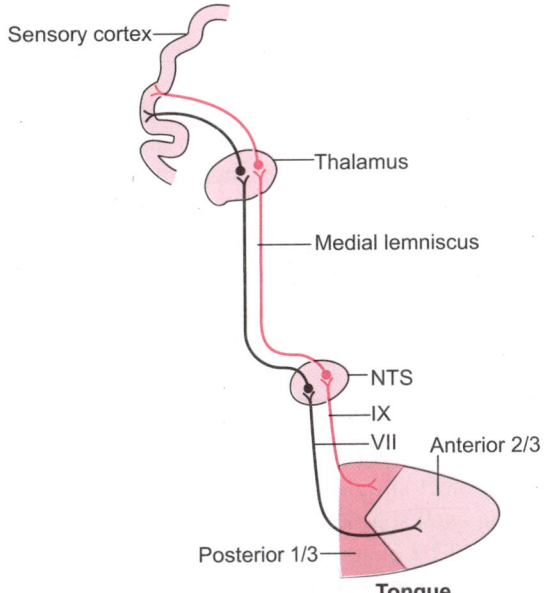

Fig. 48.1 Pathway for taste sensation (NTS: nucleus tractus solitarius; IX: ninth cranial nerve; VII: seventh cranial nerve).

METHODS OF ASSESSING TASTE

Principle

Taste receptors for different taste modalities are present in the tongue. These perceive the testants applied to the surface of the tongue.

Materials Required

The following materials will be required:

1. Strong solutions of **sucrose (10-%)**, **sodium chloride (15-%)** and **weak solutions of acetic acid (1-%)**, and **quinine sulphate (0.1-%)**, all kept in drop bottles
2. A hand lens
3. Small cotton swabs or toothpicks; gauze
4. Four cards with sweet, salt, sour, and bitter printed on them.

Procedure

1. Ask the subject to sit comfortably on a chair near to the worktable and instruct him to **point to a card** to indicate the taste he experiences.
2. Ask the subject to protrude his tongue. Using the hand lens, examine and identify the areas that have large concentrations of papillae and taste buds. Locate the fungiform and circumvallate papillae.
3. Ask the subject to rinse his mouth and then dry it with gauze. Moisten a swab with a few drops of sugar solution, apply it to the tip of the subject's tongue, and ask him to indicate, without withdrawing the tongue, the taste experienced by him.
4. Ask him to rinse his mouth again. Then, dry the tongue with gauze and repeat the procedure with the salt solution.
5. Repeat the same procedure with all four substances, one by one, on the sides, near the tip, the anterior two-thirds, and the posterior one-third of the dorsum of the tongue, taking care that the test solution does not spread across the midline. The tip of the tongue may be held with gauze while testing.

Precautions

1. Ensure that the tasting solutions are well prepared and eliciting the proper taste sensations.
2. The subject should rinse his mouth thoroughly after tasting each solution.
3. It should be ensured that the taste solutions do not spread to areas beyond the area of application of the solution.

Observation and Results

1. Record the results. Note whether the subject is able to perceive the taste sensations.

2. Note which area of the tongue has maximum perception for each taste modality.
3. Grade the intensity of taste sensation as: intense (+ + + +), moderate (+ + +), mild (+ +), slight (+), or absent (0).

DISCUSSION

Factors Affecting Taste Sensation

1. **Age:** The taste sensation decreases after the age of 50. The **number of taste buds starts decreasing** due to the enhanced degeneration process.
2. **Gender:** Generally, **women** are less sensitive to sour taste and *more sensitive to sweet and salt tastes.*
3. **Concentration of the tastants:** The intensity of the taste sensation depends on the concentration of the tastant solution. A concentrated solution elicits a stronger taste sensation than a diluted one.
4. **Area of stimulation:** The intensity of the taste sensation depends on the **number of taste buds** stimulated.
   - When a tastant solution is applied to a small area of the tongue, it produces a weaker sensation.
   - Application of the same solution to a larger area of the tongue produces a more intense sensation. This is due to the activation of a *greater number of afferent fibres.*
5. **Temperature of the tastants:** Increased temperature over some ranges tends to enhance the perceived taste sensitivity, especially for cooked food and spicy food. For example, the perception of sweet taste is increased when the food is not warm.
6. **Duration of stimulation:** The taste receptors show a slow but definite **adaptation.**
   - If a tastant solution is applied to one area of the tongue for a longer duration, the intensity of the taste sensation gradually decreases.
   - This occurs due to a **decrease in the discharge of afferent nerve fibres over time**.
7. **Effect of other tastants:** When two or more stimuli are applied simultaneously, or one after the other, one taste may affect the perception of the other.
   - This is due to **facilitation or blockade at the receptor level**.
   - For example, sweet taste is enhanced with a little bit of salt; salty taste can be reduced by mixing it with sour; and sour taste decreases when taken with sugar.
   - Also, when a bitter stimulus is applied before any other tastants, the bitter taste lingers and dominates over other tastes.
8. **Effects of taste-modifying substances:** A plant protein known as **miraculin** changes the taste of acids from sour to sweet.

- **Gymnemic acid,** when applied to the tongue, abolishes the sensation of sweet, but does not affect other taste sensations.

9. **Effects of drugs:** Some drugs **containing sulfhydryl groups**, such as captopril and penicillamine, tend to cause a temporary loss of taste.

10. **Nutrient deficiencies:** The preference for salty food arises in salt deficiency, and calorie deficiency produces a preference for sweet food.

11. **Culture and habits:** As food habits are different in different cultures, habits that a person has grown up with also affect his taste.

12. **After-effects:** If a person gets *ill after ingesting a new type of food*, he develops an aversion towards that food. This may be due to structural and functional alterations in higher-order and cortical neurons that are part of a central phenomenon.

Clinical Importance

Ageusia and hypogeusia

Absence of the sense of taste is known as **ageusia**, and diminished taste sensitivity is known as **hypogeusia**. These conditions can occur due to the following causes:

1. **Xerostomia (dryness of the mouth):** Due to the lack of salivary secretion, the chemicals in food do not get dissolved in saliva and therefore cannot reach the receptor cells. In **Sjögren's syndrome**, an autoimmune inflammatory disease, there is a progressive destruction of the salivary glands.

2. **Drugs:** Certain medications, such as captopril, cisplatin, and penicillamine are known to reduce taste perception.

3. **Tobacco use:** Prolonged use of tobacco adversely affects the taste sensation.

4. **Nutritional deficiencies:** Deficiency of vitamin B3 (niacin) or zinc may lead to impaired taste perception.

5. **Damage to receptor cells:** This may occur due to ageing, radiation therapy, or viral infections such as herpes.

6. **Injury to gustatory pathway neurons:** Injury may result from trauma, neoplasm, stroke, or systemic diseases such as diabetes mellitus and hypothyroidism.

7. **Selective taste blindness:** Some individuals exhibit insensitivity to the taste of specific substances while the perception of other tastants remains unaltered. This condition is termed **selective taste blindness**. For example, certain individuals are unable to detect the bitter taste of phenylthiocarbamide (PTC), although their perception of sweet, sour, salt, and other bitter substances is unaffected. This condition is *inherited as an autosomal recessive trait* and may be attributed to the lack of synthesis of a specific receptor protein.

Dysgeusia

Distortion of the sense of taste is known as **dysgeusia or parageusia**, in which the perception of taste is different from what is being presented (for example, salty food may taste bitter), or there is a perception of a taste without any tastants in the oral cavity (**hallucination of taste**). Dysgeusia is a feature of **temporal lobe epilepsy**.

SENSATION OF SMELL

INTRODUCTION

The sensation of smell is more developed in animals (macrosmatic) and less developed in humans (microsmatic). Receptors are present in the olfactory mucosa. This is the only part of the central nervous system that is exposed to the external world.

Olfactory Mucous Membrane and Receptors

The olfactory mucous membrane, having a surface area of approximately 5 cm², is located in the nasal cavity. This membrane contains **10–20 million sensory receptor cells**, which are bipolar neurons. Here, the *nervous system lies closest to the external environment*. The receptor cells are scattered among supporting cells and basal cells. The dendritic ends of the receptor cells are expanded to form olfactory rods, which contain cilia and vesicles. Unlike most neurons, olfactory receptor cells are constantly replaced.

Odorants: Unlike primary colours or primary tastes, there are *no definitely known primary odours*, though **seven such odours** are described: peppermint, camphoreous, floral, ethereal, musky, pungent, and putrid.

Olfactory adaptation: The olfactory sensation decreases with continued exposure to an odorant. It occurs within seconds or minutes, depending on the nature of the odorant. This is also called *olfactory fatigue*.

Olfactory Pathway

The **first-order neurons** carrying the olfactory sensation pierce the cribriform plate of the ethmoid bone to reach the *olfactory bulb*. In the olfactory bulb, they synapse with the dendrites of the mitral and tufted cells to form the *olfactory glomeruli*. The glomeruli also receive inputs from the granule cells, which can modulate the output from the olfactory bulb. The **second-order neurons** (axons of the mitral cells) form the **olfactory tract** that divides into the *medial and lateral pathways*.

Medial pathways: The fibres in the lateral division project to the *olfactory lobe of the same side* to terminate in the *centres for olfaction* (pre-pyriform cortex, amygdala, and pre-amygdaloid areas).

Lateral pathways: The fibres in the medial division project to the *opposite olfactory tubercle,* from where they go to the dorsomedial nucleus of the thalamus and the *orbitofrontal cortex* (Fig. 48.2).

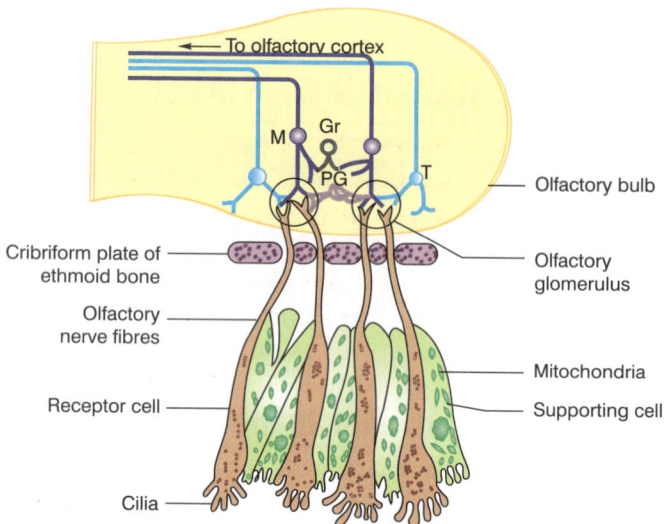

Fig. 48.2   Olfactory receptor cells and the olfactory pathway.

METHOD OF ASSESSING SMELL

Principle

The olfactory nerve carries the sensation of smell. Therefore, this nerve is tested by various olfactory stimuli.

Requirements

One small bottle each of clove oil, peppermint oil or camphor, and coffee powder (Fig. 48.3).

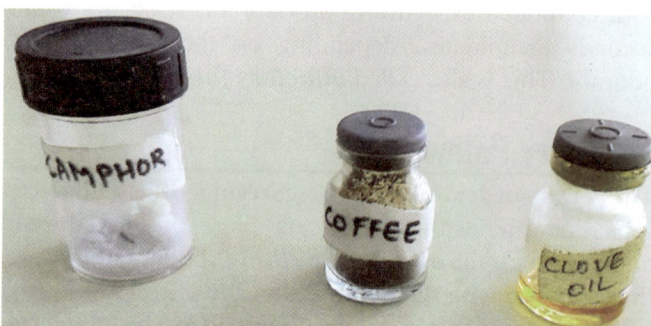

Fig. 48.3   Three solutions in bottles for testing the sensation of smell.

Procedure

1. Ask the subject to sit comfortably on a stool.
2. Make sure that both nostrils are patent and there is no inflammation of the nasal mucosa (no nasal obstruction due to a common cold).
3. Ask the subject to close his eyes and one of his nostrils.
4. Remove the cap of the bottle containing clove oil and take the bottle close to the open nostril.
5. Ask the subject whether he correctly perceives the smell.
6. Repeat the procedure with peppermint oil.
7. Ask the subject to close this nostril, and open the other nostril, and repeat the procedure.
8. Compare the results of both nostrils.
9. Ask the subject if he has any hallucinations of smell.
10. Note your result. Express the result as 'smell normal/reduced/absent/perverted', separately for each nostril.

Observation and Results

1. Observe your result for each odorant bottle (olfactory stimulant).
2. Note the results for both nostrils separately.
3. Express the result as 'smell normal/reduced/absent/perverted', separately for each nostril.

Precautions

1. The subject should close his eyes during each testing.
2. The subject must be familiar (have prior knowledge) with the odorant tested upon.
3. Both the nostrils should be examined separately.
4. One nostril should be closed when the other is examined.

DISCUSSION

Abnormalities of Smell Sensation

Anosmia

Definition: Complete abolition of the sense of smell is called anosmia.

Causes: Unilateral and bilateral anosmia could have different causes.

Unilateral anosmia
1. Tumour of the olfactory bulb
2. Tumour of the frontal lobe
3. Meningiomas pressing on the olfactory bulb or olfactory tract

Bilateral anosmia
1. Common cold
2. Head injuries in which the cribriform plate of the ethmoid bone is fractured
3. Atrophic rhinitis

Hyposmia

Definition: Decreased sensation of smell is called hyposmia.

Causes: Same as anosmia.

Parosmia

Definition: When the sensation of smell is perverted, it is known as parosmia. The offensive smell may seem like a pleasant odour or vice versa. This is also called cacosmia.

Causes: It could be due to:

1. Mental disorders
2. Can occur as an aura in epilepsy
3. Sometimes in head injury

Olfactory Hallucination

Definition: When the sensation of smell is perceived without actual presence of any odour.

Cause: It is typically seen as an aura of temporal lobe epilepsy.

VIVA

1. *What are the primary taste modalities?* (Ans. Refer to page 313, under the heading 'Introduction'.)
2. *What is umami? How is it perceived by the receptors?* (Ans. Refer to page 313, under the heading 'Introduction'.)
3. *What is the distribution pattern of receptors for primary tastes in the tongue?* (Ans. Refer to page 313, under the heading 'Basic Taste Modalities'.)
4. *What is the pathway for the taste sensation?* (Ans. Refer to page 313, under the heading 'Taste Pathway'.)
5. *What are the precautions to take while testing the taste sensation?* (Ans. Refer to page 314, under the heading 'Methods' and the subheading 'Precautions'.)
6. *What are the factors that affect taste sensation?* (Ans. Refer to page 314, under the heading 'Discussion' and the subheading 'Factors Affecting...'.)
7. *What are the abnormalities of taste sensation?* (Ans. Refer to page 315, under the heading 'Clinical Application'.)
8. *What are the specialties of olfactory receptors?* (Ans. Refer to page 315, under the heading 'Sensation of Smell' and the subheading 'Introduction'.)
9. *What is olfactory adaptation?* (Ans. Refer to page 315, under the heading 'Introduction' and the subheading 'Olfactory mucus membrane'.)
10. *What is the pathway for the sensation of smell?* (Ans. Refer to page 315, under the heading 'Olfactory Pathway').
11. *What are the abnormalities of the sensation of smell? What are its causes?* (Ans. Refer to page 316, under the heading 'Abnormalities of Smell Sensation'.)

49 | Semen Analysis

Learning Objectives

After completing this practical, you will be able to (MUST KNOW):

1. Describe the importance of semen analysis in clinical practice.
2. List the indications for semen analysis.
3. State the composition of normal semen.
4. Appreciate the morphology and motility of sperm under the microscope.
5. List the precautions taken for semen analysis.
6. Correlate the abnormal findings, if detected, with the clinical problem.

PY9.9: Interpret a normal semen analysis report including: (a) sperm count, (b) sperm morphology, and (c) sperm motility, as per the WHO guidelines and discuss the results.

INTRODUCTION

Semen analysis is the most important test for the **evaluation of male fertility**. It is routinely ordered in clinical practice to determine whether infertility is due to a defect in the semen. It is also performed *after a vasectomy* to ascertain the *completeness of the surgical procedure*. It reveals the quality and quantity of sperm in semen to identify potential **reproductive health issues in men**. It reflects the activity of the testes and accessory sex organs.

Normal semen is creamy white with a volume of ≥1.4 ml per ejaculation. It has a pH of 7.2–8.0 and liquefies within 20–30 minutes. It normally contains ≥16 million/ml sperm (≥39 million/ejaculate), with ≥42% motility, ≥4% normal morphology. Fructose is normally present (detailed description under 'Discussion').

METHODS OF ANALYSING SEMEN

Principle

The analysis of a freshly collected sample of semen provides information about male fertility, which is detected by examining the sample under the microscope.

Requirements

1. Microscope
2. Viscometer
3. Neubauer chamber and WBC pipette
4. Freshly collected sample of semen

Procedure

1. Collect semen from the person after a **minimum period of two days of sexual abstinence**.

Note: The 48-hour abstinence is recommended to allow for proper sperm maturation and ensure a more accurate assessment of sperm count and quality.

2. Perform semen analysis **30 minutes after the collection** of the sample.

Note: Immediately after collection, semen coagulates and liquefies after 15–20 minutes. Therefore, the sample is examined 30 minutes after collection. Semen contains fibrinogen, which is converted to fibrin by an unknown mechanism on exposure to the atmosphere, and coagulates the sample. Plasmin is also present in semen and is activated in 30 minutes, after which it liquefies the sample.

3. Measure the volume of the sample.
4. Observe whether the sample has been uniformly liquefied.
5. Examine the motility and morphology of the sperm, first under the low-power and then under the high-power objective of the microscope (Fig. 49.1).
6. Count the sperm by using a WBC pipette and a **Neubauer chamber**.

Note: Seminal fluid is drawn up to the 0.5 mark of the WBC pipette and then diluted up to the 11 mark by using 4% sodium bicarbonate in 1% phenol. Then, the Neubauer chamber is charged, and the sperm in the WBC squares are counted. n×50 (for details, see Chapter 9) gives the sperm count in mm³ of fluid. n×50,000 gives the sperm count per ml of fluid.

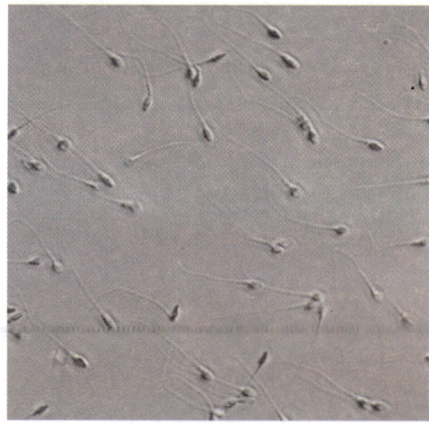

Fig. 49.1 Note the normal morphology of sperm as seen under the microscopic lens. (*Courtesy: Wikimedia*)

7. Determine the pH of the sample.
8. Determine the viscosity of the sample by using the viscometer.
9. Estimate the sugar (fructose) content of the sample using appropriate biochemical tests.

Observations and Results

1. Calculate the sperm count using the formula n x 50,000 to express it per ml of fluid.
2. Note your observations on the volume, liquefaction time, morphology, pH, fructose content, and % motility.
3. Record your comments on the semen analysis.

Precautions

1. The sample should be collected after a minimum of 48 hours of abstinence.
2. The sample should be analysed **30 minutes after collection**.
3. The analysis should ideally be **done within 6 hours of collection**. If the analysis is likely to be delayed, the sample should be stored in the refrigerator, and before analysis, the temperature of the sample should be brought to normal room temperature.

Note: Semen analysis should ideally be done within 1 to 2 hours, but not more than 6 hours after collection to ensure accurate results. Sperm motility, concentration, and morphology are affected by the time elapsed between collection and analysis. Motility and viability decline with the lapse of time.

4. While counting sperms, all the precautions taken for hemocytometry should be followed.

DISCUSSION
Details of Semen Analysis
Normal semen parameters
(Based on the *WHO Laboratory Manual for the Examination and Processing of Human Semen*, 2021, 5th Edition.)

■ **Physical examination**
1. Colour: Creamy white
2. Semen volume: ≥1.4 ml (1.4 to 5 ml)
3. pH: ≥7.4 (7.2–8.0)
4. Viscosity: 1–2 cm
5. Liquefaction time: (20–60 minutes)

■ **Microscopic examination**
1. Sperm concentration (using semen diluting fluid): ≥ 16 million/ml (16–213 million/ml)
2. Total sperm count: ≥39 million/ejaculate (39–928 million/ejaculate)

3. Motility:
   • Progressive motility (PR): ≥30%
   • Non-progressive motility (NP): ≥ 12
   • Total motility (PR NP): ≥42% (should be checked within 1 hour, as soon as semen liquefies)
4. Vitality (using eosin–nigrosin stain): ≥54% live sperm (should be checked within 1 hour)
5. Agglutination: Normally absent (if present, grades are I, II, III, IV)
6. RBC: Nil
7. Epithelial cells: Nil
8. Morphology (using eosin–nigrosin stain or Papanicolaou stain): ≥4%
9. Leucocyte concentration (using methylene blue stain): ≤ 1 million/ml or 4 WBCs/high-power field (40X)

■ **Biochemical examination**
Seliwanoff's test: Cherry red colour represents fructose present in semen (this is used to differentiate between obstructive and non-obstructive azoospermia).

Volume
A low volume of semen might suggest an anatomical or functional defect or an inflammatory condition of the genital tract.

Motility
In a normal sample, at least 42% of the sperm should show good forward motility within the first three hours of collecting the specimen. Motility **less than 42% suggests a possibility of infertility**.

Count
Sperm concentration **below 16 million/ml (<39 million/ejaculate) indicates sterility**.

Liquefaction
Delayed liquefaction of more than 2 hours suggests inflammation of the accessory glands or enzyme defects in the secretory products of the glands. Liquefaction occurs **due to the presence of plasmin** in the prostatic fluid.

Morphology
A normal sperm has an oval head, a slender midpiece, and a long tail. A healthy semen sample generally needs at least 4% of the sperm to have normal morphology, according to the WHO criteria. ***Abnormalities of more than 4% indicate pathology***. These may occur in the form of abnormal shapes and poorly formed heads or tails. An

abnormal sperm may have a bifurcated tail, bifid head, spirally coiled tail, or no head at all.

pH

Normal pH seminal fluid 7.2–8. A pH below 7.0 indicates that the semen primarily contains prostatic fluid, which may be due to a congenital absence of seminal vesicles or excessive secretion of the prostatic fluid.

Fructose

Sugar is usually present in semen. Its absence indicates obstruction or absence of the ejaculatory ducts or seminal vesicle.

Clinical Applications

Semen count is mandatory in the investigation of infertility. A normal report of semen analysis does not guarantee fertility. However, grossly reduced sperm count and motility or the presence of large numbers of abnormal sperm definitely suggest that the person is sterile. Semen analysis is performed in the following conditions:

1. **Fertility assessment:** Semen analysis helps determine if a man's sperm count, motility, and morphology are within the normal ranges, which is crucial for successful conception.
2. **Infertility evaluation:** If a couple is experiencing difficulty conceiving, a semen analysis can help identify potential **male-factor infertility issues**.
3. **Vasectomy follow-up:** Semen analysis is used to confirm the *effectiveness of a vasectomy* by checking for the presence of sperm in the semen.
4. **Assessing sperm health:** It provides information about the overall health and quality of a man's sperm.
5. **Research in reproductive biology:** Semen analysis is an essential investigation in fertility or infertility research.

VIVA

1. *What is the normal composition of the semen?* (Ans. Refer to page 318, under the heading 'Introduction'.)
2. *What is the importance of semen analysis in clinical practice?* (Ans. Refer to page 318, under the heading 'Introduction'.)
3. *When is a person considered sterile?* (Ans. Refer to page 319, under the heading 'Discussion' and the subheading 'Count'.)
4. *Why is there a need for 48 hours of abstinence before collecting the sample?* (Ans. Refer to page 319, under the heading 'Procedure', read point no. 1.)
5. *Why should the semen analysis be done after 30 minutes of collection of the sample?* (Ans. Refer to page 318, under the heading 'Procedure' read the note under point no. 2.)
6. *Why should semen analysis be done within 6 hours of collection of the sample?* (Ans. Refer to page 319, under the heading 'Precautions'.)
7. *What is the mechanism of coagulation and liquefaction of seminal fluid?* (Ans. Refer to page 318, under the heading 'Procedure'.)
8. *What is the normal sperm count?* (Ans. Refer to page 319, under the heading 'Discussion' and the subheading 'Details of semen analysis'.)
9. *What are the normal levels of various semen parameters according to which a man is said to be infertile?* (Ans. Refer to page 319, under the heading 'Discussion' and the subheading 'Details of semen analysis'.)
10. *What are the clinical uses of semen analysis?* (Ans. Refer to page 319, under the heading 'Discussion' and the subheading 'Clinical Applications'.)

50 | Pregnancy Diagnostic Tests

Learning Objectives

After completing this practical, you will be able to (MUST KNOW):
1. Describe the clinical significance of pregnancy diagnostic tests (PDTs).
2. Name the different pregnancy diagnostic tests.
3. State the principles of biological and immunological PDTs.
4. Compare the merits and demerits of various PDTs.
5. Explain the role of various hormones in the maintenance of pregnancy.

PY9.10: Discuss the physiological basis of various pregnancy tests.

INTRODUCTION

Most laboratory tests for pregnancy are based on the **demonstration of human chorionic gonadotropin** (hCG) in the urine of the pregnant woman. Since hCG appears in the urine within two weeks of pregnancy, it is the earliest diagnostic marker of pregnancy.

Pregnancy tests are classified into **biological tests, immunological tests and other tests**. The biological tests are not routinely performed in clinical practice as these are time-consuming and expensive. Moreover, the interpretation of these tests requires knowledge of the histological study of the gonadal tissues. The **immunological tests are most commonly used** to diagnose pregnancy because they can be performed quickly and can detect pregnancy as early as the seventh day of gestation. However, in recent times, **ultrasonographic detection** of pregnancy has virtually replaced the other tests of pregnancy.

METHODS OF DIAGNOSIS PREGNANCY

All pregnancy tests are based on the principle that hCG is excreted in the urine of pregnant women as early as 8–12 days after conception. The detection of hCG in urine permits early diagnosis of pregnancy.

In **biological tests**, the urine of the pregnant woman is injected into female animals, and its action on ovarian morphology is studied to confirm the presence of pregnancy. Various types of biological tests are available, including the following:
1. Aschheim–Zondek test
2. Kupperman test
3. Friedman test
4. Hogben test
5. Galli–Mainini test

In **immunological tests**, hCG is detected in the urine or serum of the pregnant woman by its reaction with specific antibodies to hCG.

Aschheim–Zondek Test

Procedure

Immature female mice weighing 6–10 g (20–30 days old) are used. The woman's urine is injected intraperitoneally or subcutaneously into five mice in varying doses (0.2–0.4 ml), thrice daily for two days. The abdomens of the mice are opened after 100 hours, and ovarian changes are observed. A positive test is indicated by enlarged and hyperemic ovaries and the presence of recent corpus luteum.

Accuracy

The accuracy rate of this test is about 90 per cent.

Disadvantages

1. It takes at least one week to report the findings.
2. A large number of animals is required for the test.
3. It is expensive.
4. Knowledge of histology is essential to detect the corpus luteum in sections of the ovary.
5. Microscopic study is required to interpret the results.

Kupperman Test

Procedure

Immature female rats are used for this test. The urine of the pregnant woman is injected subcutaneously into the rats. A positive test is indicated by marked hyperemia of the ovaries after 6 hours of injection.

Accuracy

The accuracy of this test is up to 90 per cent.

Disadvantages

1. The test is expensive.
2. It requires animals.
3. It requires skill/experience.

Friedman Test

Procedure

Adult female rabbits are used for this experiment. Urine (15 ml) from the pregnant woman is injected intravenously into the rabbit. A positive test is indicated by the presence of fresh corpus luteum and corpus hemorrhagica in the ovary, 36–48 hours after the injection.

Disadvantages
1. The test is expensive.
2. It requires animals.
3. It requires skill/experience.

Hogben Test
Procedure
Adult female toads (*Xenopus laevis*) are used for this experiment. The urine of the pregnant woman is injected into the lymph space of the toad. Positivity is indicated by ovulation (extrusion of eggs) within 18 hours of injection.

Disadvantages
1. The test requires animals.
2. It requires skill/experience.

Galli–Mainini Test
Procedure
Male toads (*Bufo bufo*) are used for this experiment. The urine of the pregnant woman is injected into the toad. Positivity is indicated by the release of sperm, which are collected from the cloaca of the test animal 3 hours after injection.

Immunological Test
Principle
The hCG secreted from the syncytiotrophoblast has antigenic properties. Its presence in the serum or in the urine can be detected using specific antibodies against hCG.

Procedure
Selection of time: The approximate level of hCG in urine for sensitivity is **1.5–3.5 IU/ml** in the slide test and 0.2–1.2 IU/ml in the tube test. This concentration of hCG is usually reached after the **eighth day of pregnancy**. Therefore, the test can be performed any time after the eighth day of pregnancy. It is ideally performed after 14 days of a missed period.

Collection of urine: The subject is advised to restrict water intake from the evening before the test. The first urine sample on the next morning is collected in a clean container. The test should be performed within 12 hours of the collection of urine. The specific gravity of the urine should be at least 1.015 and it should be protein-free.

Brief methodology: When urine containing hCG is added to the hCG antisera, the hCG will combine with

its antibody and neutralise it. If hCG-coated tanned red cells or latex particles are then added, no agglutination occurs. A **positive test is indicated by the absence of agglutination**. If the urine to which hCG antisera is added does not contain hCG, the antibody will remain available to agglutinate with the added hCG-coated particle (tanned red cells or latex particles); **agglutination occurs**, which indicates a *negative result for pregnancy*.

Tests performed: The two standard immunological tests performed are:
1. Latex agglutination inhibition (LAI) test: **Gravindex test**
2. Hemagglutination inhibition (HAI) test: **Pregnosticon test**

The required materials are supplied in **kits** containing all the reagents needed for the test.

Inference
LAI test: The test is performed on a glass slide, and the result is observed after 2 minutes. Positivity is suggested by the absence of agglutination, and negativity is suggested by the presence of agglutination.

HAI test: The test is done in a test tube, and the result is observed after 2 hours. A positive pregnancy test is indicated by the formation of a sharply demarcated brown ring at the bottom of the tube; a negative test is suggested by the absence of the ring.

Accuracy
The LAI test is 98 per cent accurate. The HAI test is 99 per cent accurate.

Advantages
1. The result is available in a short time.
2. It is simple to perform.
3. It is more accurate than biological tests.

Other Tests
Radioimmunoassay
This is a more sensitive method and can be used to detect the presence of hCG in the serum as early as 7–10 days after fertilisation. The assay can detect even 0.003 IU/ml of the β subunit and 0.001 IU/ml of the α subunit of hCG in serum. However, it has limited availability in developing countries.

Ultrasonography (USG)
The gestational ring is detected by ultrasound as early as the fifth week of pregnancy. This real-time method detects cardiac pulsation by the tenth week and fetal movement by the twelfth week. USG is a safe and painless procedure that plays a crucial role in prenatal care.

Principle

In pregnancy, USG is an accurate diagnostic test that uses sound waves to create images of the fetus and other internal structures, helping to confirm pregnancy, determine gestational age, and assess fetal development.

Uses of USG during pregnancy

1. **Confirming pregnancy:** USG can be used early in the first trimester to confirm the presence of a gestational sac and fetal heart activity.
2. **Determining gestational age and due date:** USG helps in estimating the baby's age and due date by measuring fetal measurements.
3. **Checking fetal development:** USG is used to monitor fetal growth, assess the development of organs, and check for abnormalities.
4. **Identifying multiple pregnancies:** USG can help detect whether a woman is carrying twins or triplets.
5. **Evaluating placental location:** USG is used to determine the location of the placenta and check for conditions like placenta previa (placenta covering the cervix).
6. **Assessing amniotic fluid:** USG can help assess the amount of amniotic fluid surrounding the fetus.
7. **Screening for genetic and congenital anomalies:** USG can screen for some genetic and congenital anomalies, such as Down syndrome.
8. **Guiding invasive procedures:** USG can guide the placement of needles during procedures like amniocentesis and chorionic villus sampling (CVS).

Types of USG

1. **Transabdominal USG:** This is the most common type, performed by placing a probe on the abdomen.
2. **Transvaginal USG:** This type is used in early pregnancy to obtain a clearer image of the fetus.
3. **4D USG:** This type provides more detailed images of the fetus, including facial features.

Use of USG in different trimesters

1. **First trimester:** To confirm pregnancy, determine gestational age, and screen for early pregnancy complications.
2. **Second trimester:** To assess fetal development, monitor placental location, and determine fetal sex (if desired).
3. **Third trimester:** To monitor fetal growth, check placental position, and assess fetal well-being.

DISCUSSION
Clinical Significance

Pregnancy diagnostic tests are performed for the **early detection of pregnancy**. Early pregnancy tests detect **tiny amounts of hCG in urine**. hCG appears in urine at **7–10 days** of fertilisation.

Several test kits are available, especially for immunological tests. Though these tests are sensitive and accurate and are used in many hospitals, **false negative and false positive results** can occur.

1. A **false negative result** (the test is negative, but the woman is pregnant) may occur from testing too early or from an ectopic pregnancy.
2. A **false positive result** (the test is positive, but the woman is not pregnant) may be due to excess protein or blood in urine or hCG production from other sources like choriocarcinoma and hydatidiform mole.

Thiazide diuretics, steroids, and thyroid drugs may also affect the outcome of the tests.

Ultrasonography (USG)

The earliest an ultrasound can detect pregnancy is usually **5-6 weeks after the LMP** (last menstrual period). USG is a safe and painless procedure that plays a crucial role in prenatal care.

Advantages of USG

1. USG is non-invasive and painless.
2. Provides details of the morphology of the fetus.
3. It detects abnormalities, if present.
4. It shows the amount of liquor present.
5. USG is easy to repeat.
6. It does not pose a risk of harm to the fetus or the mother.
7. When performed by an expert, it does not take too much time.

Hormones of Pregnancy

hCG: The chorion of the placenta secretes hCG. It mimics the luteinizing hormone (LH). The ***primary function of hCG*** is to rescue the corpus luteum from degeneration and to stimulate the continued production of estrogen and progesterone, which are necessary to prevent menstruation and facilitate the attachment of the embryo and fetus to the lining of the uterus. hCG appears **as early as the sixth day** after fertilisation in blood and the eighth day after fertilisation in urine, reaching a peak at the ninth week of pregnancy. The level then sharply decreases during the fourth and fifth months.

hCS: The human chorionic somatomammotropin (hCS) is ***secreted from the placenta***. It helps in preparing the mammary glands for lactation, enhances the growth of the fetus by increasing protein synthesis, causes nitrogen, potassium, and calcium retention and lipolysis and decreases glucose utilisation. ***Decreased concentration*** of hCS is *a sign of placental insufficiency.*

Relaxin: It is secreted from **the placenta**. It relaxes the uterus and helps in the **continuation of pregnancy**. In the latter part of pregnancy, it *relaxes the pubic symphysis and dilates the uterine cervix.*

Progesterone: It is secreted by the ***corpus luteum*** during early pregnancy and later by the placenta. It **relaxes the uterus** and helps in the continuation of the pregnancy.

Along with estrogen, it maintains the endometrium during pregnancy and prepares the mammary glands for lactation. **Estrogen:** It is secreted by the ***corpus luteum*** in the earlier stages and later by the placenta. The secretion of estrogen is less in early pregnancy, but the concentration *increases towards term*. Estrogen prepares the mammary glands for lactation and the mother's body for parturition.

VIVA

1. *Classify pregnancy diagnosis tests.* (Ans. Refer to page 321, under the heading 'Introduction'.)
2. *Name the biological pregnancy diagnostic tests.* (Ans. Refer to page 321, under the heading 'Methods' and the subheading 'Biological tests'.)
3. *What is the principle of the different biological tests for the detection of pregnancy?* (Ans. Refer to page 321, under the heading 'Methods' and the subheading 'Biological tests'.)
4. *What is the principle of the immunological tests for the detection of pregnancy?* (Ans. Refer to page 322, under the heading 'Immunological Tests'.)
5. *Explain the procedure and inference of immunological tests.* (Ans. Refer to page 322, under the heading 'Immunological Tests'.)
6. *What are the advantages of immunological tests?* (Ans. Refer to page 322, under the heading 'Immunological Tests' and the subheading 'Advantages'.)
7. *What are the advantages of radioimmunoassay for the detection of pregnancy?* (Ans. Refer to page 322, under the heading 'Radioimmunoassay'.)
8. *What is the earliest week that pregnancy can be detected by ultrasound (USG), and what is the underlying principle of ultrasound imaging?* (Ans. Refer to page 323, under the heading 'Ultrasonography'.)
9. *What are the uses of USG in pregnancy?* (Ans. Refer to page 323, under the heading 'Ultrasonography' and the subheading 'Uses of USG'.)
10. *What are the advantages of ultrasonography in the detection of pregnancy?* (Ans. Refer to page 323, under the heading 'Discussion' and the subheading 'Advantages of USG'.)
11. *What are the hormones secreted by the placenta during pregnancy?* (Ans. Refer to page 323, under the heading 'Discussion' and the subheading 'The hormones of pregnancy'.)
12. *What are the functions of different hormones during pregnancy?* (Ans. Refer to page 323–324, under the heading 'Discussion' and the subheading 'The hormones of pregnancy'.)

51 | Birth Control Methods

Learning Objectives

After completing this practical, you will be able to (MUST KNOW):
1. Classify contraceptives used for males and females.
2. Name the temporary and permanent methods of contraception in males and females.
3. Explain the mechanism of action of OCPs and IUCDs.

4. List the merits and demerits of each intrauterine contraceptive device.
5. List the merits and demerits of other types of contraceptives.

You may also be able to (DESIRABLE TO KNOW):
1. Describe the mechanisms and the merits and demerits of different types of contraceptives.

PY9.6: Enumerate contraceptive methods for males and females. Discuss the advantages and disadvantages of these methods.

INTRODUCTION

India is a highly populous nation. One of the major problems India has been facing in recent years is birth control. In April 1976, India formulated its first 'National Population Policy', of which 'National Population Policy–2000' is the latest. These policies primarily aim at reducing the birth rate.

When **birth control procedures** work prior to the implantation of the fertilised egg, they are called **contraceptives**, and when they work after implantation (causing the death of the embryo), they are termed as **abortifacients**.

Classification of Birth Control Methods

Contraceptive methods are classified into the following categories (Fig. 51.1):

1. Barrier methods
   - Physical methods
   - Chemical methods
2. Intrauterine devices
3. Hormonal methods
4. Post-conceptional methods
5. Permanent methods

Contraceptive methods may also be classified as temporary and permanent methods.

METHODS OF BIRTH CONTROL

Physical Methods

In males

The **condom** is the most widely used barrier device among males. It prevents sperm from being deposited in the vagina. The biggest advantage of this method is that it also provides **protection against sexually transmitted diseases**.

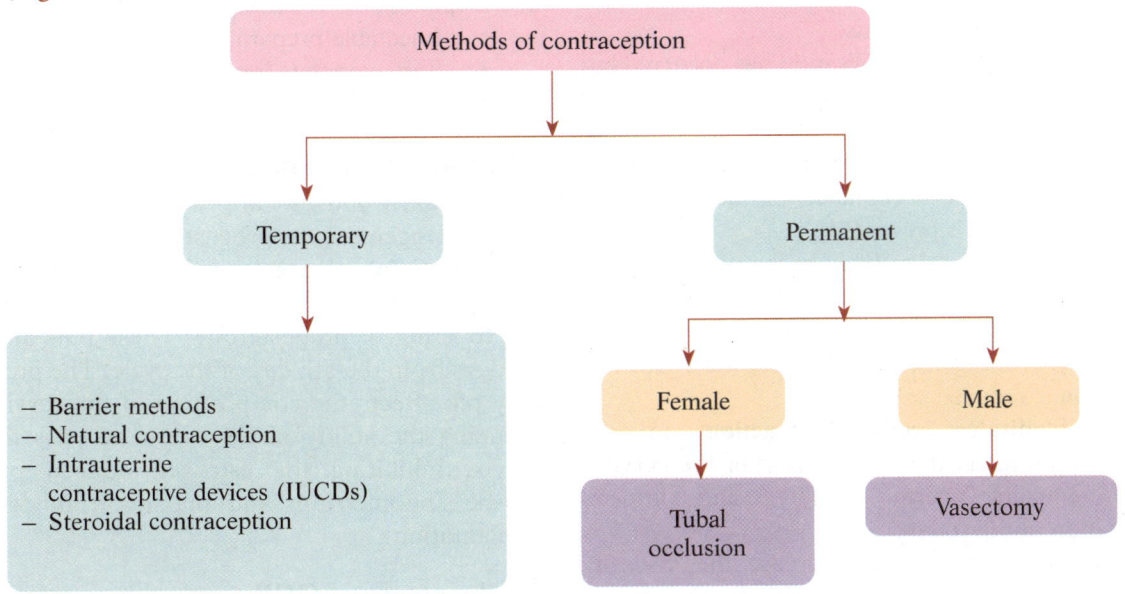

Fig. 51.1 Methods of contraception.

In females

The **diaphragm** is the most commonly used vaginal barrier. **Spermicidal jelly** is usually used along with the diaphragm. Another female barrier device is the **vaginal sponge**.

Chemical Methods

Various spermicidal agents like foams, creams, and suppositories are inserted manually into the vagina before intercourse. These act as 'surface-active agents' that attach themselves to sperm and decrease their oxygen uptake, thereby killing them. These methods are not commonly used due to their high failure rate.

Intrauterine Devices

Intrauterine devices (IUDs) are the most effective contraceptive devices for parous women (who have borne at least one child).

Types

There are **three generations** of IUDs:
1. **First-generation IUD**
   - Lippes loop
2. **Second-generation IUD**
   - **Earlier devices**—Copper-7; Copper T-200
   - **Newer devices**—Copper T variants (T-Cu 220C; T-Cu 380A; T-Cu 380Ag)
3. **Third-generation IUD** (with hormonal preparation)
   - **Progestasert**—a T-shaped device filled with 38 mg of progesterone
   - **Levonorgestrel-20 (LNG-20)**—a T-shaped IUD releasing 20 mcg of levonorgestrel, a synthetic steroid

Mechanism of action

IUDs employ various mechanisms.
1. Usually, they work after fertilisation has occurred but before the implantation is completed. The presence of these small objects in the uterus brings about uterine changes that *interfere with the endometrial preparation* for the acceptance of the blastocyst. Thus, implantation is prevented.
2. They also act as a **foreign body** in the uterine cavity, causing cellular and biochemical changes in the endometrium and the uterine fluid, which impair the viability of the gamete. Therefore, the chance of fertilisation is reduced.
3. **Copper facilitates cellular reaction** in the endometrium, alters the composition of the cervical mucus, impairs sperm motility, and impairs capacitation of the sperm.
4. **Hormone-releasing devices** increase the viscosity of the cervical mucus by releasing progesterone. They **thicken the mucus** and thus prevent the entry of the sperm into the uterus. They also make the endometrium unfavourable for implantation.

Merits and demerits

The merits and demerits of IUDs are summarised in Table 51.1.

Table 51.1   Merits and demerits of IUDs (Cu devices and hormone-releasing IUDs).

Advantages	Disadvantages
• Inexpensive—Cu-T is distributed free of cost through government channels • Simplicity in techniques of insertion and most cost-effective of all methods • Prolonged contraceptive protection after insertion (5–10) years and suitable for the rural population of developing countries • Systemic side effects are nil. Suitable for hypertensives, breastfeeding women, and epileptics • Reversibility to fertility is prompt after removal	• Require motivation • Limitation in its use • Adverse local reactions manifested by menstrual abnormalities, PID, pelvic pain, and heavy periods There are fewer side effects with third-generation IUDs • Risk of ectopic pregnancy

Hormonal Contraceptives

1. **Oral contraceptive pills**
   - Combined pill
   - Progestogen-only pill
   - Post-coital pill
   - Once-a-month pill
   - Male pill
2. **Depots** (slow-releasing formulations)
   - Injectable preparations
   - Subcutaneous implants
   - Vaginal rings

Oral contraceptive pills (OCPs)

Oral contraceptives are based on the principle that estrogen and progesterone **inhibit pituitary gonadotropin release**, thereby **preventing ovulation**. Presently, OCPs contain 30–35 mcg of estrogen and 0.5 to 1 mg of progesterone. These pills are taken for 21 days from the 5th day of the cycle. The progesterone-only pill affects the composition of the cervical mucus, reducing the ability of the sperm to pass through the cervix, inhibiting the estrogen-induced proliferation of the endometrium and making it inhospitable for implantation.

■ Advantages of OCPs

1. Very effective in preventing pregnancy.

2. Reduce the risk of endometrial and ovarian cancer.
3. Protect against acute pelvic inflammatory disease.
4. Prevent ectopic pregnancies.
5. Easy to administer (self-intake) and monitor.

■ Side effects (disadvantages) of OCPs

Though OCPs are 100% effective in preventing pregnancy, they have a few side effects, especially when consumed for many years.

1. **Increased risk of cardiovascular diseases: Myocardial infarction, cerebral thrombosis, venous thrombosis,** and **hypertension** have been reported. These side effects are more common in aged (>35 years) women and smokers.
2. **Carcinogenesis:** Increased risk of cervical cancer and breast neoplasia has been reported. Hepatic tumours occur rarely.
3. **Metabolic side effects:** OCPs **decrease HDL** and alter blood coagulability. These two factors **facilitate atherosclerosis** and proneness to myocardial infarction and stroke. They also cause **glucose intolerance** and insulin resistance.
4. **Miscellaneous:** Other side effects include *cholestatic jaundice, breast tenderness, weight gain, and migraine*.

■ Post-conceptional pills

Contraceptives can be used **within 72 hours** after intercourse (post-coital contraception).

1. These pills interfere with ovulation, the transport of the conceptus to the uterus, or implantation.
2. Usually, a high dose of estrogen or two large doses (12 hours apart) of a combined estrogen–progestin oral preparation are prescribed.
3. The method that is most effective and has the least side effects is the RU 486 (mifepristone) pill, which antagonises progesterone activity by binding competitively with progesterone receptors in the uterus.
4. This causes the endometrium to erode and the contractions of the fallopian tubes and myometrium to increase.

Depots

Subcutaneous implants are contraceptive (progestogen) capsules (Norplant) implanted beneath the skin, which release the hormone slowly and last for five years. Injectable forms (intramuscular injection of progestogen substances like Depo-Provera every three months) are also available. Vaginal rings containing levonorgestrel have been found to be effective.

Other Methods

The rhythm (safe period) method

The rhythm method is the **abstinence from sexual intercourse during the fertile period** of the cycle (near the time of ovulation).

1. In regular cycles (28 days), ovulation normally occurs between the 12th and 16th days (usually on the 14th day). Functionally, sperm can survive for two days, and an ovum for 3 days.
2. Therefore, unprotected intercourse should be avoided during the **fertile period** of the cycle, which will fall between 2 days before and 3 days after ovulation, i.e., from the 10th day to the 19th day of the cycle. The rest of the cycle is considered to be the **safe period**.
3. However, the day of ovulation is not always fixed even in regular cycles, and cycle length is also not always regular. Moreover, only the **length of the luteal phase is constant**, which is 14 days from the day of ovulation; practically, it is difficult to determine the day of ovulation.
4. Therefore, in practice, the **shortest cycle minus 18 days gives** the first day of the fertile period, and the **longest cycle minus 10 days** gives the last day of the fertile period. For example, if the duration of the shortest cycle is 25 days (25 − 18 = 7th day), and the duration of the longest cycle is 32 days (32 − 10 = 22nd day), **unprotected intercourse** should be **avoided between the 7th and 22nd days** of any cycle.
5. However, pregnancy has been documented due to intercourse on any day of the cycle. Therefore, it is believed that no period in any cycle, even the bleeding phase, is absolutely safe.

Coitus interruptus

In this method, during the fertile period, the male partner withdraws his penis from the vagina before ejaculation. Thus, sperm is not deposited in the female genital tract in the fertile period.

Breastfeeding

Ovulation is suppressed as long as the mother continues to breastfeed her baby. This occurs because prolactin, which is released during lactation, inhibits the secretion of GnRH, leading to **lactational amenorrhea**.

Family Planning Operations

The Government of India promotes family planning through various incentives, encouraging couples to undergo sterilisation after having one child, in line with the "We two – ours one" policy. Sterilisation can be performed on either the male or female partner.

Male Sterilisation

Male sterilization is performed by **vasectomy**. In this procedure, bilateral ligation of the vas deferens is performed instead of sectioning the vas because recanalization can be taken up in future whenever needed. However, antibodies developed against spermatozoa following vasectomy cause infertility after restoration of the patency of the vas.

▌Advantages
1. Most effective as a contraceptive method
2. Minimal invasiveness and quick recovery
3. Cost-effectiveness
4. No long-term side effects
5. Reduces the risk of unwanted pregnancies
6. Permanent, though reversal is possible but challenging

▌Disadvantages
1. Potential short-term surgical complications
2. Psychological impact of permanently being sterilised
3. Persistent pain in the surgical incision area
4. Fluid accumulation in the testicles
5. Swelling and inflammation may sometimes occur due to leakage of sperm

6. Rarely, pregnancy may occur, if the vasectomy has not been performed properly
7. Spermatocele may appear in the epididymis

Female sterilisation

Female sterilisation involves **bilateral tubal ligation**, where both fallopian tubes are sealed to prevent fertilisation. Tubal recanalization can also be performed later whenever needed.

▌Advantages
1. The procedure ensures secrecy unless disclosed by the woman
2. Does not interfere with sexual activity
3. No long-term health effects
4. Hormonal levels and sex drive remain unaffected
5. Highly reliable permanent method
6. Reversal (recanalization) is an option in the future

▌Disadvantages
1. Possible menstrual irregularities
2. Risk of hormonal fluctuations
3. Pain in the pelvic and lower abdominal region
4. Occurrence of hot flashes
5. Risk of ectopic pregnancy
6. Potential for pelvic infections or inflammation

VIVA

1. *Classify birth control methods.* (Ans. Refer to page 325, under the heading 'Classification ...')
2. *What are the temporary and permanent methods of contraception in males and females?* (Ans. Refer to page 325, see 'Fig. 51.1')
3. *What is the mechanism of action of IUCDs?* (Ans. Refer to page 326, under the heading 'Intrauterine Devices'.)
4. *What is the mechanism of action of OCPs?* (Ans. Refer to page 326, under the heading 'Oral Contraceptive Pills'.)
5. *List the merits and demerits of each intrauterine contraceptive device.* (Ans. Refer to page 326, see 'Table 50.1'.)
6. *List the merits and demerits of OCPs.* (Ans. Refer to page 326, under the heading 'Oral Contraceptive Pills'.)
7. *What is the post-conceptional pill? How does it work?* (Ans. Refer to page 327, under the heading 'Post-conceptional Pills'.)
8. *What is the mechanism of the rhythm (safe period) method?* (Ans. Refer to page 327, under the heading 'The rhythm (safe period) method'.)
9. *What are the advantages and disadvantages of male sterilisation?* (Ans. Refer to page 328, under the heading 'Male sterilisation'.)
10. *What are the advantages and disadvantages of female sterilisation?* (Ans. Refer to page 328, under the heading 'Female sterilisation'.)

52 | History Taking and General Examination

Learning Objectives

After completing this practical, you will be able to (MUST KNOW):

1. Describe the importance of a general examination in clinical physiology.
2. List the parameters (signs) to be examined in the general examination.
3. Examine and elicit different signs in the general examination.
4. List the common causes of abnormalities of these signs.

You may also be able to (DESIRABLE TO KNOW):

1. Explain the physiological basis of the development of abnormal signs.
2. Correlate the abnormal signs with the pathophysiology of the disease processes.

PY11.13: Obtain history and perform general examination on the volunteer/in a simulated environment.

INTRODUCTION

A detailed history-taking and a thorough general examination are essential parts of the clinical examination of a patient and should be **performed prior to any systemic clinical examination**. If meticulously performed, the history-taking and general examination provide adequate clues to the diagnosis.

History-Taking

History-taking is an important part of the clinical examination of a patient. It is performed **before the general physical examination**. History-taking includes the following:

1. Name, age, and address
2. Marital status and religion
3. **Personal, occupational, and social history** (including history of smoking and alcohol intake)
4. **History of past illness**
5. **Family history** (of similar or related problems or illness, especially among first-degree relatives)
6. History of the **present illness**
7. Treatment history (and use of drugs)
8. Presenting complaints
9. In addition, *for women*, **menstrual and obstetric history**

General Examination

Prerequisites

1. The examination should be conducted in a comfortable, private, and quiet area.

2. The examination should preferably be conducted **in daylight** because skin changes are better appreciated in natural light. Artificial light should be avoided.

3. Generally, patients feel apprehensive about being examined, especially when the environment is unfamiliar. Reassure the patient about the need for the examination in order to diagnose the disease.

4. A thorough general examination requires the subject to be **adequately exposed**. The patient should be asked to undress maximally.

5. When a male doctor is required to examine a female patient, especially if the private parts are to be examined, a **chaperone**, such as a *female attendant or nurse*, should always be present. This helps to reassure the patient and also protects the doctor from any allegations of inappropriate behaviour.

6. If it is necessary to examine covered or private areas as part of the clinical assessment, there should be no **hesitation in uncovering these regions** to perform a proper examination.

7. At any time, **only the area being examined should be exposed**. The parts of the body that have already been examined should be covered as the examiner proceeds to the next area.

8. The subject/patient should stand on the examiner's right-hand side as it is easy to examine the abdominal viscera, jugular vein, and apex beat from the right side. However, if the patient is bedridden (unable to stand), the examiner should stand on the right side of the patient to carry out the examination.

9. Careful attention must be paid to the **patient's comfort**, especially when examining elderly individuals. For example, adjusting the pillow, which often becomes displaced during the examination, can help reassure the patient.

10. A quick assessment of the patient's illness should be made. If the patient is very sick, the detailed examination may be postponed until the acute problem has been attended to. The examination should not distress an already ill patient.

Steps of examination

The general examination begins the moment the patient is seen. It should be performed without causing unnecessary embarrassment and discomfort to the patient. Ideally, the examination should be performed in daylight.

General examination is carried out under the following headings:

I.   General appearance
II. Mental state and intelligence
III. Consciousness and cooperation

General physical examination

1. Build
2. Development (height, weight and sexual maturity)
3. State of nutrition
4. Pallor (anemia)
5. Icterus (jaundice)
6. Cyanosis
7. Clubbing
8. Edema
9. Lymphadenopathy
10. Skin condition
11. **Vital signs:** Temperature, pulse, respiration, blood pressure

PICCLE (acronym 'PICKLE'): Refers to the six cardinal physical examinations (points 4–9 in the list above)—pallor, icterus, cyanosis, clubbing, edema, and lymphadenopathy—performed by a physician while examining a patient.

GENERAL APPEARANCE

Look at the subject, and observe whether he looks healthy, unwell or ill. If he looks ill, assess the severity of the illness: whether the patient is ill, very ill, or in distress.

MENTAL STATE AND INTELLIGENCE

Evaluate the patient's **mood** and study **his state of mind**. Observe the way the patient describes his emotional state.

The patient's **level of intelligence** is one of the important pieces of information to be obtained from the interview. This helps to determine the treatment that is most suitable. An approximate assessment of intelligence is obtained from the **educational and occupational history** and from an assessment of his **general knowledge**.

CONSCIOUSNESS AND COOPERATION

It is important to ascertain the **level of consciousness** of the patient, which can be described as—*clear sensorium, drowsiness, stupor, semi-coma, or coma*. If the patient is fully conscious, assess whether he is cooperative enough to provide all the required information.

BUILD

Build refers to the **skeletal structure** of a person. It is assessed in relation to the age and sex of the individual as compared to that of a normal individual from the same demographic group. The examiner should note whether the patient is *tall or short, lean or fat, and muscular or asthenic*.

DEVELOPMENT

Height

The height of every patient should be measured to find out whether he is of average height for his age and sex. If he is too tall or short, details of the **measurement of span** (from the tip of the middle finger of one side to the tip of the middle finger of the other side of outstretched upper limbs), **upper segment** (crown to the pubic symphysis), and the **lower segment** (pubic symphysis to foot) should be taken.

> **Note:** Normally, in adults, the arm-span is equal to the height of the person, and the upper segment is equal to the length of the lower segment.

Weight

The weight should ideally be recorded on an empty stomach without shoes and **with minimum clothing on**. It should be ascertained whether the patient's weight is **normal for their age and sex**, or if he is underweight or overweight.

Body mass index

Body mass index (BMI) is an important index of the physical development of an individual. It is assessed by the **Quetlet formula:**

$$BMI = \frac{\text{Weight (in kg)}}{\text{Height (in metres}^2)}$$

Though there are many other anthropometric indices such as waist circumference, waist–hip ratio, waist–height ratio, skin fold thickness, neck circumference, etc., BMI is the commonly used parameter for the assessment of **adiposity and cardiovascular (CV) risk**, as degrees of obesity have traditionally been calculated on the basis of BMI. As the Asian population is more prone to CV risks even at lower ranges of BMI compared to European, African, American, and other populations, the BMI range for grading obesity in the Asian population is different.

The BMI range for the Asian population is as follows:
Normal BMI: 18.5–22.99 (below 18.5 is underweight)
Overweight (Pre-obese): 23–24.99
Obesity: 25 or above
Underweight: <18.5

Sexual Development

Efforts should be made to assess the development of secondary sexual characteristics.

In males, the *secondary sexual characteristics* develop between *13 and 18 years*. Hair grows on the face, trunk, axillae, and pubic region. The *pubic hair* develops with the upper border convex upwards and may extend up to the umbilicus. Laryngeal growth results in a thick voice. Considerable *muscular development* occurs.

In females, the *secondary sexual characteristics* develop between *11 and 15 years*. There is *development of breasts*, and the *female distribution of fat* gives the body its characteristic curves. Hair also grows in the axillae and pubis. The *pubic hair* exhibits an upper margin, which is concave upwards.

NUTRITION

Assessment of the patient's nutritional state is an important part of the general examination. It is done by taking the dietary history and by performing a physical examination, including anthropometric measurements.

1. The **physical examination** includes measurement of the **bulk of the muscles** and body fat (**skin fold thickness**).
2. **Anthropometric measurements** include recordings of **height and weight**.

This evaluation is performed to ascertain whether the patient is well nourished or malnourished. **Malnutrition** may be due to starvation, maldigestion of food, or malabsorption of nutrients from the gastrointestinal tract.

PALLOR

Pallor refers to the *paleness of the skin and mucous membrane*. It depends on the thickness and quality of the skin, and the amount and quality of the blood in the capillaries. Thus, pallor is seen in persons with thick or opaque skin, in conditions where blood flow in the capillaries is diminished, such as shock, or when the

hemoglobin content in the blood is decreased. It is usually detected by **examining the lower palpebral conjunctiva** (Fig. 52.1).

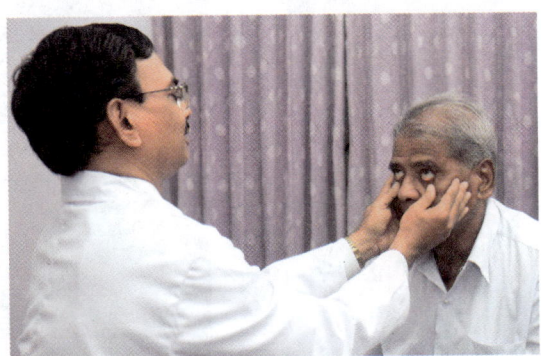

Fig. 52.1 Detection of pallor. Note that the lower eyelids are retracted downward to assess the paleness of the lower palpebral conjunctiva.

> **Note:** The tip and dorsum of the tongue, soft palate, palms, and nails should also be examined to assess pallor.

The degree of pallor is expressed as **plus 1 to plus 3** (Fig. 52.2).
1. Pallor 0: No anemia
2. Pallor +: Mild anemia
3. Pallor ++: Moderate anemia
4. Pallor +++: Severe anemia

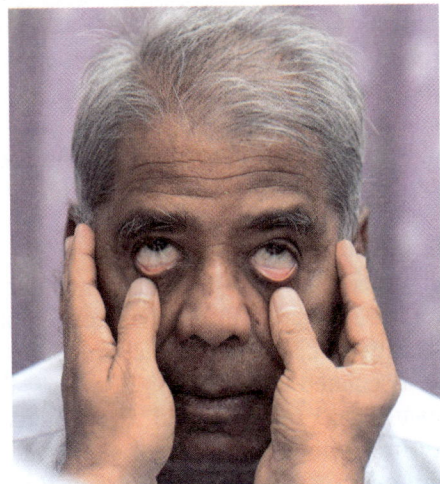

Fig. 52.2 Note the pallor as + (mild anemia) in this subject.

JAUNDICE

Jaundice is the *yellow discolouration of the sclera* (Fig. 52.3), skin and mucous membranes of the body due to the presence of excess bilirubin in the blood. The **normal serum bilirubin** concentration is *0.2–0.8 mg/100 ml* of blood. When the bilirubin level *exceeds 2 mg per cent*, jaundice appears clinically (Fig. 52.4). Hyperbilirubinemia between *0.8 and 2 mg%* is called **subclinical or latent jaundice**.

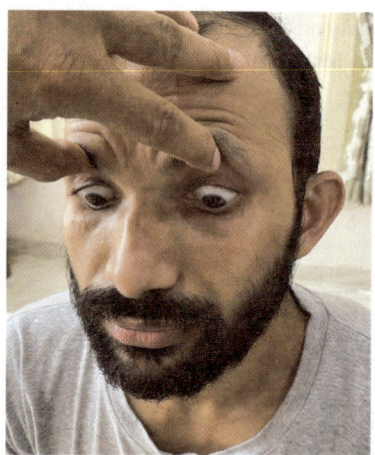

Fig. 52.3 Method of detection of icterus. Note that the upper eyelids are retracted upwards and the subject is asked to look downward to assess the yellow discolouration of the sclera.

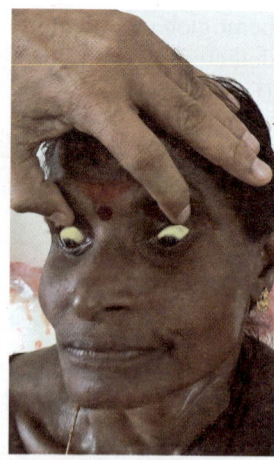

Fig. 52.4 A patient having mild jaundice. Note the yellow discolouration of the sclera.

Types of jaundice

Jaundice is classified clinically into **three types:** prehepatic, hepatic, and post-hepatic.

▌Prehepatic jaundice

Prehepatic jaundice occurs due to excessive destruction of red cells. Therefore, it is also called **hemolytic jaundice**. This type of jaundice is usually *mild to moderate*, and bilirubin is *mostly unconjugated*. Fecal stercobilinogen and urinary urobilinogen are increased. *Excretion of bilirubin in urine is absent* (**acholuric jaundice**) because the excess unconjugated bilirubin in the blood combines with albumin and therefore, cannot be filtered in the kidneys. The *van den Bergh test is indirect positive*.

▌Hepatic jaundice

This usually occurs due to hepatitis or damage to liver cells. Therefore, it is also called hepatic or **hepatocellular jaundice**. This type of jaundice is usually moderate to severe and may be associated with bleeding disorders. Bilirubin is both conjugated and unconjugated. Fecal stercobilinogen and urinary urobilinogen are normal or raised. Bilirubins exhibit a *biphasic reaction to the van den Bergh test*.

▌Post-hepatic jaundice

This occurs due to obstructions in the biliary tract. Therefore, it is called **obstructive jaundice**. Because of the obstruction, *bilirubin does not reach the intestine*. Hence, fecal stercobilinogen and urinary urobilinogen are absent. The bilirubin is conjugated and appears in the urine. The *van den Bergh test is direct positive*.

Causes of yellow discolouration of skin

1. Jaundice
2. Carotenemia

3. Hemochromatosis
4. Picrates
5. Mephacrine

CYANOSIS

Cyanosis is the *bluish discolouration of the skin and mucous membranes* of the body due to the presence of **reduced hemoglobin in more than 5 g%** in the blood.

Physiological Basis

Hemoglobin in the arterial blood is 95 per cent saturated with oxygen. Therefore, in a normal adult, about 14.25 g (taking 15 g% of hemoglobin as the standard) of the total hemoglobin **in the arterial blood** is oxyhemoglobin, and only *0.75 g is reduced hemoglobin*. In **mixed venous blood**, about 70 per cent of hemoglobin is saturated with oxygen. Hence, 10.5 g of the 15 g% of hemoglobin in the venous blood is oxyhemoglobin and *4.5 g is reduced hemoglobin*. The amount of reduced hemoglobin in capillary blood is assumed to be the mean of the arterial and venous content of reduced hemoglobin. Thus, in a normal individual at rest, *capillary blood contains 2.6 g%* (0.75 + 4.5/2) of reduced hemoglobin. Therefore, the colour of normal skin and mucous membrane is pink.

1. *When the concentration of reduced hemoglobin is more than 5 g per cent,* the skin and mucous membrane become blue because of the dark colour of the reduced hemoglobin.
2. The presence of an excess of other hemoglobin complexes like **methemoglobin and sulfhemoglobin** in the blood also produces cyanosis because of their dark colour.

Note:
1. Patients suffering from **severe anemia** with hemoglobin content less than 5 g per cent **may not show cyanosis** (because the total hemoglobin is less than 5 g%).
2. Cyanosis *may not be seen in carbon monoxide poisoning* because carboxyhemoglobin prevents the reduction of oxyhemoglobin, and the colour of carboxyhemoglobin is cherry red.

Types of Cyanosis

Cyanosis is of **three types:** peripheral, central, and mixed. There is another special category of cyanosis, called **differential cyanosis.**

Peripheral cyanosis

This occurs due to **slowing of the flow of blood through the tissues**, thereby allowing more time for the removal of oxygen by the tissues.

Causes

1. Decreased cardiac output, e.g., due to heart failure
2. Local vasoconstriction, e.g., due to extreme cold
3. Venous obstruction, e.g., superior venacaval obstruction
4. Increased viscosity of blood, e.g., polycythemia

Central cyanosis

When reduced hemoglobin concentration is more than 5 g% due to **mixing of arterial blood with venous blood** or **inadequate oxygenation** of the arterial blood, central cyanosis results. In the early stage, cyanosis manifests in the palate, tongue, and inner side of the lips. When the amount of reduced hemoglobin becomes very high, cyanosis appears in different peripheral sites too.

Causes

1. Due to the admixture of venous and arterial blood

This occurs in the *right to left shunt,* in which venous blood bypasses the pulmonary circulation and directly enters the systemic circulation. It is seen in the following conditions:

i. Fallot's tetralogy
ii. Pulmonary arteriovenous fistula
iii. Patent truncus arteriosus
iv. Transposition of great vessels

2. Due to inadequate oxygenation of arterial blood

i. Low atmospheric oxygen, e.g., at high altitudes
ii. Inadequate ventilation, e.g., due to lung collapse or airway obstruction
iii. Decreased gaseous exchange through the pulmonary membrane, e.g., hyaline membrane disease

Mixed cyanosis

In this type of cyanosis, **both central and peripheral mechanisms** operate. The most common example is chronic cor pulmonale due to emphysema.

Differential cyanosis

This is a condition in which cyanosis **appears only in one half of the body.** For example, in patent ductus arteriosus with reversal of shunt due to pulmonary hypertension, cyanosis is seen only in the lower limbs; both upper limbs are spared.

CLUBBING

Bulbous enlargement of the soft parts of the terminal phalanges with *over-curving of the nails,* both transversely and longitudinally, is called clubbing.

Detection

Clubbing is diagnosed by the presence of any of the following five signs.

1. **Fluctuation test (nail bed fluctuation):** Normally, the nail bed fluctuates very slightly. Fluctuation increases in clubbing. This is elicited by assessing fluctuation of the nail base. The examiner holds the base of the nail from both sides and gently presses the tip (Fig. 52.5) to elicit nail bed fluctuation, if present. *Alternatively,* fluctuation test can be elicited by firmly holding and fixing the patient's finger with the middle fingers and thumbs of the examiner and testing the nail bed fluctuation by pressing it alternatively from the two sides with the index fingers (Fig. 52.6).

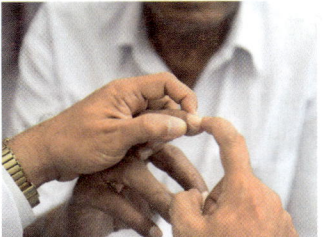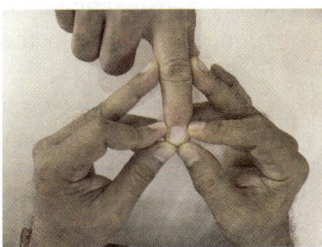

Fig. 52.5 Fluctuation test for assessing clubbing. The examiner holds the base of the nail and gently presses the tip to assess fluctuation of the nail bed.

Fig. 52.6 Alternative method of fluctuation (nail bed fluctuation) test for assessing the presence of clubbing.

2. **Curving of nails:** In clubbing, the nails curve in both transverse and longitudinal directions. This curving is due to hypertrophy of the nail bed tissue.
3. **Profile sign:** The presence of a transverse ridge at the root of the nail due to the thickening of the fibroelastic tissue is called the profile sign.
4. **Schamroth's sign:** When two fingers are held together with the nails facing each other, a space is seen at the nail folds (Fig. 52.7). This space is lost in clubbing (positive Schamroth's sign).

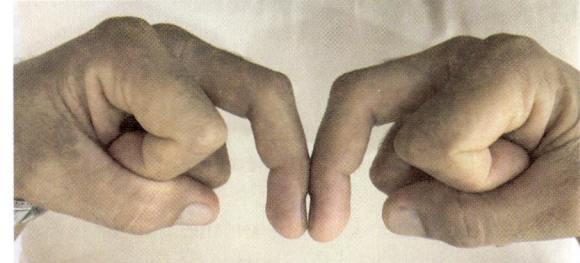

Fig. 52.7 Normal space is seen at the nail folds when nails are apposed and facing each other. This is a negative Schamroth's sign.

5. **Base angle:** In a normal finger, the angle between **the base of the nail and the adjacent portion of**

the dorsum of the terminal phalanx is around **160°** **(obtuse angle)**. In clubbing, this angle gets obliterated in the outward direction and becomes 180° or more. This is best viewed vertically from the side.

Physiological Basis

The exact physiological basis of clubbing is not known. It may occur due to any of the following causes:

1. **Dilatation of AV anastomosis:** The AV (arteriovenous) anastomotic channels are dilated in the fingers (the cause is not known). This causes hypertrophy of the tissues in the nail bed.
2. **Increased pressure gradient:** An increase in the pressure gradient between the radial artery and digital artery causes edema and increased cellularity of the connective tissue in the finger. This predisposes the finger to clubbing.
3. **Capillary stasis:** Capillary stasis results from back pressure, which may cause clubbing.
4. **Vitamin deficiency and hormonal disorders:** These are thought to be involved in the genesis of clubbing.

Causes

1. Bronchopulmonary diseases
   i. Bronchiectasis
   ii. Lung abscess
   iii. Bronchogenic carcinoma
   iv. Emphysema
2. Cardiac diseases
   i. Congenital cyanotic heart disease
   ii. Subacute bacterial endocarditis
3. Gastrointestinal diseases
   i. Ulcerative colitis
   ii. Biliary cirrhosis of the liver
4. Endocrine disorders
   i. Thyrotoxicosis
   ii. Acromegaly
5. Heredity

Degrees of Clubbing

1. **First degree:** Only increased fluctuation of the nail bed is present.
2. **Second degree:** Curving of the nail is present in addition to increased fluctuation of the nail bed.
3. **Third degree:** Increased fluctuation, increased curving, and obliteration of the base angle of the nails occur together.
4. **Fourth degree:** A combination of the above changes plus subperiosteal thickening of the wrist and ankle bones with the presence of a definite transverse ridge at the root of the nails.

EDEMA

Edema refers to swelling of the skin and subcutaneous tissues due to the excessive **accumulation of free fluid** in the interstitial tissue space.

Types of Edema

Edema is classified as **localised or generalised** and **pitting or non-pitting**.

Detection of Edema

Edema is diagnosed by pressing the skin against the bones in the dependent parts (Fig. 52.8), which leaves a *pit or depression* in the case of **pitting edema** (Fig. 52.9). Edema may be **non-pitting** as seen in filariasis.

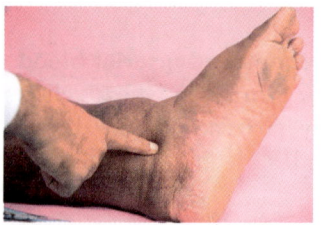 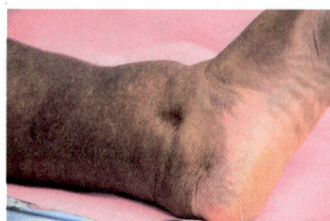

Fig. 52.8 Assessment of edema. Note that the skin against the medial malleolus (dependent part of this subject) is pressed for about 20 seconds.

Fig. 52.9 Pitting edema. Note the presence of pit (depression) in the ankle following putting pressure over the area.

Common Causes

1. Cardiac causes
   i. Congestive heart failure
   ii. Constrictive pericarditis
2. Hepatic causes
   i. Cirrhosis of the liver
   ii. Carcinoma of the liver
3. Renal causes
   i. Nephrotic syndrome
   ii. Acute nephritis
4. Anemia and hypoproteinemia

Special Features

Cardiac edema: It is usually seen in the dependent parts of the body. Dyspnea at rest is one of the associated features.

Hepatic edema: Edema is prominent on the abdomen. Ascites is one of the associated features.

Renal edema: Edema first appears in the face. Puffiness of the lower eyelid in the morning is a characteristic feature.

Anemia and hypoproteinemia: Edema is generalised from the beginning. Severe pallor is one of the associated features.

Physiological Basis

Edema occurs due to **excess accumulation of fluid in the interstitial tissue space**. Interstitial fluid is formed by filtration through the capillary walls. The capillary wall is regarded as a semi-permeable membrane. The major driving forces behind the filtration of fluid through the capillaries are hydrostatic pressure within the capillaries and **oncotic pressure** (osmotic pressure exerted by the plasma proteins). **Hydrostatic pressure** favours filtration, whereas oncotic pressure opposes it. Therefore, when *hydrostatic pressure increases* or *oncotic pressure decreases*, there is excess filtration of fluid into the interstitial tissue space. Normally, the fluid from the interstitial space is removed by the lymphatics. When excess filtration of fluid occurs, the *lymphatics cannot remove* all the fluid. As a result, the excess fluid accumulates in the interstitial tissue space. This leads to the development of edema.

Physiological Mechanisms

In cardiac failure

In congestive cardiac failure, edema develops in the dependent parts of the body due to the following mechanisms:

1. Decreased cardiac output decreases blood volume and pressure, which **increases renin release** from the kidney. Renin forms angiotensin II, which **increases aldosterone secretion** from the adrenal cortex. Aldosterone increases the reabsorption of sodium and water from the kidney. This increases total body sodium and water, which results in edema formation.
2. Decreased cardiac output also **stimulates sympathetic activity,** which causes renal vasoconstriction. Constriction of the renal artery causes the release of renin, which activates the renin–angiotensin–aldosterone axis.
3. In congestive cardiac failure, due to the failure of the right ventricle (backward failure), pressure in the systemic veins increases. This **increases hydrostatic pressure** in the capillaries, which results in edema formation.

In nephrotic syndrome

The primary cause of edema formation in nephrotic syndrome is the **loss of protein in the urine**. Protein passes from the glomerulus into the tubular fluid, which results in proteinuria. Loss of protein from the kidney *decreases oncotic pressure* because of hypoproteinemia and results in edema formation.

In cirrhosis of the liver

In cirrhosis of the liver, there is a loss of liver tissue. There is a decrease in the synthesis of protein by the liver, which results in **hypoproteinemia.** This causes decreased oncotic pressure and edema formation.

In anemia and hypoproteinemia

In anemia, hypoxia of the capillaries increases capillary permeability, which results in edema formation. However, the main cause of edema in anemia is hypoproteinemia.

LYMPHADENOPATHY

The **neck, axilla, inguinal region, and supratrochlear areas** of both sides should be examined thoroughly to check for enlargement of lymph nodes. Cervical, axillary, and inguinal lymph nodes are commonly enlarged in various infections, inflammations, and malignancies.

The **lymph nodes in the neck** should be *examined by standing behind the subject* and with the *patient's head slightly flexed* (Fig. 52.10). The glands should be examined in proper order starting from the submental group and proceeding to the submandibular, cervical, posterior auricular, and the occipital groups.

The **lymph nodes in the axilla** should also be examined by standing behind the subject and with the patient's arm slightly abducted. In the axilla, the anterior, posterior, apical, and lateral groups of lymph nodes are examined.

The lymph nodes in the **inguinal region** are examined with the patient in a supine position with their thighs extended.

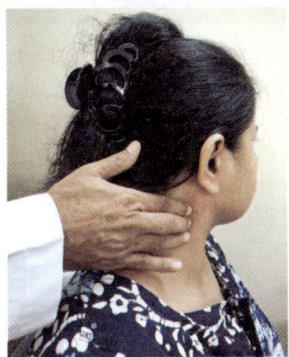

Fig. 52.10 Examination of the cervical lymph nodes.

Procedure of Examination

Lymph nodes are palpated to check their **size and shape, consistency, mobility, and tenderness**.

1. **Size and shape:** The size of the enlarged lymph node is expressed in **centimetres of its longest diameter**. The *surface of the enlarged nodes* may be *smooth, irregular, or lobulated*. Malignant lymph nodes are often irregular.
2. **Consistency:** Lymph nodes are often *elastic and rubbery*. They are *firm in tuberculosis*, firm and shotty in syphilis, and *hard in carcinoma*.
3. **Mobility:** Nodes may be **mobile or fixed**. In **benign conditions**, nodes are usually **separated and mobile**. In **tuberculosis**, the nodes are *often matted*. In **malignant conditions**, the nodes are *usually fixed* to the skin and surrounding tissues.

4. **Tenderness:** While palpating the lymph nodes, the patient may complain of pain or may grimace. This indicates that the lymph nodes are tender. Usually, lymph nodes are *tender in inflammatory conditions* and non-tender *(painless) in malignant diseases*.

Causes

1. Neoplastic
   i. *Hematologic:* Lymphomas (Hodgkin and non-Hodgkin), acute leukemia, chronic lymphocytic leukemia
   ii. *Non-hematologic:* Carcinoma of the breast, carcinoma of the lungs
2. Inflammatory
   i. *Infections:* Tuberculosis, syphilis, filariasis, infectious mononucleosis
   ii. *Connective tissue diseases:* Systemic lupus erythematosus, sarcoidosis
3. Endocrine diseases: Hyperthyroidism, Addison's disease
4. Drugs: Carbamazepine, cephaloridine, meprobamate, phenylbutazone, phenytoin

THE SKIN

The skin is examined carefully, preferably in daylight. The maximum surface of the body should be exposed while examining. The skin is examined for the **colour, pigmentation, eruptions, and secondary lesions**.
Colour: Pallor of the skin is seen in anemia. Yellow skin is seen in jaundice. Blue skin is seen in cyanosis.
Pigmentation: The skin looks white in albinism. Patches of white and black pigments are seen in vitiligo. The skin is dark in Addison's disease.
Eruptions: Different skin eruptions like macules, papules, vesicles, pustules, and petechiae are seen in different clinical conditions.
Secondary lesions: Scales, crusts, excoriations, fissures, ulcers, and scars occur in different conditions.

VITAL SIGNS

There are **four vital signs** that must always be checked in general examination. These are temperature, pulse, blood pressure (BP), and respiration. However, just as an acronym to remember it, it is referred to as '**BPTPR**' in routine practice.

Temperature

Body temperature is usually recorded using a clinical thermometer. The thermometer is placed either in the patient's mouth or axilla for at least one minute. The thermometer can also be placed in the rectum—this is done for infants and collapsed patients. The body temperature is usually expressed in Fahrenheit or in Centigrade.

Normal value

The normal body temperature at rest is **98–99°F** (36.6–37.2°C).
1. Febrile: >37.2°C (99°F or above)
2. Mild fever: 37.2–38.3°C (99–101°F)
3. Moderate fever: 38.3–40°C (101–104°F)
4. High fever: 40–41.2°C (104–106°F)
5. Hyperpyrexia: >41.6°C (>107°F)
6. Subnormal: <36.6°C (<98°F)
7. Hypothermia: <35°C (< 95°F)

Fever

Increase in the diurnal variation of body temperature by more than 1°C (1.5°F) or rise in temperature above the maximum normal temperature is called fever.

■ Types of fever

Typically, **three classical types** of fever are seen in clinical practice. These are **continued, remittent, and intermittent fever**.
Continued fever: The temperature remains high throughout the day; at no time does it touch the baseline, and the diurnal variation of temperature is not more than 1°C. This is commonly seen in:
1. Typhoid
2. Subacute bacterial endocarditis
3. Urinary tract infection
4. Brucellosis
5. Glandular fever

Remittent fever: The temperature remains raised throughout the day; at no time does it touch the baseline, but the diurnal variation is more than 2°C.
Intermittent fever: Fever is present only for several hours during the day, and the temperature returns to normal for the rest of the day. Intermittent fever may be quotidian, tertian, quartan, or irregular intermittent.
1. *Quotidian:* When the paroxysm of intermittent fever occurs every day.
2. *Tertian:* When the paroxysm of fever occurs on alternate days.
3. *Quartan:* When there is a gap of two days between consecutive attacks.
4. *Irregular intermittent:* The paroxysm of fever occurs irregularly.

■ Causes of fever

1. **Infections:** Bacterial, viral, rickettsial, fungal, or parasitic

2. **Immunologic:** Rheumatic fever, rheumatoid arthritis, other collagen diseases
3. **Neoplastic:** Carcinoma of any organ, leukemia
4. **Metabolic:** Gout, porphyria, Addison's disease
5. **Physical agents:** Heat stroke, radiation sickness
6. **Drug-induced fever**

Hypothermia

Hypothermia is a condition in which the body temperature decreases below the normal range.

■ Causes of hypothermia

1. Prolonged exposure to cold
2. Myxedema
3. Hypopituitarism
4. Hypoglycemia
5. Hypnosedative poisoning

■ Physiological effects

Hypothermia causes bradycardia, hypotension, shallow respiration and, in severe cases, confusion, stupor, and coma. The brain is probably protected by the low temperature.

Pulse

The **radial pulse** is counted for one minute when the subject is at rest. Examination of the pulse is not only performed as part of the examination of the cardiovascular system, but also routinely in general examination because it provides information about the functioning of the heart.

The pulse is palpated by the three middle fingers with the patient's forearm semipronated and wrist slightly flexed. The pulse is examined **for rate, rhythm, volume, character, and condition of the arterial wall**. A normal pulse rate is **60–100 per minute**, regular in rhythm, and normal in volume and character. The arterial wall is neither thickened nor tortuous. (Details of the procedure and abnormalities of the pulse are given in Chapter 27.)

Blood Pressure

The blood pressure is recorded using an **aneroid sphygmomanometer**, first by the palpatory and then by the auscultatory method. The normal range of blood pressure in adults is as follows:

1. Systolic: **100–119 mmHg**
2. Diastolic: **60–79 mmHg**

(Details of blood pressure recording and the conditions affecting blood pressure are given in Chapter 28).

Respiration

The **rate of respiration** is counted for a minute. It should preferably be counted when the subject's attention is distracted from his breathing. **Rhythm and type of respiration** are also noted. The normal rate of respiration in an adult is **12–20 per minute**. (Details of change in respiration in different conditions are given in Chapter 53).

OBSERVATION AND RESULTS

Note your observations and the results of the general examination in a tabular format as shown below.

Patient details and parameters	Observations and examination findings
Patient name, age, sex	Murugan, 58 yrs, male
1. General appearance	
2. Mental state and intelligence	
3. Consciousness and cooperation	
4. **General Physical Examination Findings** 　i)　Build 　ii)　Development (height, weight, and sexual maturity) 　iii)　State of nutrition 　iv)　Pallor (anemia) 　v)　Icterus (jaundice) 　vi)　Cyanosis 　vii)　Clubbing 　viii)　Edema 　ix)　Lymphadenopathy (describe each group of lymph nodes) 　x)　Skin condition	
5. **Vital signs** 　i)　Temperature 　ii)　Pulse 　iii)　Blood pressure 　iv)　Respiration	

VIVA

1. *What is the importance of general examination in clinical medicine? What are the prerequisites for it?* (**Ans.** Refer to page 329, under the heading 'Introduction'.)
2. *What types of history are taken from the patient before the general examination?* (**Ans.** Refer to page 329, under the heading 'Introduction' and the subheading 'History-taking'.)
3. *What are the parameters that are looked for in general examination?* (**Ans.** Refer to page 330, under the heading 'Steps of Examination'.)

4. *How do you assess the development of the subject?* (Ans. Refer to page 330, under the heading 'Development'.)
5. *How do you assess the nutritional status of the subject?* (Ans. Refer to page 331, under the heading 'Nutrition'.)
6. *Where do you look to confirm pallor clinically?* (Ans. Refer to page 331, under the heading 'Pallor' and Fig. 52.1 and 52.2.)
7. *What is jaundice? What is latent jaundice?* (Ans. Refer to page 332, under the heading 'Jaundice'.)
8. *Where do you look to detect jaundice clinically?* (Ans. Refer to page 333, under the heading 'Jaundice', Fig. 52.3 and 52.4.)
9. *What are the types of jaundice? How do you differentiate between them?* (Ans. Refer to page 333, under the heading 'Jaundice'.)
10. *What are the causes of yellow discolouration of the skin?* (Ans. Refer to page 333, under the heading 'Causes of Yellow Colouration of Skin'.)
11. *What is cyanosis?* (Ans. Refer to page 332, under the heading 'Cyanosis'.)
12. *What are the types of cyanosis? How do you differentiate between them?* (Ans. Refer to page 332, under the heading 'Cyanosis'.)
13. *What is the physiological basis of cyanosis?* (Ans. Refer to page 333, under the heading 'Cyanosis' and the subheading 'Physiological basis'.)
14. *What is clubbing? What is its physiological basis?* (Ans. Refer to page 333, under the heading 'Clubbing'.)
15. *What are the causes of clubbing?* (Ans. Refer to page 333, under the heading 'Clubbing'.)
16. *How do you detect clubbing?* (Ans. Refer to page 333, under the heading 'Clubbing' and the subheading 'Detection', Fig. 52.5, 52.6, and 52.7.)
17. *Define edema.* (Ans. Refer to page 334, under the heading 'Edema'.)
18. *What are the types of edema? What are the main causes of edema?* (Ans. Refer to page 333, under the heading 'Edema'.)
19. *What is the physiological basis of edema in heart failure, nephrotic syndrome, and cirrhosis of the liver?* (Ans. Refer to page 334, under the heading 'Edema' and the subheading 'Physiological basis'.)
20. *Which regions of the body are specially checked for lymph node enlargement? Why?* (Ans. Refer to page 335, under the heading 'Lymphadenopathy'.)
21. *What are the common causes of lymphadenopathy?* (Ans. Refer to page 335, under the heading 'Lymphadenopathy' and the subheading 'Causes'.)
22. *What are the important features looked in for skin examination?* (Ans. Refer to page 336, under the heading 'The Skin'.)
23. *What are the vital signs?* (Ans. Refer to page 336, under the heading 'Vital Signs'.)
24. *What is the normal body temperature?* (Ans. Refer to page 336, under the heading 'Temperature'.)
25. *What is fever?* (Ans. Refer to page 336, under the heading 'Fever'.)
26. *What are the types of fever?* (Ans. Refer to page 337, under the heading 'Fever' and the subheading 'Types'.)
27. *How do you differentiate between various types of fever?* (Ans. Refer to page 336, under the heading 'Fever' and the subheading 'Types'.)
28. *What are the common causes of fever?* (Ans. Refer to page 332, under the heading 'Fever' and the subheading 'Causes'.)
29. *What is hypothermia? What are its causes?* (Ans. Refer to page 337, under the heading 'Hypothermia'.)
30. *What is the importance of the examination of pulse in general examination?* (Ans. Refer to page 337, under the heading 'Pulse'.)
31. *What is the normal rate of respiration in adults?* (Ans. Refer to page 337, under the heading 'Respiration'.)
32. *What is the normal systolic and diastolic pressure in adults?* (Ans. Refer to page 337, under the heading 'Blood Pressure'.)

53 | Clinical Examination of the Respiratory System

Learning Objectives

After completing this practical, you will be able to (MUST KNOW):

1. Trace the different lines, prominences, lung fissures, and borders on the surface of the chest.
2. Perform a clinical examination of the respiratory system, proceeding in the proper sequence.
3. List the different abnormalities of the shape of the chest.
4. Name the different types and causes of abnormal respiration.
5. State the causes of unilateral and bilateral restriction of chest movements.
6. State the causes of increased and decreased vocal fremitus.
7. List the rules of percussion.
8. List the differences between vesicular and bronchial breath sounds.

You may also be able to (DESIRABLE TO KNOW):

1. Explain the common abnormalities observed in different parameters of the examination of the respiratory system.
2. Explain the differences between vesicular and bronchial breathing.
3. Describe the types and causes of bronchial breathing.
4. List the reasons for the production of different bronchial breath sounds.

PY6.9: Demonstrate the correct clinical examination of the respiratory system in a normal volunteer or in a simulated environment.

INTRODUCTION

Clinical examination of the respiratory system is performed to assess the functional status of the respiratory tract and lungs. It should be carried out meticulously and methodically in a patient suffering from lung disease. The clinical examination can provide sufficient information to diagnose the exact nature of pathology in the lungs. For interpretation and correlation of the findings of the clinical examination with the disease process, one should have adequate knowledge of the functional anatomy of the lungs.

Anatomical Landmarks

Different lines

The different lines that are drawn on the chest (Fig. 53.1) for denoting areas of clinical examination of the respiratory system are as follows:

1. **Midsternal line:** This is a vertical line drawn through the centre of the sternum and xiphoid.
2. **Midclavicular line:** This is a vertical line, parallel to the midsternal line, which extends downwards from the centre of each clavicle. The centre of the clavicle is located between the middle of the suprasternal notch and the tip of the acromion.
3. **Anterior axillary line:** This is a vertical line extending downwards from the anterior axillary fold.
4. **Posterior axillary line:** This is a vertical line extending downwards from the posterior axillary fold.
5. **Midaxillary line:** This is a vertical line originating at a point midway between the anterior and posterior axillary lines.
6. **Midspinal line:** This is a vertical line that passes through the centre of the back as defined by the spinal processes. This is also called the **vertebral line**.
7. **Midscapular line:** This is a vertical line on the posterior aspect of the chest, which runs parallel to the midspinal line and extends through the apices of the scapula.

Different prominences

1. **Sternal angle:** This is a transverse bony ridge at the junction of the body of the sternum and the manubrium. This is also known as the **angle of Louis** or **Ludwig's angle**.

Significance of the sternal angle:

- The second costal cartilage articulates the sternum at this point. Therefore, the *rib that corresponds* to this point is the **second rib**. The intercostal space below this is the second intercostal space. The sternal angle **helps in identifying all the intercostal spaces**.
- The **trachea bifurcates** into two main bronchi at this point.
- The level of the **upper border of the atria** of the heart coincides with this point.
- The anterior borders of the lungs meet in the midline here.
- The **disc between the fourth and fifth thoracic vertebrae** in the back coincides with this.

2. **Suprasternal notch:** This is the top of the manubrium.

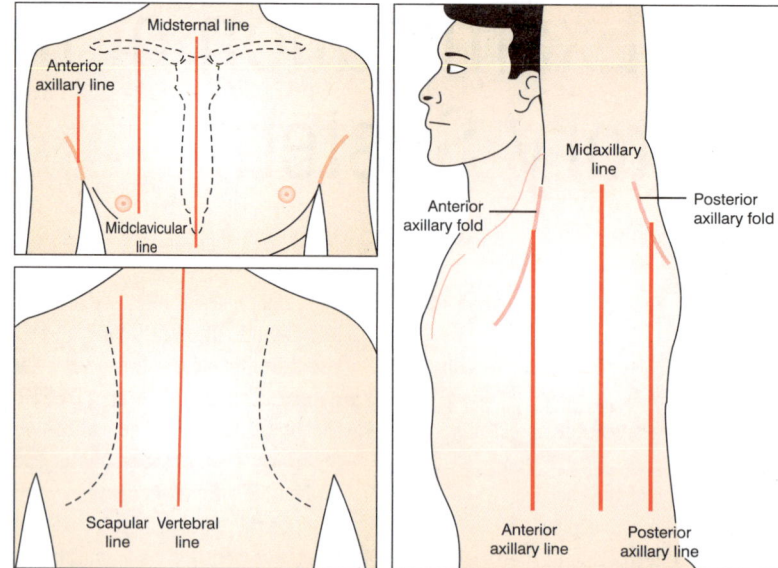

Fig. 53.1   Different lines drawn on the chest denoting areas of clinical examination of the respiratory system.

3. **Vertebral prominence:** The spinous process of the seventh cervical vertebra is the most prominent on the back and is easily seen and felt.

Lung Fissures and Borders

1. **Oblique fissure (major interlobar fissure):** It starts from the second thoracic spine posteriorly and extends obliquely downwards and forwards to the sixth costochondral junction anteriorly.
2. **Horizontal fissure (minor interlobar fissure):** It starts from the right fourth costochondral junction and passes horizontally to meet the oblique fissure in the midaxillary line.

> **Note:** The lower lobe lies below the oblique fissure on either side. Above it, lies the upper lobe on the left side. On the right side, the upper lobe lies above the horizontal fissure. Between the oblique and the horizontal fissures lies the middle lobe of the right lung. The *greater part of the back of the chest* is occupied by the *lower lobe*. The anterior aspect of the chest is occupied by the *upper lobe on the left* and *upper and middle lobe on the right*.

3. **Upper border of the lung:** It is limited to a level 5 cm above the sternoclavicular joint.
4. **Lower border of the lung:** It lies on the sixth rib on the midclavicular line, on the eighth rib on the midaxillary line, and on the tenth rib on the posterior scapular line.

METHODS OF EXAMINING THE RESPIRATORY SYSTEM

Principle

The examination of the respiratory system is carried out by inspection, palpation, percussion, and auscultation of the chest. **Inspection** shows the configuration, the degree of movement of the chest, and the type and rate of respiration. **Palpation** confirms the movement of the chest and detects abnormal pulsation, areas of tenderness, and the degree of vocal fremitus. **Percussion** demonstrates the nature of changes (if any) of the lung tissues, bronchi and the pleura, and helps ascertain whether the lung tissues contain less or more air than normal and whether the pleura contains less or more fluid than normal. **Auscultation** detects the type, intensity, and nature of breath sounds and the presence of any other sound.

Requirements

1.   Measuring tape
2.   Stethoscope

Procedure

It consists of the examination of the chest, which follows the observation of a few particular signs in general examination that are relevant to this system. It is best accomplished when the patient is standing or comfortably seated in an erect position after complete exposure of the chest in good light.

General examination

1. **Pallor:** Anemia is common in patients with *chronic hemoptysis*.
2. **Cyanosis:** It occurs due to the presence of excess *deoxygenated hemoglobin (>5 g%)*. Cyanosis may occur due to *inadequate ventilation* of perfused lung areas (as in pneumonia) or due to a decrease in the *total amount of air* ventilating the lungs (as seen in poliomyelitis).

3. **Clubbing:** Clubbing is recognised by the bulbousness of the soft, terminal portions of the fingers and by an excessive curvature of the nail in both the longitudinal and lateral planes. It is seen in **bronchogenic carcinoma and chronic suppurative diseases** of the lung like bronchiectasis, empyema, and lung abscess.

4. **Lymph node enlargement:** The **neck and supraclavicular region** should be particularly examined to check for enlargement of the lymph nodes.

5. **Vital signs:** Record and note the **temperature, pulse, BP, and respiration** (details of respiration are given below).

Examination of the chest
Inspection
Inspection of the chest should be done with the subject in the supine posture on a couch or sitting comfortably on a chair, with the chest region fully exposed. As the ribs on both sides of the chest extend downward to almost the middle of the abdomen, the **trunk should be exposed up to the umbilicus level** (Fig. 53.2).

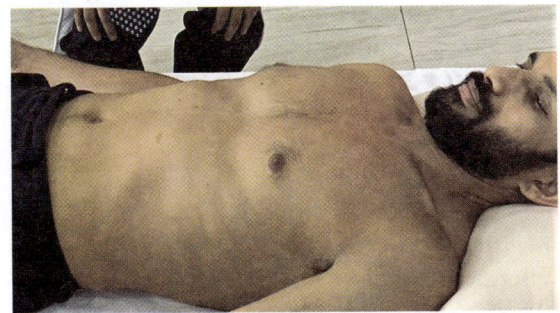

Fig. 53.2 Inspection of the chest. Note that the chest is exposed fully, and the trunk is exposed up to the level of the umbilicus. This is because the ribs on both sides of the chest extend downward almost to the middle of the abdomen.

1. **Shape:** Examine the shape of the chest. The chest of a normal, healthy adult is bilaterally symmetrical. The transverse diameter is greater than the anteroposterior diameter, **the ratio being 7:5**. Check for abnormalities of the chest.

2. **Symmetry:** Look for symmetry of the chest, comparing the two sides. The chest may bulge or be depressed either on one or both sides.

3. **Movement:** Observe whether the chest moves normally and symmetrically and equally on both sides with respiration and whether a difference exists in the movement of the upper and lower parts of the chest.

Note: Normally, the movements are equal on both sides and are more pronounced at the base of the lungs than at the apex. However, one should keep in mind that if lesions are present in both lungs, the movement may be equally affected on both sides.

4. **Respiratory movement:** Look for the following points while observing the movements of the chest with respiration.
   - **Rate:** The normal rate of respiration in adults is **12–18 breaths per minute;** it is higher in children. Increased rate of respiration is called tachypnea, and the decreased rate of respiration is called bradypnea.
   - **Rhythm:** Determine whether the respiration is regular or irregular.
   - **Depth:** Look for the depth (degree) of respiration. The respiration may be decreased unilaterally or on both sides.
   - **Type:** Note whether the respiration is predominantly thoracic or abdominal. In men, respiration is **abdominothoracic** and in women, the respiration is **thoracoabdominal**.

Palpation
1. **Expansion of the chest:** Expansion of the chest is assessed by placing the two palms firmly on both sides of the chest and apposing the thumbs in the midline anteriorly (Fig. 53.3A). The subject is asked to take a deep breath, and the movement of the thumbs away from the midline is observed (Fig. 53.3B). This indicates the extent of expansion of the chest. Normally, the **expansion is more than 5 cm at the base** of the lungs in adults, which can be elicited both in the front of the chest (Fig. 53.4A and B) and back of the chest (Fig. 53.5A and B). The expansion is less

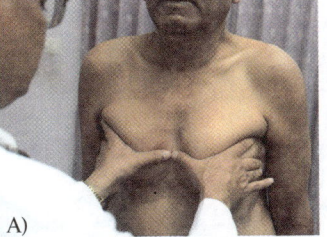
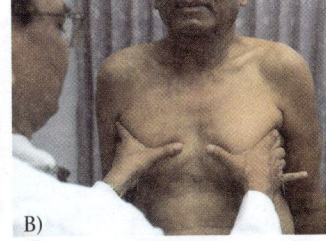

A)   B)

Fig. 53.3 Demonstration of chest expansion. **(A)** Chest expansion is performed by firmly holding the chest with both the palms and apposing the thumbs at the centre; **(B)** The subject is asked to take the maximum inspiration possible, with which thumbs move apart. The distance between the thumbs is noted as the degree of chest expansion.

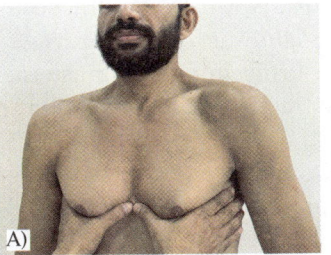
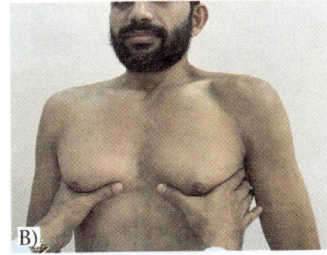

A)   B)

Fig. 53.4 Demonstration of chest expansion for the base of the lung, anteriorly: **(A)** Before expansion and **(B)** after expansion.

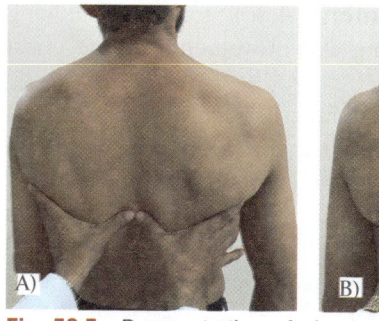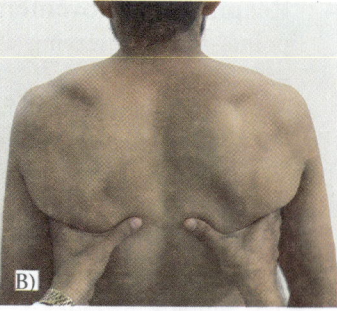

Fig. 53.5 Demonstration of chest expansion for the base of the lung, posteriorly: **(A)** Before expansion and **(B)** after expansion.

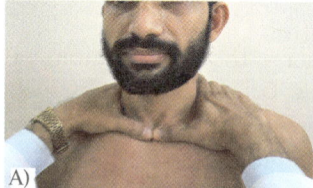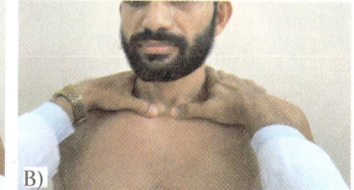

Fig. 53.6 Demonstration of chest expansion at the apex of the lung, anteriorly: **(A)** Before expansion and **(B)** after expansion.

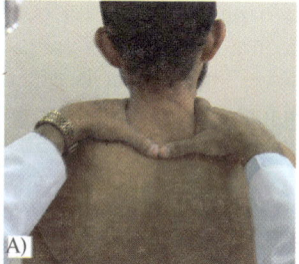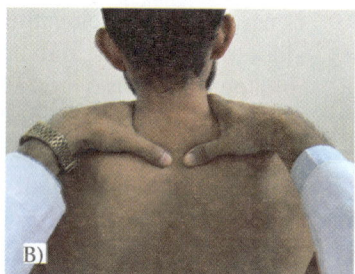

Fig. 53.7 Demonstration of chest expansion at the apex of the lung, posteriorly: **(A)** Before expansion and **(B)** after expansion.

marked at the apex of the lungs, which can be elicited both in front of the chest (Fig. 53.6A and B) and the back of the chest (Fig. 53.7A and B). Expansion may be less on the side where the lung is affected by disease.

2. **Position of the trachea:** The position of the trachea can be detected in **three ways**.
   - Place the tip of the index and ring finger of the right hand on the sternoclavicular joints (sternal ends of the clavicles) on either side and place the middle finger on the suprasternal notch. Then, gently push the middle finger forward to feel the tracheal rings (Fig. 53.8). The position of the trachea is determined by observing the *spaces between the fingertips*. Normally, the trachea is *centrally placed* or *slightly deviated to the right*.
   - Place the index finger firmly into the suprasternal notch and locate the tracheal rings in relation to the sternum.
   - Find the space between the anterior border of the sternomastoid muscle and the trachea. If the trachea has deviated to one side, the space becomes narrow on that side.

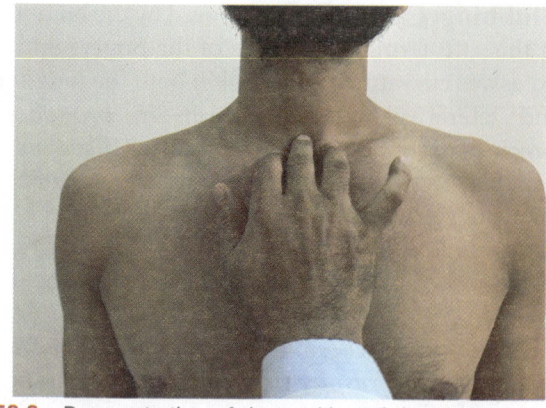

Fig. 53.8 Demonstration of the position of the trachea. Note that the tips of the index and ring finger of the right hand are placed on the sternal ends of the clavicles and the tip of the middle finger is placed on the suprasternal notch, which is then gently pushed forward to feel the tracheal rings.

3. **Position of the apex beat:** Locate the position of the apex beat (details in Chapter 54). Displacement of the apex of the heart and the trachea to one side indicates the *shifting of the mediastinum* to that side.

4. **Vocal fremitus (VF):** Ask the subject to repeatedly say 'ninety-nine' or 'one-two-three' and feel the vibration from the surface of the chest by placing the ulnar border of the hand on the surface of the chest in the intercostal space (Fig. 53.9). To compare the two sides (diseased and normal sides), examine the opposite side of the chest in the same intercostal space immediately. Note whether *VF is normal, diminished, or increased* (details in the 'Discussion' section).

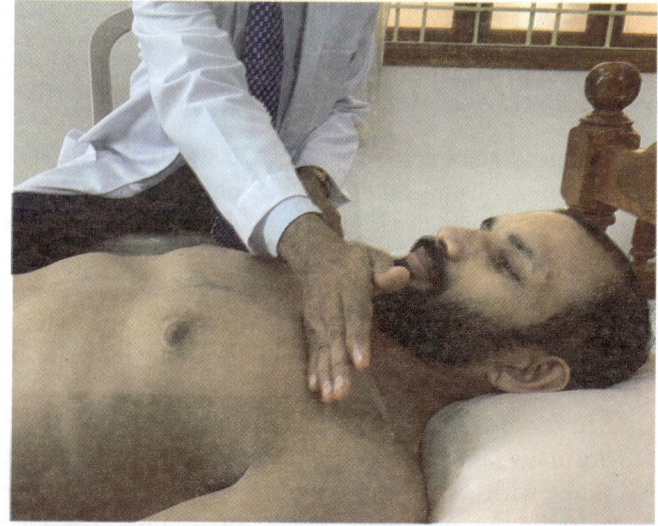

Fig. 53.9 Method of eliciting vocal fremitus (VF). Note that while the subject is saying '99' or '1-2-3', the examiner feels the vibration from the surface of the chest by placing the ulnar border of his hand firmly in the intercostal space. The opposite side of the chest in the same intercostal space is examined immediately.

Note: The vibration transmitted to the chest wall from the respiratory passages represents VF. The vibration is conducted from the larynx by the trachea and bronchi to the smaller tubes within the lungs, and then through the lung tissues to the chest wall. It should be elicited over symmetrical areas on both sides of the chest alternately. It may be **normal, increased, reduced, or absent**.

5. **Tenderness:** Palpate all the regions of the chest wall to elicit tenderness, if present. Tenderness may be seen in **injury to the chest wall, inflammatory conditions** of the ribs and intercostal muscles, **malignant deposits** in the ribs, pleurisy, a painful lung infection, and so on.

▌Percussion

Percuss **different areas** (supraclavicular, infraclavicular, mammary, inframammary, axillary, infra-axillary, suprascapular, interscapular, and infrascapular) **on both sides** of the chest.

1. While percussing the subject's back, ask him to cross his arms in front of his chest, the left hand touching the right shoulder and vice versa, and to slightly lean forward.
2. While percussing the axillary region, ask the subject to lift his hands to his head. The axillary areas are percussed with the pleximeter finger in the intercostal spaces.
3. The clavicle should be percussed directly by the percussing finger without using the pleximeter finger.

   Percussion of *corresponding regions on both sides* should be performed and compared simultaneously.

Rules of percussion:

1. Apply the pleximeter finger firmly on the surface of the chest (Fig. 53.10).
2. The percussing finger should strike the middle phalanx of the pleximeter finger perpendicularly (vertically).

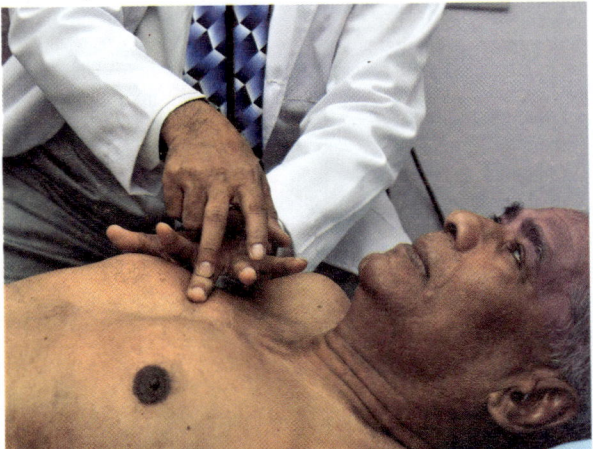

Fig. 53.10 Demonstration of percussion of the anterior aspect of the chest. Note that the pleximeter finger is placed firmly on the anterior surface of the chest in the intercostal space. The percussing finger strokes the pleximeter finger at a right angle.

3. The strokes should be delivered from the wrist and finger joints, not from the elbow.
4. The percussing finger should be lifted immediately after striking the pleximeter finger.
5. The long axis of the pleximeter finger should be parallel to the edge of the organ being percussed.
6. Percussion should be carried out from the more resonant to the less resonant area.

Note the **character of the sounds** produced by percussion, whether they are of **normal resonance, hyper-resonance, dull, stony dull, or tympanic** (details under 'Discussion').

▌Auscultation

While auscultating, place the chest piece of the stethoscope firmly over the chest and ask the patient to breathe regularly and deeply with his mouth slightly open (Fig. 53.11).

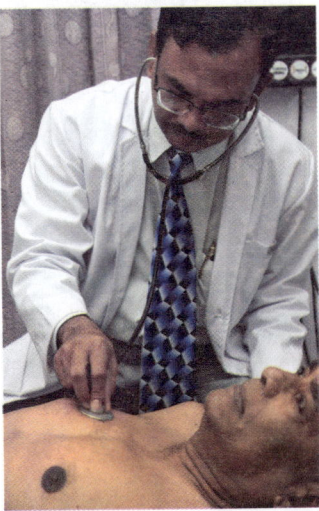

Fig. 53.11 Auscultation of breath sounds. Note that the stethoscope is firmly placed over the chest surface. If the stethoscope is placed loosely, chest movements during respiration cause rubbing of the skin against the diaphragm of the stethoscope and produce false adventitious sounds.

Auscultate **all the areas of the chest in front** (supraclavicular, infraclavicular, mammary, and inframammary), all the areas on the **side of the chest** (axillary and infra-axillary), and all the areas **on the back** such as the suprascapular (Fig. 53.12), interscapular

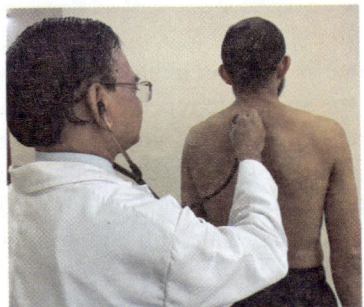

Fig. 53.12 Auscultation of breath sounds in the suprascapular region.

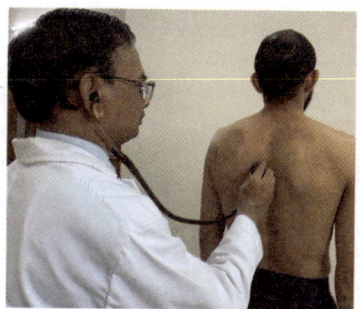

Fig. 53.13   Auscultation of breath sounds in the interscapular region.

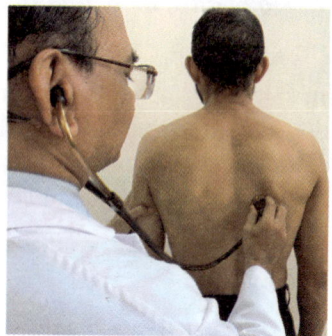

Fig. 53.14   Auscultation of breath sounds in the infrascapular region.

(Fig. 53.13), and infrascapular (Fig. 53.14) regions, and compare the two sides immediately. Usually, breath sounds are clearer and louder on the infrascapular region.

> **Note:** The purpose of auscultation is to obtain information over and above what the preceding three steps (inspection, palpation, and percussion) of physical examination furnish. Auscultation is performed to detect the type of breath sound, the intensity and character of vocal resonance, and presence of any adventitious sounds.

Breath sounds

Auscultate all the areas over the chest for breath sounds. Use the diaphragm of the stethoscope to auscultate breath sounds. Try to note the *intensity, character of breath sounds, and type of breath sounds, i.e., vesicular or bronchial*. Try to differentiate between vesicular and bronchial breath sounds. To appreciate the bronchial breath sound, place the diaphragm of the stethoscope on the trachea (Fig. 53.15). The details of differences between vesicular and bronchial breath sounds are detailed in the 'Discussion' section.

Vocal resonance

Vocal resonance is the auscultatory counterpart of vocal fremitus. Ask the subject to repeatedly say 'ninety-nine' or 'one-two-three' at a constant volume and auscultate the *symmetrical areas of the two sides* of the chest. The intensity of vocal resonance **depends on** the *loudness and depth* of the subject's voice and the conductivity of the lungs. It may be **normal, decreased, or increased** (details in 'Discussion'). Vocal resonance of **normal intensity** conveys the impression of being produced just at the chest piece of the stethoscope and is *heard as a soft sound*.

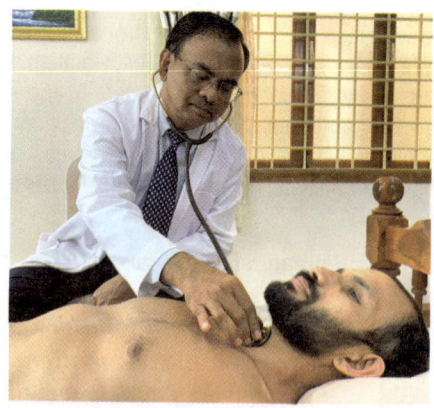

Fig. 53.15   Auscultation of breath sounds on the trachea. Note that normally, tracheal sounds (produced by the flow of air through the trachea) resemble bronchial breath sounds.

Adventitious (added) sounds

Note the presence of any adventitious sounds such as crepitations, pleural rub, rhonchi, etc.

Observation and Results

1. Note your observations in a tabular format as given below.

Parameters	Observation / Findings	
Patient's name, age, gender, height, body weight		
General Examination i. Pallor ii. Cyanosis iii. Clubbing iv. L.N. enlargement v. Vital Signs		
Examination of chest	Left side	Right side
Inspection i. Shape of chest ii. Symmetry of chest iii. Movement of chest iv. Respiratory movement		
Palpation i. Expansion of chest ii. Position of trachea iii. Position of apex beat iv. Vocal fremitus v. Tenderness		
Percussion: Percuss and note the character of percussion sounds in the following areas: i. Supraclavicular ii. Infraclavicular iii. Mammary iv. Inframammary v. Axillary vi. Infra-axillary vii. Suprascapular viii. Interscapular ix. Infrascapular		

Auscultation		
i. Breath sounds (auscultate area-wise as described above for percussion) ii. Vocal resonance iii. Added sounds		

2. Analyse the results and report the findings with your comments on respiratory functions.

Precautions

1. The examination should be carried out with the subject standing or seated comfortably with their chest fully exposed.
2. General examination should be carried out before examining the chest.
3. Inspection of the chest should be performed without touching the subject.
4. While assessing chest expansion, the subject should be instructed to expand his chest as much as possible.
5. While evaluating the position of the trachea, the tracheal rings should be palpated gently. Excessive pressure will cause discomfort to the subject.
6. Both VF and VR should be elicited on symmetrical areas of the two sides simultaneously and compared.
7. During percussion, the rules of percussion should be adhered to strictly and the procedure should be performed simultaneously on both sides, and the findings should be compared.
8. For eliciting VR on different areas of the chest, the subject should be instructed to speak at a steady pitch and volume throughout the examination to maintain uniformity.

DISCUSSION

Inspectory Findings

Shape of the chest

The chest of a normal, healthy adult is bilaterally symmetrical, and the transverse diameter is greater than the anteroposterior diameter, the **ratio being 7:5**. The following abnormalities should be looked for during the inspection (Fig. 53.16).

▐ Flat chest

This is usually associated with a long neck, prominent larynx and clavicle, and a long, narrow chest.
Features:
1. Exaggerated supra- and infraclavicular fossa
2. Narrow intercostal spaces
3. Acute subcostal angle
Causes: It is seen in healthy people, but may be associated with the following:

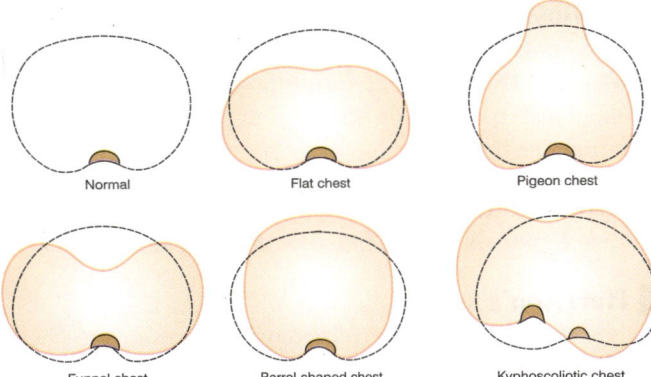

Fig. 53.16   Types (shapes) of chests. The normal shape of the chest is marked by dotted lines. Note that the ratio of the transverse to the anteroposterior diameter of the normal adult chest is 7:5.

1. Rickets in childhood
2. Chronic nasal obstruction from hypertrophied adenoid
3. Bilateral tuberculosis

▐ Pigeon chest *(pectus carinatum)*

The sternum is unduly prominent and projects beyond the plane of the front of the abdomen. It is **seen in:**
1. Children with rickets
2. Recurrent lung infection in children

▐ Funnel chest *(pectus excavatum)*

Features:
1. Depression at the lower end of the sternum
2. Prominent costochondral junction
3. Diminished anteroposterior diameter of the chest
Causes: It could be due to rickets or congenital.

▐ Barrel-shaped chest

Features:
1. Increased anteroposterior diameter of the chest.
2. The ribs are wide apart and tend to be horizontal.
3. The spine is unduly concave.
4. The sternum is more arched.
5. The angle of Louis is more prominent.
6. Fullness of supraclavicular fossae.
Cause: The usual cause is chronic obstructive emphysema.

▐ Kyphosis

This refers to **the backward bending of the vertebral column** resulting in convexity posteriorly and concavity anteriorly. It causes the shortening of the chest and undue prominence of the vertebrae.
Causes:
1. Caries spine
2. Osteoarthritis
3. Secondary osteoporosis
4. Chronic obstructive emphysema
5. Ankylosing spondylitis

Scoliosis

This refers to the **lateral bending of the spine and rotation of the vertebrae** resulting in undue prominence of the chest and scapula on the side of the convexity and flattening of the chest.

Kyphoscoliosis

In this, **kyphosis is associated with scoliosis**.

Harrison's sulcus

This is a **transverse groove or constriction** in the chest, which begins at the xiphisternum and passes outwards and slightly downwards, sometimes, reaching the midaxillary line. It is seen in **rickets**.

Rickety rosary

This is characterised by the presence of a number of **rounded or knob-like projections** at the costochondral junctions. It is usually seen in **rickets**.

Symmetry of the chest

The chest may bulge or be depressed, either on one side or on both sides.

Localised or unilateral fullness (bulging)

1.   Pleural effusion
2.   Pneumothorax
3.   Intrathoracic tumours

Symmetrical or bilateral fullness

1.   Emphysema
2.   Bilateral pleural effusion
3.   Bilateral pneumothorax

Unilateral depression

1.   Fibrosis
2.   Collapse

Bilateral depression

1.   Bilateral fibrosis
2.   Bilateral collapse

Respiratory movements

Rate

The normal rate of respiration in adults is **12–18 breaths per minute**. The respiration rate is greater in children than in adults. Increased rate of respiration is called *tachypnea*, and decreased rate of respiration is called *bradypnea*.

Causes of tachypnea:
I.   Physiological conditions
1.   Newborns and infants
2.   Children
3.   Gender (rate of respiration is higher in women)
4.   Exercise

5.   Excitement and emotion
6.   Nervousness

II.   **Pathological conditions**
Different disease conditions that produce hypoxia; for example, pneumonia causes tachypnea.

Causes of bradypnea: Bradypnea is not a common occurrence. It is usually seen in conditions of CNS depression, such as narcotic poisoning.

Rhythm

Irregular respiration is commonly seen in intracranial lesions.

Depth

The respiration may be decreased unilaterally or on both sides.

Unilateral restriction of movement:
1.   Pleural effusion
2.   Pneumothorax
3.   Fibrosis
4.   Collapse
5.   Consolidation

Bilateral restriction of movement:
1.   Emphysema
2.   Bilateral pleural effusion
3.   Bilateral consolidation

Type

Respiration may be predominantly thoracic or abdominal. In men, respiration is abdominothoracic; in women, respiration is thoracoabdominal.

Types of abnormal respiration

1.   **Kussmaul respiration:** Characterised by increased rate and depth of respiration (air hunger). It is seen in *metabolic acidosis,* such as *diabetic ketoacidosis.*
2.   **Cheyne–Stokes respiration:** In this type of respiration, a period of **hyperpnea is followed by apnea**. It is seen in physiological conditions like sleep (especially in infants), at high altitudes, following hyperventilation, and in pathological conditions like *cardiac failure, renal failure, brain tumour, and narcotic poisoning*.
3.   **Biot's respiration:** Breathing is irregular in both depth and rhythm, with irregular pauses and occasional sighs. It is seen in **meningitis**.

Palpatory Findings

Expansion of the chest

Normally, the expansion is **more than 5 cm at the base** of the lungs in adults. The expansion is *less towards the apex* of the lungs. *Maximum* chest expansion is detected at the *fourth intercostal space*. It is always less on the side of the chest that is affected by a disease of the chest wall or lung.

Position of apex and trachea

Displacement of the apex and trachea to one side indicates the *shifting of the mediastinum* to that side. However, displacement of the apex may occur without displacement of the trachea; alternatively, the apex and trachea may displace in opposite directions depending on the nature of pathology.

Shifting of the mediastinum

1. The mediastinum **shifts to the side of the** *collapsed and fibrosed lung*.
2. It **shifts to the opposite side** in cases of *pleural effusion, pneumothorax, hydropneumothorax, or a mass* (e.g., tumour) in the thorax.

Vocal fremitus (VF)

VF may be **normal, increased, reduced, or absent**.
VF is increased in:
1. Consolidation of the lungs, e.g., lobar pneumonia
2. Large cavity near the chest surface
VF is diminished in:
1. Bronchial obstruction
2. Collapse
3. Fibrosis
4. Thickened pleura
5. Emphysema
VF is absent in: VF may be completely absent when the lung is separated from the chest wall by massive pleural effusion or pneumothorax.

Tenderness

Tenderness may be present due to an *injury to the chest wall, inflammatory conditions of the ribs* and intercostal muscles, *malignant deposits* in the ribs, pleurisy, or *painful lesions* of the lungs.

Percussion Findings

Significance

Percussion is carried out to detect the limit of lung resonance and the presence of any pathology in the lungs. Percussion over a **normal lung produces a resonant note**. '*Resonant*' is a relative term since there is no absolute standard.
1. **Cardiac dullness** is noted on the left side between the third and fifth spaces.
2. **Hepatic dullness** is noted on the right side from the fifth rib downwards in the midclavicular line, from the eighth rib downwards in the midaxillary line, and from the tenth rib downwards in the midscapular line.
3. One should keep in mind that lesions more than **5 cm away from the chest wall** or lesions **less than 2–3 cm**

in diameter will not alter the percussion note. The percussion note is expressed as **normal resonance, hyper-resonance, impaired resonance or dullness**, and **stony dullness**.
4. When the dullness shifts from one part of the chest to the other, it is called **shifting dullness**.

Hyper-resonance

Hyper-resonance occurs when the **amount of air in the lungs or chest cavity is increased**. This occurs in the following conditions:
1. Emphysema
2. Pneumothorax
3. Over an emphysematous bulla
4. Over a large superficial cavity

Dullness or impaired resonance

Dullness or impaired resonance results from any condition that *interferes with the production of normal resonant vibrations* within the lungs or the *transmission of these vibrations* to the chest wall. This is seen in the following conditions:
1. Consolidation
2. Thickened pleura
3. Fibrosis and collapse
4. Atelectasis

Stony dullness

When the percussion note is **very dull**, it is called stony dullness. It is seen in **pleural effusion**.

Shifting dullness

If the dullness shifts when the **patient changes positions**, it is called shifting dullness. It is one of the important tests to detect the presence of air and fluid in the pleural cavity. It is a reliable sign of **hydropneumothorax**.

Tidal percussion

A dull note obtained above the upper border of liver dullness may be due to **liver enlargement** or a **disorder either in the lungs or pleura**. Tidal percussion is performed to *ascertain the pathology*. Normally, there is an increase in the area of resonance downwards by 4–6 cm during full inspiration due to the movement of the diaphragm, lungs, and liver downwards. **In upward enlargement of the liver**, the increase in the area of resonance in deep inspiration (in tidal percussion) *remains within normal limits*. **In lung pathology**, the area of resonance decreases on tidal percussion.

Auscultatory Findings

Auscultation is performed to detect the type of breath sound, the intensity and character of vocal resonance, and the presence of any adventitious sounds.

Breath bounds

Breath sounds originate in the large airways due to turbulent airflow during breathing. Sounds produced in the large airways (**bronchial breath sounds**) are of *higher frequencies* of above 600 Hz. These sounds are transmitted to the lung tissue, which acts as a low-pass filter, filtering out high-frequency sounds and converting them into low-frequency sounds (**vesicular sounds**) that are transmitted to the chest wall. Therefore, sounds auscultated from the chest wall in normal people are vesicular breath sounds, though the sounds originate in the large airways (bronchi).

Puerile breathing: In children, breath sounds are normally louder and harsher than in adults—a pattern known as puerile breathing. Sometimes, during exercise, a similar kind of breathing may be noted.

Intensity

Breath sounds are produced by the repetitive movement of air into and out of the ventilated alveoli. The intensity of the sound is directly proportional to the amount of air entering the alveoli. It may be normal, reduced, or increased.

Reduced intensity: Breath sounds decrease in intensity when there is localised airway narrowing, if the lung is extensively damaged by the disease process, or if there is *interference in the transmission of sound from the lung tissue to the chest wall*.

1. **Airway narrowing**
   - Bronchial obstruction with or without collapse of the lung
   - Consolidation with an obstructed bronchus (obstructive pneumonia)
2. **Damage to lung tissue**
   - Fibrosis
   - Atelectasis
3. **Interference in transmission of sounds**
   - Thickened pleura
   - Pleural effusion
   - Pneumothorax
   - Emphysema

Increased intensity: The intensity of breath sounds may be increased in thin subjects or when the *ventilation of the lung tissue is increased* (e.g. in *compensatory emphysema*). Loud breath sounds should not be confused with bronchial breath sounds.

Character

On the basis of character, breath sounds are divided into **two types**: vesicular and bronchial (Fig. 53.17A and B).

■ Vesicular breath sounds

The normal character of breath sounds is vesicular. These sounds originate in the large airways, but when

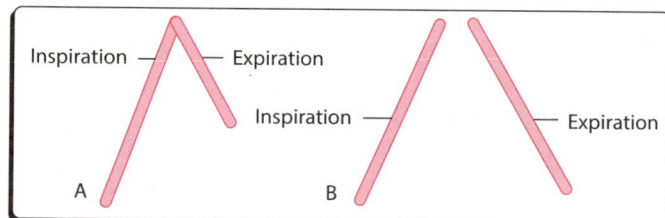

Fig. 53.17 Breath sounds: **(A)** Vesicular and **(B)** bronchial.

transmitted through the lung tissue to the chest wall, they become low-pitched vesicular sounds. These sounds have the *following characteristics:*

1. Duration of inspiration is more than that of expiration.
2. Intensity of inspiration is greater than that of expiration.
3. There is no gap between inspiration and expiration.
4. Sounds are rustling in nature.
5. They are low-pitched, with frequencies in the range of 200–600 Hz.

Vesicular breath sound with prolonged expiration: In some diseases, the breath sound is normal in character (vesicular), but the duration of expiration is either equal to or more than that of inspiration. There will be no gap between expiration and inspiration. This is seen when there is *partial obstruction of the bronchi* as in asthma.

■ Bronchial breath sounds

Bronchial breath sounds *originate in the larger airways* and are **transmitted directly to the chest wall** without passing through the alveoli. The sound passing through the lung tissue is not modified and auscultated like bronchial sounds from the chest walls. This sound resembles the sound obtained by listening over the trachea by directly placing a stethoscope on the trachea (**tracheal breath sounds**).

> **Note:** Bronchial breath sounds are **demonstrated to students by auscultating over the trachea**. Bronchial breath sounds are also sometimes heard in the upper interscapular region and at the apex of the right lung because the trachea and bronchi lie close to the surface in these areas.

The following are the **characteristics of bronchial breath sounds** (Table 53.1):

1. Then duration of expiration is equal to or longer than that of inspiration.
2. The intensity of expiration is more than that of inspiration.
3. There is a definite gap between inspiration and expiration (Fig. 53.17B).
4. Sounds are harsh or aspirate in nature.
5. They are high-pitched with frequencies above 600 Hz.

Table 53.1 Differences between vesicular and bronchial breath sounds.

	Vesicular breath sounds	Bronchial breath sounds
Origin	Larger airways, filled with normal air in healthy lung tissues	Larger airways, but the lung tissue is diseased by infiltration of inflammatory material, resulting in consolidation or there is fibrosis or lung collapse
Location	Heard over the healthy lung fields	Normally heard over the trachea (tracheal sound mimics bronchial breath sounds) In diseases in which the bronchus is patent, but the alveoli are not filled with air
Character	Low-pitched and soft No pause between the end of inspiration and the beginning of expiration	High-pitched, louder and harsh Definitive gap between the end of inspiration and the beginning of expiration
Relative duration	Expiration is less than inspiration	Both inspiration and expiration are equal

Types of bronchial breath sounds: Bronchial breath sounds are of **three types**: tubular, cavernous, and amphoric.

1. **Tubular bronchial breath sound** is a *high-pitched sound* resulting from the passage of vibrations produced in the small bronchi directly to the chest wall *through solid lung tissue*. This is seen when the *lung parenchyma becomes a solid mass*, as seen in *consolidation*.
2. **Cavernous bronchial breath sound** is a *low-pitched* bronchial breath sound *heard over a cavity*, which is situated superficially and communicated to a patent bronchus. The size of the cavity *should be more than 2 cm in diameter to produce a cavernous breath sound*.
3. **Amphoric bronchial breath sound** is a *high-pitched* bronchial sound that resembles the sound produced by blowing air into a wide-mouthed bottle. This is heard over *a very large cavity* communicating with a pneumothorax. It is also seen in *large pulmonary cysts* that communicate with a patent bronchus.

Vocal resonance

Vocal resonance is the auscultatory counterpart of vocal fremitus. The intensity of vocal resonance depends on the **loudness and depth of the subject's voice** and the **conductivity of the lungs**. It may be *normal, decreased, or increased*.

Increased vocal resonance

When the sounds appear to be nearer to the ear than the chestpiece and louder than normal, the vocal resonance

is said to be increased. The **three types** of increased vocal resonance are bronchophony, aegophony, and whispering pectoriloquy.

1. **Bronchophony:** If the vocal resonance is increased and appears to **arise from the earpiece of the stethoscope**, it is described as bronchophony. It is seen in **consolidation of the lungs**, e.g., in lobar pneumonia.
2. **Aegophony:** When the increased vocal resonance is **high-pitched,** giving a nasal intonation or having a bleating character ('goat voice'), it is called aegophony.
3. **Whispering pectoriloquy:** If the vocal resonance is increased to such an extent that the sounds become very clear and seem to be **spoken (whispering) right into the listener's ear**, it is called whispering pectoriloquy. This is tested by asking the patient to whisper instead of speaking loudly. It is seen in **consolidation** and over a **large superficial cavity** communicating with a patent bronchus.

Diminished vocal resonance

Vocal resonance decreases in the following conditions:
1. Pleural effusion
2. Pneumothorax
3. Collapse
4. Thickened pleura
5. Emphysema

Adventitious (added) sounds

These sounds may arise from the **lungs and bronchi or the pleura**. The sounds that arise from the lungs and bronchi are ronchi, wheeze, stridor, and crepitations; the ones originating from the pleura are called the pleural rub.

Ronchi

These are **prolonged, uninterrupted musical sounds** that occur due to partial obstruction of the flow of air in a **narrowed bronchus or bronchiole**. The narrowing of the lumen of the airway may occur due to mucosal swelling, viscid thick secretion, spasm, or infiltration of the wall. Ronchi are of **two types**: sibilant and sonorous. **Sibilant ronchi** are high-pitched and are produced in the smaller bronchi. **Sonorous ronchi** are low-pitched and are produced in the large bronchi.

Causes:
1. Bronchitis
2. Bronchial asthma
3. Obstruction of the bronchial tube by a tumour or foreign body

Wheeze

Wheeze is a **high-pitched musical sound**, which results from **partial airway obstruction**. It is louder and more persistent during expiration. Sometimes, the sound is so loud that it can be heard without the aid of a stethoscope. It is heard during *attacks of asthma*.

Stridor

This is a **jerky, high-pitched and coarse sound** usually heard during inspiration. It occurs due to *obstruction to inspiratory airflow* due to airway obstruction. It is commonly heard in:

1. Foreign body impaction
2. Tumour (pressing the airway from outside)
3. Diphtheria (diphtheric membrane)

Crepitations

These are **moist, discontinuous, and crackling or bubbling sounds** produced either in the alveoli, bronchi, or in cavities. These are produced only in the presence of fluid or secretions.

Crepitations are of **two types**: fine and coarse.

1. **Fine crepitations:** These are caused by the **opening of collapsed alveoli**. It occurs at the end of an inspiration and indicates the presence of exudate in the alveoli. When collapsed alveoli open, the separation of the alveolar wall produces a crackling sound. These are heard in the *early stages of pneumonia, localised tuberculosis*, and at the base of the lungs *in heart failure*.
2. **Coarse crepitations:** These are heard in any phase of respiration and indicate the presence of secretion in the bronchi or bronchioles. It is heard in bronchitis, polycystic diseases of the lungs, resolving stage of pneumonia, and bronchiectasis.

Pleural rub

This is a **rough, harsh crackling sound** produced by the rubbing of the visceral and parietal pleura against each other during respiration. It indicates *inflammation of the pleura* and the presence of inflammatory exudates. It can be confused with coarse crepitations. It *disappears when the subject is asked to hold his breath* and remains unaffected by coughing.

OSPE

I.   Clinically assess the expansion of the lower part of the chest.

Steps

1. Provide proper instructions to the subject.
2. Place both palms on both sides of the lower part of the chest, in such a way that the thumbs remain in the front and other fingers on the sides of the chest.
3. Try to bring the thumbs close to the midline in the front of the chest in such a way that the tips of the thumbs just touch each other.
4. Ask the subject to take a deep breath.
5. Note the expansion of the chest by observing the movement of the thumbs away from the midline on both sides.

II.   Elicit vocal fremitus from the infraclavicular region of the chest of the given subject and report your findings.

Steps

1. Provide proper instructions to the subject.
2. Place the ulnar border of your hand on the infraclavicular region of one side of the chest.
3. Ask the subject to say "1-2-3" or "99".
4. Feel for the vibration on the chest wall.
5. Repeat the same on the opposite side and compare.
6. Report the findings.

III.   Elicit vocal resonance from the infraclavicular region of the chest of the given subject.

Steps

1. Provide appropriate instructions to the subject.
2. Place the diaphragm of the stethoscope on the infraclavicular region of one side of the chest.
3. Ask the subject to say "1-2-3" or "99".
4. Listen to the sounds on the chest wall.
5. Repeat the same on the opposite side and compare.
6. Report the findings.

IV.   Percuss the infraclavicular region of the chest of the given subject and report your findings.

Steps

1. Provide proper instructions to the subject.
2. Place the pleximeter finger (middle finger of the left hand) firmly on an intercostal space, keeping the other fingers elevated and off the chest wall.
3. Using the middle finger of the right hand as the percussing finger, strike the pleximeter finger sharply with a wrist movement, lifting the percussing finger immediately after each stroke.
4. Percuss over all intercostal spaces on one side, noting the quality of the percussion note.
5. Repeat on the opposite side.
6. Compare both sides and record your observations.

V.   Percuss the infraclavicular region of the chest of the given subject and report your findings.

Steps

1. Provide proper instructions to the subject.
2. Place the pleximeter (middle finger of the left hand) firmly on the intercostal space horizontal to the ribs with the other fingers not touching the chest wall, on one side of the chest.
3. Strike the pleximeter finger with the percussing finger (middle finger of the right hand) by moving the wrist joint and after each stroke immediately lift the percussing finger.
4. Percuss all the intercostal spaces and note the resonant sounds.
5. Percuss the opposite side of the chest and compare.
6. Report the findings.

VIVA

1. *How do you draw the midsternal, midclavicular, anterior-axillary, posterior-axillary, midaxillary, midspinal, and midscapular lines?* (**Ans.** Refer to page 339, under the heading 'Anatomical Landmarks' and the subheading 'Different Lines'.)
2. *How do you locate the sternal angle? What is its significance?* (**Ans.** Refer to page 339, under the heading 'Different Prominences' and the subheading 'Sternal angle'.)
3. *How do you trace the surface anatomy of major interlobar and horizontal fissures of the lungs?* (**Ans.** Refer to page 340, under the heading 'Lung Fissure and Borders'.)
4. *How do you determine the lower border of the lungs on the chest?* (**Ans.** Refer to page 340, under the heading 'Lung Fissure and Borders', read No. 4 'Lower Border...'.)
5. *What is the significance of looking for clubbing and cyanosis before examining the chest?* (**Ans.** Refer to page 341, under the heading 'General Examination' and the subheading 'Cyanosis and clubbing'.)
6. *What are the common abnormalities of the shape of the chest?* (**Ans.** Refer to page 345, under the heading 'Discussion' and the subheading 'Inspectory Findings...Shape of the Chest'.)
7. *What are the features of the flat chest? In what conditions is it observed?* (**Ans.** Refer to page 345, under the heading 'Shape of the Chest' and the subheading 'Flat chest'.)
8. *What is 'pigeon chest'? In what conditions is it observed?* (**Ans.** Refer to page 345, under the heading 'Shape of the Chest' and the subheading 'Pigeon chest'.)
9. *What is 'barrel-shaped chest'? In what conditions is it observed?* (**Ans.** Refer to page 345, under the heading 'Shape of the Chest' and the subheading 'Barrel-shaped chest'.)
10. *What is kyphoscoliosis? In what conditions is it observed?* (**Ans.** Refer to page 346, under the heading 'Shape of the Chest' and the subheading 'Kyphoscoliosis'.)
11. *What is 'rickety rosary'? In what conditions is it observed?* (**Ans.** Refer to page 346, under the heading 'Shape of the Chest' and the subheading 'Rickety rosary'.)
12. *What are the causes of unilateral bulging of the chest?* (**Ans.** Refer to page 346, under the heading 'Shape of the Chest' and the subheading 'Localised or unilateral fullness'.)
13. *What are the causes of tachypnea?* (**Ans.** Refer to page 346, under the heading 'Respiratory Movements' and the subheading 'Rate'.)
14. *What are the causes of unilateral restriction of movement of the chest?* (**Ans.** Refer to page 346, under the heading 'Respiratory Movements' and the subheadings 'Depth', 'Unilateral Restriction...'.)
15. *What are the types of abnormal respiration?* (**Ans.** Refer to page 346, under the heading 'Respiratory Movements' and the subheading 'Types of abnormal respiration'.)
16. *What is Cheyne–Stokes respiration? What are the causes of this abnormal respiration?* (**Ans.** Refer to page 346, under the heading 'Types of Abnormal Respiration' and the subheading 'Cheyne–Stokes respiration'.)
17. *How do you clinically determine the expansion of the chest?* (**Ans.** Refer to page 341-342, under the heading 'Palpation' and the subheading 'Expansion of the chest', Fig. 52.3 to 52.7.)
18. *How do you clinically determine the position of the trachea?* (**Ans.** Refer to page 342, under the heading 'Palpation' and the subheading 'Position of trachea' and Fig. 52.8.)
19. *What are the causes of shifting of the mediastinum?* (**Ans.** Refer to page 347, under the heading 'Palpatory Findings' and the subheading 'Shifting of mediastinum'.)
20. *What are the causes of increased and decreased vocal fremitus?* (**Ans.** Refer to page 347, under the heading 'Palpatory Findings' and the subheading 'Vocal fremitus'.)
21. *What are the rules of percussion?* (**Ans.** Refer to page 347, under the heading 'Rules of Percussion'.)
22. *What are the causes of hyper-resonance of the lungs?* (**Ans.** Refer to page 347, under the heading 'Percussion Findings' and the subheading 'Hyper-resonance'.)
23. *What are the causes of dullness of the lungs?* (**Ans.** Refer to page 347, under the heading 'Percussion Findings' and the subheading 'Dullness...'.)
24. *What is stony dullness? In what conditions does it occur?* (**Ans.** Refer to page 347, under the heading 'Percussion Findings' and the subheading 'Stony dullness'.)
25. *What is shifting dullness? In what conditions does it occur?* (**Ans.** Refer to page 347, under the heading 'Percussion Findings' and the subheading 'Shifting dullness'.)
26. *What is tidal percussion? What is its significance?* (**Ans.** Refer to page 347, under the heading 'Percussion Findings' and the subheading 'Tidal percussion'.)
27. *What are the types of breath sounds? How do you differentiate between them?* (**Ans.** Refer to page 348, under the heading 'Breath Sounds' and the subheading 'Table 53.1'.)

28. *What conditions lead to reduced breath sound intensity?* (Ans. Refer to page 348, under the heading 'Breath Sounds' and the subheading 'Reduced intensity'.)
29. *What are the features of bronchial breath sounds?* (Ans. Refer to page 348, under the heading 'Character' and the subheading 'Bronchial breath sounds'.)
30. *What are the types of bronchial breath sounds, and how are they produced?* (Ans. Refer to page 348, under the heading 'Bronchial Breath Sounds' and the subheading 'Types of...'.)
31. *What do you mean by vocal resonance?* (Ans. Refer to page 348, under the heading 'Vocal Resonance'.)
32. *Name the conditions in which vocal resonance is increased and those in which it is decreased.* (Ans. Refer to page 344, under the heading 'Vocal Resonance' and the subheading 'Increased and decreased vocal resonance'.)
33. *What is bronchophony, and in what conditions is it seen?* (Ans. Refer to page 349, under the heading 'Vocal Resonance' and the subheading 'Bronchophony'.)
34. *What is aegophony? In what conditions is it seen?* (Ans. Refer to page 349, under the heading 'Vocal Resonance' and the subheading 'Aegophony'.)
35. *What does whispering pectoriloquy indicate?* (Ans. Refer to page 349, under the heading 'Vocal Resonance' and the subheading 'Whispering pectoriloquy'.)
36. *What are adventitious breath sounds?* (Ans. Refer to page 349, under the heading 'Adventitious Sounds'.)
37. *What is the mechanism of production of ronchi? In what conditions is it seen?* (Ans. Refer to page 349, under the heading 'Adventitious Sounds' and the subheading 'Ronchi'.)
38. *What is a wheeze?* (Ans. Refer to page 349, under the heading 'Adventitious Sounds' and the subheading 'Wheeze'.)
39. *What are the types and causes of crepitations?* (Ans. Refer to page 350, under the heading 'Adventitious Sounds' and the subheading 'Crepitations'.)
40. *What is the mechanism of production of crepitations?* (Ans. Refer to page 350, under the heading 'Adventitious Sounds' and the subheading 'Crepitations'.)
41. *What do you mean by pleural rub, and in what conditions is it seen?* (Ans. Refer to page 350, see 'Adventitious Sounds' and the subheading 'Pleural rub'.)

54 | Clinical Examination of the Cardiovascular System

Learning Objectives

After completing this practical, you will be able to (MUST KNOW):

1. Appreciate the importance of the examination of the cardiovascular system (CVS) in clinical physiology.
2. List the parameters to be examined in the clinical examination of the CVS.
3. Define precordium and apex beat.
4. Draw the midclavicular line on the precordium.
5. Localise the apex of the subject.
6. Locate the different auscultatory areas on the precordium.
7. Auscultate the heart sounds.
8. Examine the neck veins.
9. List the common causes of impalpable apex beat.
10. Enumerate the types and causes of heart sounds.
11. Name the waves in JVP and their mechanism of production.

You may also be able to (DESIRABLE TO KNOW):

1. Draw different anatomical lines and borders of the heart.
2. Locate the position of the heart valves and auscultatory areas.
3. Elicit parasternal heave and appreciate the thrill, if present.
4. Percuss to define the border of the heart.
5. List the different conditions in which JVP is raised and prominent 'a', 'c', and 'v' waves are seen in the JVP tracing.
6. Explain the different conditions in which the apex is not palpable.
7. List the causes, character, and significance of heart sounds.
8. Elucidate the mechanism and causes of the split of first and second heart sounds.

> **PY5.15:** Demonstrate the correct clinical examination of the cardiovascular system in a normal volunteer or a simulated environment.

INTRODUCTION

The examination of the cardiovascular system (CVS) comprises the **examination of the precordium and blood vessels**. Careful *assessment of the arterial and venous pulses* should always precede examination of the precordium. Auscultation of the heart should be taken up only after the precordium has been thoroughly examined.

Anatomical Landmarks

The **precordium** is defined as the *anterior aspect of the chest wall, which overlies the heart*. Different borders of the heart and the positions of the valves are demarcated on the precordium to make the clinical examination of the cardiovascular system convenient.

Different lines

(Refer to Fig. 53.1, Chapter 53.)

Midclavicular line: This is defined as the **vertical line dropped from the centre of the clavicle**. The midpoint of the clavicle is determined by taking a point on the clavicle midway between the middle of the suprasternal notch and the tip of the acromion.

Anterior axillary line: This is defined as the vertical line descending from the anterior border of the axilla.

Midaxillary line: This is defined as the vertical line descending from the centre of the axilla.

Posterior axillary line: This is defined as the vertical line descending from the posterior border of the axilla.

Parasternal line : This is defined as the vertical line passing through the costochondral junction close to either side of the sternum.

Borders of the heart

Base of the heart: This is represented by a line joining the right third sternocostal articulation to a point at the level of the left second intercostal space, just internal to the parasternal line.

Right border of the heart: This extends from the right third sternocostal articulation above to the right seventh intercostal articulation below. It is slightly curved with convexity to the right.

Left border of the heart: This is traced by a line joining the point at the level of the left second intercostal space just internal to the parasternal line above and the apex beat below.

Position of the heart valves

Mitral valve: This is obliquely placed behind the inner end of the left fourth costal cartilage and the adjoining part of the sternum.

Tricuspid valve: This is situated obliquely behind the right fifth costal cartilage.

Pulmonary valve: This is placed horizontally at the upper border of the left third costal cartilage.

Aortic valve: This lies obliquely across the left half of the sternum at the level of the lower border of the left third costal cartilage.

Auscultatory areas

Mitral area: This area corresponds to the **apex beat of the heart**. The **first *heart sound is best heard*** over the mitral area. Normally, this is present in the left fifth intercostal space, half an inch medial to the midclavicular line (Fig. 54.1). However, in different pathological conditions, the position of the apex changes. Therefore, the auscultatory area of the mitral valve changes with the position of the apex.

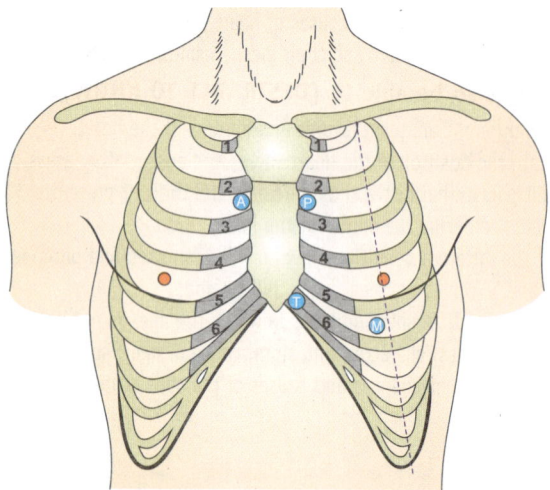

Fig. 54.1   Auscultatory areas on the precordium (**A:** aortic area; **P:** pulmonary area; **T:** tricuspid area; **M:** mitral area [apex of the heart]). The vertical dotted line drawn on the left side is the midclavicular line. Note that the second rib is attached to the manubrium sterni.

Pulmonary area: This area is half an inch in diameter with its centre in the left second intercostal space, close to the parasternal line.

Aortic area: This area is half an inch in diameter with its centre in the right second intercostal space, close to the parasternal line.

Aortic murmurs are often best heard in the left third intercostal space, close to the sternum. Therefore, this area is called the second aortic area or **Erb's point**.

Tricuspid area: This area is half an inch in diameter with its centre on the left side, close to the sternum, towards its lower end.

METHODS OF EXAMINING THE CARDIOVASCULAR SYSTEM

Principle

The process of examination of the cardiovascular system consists of **inspection, palpation, percussion, and auscultation** of the precordium, which follow the examination of arterial and venous pulses, recording of blood pressure, and a brief general examination of the subject. The functions or any alteration in functions of the CVS are detected by thorough examination of the precordium and blood vessels.

Requirements

1. **Stethoscope** (an octopus stethoscope should be available for students to learn)

   Octopus stethoscope: This is a specially designed stethoscope in which the **master stethoscope** (longer and bigger diameter tube, marked with a band at the centre) originates from the top of a central cabinet (Fig. 54.2). Another long tube that originates below the cabinet is attached to the chest piece (diaphragm) of the stethoscope, used for placing the diaphragm on the chest for auscultation. From the peripheral side of the central cabinet, six tubes originate and branch out to connect to their respective ear knobs (called **daughter stethoscopes,** which are slightly shorter in length and have tubes of smaller diameters). The instructor (teacher) who demonstrates heart sounds to the students (learners), uses the master stethoscope and learners use the daughter stethoscopes simultaneously. The octopus stethoscope makes it possible for six learners to simultaneously follow the demonstration and identify the types of heart sounds and their qualities, especially the murmurs.

2. **Cardiac bed** or a couch with provisions to lift the head end of the bed (Fig. 54.3).

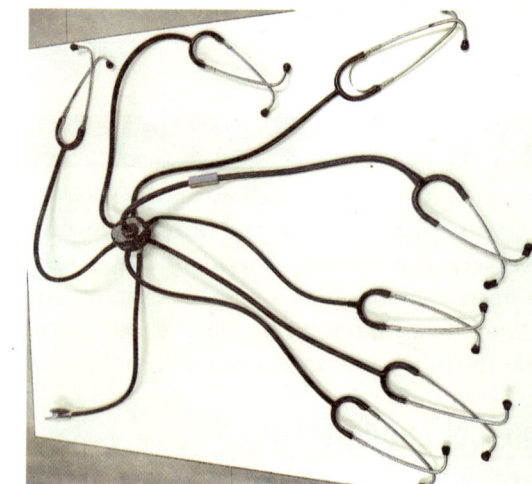

Fig. 54.2   Octopus stethoscope.

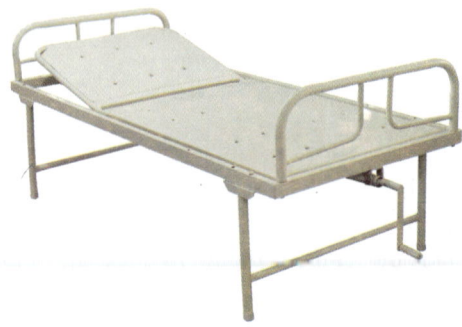

Fig. 54.3   Cardiac bed with provisions to raise the head end. This arrangement to lift the head helps in the examination of the jugular venous pulse (JVP) in the neck in the reclined position. With the patient's head at 45° to his body, the demonstration of JVP becomes easier.

Note: This type of bed is used for cardiac patients, which helps in the examination of the jugular venous pulse (JVP) in the neck. With the head of the patient at a 45° angle to his body, demonstration of JVP becomes easier.

Procedure

Examination of the CVS includes: (1) **general examination** (emphasising a few particular signs) including examination of the radial pulse and blood pressure, (2) **examination of the neck veins**, and (3) **examination of the precordium**.

General examination in relation to CVS
Anemia
Check for the degree of pallor. The degree of anemia gives a rough idea of the dynamics of circulation, heart rate, and blood pressure.

Cyanosis
Check for the presence of cyanosis. This may be present in conditions where there is **mixing of arterial blood with venous blood**, as seen in Fallot's tetralogy or patent truncus arteriosus.

Edema
Check for the presence of edema in the **dependent parts of the body**. In cardiac patients, the location of edema depends on the posture of the patient. It is detected by applying pressure over the distal end of the tibia if the patient is mobile. But, if the patient is confined to bed, the sacral area should be examined for the presence of edema.

Clubbing
Nail beds should be examined for the presence of clubbing. If cyanosis is present along with clubbing, this suggests right to left shunt. Clubbing may be present in congenital cyanotic heart disease and in subacute bacterial endocarditis.

Dyspnea
Breathlessness is a feature of heart failure. Dyspnea may be present even at rest.

Abdominal signs
1. **Hepatomegaly:** Tender hepatomegaly may be present in congestive cardiac failure.
2. **Splenomegaly:** The spleen may be enlarged in bacterial endocarditis.
3. **Ascites:** Ascites may be present in heart failure.
4. **Epigastric pulsation:** Epigastric pulsation may occur due to the following cardiovascular disorders:
   - Aortic pulsation—usually in thin and nervous patients
   - Aneurysm of the abdominal aorta
   - Hypertrophy of the heart (especially the right ventricle) may produce an epigastric systolic thrust

Pulse
Examine the radial pulse for **at least one minute**. The arterial pulses of both sides should be examined to check the bilateral symmetry, and the femoral arteries should be examined to detect radiofemoral delay, if present. Brachial, carotid, temporal, popliteal, posterior tibial, and dorsalis pedis arteries should also be examined (also see Chapter 27).

Blood pressure
Blood pressure (BP) should be detected by sphygmomanometry, preferably using an aneroid manometer. It should be recorded on both sides in cardiac patients. BP should also be recorded by both palpatory and auscultatory methods, especially if the patient is hypertensive (see Chapter 28).

Examination of the neck veins
Venous pulses are examined, especially in the neck region.

Examine the neck veins in daylight with the patient **reclining at an angle of about 45°**. If the patient is lying on a cardiac bed or couch (Fig. 54.3), the head end of the bed can be raised to 45° for this purpose. Otherwise, the subject's back can be supported by the examiner so that the neck muscles are relaxed and the subject reclines at an angle of 45°. Study the level of pressure in the internal jugular veins (**jugular venous pressure [JVP]**). The pressure is expressed in terms of centimetres of the vertical distance between the top of the column of blood and the sternal angle, which corresponds to the upper border of the clavicle with the subject reclining at 45° (Fig. 54.4A and B). It may be easier to recognise the pulsation in the external jugular veins, but pulsation in the *internal jugular vein is more reliable*, because it directly reflects the pressure changes in the right atrium.

External jugular veins are not reliable for the following reasons:
1. Venous valves, present in the external jugular veins, prevent the smooth conduction of venous pressure.
2. As the external jugular system passes through the fascial planes, they are likely to be affected by external compression.

Why the 45° angle of the neck?
The subject's neck is reclined to 45° because, normally, in this position, the *sternal angle comes to the level of the clavicle*. If the person is in good health, the sternal angle corresponds to the middle of the right atrium and approximately *represents the normal venous pressure*,

A)

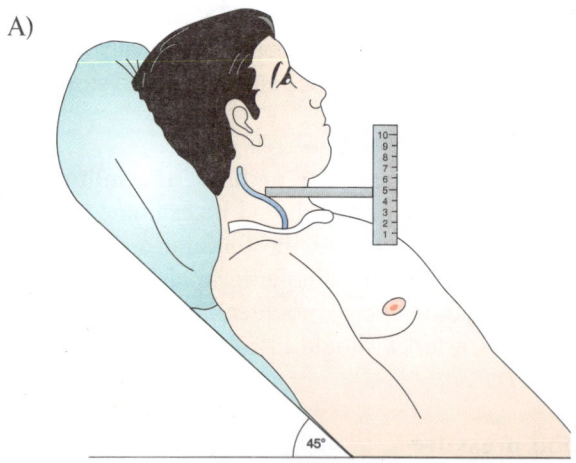

B)

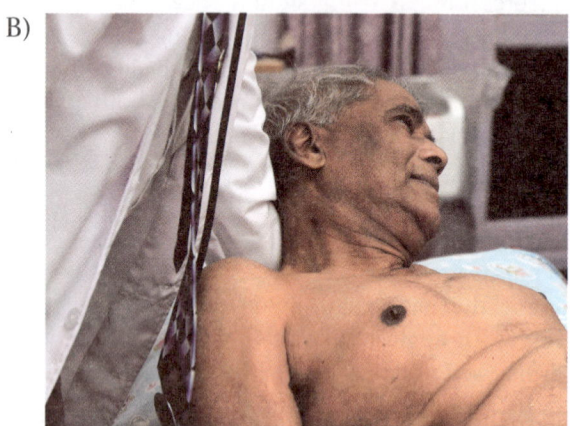

Fig. 54.4   (A) Method of clinical assessment of jugular vein pressure (JVP). It is measured as the vertical height of the JVP above the clavicle with the patient reclining at 45° and **(B)** examination of neck veins for JVP. With the support of the examiner, the subject is reclined at an angle of 45°.

whatever the position of the subject. When the subject is propped up at an angle of 45°, the venous pressure *appears just at the upper border of the clavicle*, because in this position, the sternal angle and clavicle remain at the same level horizontally. Therefore, venous pressure *above the clavicle in this position is considered as raised JVP*.

> **Note:** In the neck, the arterial pulsation may be confused with venous pulsation. The **venous pulses can be differentiated from the arterial pulses** by the following parameters.

1. The **venous pulse is better seen than felt,** whereas the arterial pulse is better felt than seen (Table 54.1).
2. The **venous pulse has a definite upper level,** which falls during inspiration when blood is drawn into the heart.
3. By exerting moderate pressure above the clavicle with a finger, the **venous pulse can be obliterated,** but not the arterial pulse.
4. If carefully observed, **two to three waves can be seen** in the venous pulse.

Examination of the precordium

The **precordium** is defined as the *anterior aspect of the chest wall, which overlies the heart*. The process of examination of the precordium consists of **inspection, palpation, percussion, and auscultation**. The subject should lie down on a couch, and the examination should be carried out in adequate daylight with the precordium fully exposed (Fig. 54.5).

▌Inspection
1. **Skeletal deformity:** Look for any precordial bulging or depression. The former is usually seen in *congenital heart diseases*.
2. **Dilated and engorged superficial veins:** Look for the presence of any dilated and engorged superficial veins over the precordium. This may be seen in *superior or inferior venacaval obstruction*.
3. **Pulsation:**
   Apical pulsation: Look for pulsation of the apex. Normally, the pulsation of the cardiac apex is visible. The presence of all other pulsations over the precordium is considered abnormal.

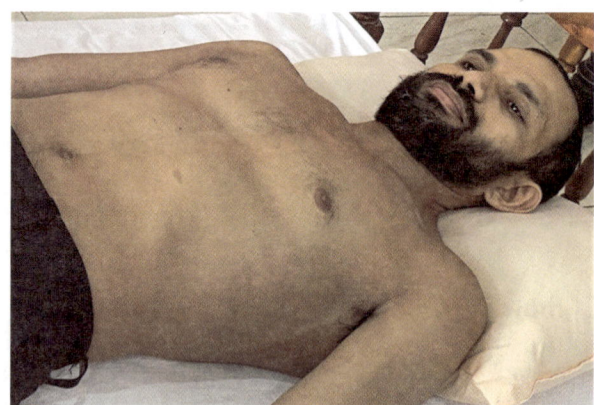

Fig. 54.5 Position of the subject for the examination of the precordium. The subject should lie down on a couch with the precordium fully exposed along with the neck area and the upper part of the abdomen (epigastrium).

Other pulsations: Look for pulsation in the other areas of the precordium, especially on the pulmonary and aortic areas and in the left parasternal area. Other pulsations are seen in the **following conditions:**
- Pulsation **on the pulmonary area** is seen in *pulmonary hypertension or pulmonary artery dilatation*.
- Pulsation **on the aortic area** may be seen in *aneurysm of the aorta*.
- Pulsation **on the left parasternal area** indicates *right ventricular hypertrophy*.
- Pulsation **over the suprasternal notch** indicates *aneurysm of the arch of the aorta or coarctation of the aorta*.

Palpation

1. **Apex beat:** The apex is defined as the *lowermost and outermost definite cardiac impulse*. Describe the **position and character** of the apex.

   Position: Locate the position of the apex of the heart. This is done by first placing the palm on the precordium to feel the apical impulse (Fig. 54.6A) and then by placing the ulnar border of the palm on the pulsation area horizontally (Fig. 54.6B). Finally, the apex is localised by the tip of the middle or index finger (Fig. 54.6C).

   - If the **apex is not palpable in the supine position**, ask the subject to *sit up, and try to locate the apex* in the sitting posture.
   - If the apex is **still not palpable**, ask the subject to *lean forward as much as he can in the sitting posture*, and try to locate the apex in the leaning position.
   - If the apex is **still not palpable**, palpate the corresponding area of the chest *on the right side* (in dextrocardia or dextroversion, the apex of the heart may shift to the right).

   Ideally, the apex **should not be palpated in the left lateral position** because it *shifts the apex laterally*, and there is *variation in shifting* as well.

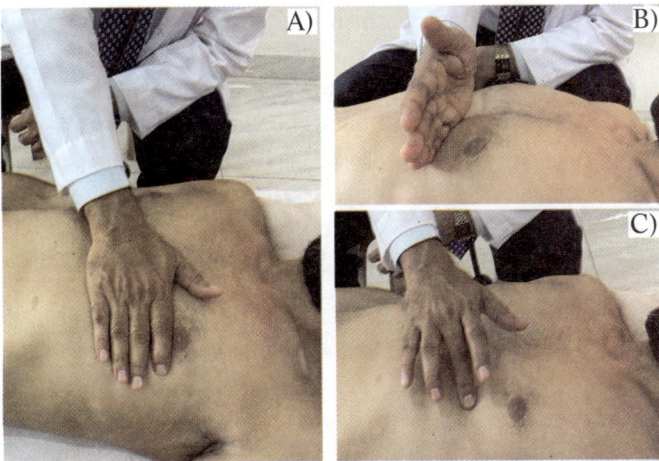

Fig. 54.6 Localisation of the apex of the heart. **(A)** The palm is gently placed on the precordium to feel the apical impulse; **(B)** the ulnar border of the palm is placed in the intercostal space to better appreciate the impulse; **(C)** finally, the apex is localised by the tip of the middle or index finger.

Note the position of the apex **in the intercostal space in relation to the midclavicular line**. The intercostal spaces are counted by palpating the manubrium sterni (the most elevated point on the sternum). The *second rib joins the manubrium sterni*. The space below the second rib is the *second intercostal space*, and accordingly, other intercostal spaces are counted.

Note:
1. The apex is defined as the **lowermost and outermost definite cardiac impulse**. Therefore, if other pulsations are present on the precordium, the apex can be easily identified.
2. The apex beat is normally located in the left fifth intercostal space, half an inch medial to the midclavicular line. *When students are asked to locate the apex, before they palpate and localise it, they start counting the intercostal spaces and put the tip of their finger medial to the midclavicular line in the fifth space to feel the apex.* **This is wrong** because the apex may not always be present exactly in that position. Moreover, you do not know if the subject has any pathology in the heart. Therefore, the apex **must first be localised** as described above, and **then its position should be identified and demarcated**.

Causes of impalpable apex:
- Left-sided pleural effusion
- Pneumothorax
- Hydropneumothorax
- Pericardial effusion
- Shift of the mediastinum to the right (right-sided lung fibrosis and collapse)
- Obesity (thick chest wall)
- Apex lying under a rib
- Dextrocardia (the apex will be palpable on the right side)

Character: Try to describe the character of the apex.

Note: Normally, the apex beat *just touches and slightly elevates* the examining finger. The **common abnormal characteristics** are:
1. **Tapping apex:** Seen in advanced mitral stenosis.
2. **Forceful and well-sustained apex:** Seen in gross left ventricular hypertrophy due to chronic systemic hypertension, which causes *pressure overload* and increases wall thickness.
3. **Forceful but ill-sustained apex:** Seen in right ventricular hypertrophy or mild to moderate left ventricular hypertrophy. In left ventricular hypertrophy, due to *volume overload* (as in aortic regurgitation), there is an increase in the ventricular cavity size rather than wall thickness. Therefore, the apex is forceful but ill-sustained.

2. **Parasternal heave:** Place the ulnar border of the palm firmly on the left parasternal line and feel for any thrust or pulsations and check whether the hand is lifted with each pulsation (Fig. 54.7).

Note: The presence of parasternal heave suggests *right ventricular hypertrophy*.

3. **Thrills:** Palpate all over the precordium for thrills.

Note: A thrill is a **palpable murmur**. Thrills are best appreciated when the patient holds his breath during an expiration. Thrills may be present in *valvular defects* or in cases of *aneurysm* of the great vessels.

4. **Tender points:** Palpate the precordium for the presence of any painful points over it.

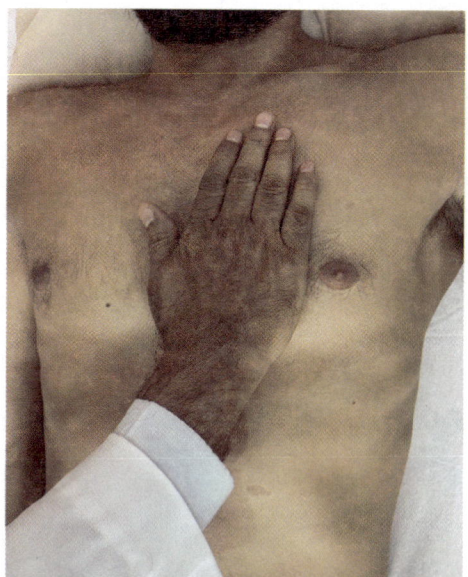

Fig. 54.7   Method of elicitation of parasternal heave. The palm is firmly placed on the left parasternal line to feel the thrust or pulsations, if any, and note whether the hand is lifted with each pulsation.

> **Note:** A tender point over the precordium may be due to *costochondritis, myalgia, fracture* of ribs, or pleuritis.

5. **Direction of flow in veins:** If the veins are dilated and engorged over the precordium, detect the direction of flow in the veins.
   - **In superior venacaval obstruction**, the direction of blood flow in the veins is from above downwards.
   - **In inferior venacaval obstruction**, the direction of blood flow in the veins is from below upwards.

> **Note:** The position of the trachea should be checked along with the position of the apex to assess the **position of the mediastinum.**

█ Percussion

Percussion is carried out to define cardiac borders in order to detect the **extent of cardiac dullness** in conditions like pericardial effusion. Cardiac dullness is detected by performing a *light percussion*. The details of the rules of percussion are discussed under the examination of the respiratory system.

█ Auscultation

With the help of the stethoscope, *auscultate the different areas* in the following sequence: **mitral area, pulmonary area, aortic area, and tricuspid area.** The diaphragm of the stethoscope should be placed firmly on different areas to hear the heart sounds (Fig. 54.8).

In each area, the following points should be noted during auscultation:

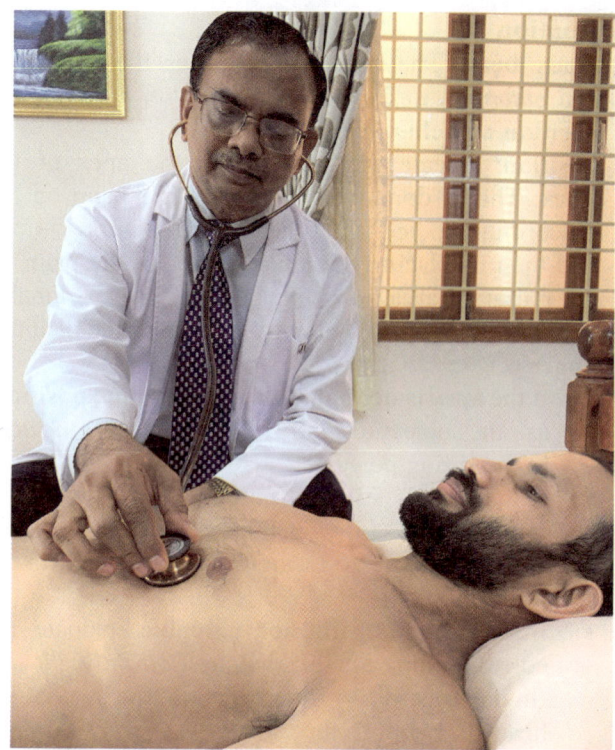

Fig. 54.8   The method of auscultation for heart sounds. Note that the diaphragm of the stethoscope is placed firmly on the apex (mitral area).

1. **First (S1) and second (S2) heart sounds:** Note their **quality, intensity, duration, and character**. S1 is heard better on the mitral area, and S2 is heard better over the pulmonary and aortic areas.

> **Note:** The first and second heart sounds can be differentiated by their **pitch and duration**. The first heart sound is heard as '**lub**' and the second sound as '**dub**'. For beginners, it is difficult to differentiate these sounds. They can *palpate the carotid artery* in the neck while auscultating the heart sounds. The heart sound that coincides with the carotid pulsation is the first heart sound and the sound that follows the pulsation is the second heart sound.

2. **Other sounds (if present):**
   - Third heart sound (S3)
   - Fourth heart sound (S4)
   - Murmurs
   - Opening snap
   - Ejection click

   If a murmur is present, note the site of origin, timing, character, radiation, and its relation with respiration.

Observation and Results

1. Note your observations in a tabular format as given on the next page.

Parameters	Observations / Findings
Patient's name, age, gender, height, body weight	
General examination	
i. Pallor ii. Cyanosis iii. Clubbing iv. Dyspnea v. Abdominal signs vi. Pulse vii. Blood pressure	
Examination of neck veins	
Examination of precordium	
Inspection i. Skeletal deformity ii. Dilated and engorged superficial veins iii. Pulsations (apical and others)	
Palpation i. Apex beat ii. Parasternal heave iii. Thrills iv. Tender points v. Direction of flow in the veins	
Percussion Lightly percuss to note the cardiac borders	
Auscultation i. S1 and S2 ii. Other sounds	

2. Analyse the results and report your findings with your comments on cardiovascular functions.

DISCUSSION

Clinical Significance

Arterial pulse

Comment on the **rate, rhythm, character, and volume** of pulse, especially if there is tachycardia or bradycardia, **irregularity in rhythm**, and if pulse is of **any specific abnormal type**. A detailed discussion on arterial pulse is given in Chapter 27.

Venous pulse

The pulsation of **internal jugular veins** in the neck is examined clinically to determine the atrial pressure activity

(Table 54.1). Jugular venous pulse (JVP) has **five waves**: three positive waves (ascents) and two negative waves (descents). The positive waves are the 'a', 'c', and 'v' waves and the negative waves are the 'x' and 'y' descents (Fig. 54.9).

a wave: Due to *atrial contraction*.

c wave: Coincides with the onset of ventricular systole and results from the *movement (bulging) of the tricuspid valve ring* into the right atrium as the right ventricular pressure rises.

v wave: *Indicates the passive rise in pressure* in the right atrium as *venous return continues* while the tricuspid valve is closed.

X descent: Caused by a fall in right atrial pressure due to relaxation of the right atrium.

Y descent: Occurs due to fall in the right atrial pressure when blood enters the right ventricle as the tricuspid valve opens.

Conditions that alter JVP
Raised JVP
1. Right ventricular failure
2. Obstruction of the superior vena cava
3. Increase in circulating blood volume
   - Pregnancy
   - Acute nephritis
   - Over-judicious treatment with IV fluids
4. Constrictive pericarditis
5. Tricuspid incompetence

Note: Persistent elevation of JVP is one of the **earliest signs of congestive cardiac failure** and is considered a **reliable sign** of the failure.

Prominent 'a' wave
1. Pulmonary stenosis
2. Pulmonary hypertension
3. Tricuspid stenosis (usually, in this condition, there is atrial fibrillation, so, the 'a' wave may not be seen)
4. Myxoma of the right atrium
5. Distended right atrium in atrial septal defects
6. Cardiomyopathy

Physiological basis: A prominent 'a' wave occurs due to increased force of right atrial contraction associated with right atrial hypertrophy or hypertrophy of the right ventricle. When the right atrium contracts against increased resistance, the 'a' wave becomes prominent.

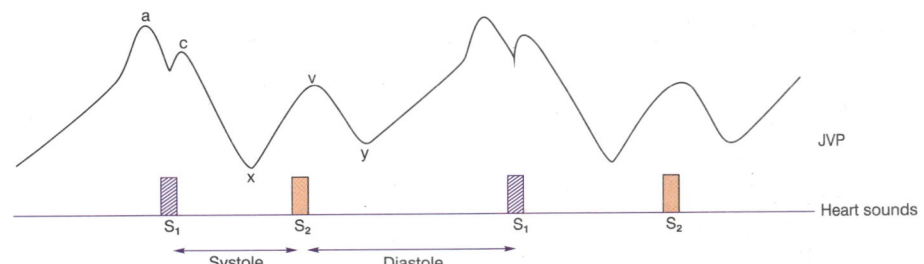

Fig. 54.9   JVP and heart sounds (JVP: jugular venous pressure; S1: first heart sound; S2: second heart sound).

Table 54.1   Differences between jugular venous pulse and carotid arterial pulse.

	Jugular venous pulse	Carotid arterial pulse
Feeling on touching the vessel	Not palpable	Palpable
Height of pulsation in relation to respiration	Varies with respiration	Independent of respiration
Propensity to be occluded	Can be easily occluded	Cannot be occluded, unless substantial pressure is exerted to occlude it
Height of pulsation in relation to abdominal pressure	Height increases with abdominal pressure	Pulse is independent of abdominal pressure
Prominence of pulse in relation to position of the patient	Best observed with the neck at 45° angle in relation to body. Prominence of pulsation varies with the position of the patient	Independent of the position of the patient
Direction of flow/pulsatility	Rapid inward movement	Rapid outward movement
Peaks in the pulse	Two visible peaks per heartbeat	One peak per heartbeat (felt but not visible)

Cannon wave (Fig. 54.10): When the amplitude of the 'a' wave is very high, it is called a cannon wave (**giant 'a' wave**). It is seen when the *right atrium contracts against a closed tricuspid valve*. It occurs in the following conditions:
1. Complete heart block when atrial and ventricular systole coincide.
2. Nodal rhythm when the atrium and ventricle are activated simultaneously.

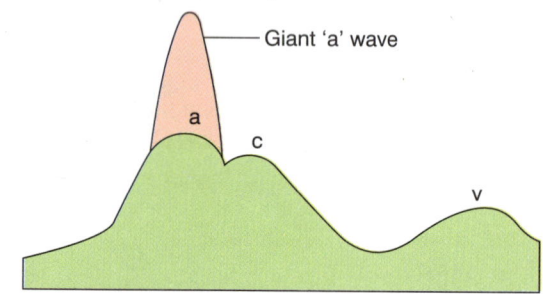

Fig. 54.10   Canon wave: Note the giant 'a' wave in JVP.

Absence of 'a' wave: The 'a' wave disappears in *atrial fibrillation*.

Prominent 'v' wave: It is seen in *tricuspid regurgitation* because when the ventricle contracts during systole, blood enters the right atrium through the incompetent tricuspid valve. It is also seen in *constrictive pericarditis* and *heart failure*.

Precordial Examination

The **two most important parameters** in precordial examination are: (1) the character and position of the apex of the heart and (2) heart sounds.

Apex of the heart

The position of the apex beat is a valuable physical sign in the examination of the CVS. The apex of the heart is **formed by the left ventricle**. Therefore, in *left ventricular hypertrophy*, the apex becomes ***more forceful***.

Displacement of the apex occurs due to ***push or pull*** from the surrounding viscera.
1. **Pushing** may be due to pleural effusion and pneumothorax, and **pulling** may be due to pulmonary fibrosis and collapse.
2. Apical displacement also occurs due to ***cardiac diseases***, such as enlargement of the left ventricle.
3. It can also occur due to ***deformities of the thoracic cage***, such as scoliosis.

Heart sounds

Four heart sounds have been described: first heart sound (S1), second heart sound (S2), third heart sound (S3), and fourth heart sound (S4). **S1 and S2 are heard normally**.

■ First heart sound

The first heart sound represents the beginning of the systole.
Causes: It occurs due to vibration set up by:
1. Sudden **closure of the AV valves**.
2. Rapid *increase in tension in the ventricular muscles* during isometric contraction acting on full ventricles.
3. *Turbulence created* in the blood due to ventricular contraction.

Character: Soft sound heard as 'lub'.
Duration: About 0.15 seconds
Frequency: 25–45 Hz
Significance: It signifies the *beginning of the ventricular systole* and AV valve closure.

1. **Accentuation of first heart sound**
   - Exercise
   - Hyperkinetic circulatory states like anemia and beri beri
   - Hypertension
2. **Diminution of first heart sound**
   - Shock
   - Acute myocardial infarction

- Constrictive pericarditis
- Pericardial effusion
- Cardiomyopathy (advanced stage)
- Obesity
- Emphysema

Splitting: The first heart sound has **two components**: *the mitral and the tricuspid components*. The mitral valve closes just before the tricuspid valve. This gives rise to splitting of the first heart sound. However, this splitting cannot normally be *detected by auscultation* because both the components are **very low-pitched and merge into each other**. Therefore, when splitting of S1 is heard, it is **considered pathological**.

Second heart sound

Causes:

1. Primarily caused by the **closure of the semilunar valves**.
2. The *rushing of blood into the ventricles* due to the opening of the AV valves also contributes.

Character: This is heard as 'dub'.

Duration: About 0.12 seconds

Frequency: 50 Hz

Significance: It signifies the end of clinical systole and closure of the semilunar valves.

1. **Loud A2** (increased aortic component)
   - Systemic hypertension
2. **Diminished A2**
   - Aortic stenosis
   - Aortic incompetence
3. **Loud P2** (increased pulmonary component)
   - Pulmonary hypertension
4. **Diminished P2**
   - Pulmonary stenosis

Splitting: Splitting of the second sound occurs due to the *gap between the aortic and pulmonary components*. It is easy to detect because aortic and pulmonary valve closure sounds are **high-pitched and can be separated**. Aortic valve closure is audible in all areas, whereas pulmonary valve closure is audible only in the pulmonary area. Splitting is most *easily heard in children* and may not be audible in elderly subjects.

Mechanism of splitting: The splitting of the second heart sound is due to the separation between the closure of aortic and pulmonary valves. The closure of the pulmonary valve always follows the closure of the aortic valve (*aortic valve closes first*). The splitting is *distinctly heard during inspiration*.

1. During inspiration, more blood is drawn into the thorax. Therefore, venous return to the right atrium increases, and *right ventricular stroke volume increases*. This increases the **duration of right ventricular systole**. Thus, P2 is slightly delayed.
2. Also, during inspiration, *left ventricular stroke volume decreases* because blood is pooled in the dilated pulmonary vessels and dilated left atrium (this dilatation occurs due to increased negative intrathoracic pressure). Therefore, **left ventricular systole is shortened** and A2 comes earlier. Therefore, during inspiration, A2 occurs earlier and P2 occurs later.

Hence, splitting of the second sound widens during inspiration. Exactly the opposite happens during expiration and splitting narrows.

Reverse splitting: This occurs when the **left ventricle takes more time to empty** than the right ventricle. It is seen in *left bundle branch block* (LBBB) and left ventricular failure.

Third heart sound

The third heart sound is *usually not heard* in many healthy individuals. Sometimes, it may be heard in children and young adults. It is usually heard in conditions in which the *circulation becomes hyperkinetic*. The third sound can arise *from either side of the heart*, but usually, it arises in the left ventricle.

Causes:

1. It is caused by the vibration set up in the ventricle during the early period of rapid ventricular filling.
2. Rebound fencing of the cusp of the valve and chordae of the respective valve due to vigorous elongation of the ventricle caused by rapid inflow of blood also contributes to this.

Character: It is best heard in the mitral area. It follows the aortic component of the second sound and is heard early in the diastole, that is, just after the second sound.

Duration: 0.1 second

Pitch: Low-pitched

Significance:

1. This is attributed to **rapid ventricular filling**. It is found in relatively hyperkinetic circulation, in young persons, and where the mitral diastolic flow is increased as in mitral regurgitation and VSD.
2. It is an important **sign of heart failure** due to any cause. In heart failure, the atrial pressure is increased, and early filling of the ventricle is rapid.
3. It may be heard shortly after *myocardial infarction* or in diseases where the *distensibility of the ventricular muscle is altered*. The sound arises from vibrations in the atrioventricular valve structures and in the ventricular muscle.

Fourth heart sound

This is also called the atrial sound because it is produced during atrial contraction. It is not heard in normal individuals. The presence of the fourth heart sound is always considered abnormal.

Causes:

1. It is caused by atrial contraction.
2. It is produced by the vibration set up within the ventricle due to inflow of blood produced by atrial systole.

Character: It occurs just before the first sound, that is, *late in the diastole*, and is *low-pitched*.

Significance:

1. It always indicates *increased stiffness* or non-compliance of the ventricles. Therefore, when a bolus of blood is delivered into the ventricle by atrial contraction, it facilitates a *sudden increase of pressure* in the ventricle.
2. It is seen in left ventricular hypertrophy due to *hypertension, myocardial infarction, pulmonary embolism, and pulmonary hypertension.*

Triple heart sound

This consists of three heart sounds: the first and second heart sounds, and either the third or fourth heart sound. The *triple rhythm* associated with a normal heart may not be a serious one, but if it is present with a *definite cardiac pathology*, it may signify a *serious condition*.

Gallop rhythm: When the heart rate increases to *more than 100 per minute*, the triple rhythm is called gallop rhythm because it produces a typical cadence of the gallop of a horse. The individual sounds cannot be identified separately. If the *gallop is due to the third heart sound*, it is called a **proto-diastolic gallop**; if it is *due to the fourth heart sound*, it is called **pre-systolic gallop**.

Murmurs

Murmurs occur due to **turbulence in the blood flow** at or near a valve or abnormal communication within the heart. Murmurs differ from normal heart sounds in the sense that they have a *longer duration and higher frequency*, whereas heart sounds have a shorter duration and lower frequency. When a murmur is present, the following points are carefully noted:

1. **Site of origin:** The area over which the murmur is maximally heard should be noted. The *point of maximal intensity* usually (but not always) indicates its site of origin.
2. **Timing and duration:** Depending on the timing of the murmur, they are classified into *systolic, diastolic, or*

continuous murmurs. Depending on the duration, it may be *early diastolic, mid-diastolic, early systolic, pan-systolic*, and so on.

3. **Character:** The murmur may be soft, blowing to harsh, rough, and rumbling. *Loud and rough murmurs* are usually associated with organic valvular and congenital lesions, for example, *murmur of mitral stenosis* is always rough and rumbling in character.
4. **Radiation (conduction):** From the site of maximum intensity, auscultation is performed in different directions to detect whether the murmur is localised or conducted to other parts. Conduction is characteristic of some murmurs, for example, the *murmur of mitral stenosis is usually localised*, whereas the *murmur of mitral incompetence* selectively **propagates towards the axilla**.
5. **Relation with respiration:** During inspiration, the stroke volume of the right ventricle increases, while that of the left decreases. Therefore, any murmur becoming *louder during inspiration* is considered to **originate from the right ventricle**, and any murmur *louder during expiration* is said to **originate from the left side** of the heart.

OSPE

I.   Locate the apex beat of the subject and report your findings.

Steps

1. Expose the precordium.
2. Inspect for the apex beat.
3. Place the palm on the precordium over the mitral area to feel apical pulsation.
4. Use the ulnar border of the hand to further confirm the pulsation.
5. Use the tip of the middle finger to finally locate the apex and mark its position.
6. Count the intercostal spaces and report the exact position of the apex.

II.   Examine the neck veins of the subject and report your findings.

Steps

1. Ask the subject to lie down on a couch and stand on the right side of the subject.
2. Elevate the head end of the bed or support the subject's back to recline him at an angle of 45°.
3. Turn the subject's head to the opposite side.
4. Ask the subject to relax his neck.
5. Look for the engorgement of the internal jugular vein.

6. If the JVP is raised, look for the upper level of the engorgement and measure the height of the pressure.

III. Auscultate the apex of the subject and report your findings

Steps
1. Expose the precordium.
2. Localise the apex of the subject.

3. Lightly place the diaphragm of the stethoscope on the apex to auscultate it.
4. Place your fingers gently on the carotid artery to differentiate the first from the second sound.
5. Check for the intensity and character of the sounds and report your findings.

VIVA

1. What are the general physical signs that are specifically looked for before commencing the clinical examination of the cardiovascular system? (Ans. Refer to page 355, under the heading 'General Examination...'.)
2. What is the importance of detecting cyanosis in the examination of the CVS? (Ans. Refer to page 355, under the heading 'General Examination...', read 'Cyanosis'.)
3. What are the characteristics of edema seen in cardiac patients? (Ans. Refer to page 355, under the heading 'General Examination...' read 'Edema'.)
4. Why should the radial pulse be examined before the examination of the precordium? (Ans. Refer to page 355, under the heading 'General Examination...' read 'Pulse'.)
5. What is the importance of recording blood pressure in the examination of a patient of CVS? (Ans. Refer to page 355, under the heading 'Blood Pressure'.)
6. Why are the neck veins usually preferred for the examination of the venous pulse, and how is it done clinically? (Ans. Refer to page 355, under the heading 'Examination of the Neck Veins', Fig. 54.4.)
7. How do you differentiate venous pulses from arterial pulses in the neck? (Ans. Refer to page 355 under the heading 'Examination of the Neck Veins', Fig. 54.4 and page 360 Table 54.1.)
8. Why are the internal jugular veins preferred to the external jugulars for examination of the neck veins? (Ans. Refer to page 355, under the heading 'Examination of the Neck Veins'.)
9. What are the waves seen in JVP, and how are they produced? (Ans. Refer to page 359, under the heading 'Discussion' and the subheading 'Venous pulse'.)
10. In what conditions does an 'a' wave become more prominent? (Ans. Refer to page 359, under the heading 'Conditions that alter JVP' and the subheading 'Prominent 'a' wave'.)
11. What is a cannon wave, and how is it produced? (Ans. Refer to page 360, under the heading 'Conditions that alter JVP' and the subheading 'Cannon wave'.)
12. In which pathological conditions can 'a' wave be absent and 'v' wave become prominent? (Ans. Refer to page 359, under the heading 'Conditions that alter JVP' and the subheadings 'Absence of 'a' wave' and 'Prominent 'v' wave'.)
13. What is the significance of raised JVP, and in which clinical conditions is it seen? (Ans. Refer to page 359, under the heading 'Conditions that alter JVP' and the subheading 'Raised JVP'.)
14. List the differences between JVP and the carotid arterial pulse. (Ans. Refer to page 360, see Table 54.1.)
15. Define precordium and explain how the precordium is examined. (Ans. Refer to page 356, under the heading 'Examination of Precordium', Fig. 54.5.)
16. What should one look for during the inspection of the precordium? (Ans. Refer to page 356, under the heading 'Examination of Precordium' and the subheading 'Inspection'.)
17. In what clinical conditions can precordial bulging occur? (Ans. Refer to page 356, under the heading 'Examination of Precordium' and the subheading 'Inspection' point no. 1.)
18. Define apex beat. (Ans. Refer to page 352, under the heading 'Palpation' and the subheading 'Apex beat'.)
19. What are the procedures to localise the apex if it is not palpable in the supine position? (Ans. Refer to page 357, under the heading 'Palpation' and the subheading 'Apex beat'.)
20. Why should the apex beat not be localised in the left lateral position? (Ans. Refer to page 357, under the heading 'Palpation' and the subheading 'Apex beat'.)
21. Name the different conditions in which the apex beat may not be palpable. (Ans. Refer to page 357, under the heading 'Causes of impalpable apex'.)
22. Name the conditions in which the apex may become forceful and well-sustained and explain the reason for this. (Ans. Refer to page 357, under the heading 'Apex beat' and the subheading 'Character'.)

23. *What do you mean by 'tapping apex', and in which condition is it seen?* (Ans. Refer to page 357, the note under the heading 'Apex beat' and the subheading 'Character'.)

24. *What is the importance of examining the position of the trachea along with the location of the apex?* (Ans. To assess the shifting of the mediastinum. If both apex and trachea are shifted to one side, the mediastinum also shifts to that side.)

25. *What is parasternal heave? In what conditions is this seen?* (Ans. Refer to page 357, under the heading 'Parasternal heave'.)

26. *What are the heart sounds? What heart sounds are normally heard?* (Ans. Refer to page 360, under the heading 'Heart Sounds'.)

27. *What are the causes of the first heart sound, and how is it confirmed clinically?* (Ans. Refer to page 360, under the heading 'Heart Sounds' and the subheading 'First heart sound'.)

28. *What are the conditions in which the first sound becomes louder?* (Ans. Refer to page 360, under the heading 'Heart Sounds' and the subheading 'First heart sound'.)

29. *What do you mean by splitting of the second sound?* Why is splitting better appreciated during inspiration? (Ans. Refer to page 361, under the heading 'Second heart sound' and the subheading 'Splitting'.)

30. *What is reverse split? In which clinical conditions is it seen?* (Ans. Refer to page 361, under the heading 'Second Heart Sound' and the subheading 'Reverse splitting'.)

31. *What is the gallop rhythm? What is its significance?* (Ans. Refer to page 362, under the heading 'Triple heart sound' and the subheading 'Gallop rhythm'.)

32. *How are murmurs produced? What are the types of murmurs?* (Ans. Refer to page 362, under the heading 'Murmurs'.)

55 | Clinical Examination of the Gastrointestinal System

Learning Objectives

After completing this practical, you will be able to (MUST KNOW):
1. Name the different quadrants of the abdomen.
2. Explain the importance of the clinical examination of the GI system.
3. Enumerate the steps of examining the GI system.
4. Demonstrate the procedures for palpation of the liver and spleen.
5. Percuss the abdomen.
6. Auscultate bowel sounds.

You may also be able to (DESIRABLE TO KNOW):
1. Explain various positive inspectory findings.
2. List the causes of hepatomegaly and splenomegaly.
3. Explain the importance of fluid thrill and shifting dullness.
4. Correlate abnormal bowel sounds with intestinal dysfunctions.

PY5.15: Demonstrate the correct clinical examination of the abdomen in a normal volunteer or simulated environment.

INTRODUCTION

Disorders of the gastrointestinal (GI) system are very common in the general population. Dyspepsia, diarrhea, dysentery, indigestion, and vomiting are routinely encountered complaints in clinical practice. Many of the causes of these dysfunctions can be easily diagnosed if the physician carries out a thorough and systematic examination of the GI system. **Examination of the abdomen** is a major part of the clinical examination of the GI system. While performing the abdominal examination, the physician should remember the **anatomical positions of the abdominal viscera**. Disorders of abdominal structures can be appropriately diagnosed because the *location of these organs is precise*. Therefore, an abnormal sign elicited from a particular region of the abdomen indicates the dysfunction *of the viscera underneath*.

Anatomical Landmarks

The abdomen is divided into **nine quadrants** by *two transverse and two vertical lines* (Fig. 55.1). The quadrants are epigastrium, right hypochondrium, left hypochondrium, umbilical, right lumbar, left lumbar, hypogastrium (suprapubic), right ileac, and left ileac.

METHODS OF EXAMINING THE GI SYSTEM

The examination of the GI system proceeds in the **following sequence.**

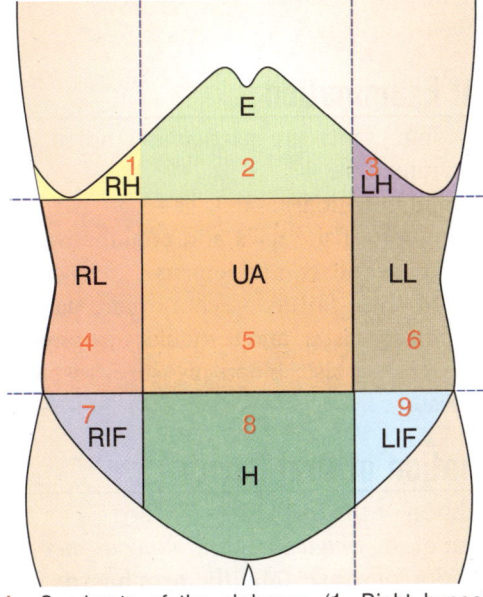

Fig. 55.1 Quadrants of the abdomen (1. Right hypochondrium (RH); 2. Epigastrium (E); 3. Left hypochondrium (LH); 4. Right lumbar (RL); 5. Umbilical (UA); 6. Left lumbar (LL); 7. Right ileac (RIF); 8. Hypogastrium (or suprapubic) (H); 9. Left ileac (LIF)).

1. History-taking
2. General examination
3. Examination of the oral cavity
4. Abdominal examination
5. Special examinations

History-Taking

In a patient with a GI disorder, the following questions should be asked (and noted in the examination record). Accurate and relevant **present and past histories** give the physician important clues to the diagnosis.
1. Does the patient have a good **appetite**, or does he have anorexia, nausea, or vomiting?

2. Is he able to swallow properly or does he have **dysphagia?**
3. Is there abnormal **flatulence?**
4. Are there frequent *acid eructations, retrosternal burning,* or water brash?
5. Are the **stools** normal, or has there been diarrhea or constipation? What is the appearance of the stool (colour, excess mucus, presence of worms)?
6. Are there any **abdominal abnormalities**—abdominal pain, swelling, or distension?
7. Is there a history of **hematemesis** (vomiting out of blood), **melena** (dark, tarry stool due to the presence of altered blood in it), or **bleeding per rectum?**
8. Is there a history of **jaundice, fever, or recent weight loss?**
9. What are the patient's habits with respect to *alcoholism* and smoking?
10. Is there a past history of tuberculosis, malaria, kala azar, hemolytic crisis (sudden onset of pallor and dyspnea), or drugs?

General Examination

The following points are particularly noted during the general examination.
1. Build and nutrition
2. Examination of the nails and conjunctiva for **pallor, clubbing, cyanosis, and icterus**
3. **Signs of liver failure**—scanty hair, palmar, spider nevi, gynecomastia, and testicular atrophy
4. **Vital signs**—pulse, blood pressure, respiration, and temperature

Examination of Oral Cavity

1. Condition of the **teeth**
2. Health of the *tongue and oral mucous membrane*
3. Condition of **tonsils and the oropharynx**

Examination of the Abdomen

Abdominal examination consists of the **following steps:**
1. Inspection
2. Palpation
3. Percussion
4. Auscultation

Inspection of the abdomen

Ask the patient to lie down comfortably on a couch **in the supine position with his arms by his side**. The room should be well lit. Stand on the right side of the patient. *Fully expose the abdomen*—the patient's clothing should be drawn up to the xiphisternum and pulled below *to the lower margin of the pubic symphysis* (sites of hernial orifice should be visible). Closely observe the abdomen for the following findings (Fig. 55.2).

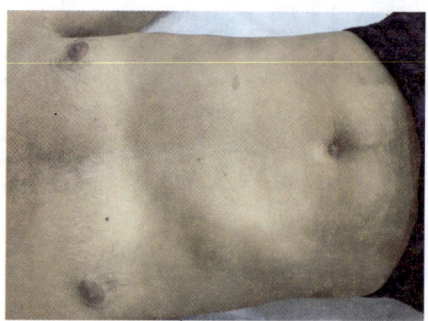

Fig. 55.2   Inspection of abdomen. Abdomen is exposed fully up to the lower level of the hypogastrium.

1. **Shape of the abdomen:** Is the abdomen normal in shape, distended, or scaphoid?
2. **Umbilicus:** Note the position of the umbilicus. Is it *central and inverted or everted*?
3. **Abdominal movements:** Observe the abdominal movements during inspiration and expiration. Are the movements free and equal on both sides, markedly diminished, or absent?
4. **Pulsations:** Is the pulsation of the abdominal aorta visible? Is there any other pulsation?
5. **Dilated veins:** Is there any dilatation of the abdominal vein?
6. **Peristalsis:** Is *gastric or intestinal peristalsis visible*? Peristalsis is best elicited by patiently observing the abdomen for some time.
7. **Hernial orifices:** Are the hernial orifices bulging *with strain or coughing*? Observe the hernial sites in the groin for the presence of swelling. If there is no swelling, ask the patient to stand up, turn his head to one side and cough. The impulse on coughing should be noted, if present.
8. **Scars:** Is there any surgical scar on the abdomen? Is the scar recent (pink or red) or old (pigmented and dark)?
9. **Surface and skin of abdomen:** Is the surface smooth? Is the skin shiny? Note any abnormal pigmentation and striae, if present.

Palpation of the abdomen

Palpation of the abdomen is an important part of the clinical examination of the GI system. Ask the subject to lie on his back with his **legs semi-flexed to relax the abdomen**. Ask him to relax and breathe quietly. Palpation should be performed for **all areas** of the abdomen. Generally, it can *start from the left ileac region* and then proceed *anticlockwise* to end in the suprapubic and umbilical regions. If the subject complains of pain in an area, that area should be palpated last.
1. Palpate lightly first and then perform **deeper palpation** (with both hands, if necessary).
2. While palpating, note the **consistency** (softness or rigidity), **tenderness** (can be observed from the

facial changes), and **guarding** of the abdomen in any particular region, if present.

3. Then palpate for the **liver**, **spleen**, **right** and **left kidneys**, gall bladder, urinary bladder, aorta and para-aortic glands.

4. **If a mass is present**, note its *location, size, surface, borders, consistency, and tenderness*.

5. **If fluid is present**, try to confirm the presence of fluid by eliciting *fluid thrill and shifting dullness*.

Palpation of the liver

Ask the subject to lie down comfortably on the couch and *flex his leg slightly*. Give proper instructions to the subject. Expose the abdomen (as described above). *Sit on the couch beside the right side of the subject.*

1. Place *both hands side-by-side and flat* on the abdomen in the **right subcostal region**, lateral to the rectus muscle, with the *fingers pointing to the ribs*.

2. Ask the subject to take a deep breath and at the height of inspiration, *press the fingers firmly inwards and upwards*.

3. If resistance is encountered, move the hand further down till the resistance disappears.

4. **If the liver is palpable**, its margin is felt as a sharp regular border that rides beneath the fingers. Note the *size* of the enlargement and the *surface, consistency, and tenderness* of the liver.

Alternate method of palpating the liver (commonly used)

1. Sit on a chair to the right side of the subject.

2. Place the *right hand below and parallel to the right subcostal margin* in such a way that the index finger remains just below it (Fig. 55.3).

3. Ask the subject to breathe deeply and at the height of inspiration, *press the index finger slightly inwards. The edge of the liver is felt against the radial border* of the index finger.

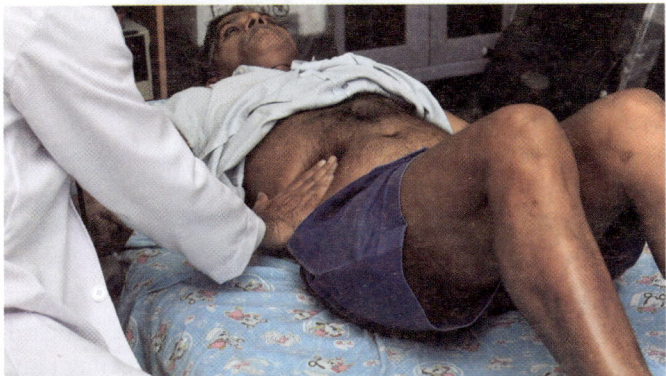

Fig. 55.3   Palpation of the liver. Note that the index finger of the right hand is pressed inwards below the right subcostal margin when the subject takes a deep breath. The legs are semi-flexed to relax the abdomen.

4. If resistance is encountered, move the hand further down till the resistance disappears.

> **Note:** The *lower limb should be semi-flexed at the knee to* relax the abdomen, which facilitates the palpation of the abdominal organs.

Palpation of the spleen

From the left subcostal margin, the *spleen enlarges downwards towards the right ileac fossa* (Fig. 55.4). Therefore, the spleen is palpated along an oblique line, starting from the right ileac fossa towards the left subcostal margin.

1. Place the *palm of the right hand on the right ileac fossa* below and to the right of the umbilicus, with the fingers close to each other and pointing towards the left subcostal margin (Fig. 55.5). Ask the subject to take a deep breath and press deep with the fingers of the right hand. **If the spleen is palpable**, it touches the tip of the fingers with each inspiration. Palpate the *surface of the spleen* and examine for *consistency and tenderness*.

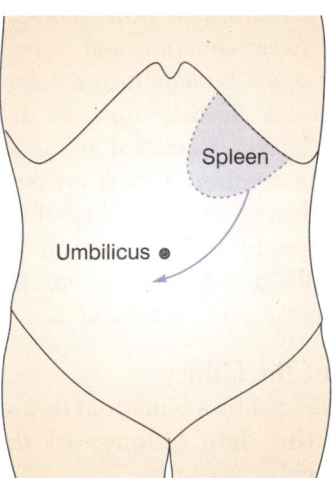

Fig. 55.4   The direction of spleen enlargement. The dotted line below the left subcostal margin depicts the surface marking of an enlarged spleen. The arrow indicates the direction of splenomegaly (towards the right ileac fossa).

2. **If the spleen is not palpable**, repeat the procedure of palpation 2 cm above, in the line of spleen enlargement, and *repeat the procedure till you reach the left subcostal margin* (Fig. 55.5).

3. **If the spleen is still not palpable**, place the flat area of the right hand beneath the left costal margin and the left hand over the lowermost rib posterolaterally on the left side of the subject. Ask the patient to take a deep breath and *press deep with the fingers of the right hand*. At the same time, exert considerable pressure medially and downward with the left hand.

4. If the spleen is **not palpable but suspected to be enlarged**, turn the patient *halfway onto his right side*

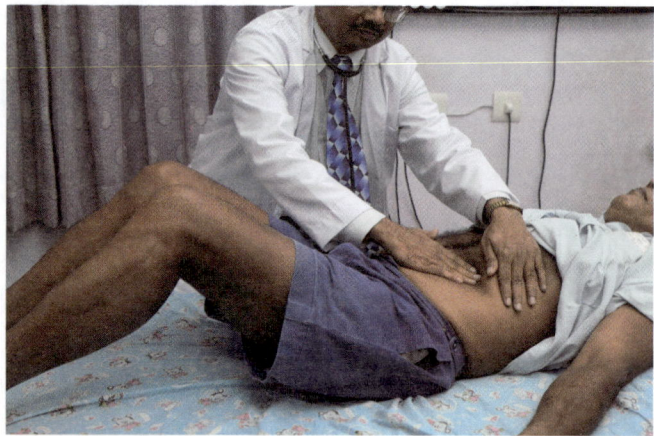

Fig. 55.5 Palpation of the spleen. The palm of the right hand is placed on the right ileac fossa below and to the right of the umbilicus with the fingers close to each other and pointing towards the left subcostal margin. While the subject takes a deep breath, the examiner presses deep with the fingers of the right hand.

and ask him to rest/lean on your left hand, and *repeat the maneuver*.

In venous engorgement: If the veins are prominently engorged, the ***direction of flow*** should be assessed to differentiate between inferior and superior vena caval obstruction (this will be taught in greater detail later, in the clinical classes). To determine the direction of flow, *a section of the vein is emptied using two fingers*, and ***each end of the emptied part is pressed*** with a finger. One finger is released, and the filling of the vein is noted. Similarly, the other finger is released, and the filling of the vein is noted. Blood ***enters more rapidly and fills the vein*** from the direction of the blood flow.

Palpation of the kidney

Kidneys are palpated by a **bimanual technique**.

Palpation of the right kidney: Ask the subject to lie down comfortably on a couch.

1. Standing or sitting on the right of the patient, place the *left hand posteriorly below the lower rib cage* and *right hand on the lower part of the upper quadrant* of the abdomen (Fig. 55.6). ***Push the two hands together firmly*** but gently as the patient breathes out.

2. Feel the lower pole as the patient breathes in deeply. Try to *trap the palpable kidney between the two hands* by delaying application pressure until the end of the inspiration. This helps in palpating the kidney as it slides up on expiration.

3. Confirm the structure of the kidney by *pushing it between the two hands* (**ballotting**) and assessing its degree of movement during respiration. Assess the size, surface, and consistency of the kidney.

Palpation of the left kidney: Standing at the same position on the right side of the subject, repeat the procedure to palpate the kidney of the left side.

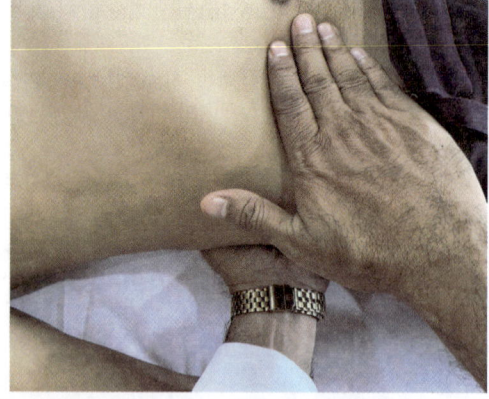

Fig. 55.6 Bimanual palpation of the right kidney.

Fluid thrill

1. Ask the subject to lie on his back. Ask the subject or an assistant to place the *ulnar border of his hand firmly on the midline* of the abdomen of the subject.

2. Sit on a chair to the right of the subject and place the *flat of your left hand on the side of the left lumbar region*.

3. Using your right hand, *tap the side of the right lumbar region* (Fig. 55.7).

4. If a large amount of ascites is present, a ***fluid thrill or a wave is felt as an impulse*** by the left hand (which is placed on the left lumbar region.

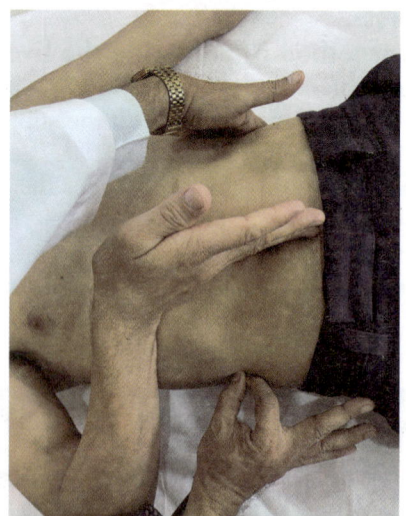

Fig. 55.7 Eliciting fluid thrill.

Percussion of the abdomen

Percuss the abdomen *lightly following the rules of percussion* as described in Chapter 53 (Fig. 55.8).

1. Normally, a ***resonant (tympanitic) note*** is heard, except over areas of liver and spleen enlargement and over a tumour, mass, or fluid.

2. The *absence of dullness* over these areas makes the diagnosis of hepatomegaly and splenomegaly or an abdominal tumour unlikely. Thus, percussion further confirms *hepatomegaly and splenomegaly*, if present.

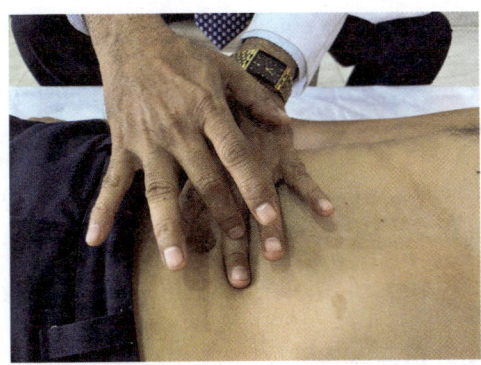

Fig. 55.8   Percussion of the abdomen.

Shifting dullness

The maneuver of shifting dullness is performed to confirm the presence fluid in the peritoneal cavity.

1. If presence of fluid is suspected, percussion should be performed first with the **patient lying on his back** (Fig. 55.9A) and then **lying alternately on each side** (Fig. 55.9B and C).
2. While the patient is lying on his side, the **upper flank will be resonant** because the fluid is pushed down by gravity to the lower flank. Hence, this is called *shifting dullness*.

    The detailed procedure is described in the caption of Fig. 55.9.

Auscultation of the abdomen

Auscultation is carried out by placing the *diaphragm of the stethoscope* on different areas of the abdomen. Auscultation is performed to **detect bowel sounds, peristaltic rub, and bruit**. Note whether bowel sounds are normal, absent, or increased. ***Normal bowel sounds*** are heard as intermittent, *low-, or medium-pitched gurgles*, occasionally interspersed with high-pitched noises.

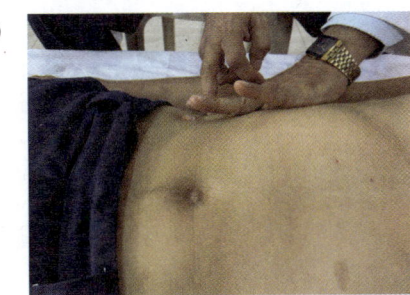

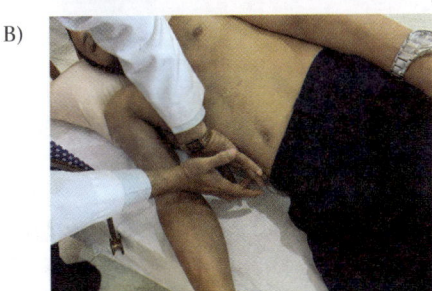

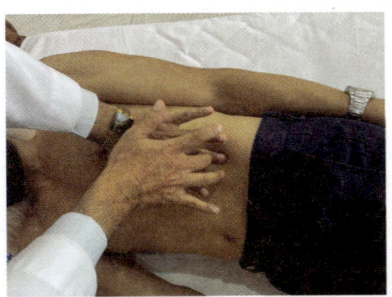

Fig. 55.9   Percussion for the demonstration of shifting dullness. **(A)** With the patient in the supine position, the abdomen is percussed from the central umbilical region to the flank, and dullness is noted in the flank if peritoneal effusion is present. **(B)** Without the examiner changing the position of the hand, the subject is asked to shift his body position to the opposite side. Now, on percussion, the dullness is absent because the fluid shifts from this upper region to the lower region on the opposite side. **(C)** The percussion on the other side (the lower side) yields more dullness due to the shift of fluid to this lower side.

Observation and Results

1. Note your observations in a tabular format as given below.

Parameters	Observation / Findings
Patient's name, age, gender, height, body weight	
History-taking	
i. H/o appetite, dysphagia (if any), acid eructation, flatulence, stool, etc. ii. H/o hematemesis, melena, bleeding P/R iii. Personal h/o smoking, alcoholism	
General examination	
i. Pallor ii. Build and nutrition iii. Clubbing, icterus iv. Signs of liver failure v. Vital signs	
Examination of oral cavity	
i. Teeth, tongue ii. Oral mucous membrane iii. Tonsil, oropharynx	
Examination of abdomen	
Inspection i. Shape of abdomen ii. Umbilicus iii. Abdominal movements iv. Pulsations v. Dilated veins vi. Peristalsis vii. Hernial orifices viii. Scar and skin surface	

Palpation i. Palpation of liver ii. Palpation of spleen iii. Palpation of right and left kidneys iv. Fluid thrill v. Direction of flow if veins are engorged	
Percussion i. General percussion ii. Shifting dullness	
Auscultation i. Bowel sounds ii. Other sounds, if any	

2. Analyse the results and report your findings with your comments on gastrointestinal functions.

Special Examinations

The following special investigations are performed in some cases:

1. Per rectum (PR) examination
2. Proctoscopy
3. Abdominal ultrasound

DISCUSSION

Inspectory Findings

Shape of the abdomen

In an individual of normal build, the abdomen typically appears **boat-shaped**. **Abdominal distension** occurs due to **six factors**, often remembered as the **6 Fs:**

1. **Fat** (abdominal obesity)
2. **Fluid** in excess in the peritoneal cavity (ascites)
3. **Flatus** (excess gas in the large intestine)
4. **Fetus** (pregnancy)
5. **Full** urinary bladder
6. **Feces** (accumulation of excess stool in the large intestine as seen in constipation)

Abdominal swelling also occurs in *tumours of abdominal organs*.

Generalised distension occurs in ascites, obesity, and patients with excessive flatus. **Localised distension** occurs in hepatomegaly (distension in the right hypochondriac region) or splenomegaly (distension in the left hypochondriac region), and in neoplasms. A full bladder and bowel produce **distension of the hypogastrium**. A **scaphoid or sunken abdomen** is seen in starvation and malignancy, especially of the stomach and esophagus.

Umbilicus

Normally, the umbilicus is **inverted and situated centrally** in the abdomen. The distance between the xiphisternum and the umbilicus is equal to the distance between the umbilicus and the symphysis pubis.

In ascites, the distance between the xiphisternum and umbilicus is more than that between the umbilicus and symphysis pubis. Conversely, **in ovarian tumours,** the distance between the xiphisternum and umbilicus is less than that between the umbilicus and symphysis pubis. In ascites, the **umbilicus is flattened or everted**, whereas in obesity, the **umbilical cleft is deeper** than normal.

Abdominal movement

Movement of the abdominal wall occurs **during respiration**. In fact, **respiratory rate is counted** by observing abdominal movement during respiration. Abdominal movement is **absent in peritonitis**.

Pulsations

Normally, pulsations are not visible over the abdomen. However, aortic pulsation may be visible in the nervous or anemic individual. *Aortic aneurysm* produces expansible pulsations.

Dilated veins

The presence of dilated veins **suggests venous obstruction**.

In **inferior vena caval obstruction**, there will be dilated veins on the sides with *flow of blood from below upwards*. This occurs because blood bypasses the inferior vena cava and travels from the lower limbs to the thorax via the veins of the abdominal wall.

In **portal vein obstruction**, the engorged veins are *centrally placed* and *may form a cluster* around the umbilicus (*caput medusa*). The blood in these veins *flows in all directions* away from the umbilicus. This represents the **opening of anastomosis** between portal and systemic veins.

Peristalsis

Peristaltic waves of the stomach (moving from left to right) are **seen in pyloric stenosis** in the epigastric and left hypochondriac regions. *Peristaltic waves of the large intestine* (transverse colon) are seen in the same region, but they move **from right to left**. Peristaltic waves of the small intestine have a **ladder pattern** and are seen below the centre of the abdomen.

Hernial sites

The *impulse observed at hernial sites* on coughing **suggests hernia**. Femoral or inguinal and direct or indirect hernia should be differentiated (to be studied in clinical classes).

Skin over the abdomen

Smooth and glossy skin indicates *abdominal distension,* whereas wrinkled skin suggests an *old distension* that has been relieved. **Abdominal striae** represent the rupture of subepidermal connective tissue because of abdominal distension. When formed first, the striae are *reddish or pink;* when the distension stabilises or regresses, the colour of the striae *fades to white.* Abdominal striae are seen commonly in **obesity, massive ascites** and following **pregnancy, or corticosteroid therapy.**

Palpatory Findings

Normally, the abdomen is soft, and no tenderness is elicited on palpation.

Abdominal tenderness

The pain felt by the patient on applying pressure is called tenderness. It is commonly found in **inflammatory lesions** of the viscera and the surrounding peritoneum. The **location of tenderness** often suggests a specific pathology. Some examples are:

1. Tenderness in the epigastrium: Peptic ulcer
2. Tenderness in the right hypochondrium: Hepatitis or cholecystitis
3. Tenderness in the right iliac fossa: appendicitis
   Purely visceral pain such as gastric or intestinal colic may not be associated with tenderness.

Guarding and rigidity

Abdominal guarding and rigidity occur due to the **contraction of the muscles** of the abdominal wall; this is often a part of the *defence mechanism over a tender region.* Abdominal rigidity usually occurs over an inflamed organ, e.g., in **pancreatitis or cholecystitis.** Generalised rigidity occurs in **peritonitis.**

Fluid thrill

The presence of fluid thrill indicates the **accumulation of a large amount of free fluid** in the peritoneal cavity (**gross ascites**).

Hepatomegaly

Hepatomegaly refers to an enlarged liver. Usually, the **liver is palpable if enlarged,** as the lower border of the liver normally lies at the right subcostal margin. The common **causes of hepatomegaly** are:

1. Infective hepatitis
2. Chronic amebiasis
3. Malaria
4. Kala azar
5. Congestive heart failure
6. Leukemias
7. Hodgkin's disease
8. Hepatic tumours
9. Portal hypertension
10. Hydatid cyst

Splenomegaly

Splenomegaly is the enlargement of the spleen. To be palpable, the **spleen has to enlarge 2.5 times** its normal size. Thus, a mildly enlarged spleen is not always palpable, and the palpable spleen is considerably enlarged. The common **causes of splenomegaly** are:

1. Malaria
2. Kala azar
3. Leukemias
4. Lymphomas
5. Hemolytic anemias
6. Portal hypertension
7. Tropical splenomegaly

Percussion Findings

The normal percussion note of the abdomen is **resonant (tympanitic).** Accumulation of excess gas yields a high tympanitic note, and accumulation of fluid yields a dull note. Since fluid first accumulates in the flanks, the areas of dullness on both sides resemble a horseshoe. Hence, it is called **horseshoe dullness,** which is **confirmed by eliciting shifting dullness.**

In addition to determining the presence of fluid, percussion helps to **delineate the border of an enlarged viscera** or abdominal tumour. Hepatomegaly, splenomegaly, and abdominal lumps or tumours can be **confirmed by eliciting the dull note** over the respective structures.

Auscultatory Findings

Bowel sounds

These are intestinal sounds generated by the contractions of the muscular walls of the gut and the resultant vibration of the gut wall produced by the movement of a gas–fluid mixture through the gut. These bowel sounds *persist in the fasting state* due to the presence of intestinal secretions and swallowed air.

1. **Loud bowel sounds** occur due to hyperperistalsis of the intestine (**peristaltic rush**).
2. **Exaggerated bowel sounds** accompanied by some degree of abdominal distension and cramp-like abdominal pain suggest **partial bowel obstruction.**
3. **Absence of bowel sounds** for at least 10 minutes suggests bowel **atony or paralytic ileus.**

Other sounds

Arterial bruit: These are variable harsh sounds that occur due to turbulences in *arterial flow.* A loud bruit suggests **aortic aneurysm and atherosclerosis** or extreme tortuosity of the aorta. Bruit over the kidneys in the flanks suggests renal artery stenosis.

Venous hum: This is *a continuous, soft, and low-pitched sound* that may be heard over the liver area and umbilicus in ***portal-systemic shunting*** of venous flow when portal flow is obstructed.

VIVA

1. *Name the various quadrants of the abdomen.* (Ans. Refer to page 365, under the heading 'Anatomical Landmarks'.)
2. *What are the important histories to be taken before examining the GIS?* (Ans. Refer to page 365, under the heading 'History-taking'.)
3. *What points should be observed in the inspection of the abdomen?* (Ans. Refer to page 366, under the heading 'Inspection'.)
4. *What are the methods of liver palpation? How is the palpation of the liver performed?* (Ans. Refer to page 367, under the heading 'Palpation of the liver'.)
5. *How is the palpation of the spleen performed?* (Ans. Refer to page 367, under the heading 'Palpation of the spleen'.)
6. *If the veins are prominent, how is superior and inferior vena caval obstruction detected?* (Ans. Refer to page 366, under the subheading 'In Venous Engorgement'.)
7. *What is the procedure for the palpation of the kidney?* (Ans. Refer to page 368, under the heading 'Palpation of the kidney'.)
8. *How is the fluid thrill test performed?* (Ans. Refer to page 368, under the heading 'Fluid thrill'.)
9. *How is shifting dullness elicited?* (Ans. Refer to page 369, under the heading 'Shifting dullness'.)
10. *What is fluid thrill? What is its importance?* (Ans. Refer to page 368, under the heading 'Fluid thrill'.)
11. *What is shifting dullness? What is its importance?* (Ans. Refer to page 371, under the heading 'Percussion Findings' and the subheading 'Horseshoe dullness'.)
12. *What are the types of bowel sounds, and how are they produced?* (Ans. Refer to page 371, under the heading 'Bowel sounds'.)
13. *What are the common causes of hepatomegaly?* (Ans. Refer to page 371, under the heading 'Hepatomegaly'.)
14. *What are the common causes of splenomegaly?* (Ans. Refer to page 371, under the heading 'Splenomegaly'.)
15. *What is the normal shape of the abdomen and how is the shape altered in different conditions?* (Ans. Refer to page 370, under the heading 'Shape of the abdomen'.)
16. *What is the importance of the position of the umbilicus?* (Ans. Refer to page 370, under the heading 'Umbilicus'.)
17. *What is the importance of abdominal venous engorgement?* (Ans. Refer to page 370, under the heading 'Dilated veins'.)
18. *What is the significance of abdominal guarding?* (Ans. Refer to page 371, under the heading 'Guarding and Rigidity'.)

56 Clinical Examination of the Nervous System I (Higher Functions and Cranial Nerves)

Learning Objectives

After completing this practical, you will be able to (MUST KNOW):
1. Describe the importance of performing this practical in clinical physiology.
2. List the functions of all the cranial nerves.
3. Perform clinical examination of all the cranial nerves.
4. List the precautions observed while examining each of the cranial nerves.
5. List the parameters to be examined for assessing higher functions and speech.
6. List the common effects of lesions of the cranial nerves.

You may also be able to (DESIRABLE TO KNOW):
1. Trace the pathway of all the cranial nerves.
2. Explain the abnormalities observed following lesions of the cranial nerves.
3. List the differences between supra- and infranuclear palsy of the 7th and 12th cranial nerves.
4. List the common problems of higher functions and name the types of aphasias.

PY5.15: Demonstrate the correct clinical examination of the nervous system: higher functions, sensory system, motor system, reflexes, and cranial nerves in a normal volunteer or simulated environment.

Clinical examination of the nervous system is generally performed in the **following sequence**:
1. Examination of the higher functions and speech
2. Examination of the cranial nerves
3. Examination of the sensory system
4. Examination of the motor system and reflexes

Each examination as listed above requires detailed description. Therefore, the first two examinations are described in this chapter and the third and fourth examinations are described subsequently in separate chapters.

CLINICAL EXAMINATION OF HIGHER FUNCTIONS AND SPEECH

HIGHER FUNCTIONS

Higher mental and intellectual functions are assessed under the following headings:
1. **Appearance and behaviour:** Observe whether the patient is **well-oriented and well-behaved** or if he appears *disturbed, agitated, or confused*. Note his **attention span**—whether it is focused, wandering, or suggestive of flight of ideas. Note *how he is dressed, his general hygiene*, and the condition of his nails, hands, and hair.

2. **Emotional state:** Assess the patient's emotional state. Assess whether his **mood seems elevated or depressed** and whether there are *notable emotional disturbances*. Enquire about the quality and duration of his sleep and the quality of his dreams.

3. **Delusions and hallucinations:** Note whether the patient is **experiencing delusions** (false beliefs, which continue to be held despite evidence to the contrary) or **hallucinations** (false impressions).

4. **Level of consciousness and memory:** Assess whether there is any **clouding of consciousness**. Also ask questions to assess for evidence of *loss of memory*, if any.

5. **Orientation of place and time:** Ask the patient about his **surroundings** (whether he is at the hospital or home) and *the time, date, month and year*. Disorientation, if present, should be noted.

6. **Level of memory:** Ask a few basic questions to assess the patient's **recent and past memory**. Loss of recent or remote memory is indicative of brain injury.

7. **General orientation and intelligence:** Assess this by asking the patient about his personal history, social history, and educational history, especially the *nature of his work and habits*.

SPEECH (LANGUAGE) FUNCTIONS

Speech is a vital phenomenon by which an individual expresses himself. The **ability to understand and express** oneself is the highest quality of the brain, and the human being is endowed with this highly developed quality. Speech has **two components**: the sensory and motor.

The **sensory or receptive part** of speech includes *vision and hearing* of the texts and related sounds.

The **motor or expressive part** includes *spoken and written speech*. Thus, the disorders of speech may be **aphasias or dysarthria**.

Assess if the subject is having **aphasias**, i.e., *loss of the ability to understand and use symbols*, which may be **sensory or fluent aphasia** that occurs due to lesions in the Wernicke's area or **motor (or nonfluent) aphasia** that occurs due to lesions in the Broca's area. The patient may also have global aphasia or **dysarthria**, which is assessed by *looking for articulation*.

CLINICAL EXAMINATION OF THE CRANIAL NERVES

INTRODUCTION

There are **twelve pairs of cranial nerves** (CN). Some of these contain only sensory fibres and are thus known as **sensory cranial nerves**. A few cranial nerves are predominantly motor in function and are therefore called **motor cranial nerves**. The remaining cranial nerves contain both sensory and motor fibres and hence, are called **mixed cranial nerves**.

CN 1, 2, and 8 are sensory; **3, 4, 6, 11 and 12 are predominantly motor**; and **5, 7, 9, and 10 are mixed**. A systematic and thorough examination of cranial nerves is *part of the clinical evaluation of a subject with a neurological deficit*. The cranial nerves may be affected by a primary disease of the cranial nerve or by a disease of the brain or the meninges, or sometimes, secondary to other systemic disorders.

Anatomical and Physiological Considerations
Olfactory or first cranial nerve

Anatomy: This nerve **arises from the olfactory mucosa**. The nasal mucous membrane contains **bipolar sensory cells** that constitute the *first order of neurons*. Their central processes pass through the olfactory foramina in the cribriform plate of the ethmoid bone and **terminate in the olfactory bulb**. From the olfactory bulb, the *second order of neurons* arises and **projects to the olfactory cortex**, which consists of the periamygdaloid and prepiriform areas of the piriform lobe (the olfactory pathway has been described in Chapter 48, under the heading 'Sensation of Smell' and in Fig. 48.2).

Function: The olfactory nerve carries the **sensation of smell** from the nasal mucosa to the olfactory cortex of the brain.

Optic or second cranial nerve

Anatomy: This is one of the most important cranial nerves because it **subserves vision**. The fibres of **the optic nerve** arise in the retina and pass through the optic foramen to **form the optic chiasma** and then **the optic tract**.

1. **At the chiasma**, the fibres from the **inner half of each retina decussate**, while those from the outer half *remain on the same side*. Thus, **each optic tract consists** of fibres from the outer half of the retina of the same side and from the inner half of the retina of the opposite side (refer to 'Visual Pathway', Fig. 44.1, Chapter 44).

2. Most of the *fibres of the optic tract* pass onto the **lateral geniculate body** (LGB) of the thalamus, and *some fibres from the optic tract* reach the **pretectal area**, which is involved in the *regulation of pupillary reflexes* and movement of the orbital muscles.

3. The fibres from the *LGB travel in the optic radiation* to reach **the visual (calcarine) cortex**. The calcarine cortex constitutes the main visual centre and *represents the opposite half* of the field of vision.

4. The area of **central or macular vision** has *extensive cortical representation* and dual blood supply from the middle and posterior cerebral arteries.

Function: The optic nerve serves the most important special sensation, **vision**. Normal vision is dependent on the integrity of the visual pathway, i.e., the receptors in the retina, optic nerve, optic chiasma, optic tract, lateral geniculate body, and visual cortex.

Oculomotor or third cranial nerve

Anatomy: This is predominantly a **motor nerve**. The nuclei of the third cranial nerve lie in the midbrain, just anterior to the cerebral aqueduct, at the level of the superior and inferior colliculi. The nerve fibres emerge at the upper border of the pons, pass through the cavernous sinus and superior orbital fissure, and supply the **four extrinsic muscles of the eyeball** (superior rectus, medial rectus, inferior rectus, and inferior oblique; Fig. 56.1). It also supplies the levator palpebrae superioris of the upper

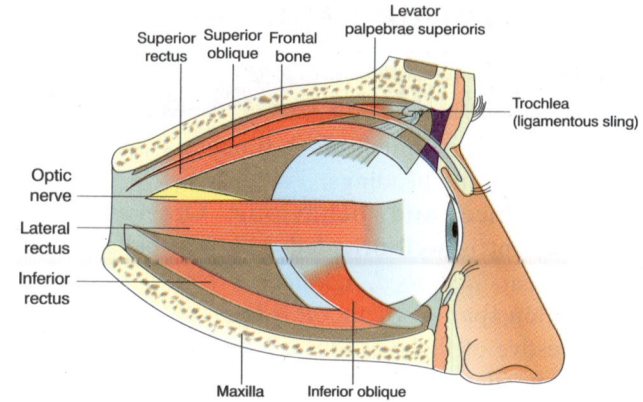

Fig. 56.1   Muscles attached to the left eye.

eyelid. The third cranial nerve carries parasympathetic innervation to the sphincter muscles of the iris (sphincter pupillae) and ciliary muscles (involved in control of accommodation).

Functions:
1. It controls all the **movements of the eyeball** *except lateral deviation* of the eye and *depression of the medially deviated eye*.
2. It controls the **size of the pupil**.
3. It is involved in the **accommodation** of vision.

Trochlear or fourth cranial nerve

Anatomy: This is primarily a **motor cranial nerve**. The nucleus of the fourth cranial nerve is located in the midbrain. The fibres decussate before emerging from the brain and enter the orbit *through the superior orbital fissure* to supply the superior oblique muscle. The fourth cranial nerve supplies the ***superior oblique muscle*** of the opposite side of the eyeball.

> **Note:** This is a peculiar nerve in the sense that it is the *only cranial nerve* that **decussates between its nuclei of origin and the point of emergence.**

Function: It causes *depression of the medially deviated eye*.

Trigeminal or fifth cranial nerve

Anatomy: This consists of both **motor and sensory fibres**. It has three subdivisions: **ophthalmic, maxillary, and mandibular**. The ophthalmic and maxillary divisions are sensory, whereas the mandibular division is both motor and sensory.

Motor component of the fifth nerve: The motor fibres originate in the pons and exit the brain through the foramen ovale to innervate the **muscles of mastication** (masseters and temporalis). The motor fibres of the fifth nerve are present only in the ***mandibular division*** of the nerve.

Sensory component of the fifth nerve: Sensory fibres of the fifth nerve are present in ***all three divisions*** of the nerve (Fig. 56.2).

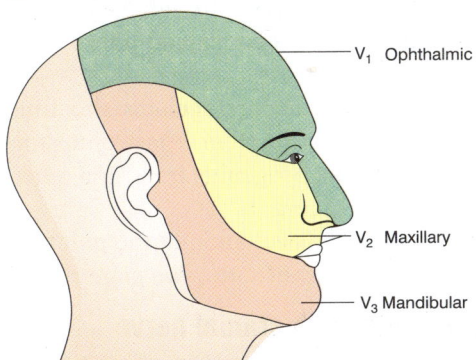

V₁ Ophthalmic

V₂ Maxillary

V₃ Mandibular

Fig. 56.2   Areas supplied by the three peripheral sensory branches of the trigeminal nerve.

Ophthalmic division: The ophthalmic division carries fibres that receive sensations from the skin over the upper eyelid, the eyeball, the lacrimal glands, the nasal cavity, the side of the nose, the conjunctival surface of the upper but not the lower lid, the forehead and the scalp as far as the vertex. These fibres *pass through the superior orbital fissure*.

Maxillary division: The maxillary division carries sensations from the upper part of the cheek, the lower eyelid and its conjunctival surface, the skin and mucous membrane of the nose, the upper lip, the upper teeth, the upper part of the pharynx, the roof of the mouth and soft palate, and the medial inferior quadrant of the cornea. The fibres in the maxillary division enter the brain *through the foramen rotundum*.

Mandibular division: Sensory fibres in the mandibular division carry sensations from the lower part of the face, the lower lip, the ear, anterior two-thirds of the tongue (not taste) and the lower teeth. These fibres pass *through the foramen ovale*.

The sensory fibres from all three divisions of the trigeminal nerve **end in the pons**.

Functions: The trigeminal nerve carries ***general sensation*** from different parts of the face and a part of the head and neck. Through its motor functions, it is involved in **mastication** (chewing).

Abducent or sixth cranial nerve

Anatomy: This is primarily **a motor nerve**. Its fibres originate in the nucleus, i.e., in the *lower part of the pons*, near the internal genu of the facial canal. After emerging from the pons, it traverses a long intracranial course to enter the orbital cavity through the *medial end of the superior orbital fissure* to supply the **lateral rectus muscle**.

> **Note:** The **long intracranial course** of this nerve makes it vulnerable to the *effects of raised intracranial pressure*.

Function: It helps in the **lateral deviation** (abduction) of the eye.

Facial or seventh cranial nerve

Anatomy: The seventh cranial nerve is a mixed nerve. It has both motor and sensory components.
1. **Motor component:** The motor fibres originate in the pons, pass through the stylomastoid foramen, and innervate the ***muscles of facial expression, scalp, and platysma*** (neck muscle).
2. **Sensory component:** Fibres arise from the taste buds present in the ***anterior two-thirds of the tongue***, pass through the stylomastoid foramen, and end in the geniculate ganglion, a nucleus in the pons from where fibres travel to the *gustatory area in the parietal lobe* of the cerebral cortex through the thalamus.

During its course, the facial nerve travels through the **facial canal** in the temporal bone. The **chorda tympani nerve**, which carries the taste sensation from the anterior two-thirds of the tongue, joins the facial nerve in the facial canal (Fig. 56.3). This part of the nerve is **vulnerable to injury and edema** because it is enclosed in a bony tube.

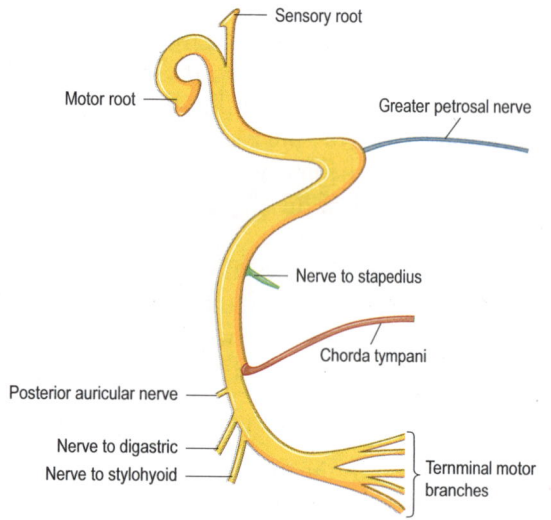

Fig. 56.3   Facial nerve: origin and branches.

Functions:
1. It supplies **all the muscles of the face** (*except the levator palpebrae superioris*) **scalp, and platysma**. Therefore, it carries out **all facial expressions**.
2. It carries the **taste sensation** from the *anterior two-thirds* of the tongue.

Vestibulocochlear or eighth cranial nerve
Anatomy: It has **two components:** the cochlear and the vestibular.
1. **The cochlear nerve:** The auditory (cochlear) fibres arise in the spiral organ (**organ of Corti**) and form the *spiral ganglion*. Fibres from the spiral ganglion pass through the internal auditory meatus to reach the **nuclei in the medulla**, from where the fibres project **to the thalamus,** and from there **to the auditory cortex** (for details, refer to Fig. 47.1 in Chapter 47).
2. **The vestibular nerve:** The vestibular fibres originate in the semicircular canals, saccule, and utricle and form the vestibular ganglion. The fibres from the vestibular ganglion terminate in the **vestibular nuclei** present in the **pons and medulla**. A good deal of projection also **reaches the cerebellum**.

Functions:
1. The **cochlear fibres** convey impulses associated with **hearing**.
2. The **vestibular fibres** convey impulses associated with **equilibrium**.

Glossopharyngeal or ninth cranial nerve
Anatomy: The glossopharyngeal nerve is a **mixed nerve**. It has *both motor and sensory components*.
1. **The motor fibres:** The fibres originate in the **nucleus ambiguous** in the medulla. They accompany *the tenth and eleventh cranial nerve* and exit the skull through the jugular foramen to supply the **middle constrictor of the pharynx** and **stylopharyngeous muscle**. They also supply parasympathetic fibres to the parotid gland.
2. **The sensory fibres:** These fibres arise from the *taste buds in the posterior third of the tongue and baroreceptors in the carotid sinus*. They carry general sensation from the nasopharynx and posterior aspect of the soft palate. These fibres terminate in the **nucleus tractus solitarius** (NTS).

Functions:
1. The ninth cranial nerve is involved in the activation of the **pharyngeal reflex**.
2. It carries the *taste sensation* from the **posterior third of the tongue**.
3. It helps in the *secretion of saliva*.
4. It is involved in the **regulation of blood pressure** (baroreceptor reflex).

Vagus or tenth cranial nerve
Anatomy: The vagus nerve is a mixed nerve. It has both motor and sensory components.
1. **The motor fibres:** These fibres originate in the **nucleus ambiguous** in the medulla. The vagus nerve exits the skull through the jugular foramen to supply the structures in the neck, thorax, and abdomen. Their function is **motor to** the soft palate (with *the exception of tensor palati*), pharynx, larynx, respiratory passages, esophagus, stomach, small intestine, and most parts of the large intestine, gall bladder, and heart. Their function is **secretomotor to most of these organs**.
2. **The sensory fibres:** These carry sensations from the **aortic arch and aortic bodies**, which mediate **baroreceptor and chemoreceptor reflexes**. They also carry sensations from the structures that they innervate. The fibres pass through the jugular foramen and terminate in the medulla and pons.

Functions:
1. The tenth cranial nerve regulates the functions of the cardiovascular system, gastrointestinal tract, respiratory system, urogenital tract, and other thoracic and abdominal viscera.
2. It is involved in the elicitation of the **palatal reflex**.
3. It subserves **laryngeal and pharyngeal functions**.

Accessory or eleventh cranial nerve
Anatomy: This is a **pure motor nerve** of cranial and spinal origin.

1. The **cranial fibres** originate in the **nucleus ambiguous** in the medulla. The **spinal fibres** emerge from the sixth cervical segment of the spinal cord, ascend through the foramen magnum into the brain and join the cranial fibres.
2. The fibres exit the skull **through the jugular foramen** and divide into the cranial and spinal parts. The **cranial part** supplies a *motor nerve to the larynx, pharynx, and soft palate*. The **spinal part** supplies the *sternomastoid and the trapezius muscle*.

Functions:
1. The **cranial portion** mediates *swallowing movements*.
2. The **spinal portion** mediates *head and shoulder movements*.

Hypoglossal or twelfth cranial nerve

Anatomy: The twelfth cranial nerve is a **pure motor nerve**. The fibres originate from its nucleus, which is present in the medulla. It exits the skull via the *hypoglossal canal* (anterior condyloid foramen) and joins the *ansa hypoglossi* in the cervical region. It supplies the **muscles of the tongue** on the same side. It also supplies the **hypoglossus, styloglossus, and genioglossus** muscles.

Functions:
1. It helps in the **movement of the tongue** and therefore, *assists in speech and swallowing*.
2. It assists in **depressing the hyoid bone**.

METHODS TO ASSESS THE CRANIAL NERVES

Assessment of the Olfactory Nerve

Principle

The olfactory nerve carries the sensation of smell. Therefore, this nerve is tested using various olfactory stimuli.

Requirements

One small bottle each of clove oil, peppermint oil or camphor, and coffee powder (refer to Fig. 48.3, Chapter 48).

Procedure

1. Ask the subject to sit comfortably on a stool and close his eyes and one of his nostrils.
2. Uncap the bottle containing clove oil, bring the bottle close to the open nostril, and ask if the **subject perceives the smell correctly.**
3. Repeat the procedure with **peppermint oil**.
4. Ask the subject to block the tested nostril, open the other nostril, and repeat the above steps.
5. Compare the results of the two nostrils.
6. Ask the subject if he experiences hallucinations of smell (for further details, refer to Chapter 48).

Results

Note down your observations. Express the results as: "Smell normal/reduced/absent/perverted", separately for each nostril.

Precautions

1. The subject should close his eyes.
2. The subject must be familiar with the odours used.
3. The two nostrils should be examined separately.
4. One nostril should be closed while the other is being examined.

Assessment of the Optic Nerve

Principle

The optic nerve carries the sensation of vision. The examination of this nerve reveals intactness of the visual pathway, field of vision, and acuity of vision.

Requirements

1. Snellen's chart
2. Lister's or Goldmann's perimeter
3. Ishihara chart

Procedure

The optic nerve is tested for **acuity of vision, field of vision,** and **colour vision**. These tests are described in detail in Chapters 44, 45, and 46, respectively.

Clinically, the field of vision is detected by the 'confrontation test' at the bedside of the patient.

▮ Confrontation test

1. Ask the subject to comfortably sit on a stool in an erect position.
2. Sit on a stool in front of the subject in such a way that your eyes and the subject's eyes remain *at the same level* and at a **distance of about 3 feet** (Fig. 56.4).
3. Ask the subject to fix her gaze at the tip of your nose.

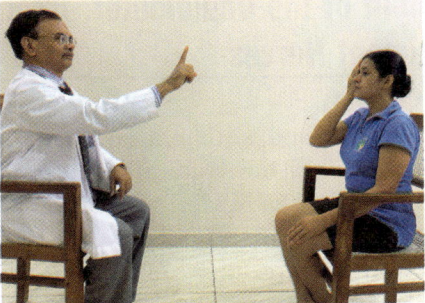

Fig. 56.4 Performing the confrontation test (the testing of eyeball movements for the assessment of oculomotor nerve function is performed in a similar manner). Note that the examiner's eyes and the subject's eyes are at approximately the same level. The subject is instructed to fix her gaze on the tip of the examiner's index finger, positioned at a distance of about 25 cm, and to follow the finger's movement.

4. Ask the subject to close one eye. Close your opposite eye.

5. Move your finger midway between yourself and the subject to **test the field of vision in the four quadrants** (upper, lower, nasal, and temporal). Bring your finger from the periphery of the four quadrants to the centre of the visual field and ask the subject to say 'yes' when she sees the finger.

> **Note:** If the subject's vision is normal, at the point at which the examiner catches sight of the moving finger, the subject should also be able to see it.

6. Compare the subject's field of vision with yours and note your observations.

7. Repeat the procedure with the other eye.

Observation and results

1. The results of acuity of vision, field of vision, and colour vision have been described in Chapters 44–46.

2. Note the approximate field of vision in the four quadrants assessed by the confrontation test and write down your comments.

Precautions

1. The distance between the examiner and the subject **should be 3 feet**.

2. The examiner's eye should *remain level* with that of the subject.

3. The examiner's field of vision should be normal.

4. The subject should fix his gaze at the centre.

5. The examiner should move his finger midway between himself and the subject.

6. While one eye is being examined, the other eye should be closed.

7. The subject *should wear glasses* during the procedure *if he uses them regularly* for refractive errors. Restriction of the field of vision due to glasses should be kept in mind.

Assessment of the Oculomotor, Trochlear and Abducent Nerves

Principle

The third, fourth, and sixth cranial nerves are tested together because they **innervate all the external ocular muscles**. The eyeball moves in different directions, and the movements are named accordingly.

1. **Horizontal movement** in an outward direction is called *abduction,* and in an inward direction is called *adduction.* **Vertical movement** in the upward direction is called *elevation,* and in the downward direction is called *depression*.

2. The eye is also capable of **rotatory movements**. The rolling movement of the eye towards the nose is called **internal rotation,** and movement away from the nose is called **external rotation**.

The *superior and inferior rectus* elevate and depress the eye when it **is in abduction**, and the *inferior and superior oblique* elevate and depress the eye when it **is in adduction** (Fig. 56.5).

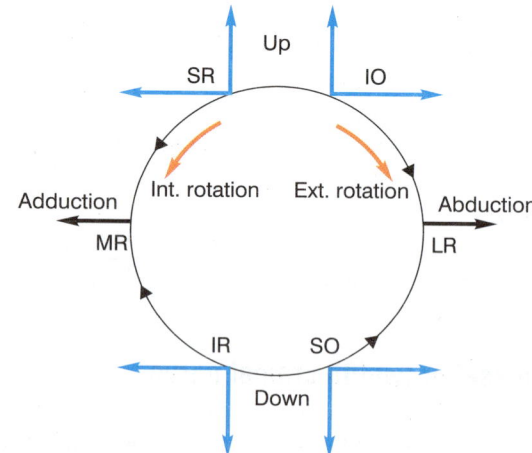

Fig. 56.5   Direction of eyeball movements based on the mechanism of action of different extraocular muscles. Accordingly, different eye movements are performed for assessing the functions of the 3rd, 4th, and 6th cranial nerves (LR: lateral rectus; MR: medial rectus; SO: superior oblique; IO: inferior oblique; SR: superior rectus; IR: inferior rectus).

Requirements

1. Torch—a pencil torch is preferred (Fig. 56.6)
2. Cardboard

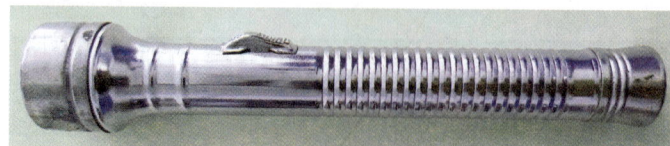

Fig. 56.6   Pencil torch (sharply focusses light onto the eye).

Procedure

1. Ask the subject to sit comfortably on a stool and yourself sit in front of the subject.

2. Examine the subject's eyes for the presence of **ptosis** (drooping of the eyelid) and **nystagmus** (rhythmic, involuntary, and jerky movement of the eyeball), if any.

3. Instruct the subject to follow the direction of the movement of your finger.

4. Bring your index finger to the front of the subject's eyes, keeping a **distance of around 25 cm** (the normal visual distance) from the subject.

5. Ask the subject to look at and follow the movements of your index finger and observe the movements of the eyeball of the subject (Fig. 56.5) while moving your finger (as depicted in Fig. 56.4).

6. First, move your finger **laterally to the right of the subject** (this tests the function of the lateral rectus of the right eye and the medial rectus of the left eye simultaneously). From there, **move your finger vertically upwards** (this tests the superior rectus of

the right eye and the inferior oblique of the left eye) **and downwards** (this tests the inferior rectus of the right eye and superior oblique of the left eye).

7. Now, move your finger **laterally to the left** (this tests the lateral rectus of the left eye and the medial rectus of the right eye). From there, **move your finger vertically upward** (this tests the superior rectus of the left eye and inferior oblique of the right eye) **and downward** (this tests the inferior rectus of the left eye and superior oblique of the right eye).

8. Examine the **pupillary reaction to light** (*light reflex*).
   - Hold a piece of cardboard between the two eyes or place your hand between the eyes (Fig. 56.7A).
   - Switch on the torch and, bringing it from the side, rapidly focus the light onto one of the subject's eyes. Look for the reactions of the pupil of that eye (**direct light reflex**) as well the pupil of the other eye (**indirect or consensual light reflex**; Fig. 56.7B).
   - Repeat the light reflex testing for the other eye (Fig. 56.7C).

9. Examine the **pupillary reaction to accommodation** (*accommodation reflex*).
   - Ask the subject to **look at a distant object**.
   - Bring the index finger of your hand to a point midway between the two eyes and *very close to the subject's eyes*. Ask the subject to *look at the tip of your index finger* (Fig. 56.8).

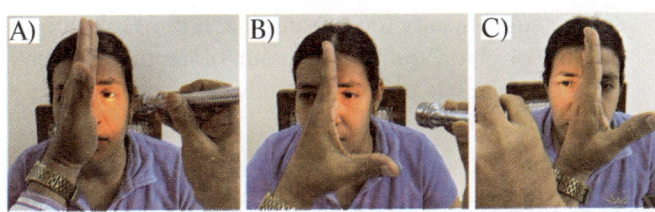

Fig. 56.7 Procedure for assessing light reflex. **(A)** The examiner, with his hand between the subject's eyes, focuses light on one eye by bringing the torch from the side and looks for pupillary constriction. **(B)** While testing direct light reflex of one eye, the examiner should also look for the pupillary reaction of the other eye (indirect or consensual light reflex). **(C)** Testing of light reflex in the opposite eye.

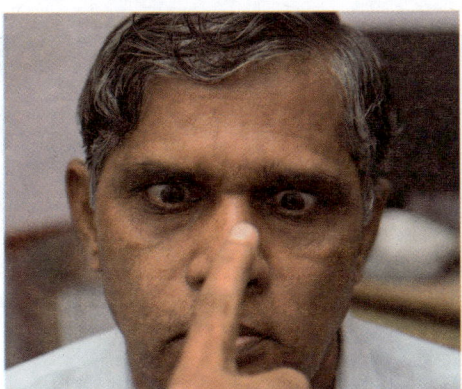

Fig. 56.8 Procedure for assessing accommodation reflex. Note the medial deviation of the subject's eye and the constriction of the pupil when he looks at the tip of the examiner's finger held close to his eyes.

- Examine for **medial deviation and pupillary constriction** of both eyes.

Observation and results

1. Note the eyeball movements in all directions and note down your opinion on the intactness of the extraocular muscles.
2. Observe the pupillary reactions to direct and indirect light reflexes, and write down your comments.
3. Note the pupillary constriction and medial deviation of the eye in response to accommodation and give your inputs.

Precautions

1. The examiner's finger should remain **about 25 cm** (the normal visual distance) from the subject's eyes while testing for eye movement.
2. The light reflexes of *both the eyes should be elicited separately* by holding a piece of cardboard between the eyes.
3. While eliciting light reflex, the light should not be projected directly from the front. Instead, it should be *brought from the side* of the eye and then quickly focused on the pupil.
4. While eliciting accommodation, the subject should *quickly shift his gaze* from a distant object onto an object very close to his eyes.

Assessment of the Trigeminal Nerve

Principle

The trigeminal nerve supplies the **muscle of mastication** and carries **sensations from the face**. The examination of the different sensations on the face and the ability of the subject to chew helps determine the intactness of the trigeminal nerve.

Requirements

1. Cotton wool
2. Pin
3. Tuning fork of 128 Hz
4. Glass tubes containing warm and cold water
5. Knee hammer

Procedure

1. Give proper instructions to the subject and explain to her the nature of the examination.
2. Ask the subject to sit comfortably on a stool.
3. **Examine all sensations** (as described in Chapter 57): Test all the sensations of the face, keeping the areas supplied by the *ophthalmic, maxillary, and mandibular divisions* in mind (refer to Fig. 56.2).
4. **Examine the motor functions:** Ask the subject to *clench her teeth* and palpate the *prominence of the temporal and masseter* on both sides by palpating the temple and the upper part of the cheek. Ask the subject to *open her mouth* and look for *deviation of the jaw*, if present.

Note: If there is paralysis of one side, the muscle on that side will fail to become prominent, and on opening the mouth, the **jaw will deviate towards the paralysed side** because it is pushed over by the lateral pterygoid muscle of the healthy side. Normally, the lateral pterygoid muscle pushes the jaw towards the midline.

5. **Test conjunctival reflex:** Bring a piece of cotton wool *from the side* (the subject should not know that you are going to touch her conjunctiva) and *immediately touch the conjunctiva* (Fig. 56.9A). Look for the response (the subject should **blink**).

6. **Test corneal reflex:** Touch the limbus, i.e., the *sclerocorneal junction* (Fig. 56.9B) of the eye with cotton wool and look for the response (**blinking**).

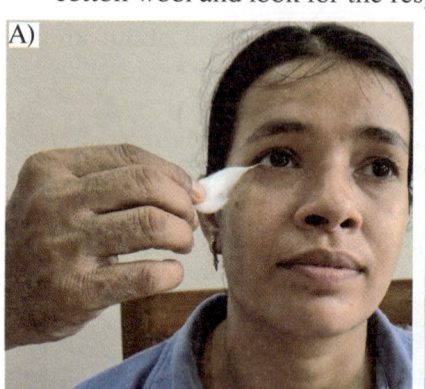 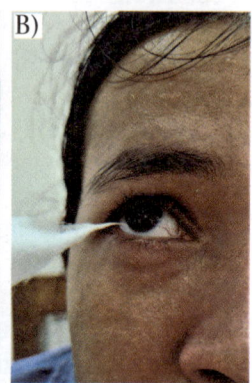

Fig. 56.9 **(A)** Elicitation of conjuctival reflex and **(B)** elicitation of corneal reflex. Note that for corneal reflex, the limbus (sclerocorneal junction) is touched but not the cornea, to avoid possible damage to the cornea.

7. **Elicit jaw jerk:** Ask the subject to *partially open her mouth.* Place your left index finger in the groove under the lower lip and *lightly tap on the nail of the finger* with the help of the knee hammer (Fig. 56.10). Observe the response (if the jerk is present, the **mouth snaps shut**).

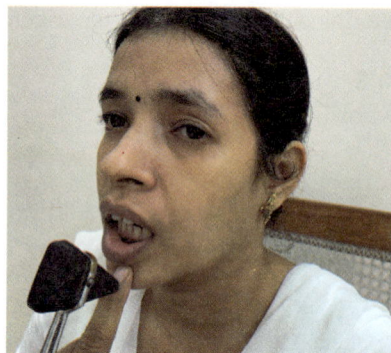

Fig. 56.10   Elicitation of jaw jerk.

Observation and results

1. Note the intactness of the sensations of all three divisions of the trigeminal nerve on the face.
2. Record the motor functions by noting the prominence of the temporal and masseter on both sides and deviation of the jaw on the opening of the mouth, if any.
3. Note the blinking of eyes in response to conjunctival and corneal reflexes.

4. Note the jaw-jerk response.
5. Summarise your comments on the tests of the fifth cranial nerve.

Precautions

1. The subject should be instructed properly.
2. All the sensations should be elicited from the face according to the distribution of the three subdivisions of the fifth nerve.
3. The masseter and temporalis should be examined on both sides and compared simultaneously.
4. While eliciting the corneal and conjunctival reflexes, the subject should not be aware of the procedure. Otherwise, she will close her eyes before the conjunctiva is touched.

Assessment of the Facial Nerve

Principle

The facial nerve carries the **taste sensation from the anterior two-thirds of the tongue** and supplies the **muscles of facial expression**. Therefore, the examination of the taste sensation of the anterior two-thirds of the tongue and the ability of the subject to **perform all facial expressions** indicate the intactness of the facial nerve.

Requirements

1. Four small vials containing strong solutions that are sweet (sugar), salty (common salt), bitter (solution of quinine or chloroquine), and sour (lime juice or weak solutions of citric acid) separately
2. Four glass rods

Procedure

1. Ask the subject to *frown or open his eyes wide* (Fig. 56.11). Look for the **wrinkling of the forehead** (to assess the frontal belly of the occipitofrontalis).
2. Ask the *subject to shut his eyes as tightly as he can.* Try to **open the eyes** while he tries to keep them closed (Fig. 56.12). This is the test for orbicularis oculi.

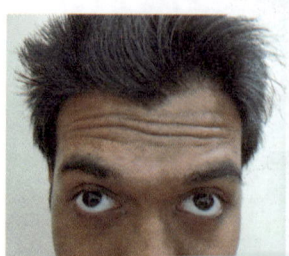 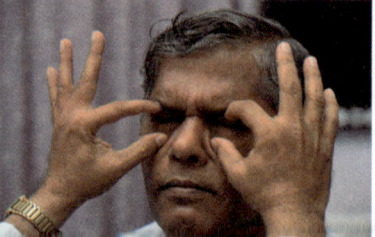

Fig. 56.11 Test for the frontal belly of occipitofrontalis. Note the wrinkling of the forehead when the subject frowns or opens his eyes wide.

Fig. 56.12 Procedure for testing the orbicularis oculi.

Note: If one side of the nerve is paralysed, the affected eye is either not closed at all, in which case the **eyeball rolls upward** to make up for the failure of the lid to descend (**Bell's phenomenon**), or if the eye is closed, the eyelashes are not buried. Bell's phenomenon is a normal phenomenon *preserved in facial palsies of the lower motor neuron type*.

3. Ask the subject to *show his teeth* (Fig. 56.13). Look for *deviation of the angle of the mouth*, if present (to test for orbicularis oris).

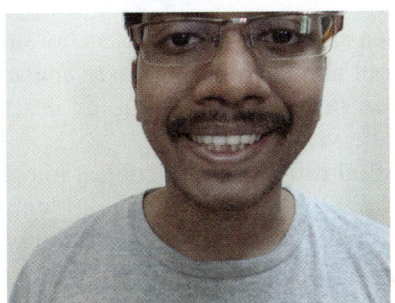

Fig. 56.13   Test for orbicularis oris. Deviation of the angle of the mouth is noted when the subject shows his teeth.

Note: If the seventh nerve is paralysed, the *angle of the mouth on the affected side becomes less prominent*. Instead of being elevated upwards and laterally, it is *drawn towards the midline* by the unopposed action of the orbicularis oris of the healthy side.

4. Ask the subject to *inflate his mouth with air and blow out his cheeks*. Tap on each inflated cheek with a finger (test for the buccinator muscle; Fig. 56.14).

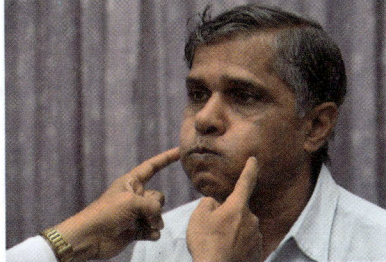

Fig. 56.14   Procedure for testing the buccinator muscle.

Note: Air escapes from the mouth more easily from the paralysed side.

5. Ask the *subject to whistle* (test for both orbicularis oris and buccinator; Fig. 56.15).

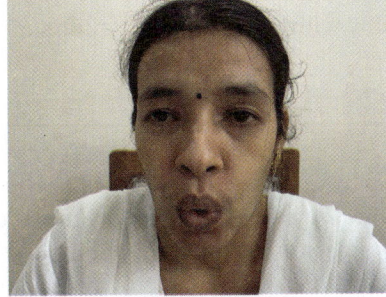

Fig. 56.15   Test for both orbicularis oris and buccinator. The ability to whistle is assessed.

6. Ask the subject to *clench his teeth* and observe the *prominence of the platysma* muscle in the neck (Fig. 56.16).

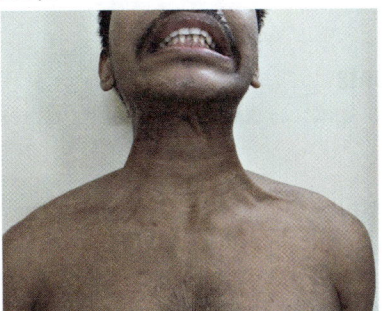

Fig. 56.16   Procedure for testing the platysma. Note the prominence of the platysma in the neck while the subject clenches his teeth.

7. Test the *taste sensations from the anterior two-thirds* of the tongue. Ask the subject to protrude his tongue. Dip one glass rod in the **sweet solution** and touch different parts of the tongue with the tip of the rod. Ask the subject what taste he senses. Repeat the procedure with the **salty, sour, and bitter** solutions using separate glass rods for each solution (for details, refer to Chapter 48).

Note: While testing for different taste sensations, the relative distribution of taste buds in the tongue for different modalities of taste should be kept in mind. The taste buds for sweetness are more concentrated at the tip, bitter at the back, and salt and sour on the sides of the tongue.

Observation and results

1. Record the responses of all facial muscles to different maneuvers.
2. Check for Bell's phenomenon (upward deviation of the eye when attempting to close the eyelids), if present.
3. Observe the prominence of the platysma in response to clenching of the teeth.
4. Note the taste sensations from the anterior 2/3rd of the tongue in response to different testants applied.
5. Comment on the intactness of the 7th cranial nerve.

Precautions

1. The subject should be properly instructed.
2. The functions the facial muscles on both sides should be tested simultaneously and compared.
3. Separate rods should be used for testing different taste solutions.
4. The sensation of bitterness should be tested last.
5. The subject should be asked to rinse their mouth after testing each solution.

Assessment of the Vestibulocochlear Nerve
Principle

The eighth nerve has two components, vestibular and cochlear. The **cochlear nerve is involved in hearing** and the **vestibular in balance and equilibrium**. Therefore, the functions of the eighth nerve are tested by performing **hearing and vestibular tests**. *Hearing tests* are described in Chapter 47.

Requirements

There are no special requirements for this test.

Procedure

1. Ask the subject whether he has **giddiness, dizziness, motion sickness, and vertigo** (sensation that external objects seem to move around him).
2. Examine the subject's eye for the presence of **nystagmus** (involuntary rhythmic and jerky movements of the eyeball).

> **Note:** Nystagmus is observed by asking the subject to look in a different direction. Clinically, it can be elicited by hyperextending the neck and then rapidly moving the head side to side.

3. Elicit nystagmus by performing the *caloric and rotation tests* (usually not done in physiology).
   - **Caloric test:** Irrigate the ear with **warm or cold water**. This sets up convection currents in the endolymph of the semicircular canals and produces nystagmus.
   - **Rotation test:** Rotate the subject in a special rotating chair (Barany's chair). **Rotation induces nystagmus**.
4. **Balance test:** Assessment of postural balance tests vestibular functions. For example, ask the subject to *walk in a straight line or stand erect with his feet together* and his **eyes open** (when the eyes are closed, the test is called the Romberg sign, which indicates postural imbalance other than that of cerebellar and vestibular origin)
5. **Electronystagmography** can be performed to assess nystagmus (if available).

Observation and results

Note the observations of tests for hearing, vertigo, nystagmus and balance, and comment on the intactness of the eighth cranial nerve.

Assessment of the Glossopharyngeal Nerve

Principle

The ninth cranial nerve carries general as well as **taste sensations from the posterior third** of the tongue and mucous membrane of the pharynx and supplies **motor fibres to the middle constrictor of the pharynx** and the **stylopharyngeous muscle**. It also carries sensations from **the carotid sinus**. Therefore, the functions of the ninth nerve are tested by eliciting *taste sensations from the* posterior third of the tongue and the pharyngeal

reflex and by testing the **heart rate and blood pressure** response to standing.

Requirements

1. Different taste solutions, as described for the seventh nerve
2. Swab stick
3. Aneroid sphygmomanometer

Procedure

1. **Taste sensation:** Ask the subject to sit comfortably on a stool and elicit all the **taste sensations in the posterior third** of the tongue as described for the seventh nerve.
2. **Pharyngeal reflex:** Ask the subject to open his mouth wide. *Tickle the back of the pharynx* with the help of a swab stick and observe the *contraction of the posterior pharyngeal wall* (pharyngeal reflex).
3. **HR and BP response to standing:** Ask the subject to lie down and record his blood pressure. Then ask him to stand up and immediately record his blood pressure (described in Chapter 37).

> **Note:** A fall in systolic BP >20 mmHg or diastolic BP >10 mmHg on standing from the supine position is considered to be **orthostatic hypotension** and may indicate dysfunction of the ninth nerve.

Observation and results

1. Note the intactness of taste sensations from the posterior third of the tongue.
2. Check for the presence of the pharyngeal reflex.
3. Note the HR and BP responses to standing and observe if there is orthostatic hypotension.
4. Comment on the functional integrity of the ninth nerve.

Precautions

1. Follow all instructions used for taste sensation testing of the seventh nerve.
2. Swab sticks should not be placed in the pharynx for a long time to elicit the pharyngeal reflex.
3. The blood pressure should be recorded immediately (preferably within 15 seconds) after standing.

Assessment of the Vagus Nerve

Principle

The vagus nerve supplies *motor fibres to the soft palate, pharynx, and larynx*. It also innervates the respiratory passage and most of the thoracic and abdominal viscera. Therefore, this nerve is tested by eliciting **palatal, pharyngeal, and laryngeal reflexes** and by assessing **visceral functions**.

Requirement

This test only requires a swab stick.

Procedure

1. Ask the subject to open his mouth wide and say "Aaah". Observe the **arch of the palate** and whether it is formed equally on both sides or whether it is flat on one or both sides.
2. Elicit the **pharyngeal reflex** as described for the ninth nerve.
3. The **laryngeal reflex** is tested by laryngoscopy.
4. *Visceral functions* of the tenth nerve can be tested separately.

Observation and results

Note the responses of palatal and pharyngeal reflexes and comment on the functional integrity of the vagus nerve.

Assessment of the Accessory Nerve

Principle

The accessory nerve supplies the **sternomastoid and trapezius muscles**. Therefore, its functions are tested by testing the actions of these muscles.

Requirements

There are no special requirements for this test.

Procedure

1. Stand behind the subject and press his shoulders. Ask the subject to **shrug his shoulders against the passive resistance** (Fig. 56.17).

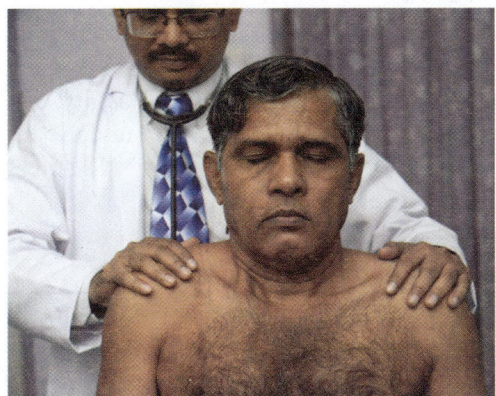

Fig. 56.17 Testing the function of the 11th cranial nerve (trapezius muscle).

Note: This test is performed to assess the function of the trapezius.

2. Ask the subject to **move her chin to one side**. Try to *prevent it by opposing the movement* (Fig. 56.18). Note the **prominence of the sternomastoid muscle** of the *opposite side*. Repeat the procedure by asking the subject to move her chin against resistance to the opposite side (Fig. 56.19). Ask the subject to

depress her chin against the resistance of your hand (Fig. 56.20).

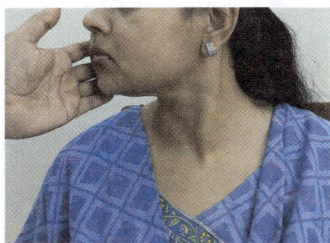

Fig. 56.18 Testing the function of the 11th cranial nerve (sternocleidomastoid muscle of one side).

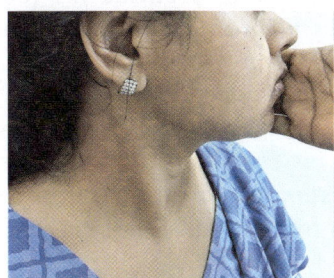

Fig. 56.19 Testing the function of the accessory nerve of the other side.

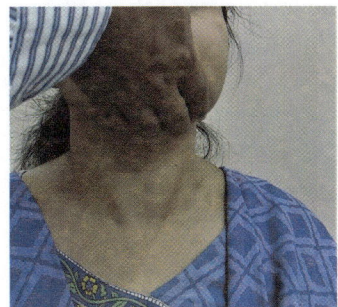

Fig. 56.20 Testing the function of the 11th cranial nerve (sternocleidomastoid muscle of both sides). Note the prominence of both sternocleidomastoid muscles while the subject depresses her chin against resistance.

Note: Movement of the chin to one side against resistance indicates the power of the sternomastoid of the opposite side. Depressing the chin against resistance indicates the power of the sternomastoid of both sides simultaneously.

Observation and results

Note the strength of the sternomastoid and trapezius muscles and comment on the intactness of the 11th cranial nerve.

Precautions

1. The examiner should stand behind the subject while testing the trapezius.
2. While testing for trapezius, press moderately on the shoulders.
3. While testing for the sternomastoid, the examiner should offer gentle resistance against the movement of the chin.

Assessment of the Hypoglossal Nerve

Principle

The hypoglossal nerve is **a pure motor nerve** that supplies the **muscles of the tongue and the depressors of the hyoid bone**. Therefore, this nerve is tested by testing the movement of the tongue and hyoid bone.

Requirements

There are no special requirements for this test.

Procedure

1. Ask the subject to protrude his tongue and note whether the **median raphe of the tongue** is straight or concave towards one side. Also observe whether *atrophy, fasciculation, or tremor* is present.
2. Ask the subject to move his tongue from side to side and *push his cheek laterally* from the inside. Now, apply **resistance against the tongue movements** by pressing it from the outside of the cheek (Fig. 56.21).

Observation and results

Note the strength and functions of the tongue muscle and comment on the intactness of the 12th cranial nerve.

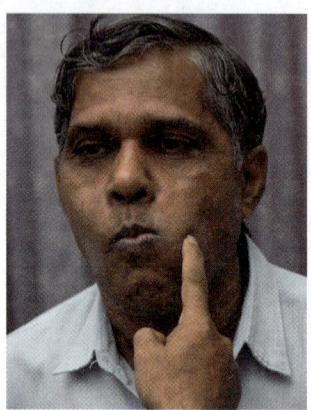

Fig. 56.21   Testing the function of the hypoglossal nerve (strength of the tongue muscle). The subject pushes out his cheek from inside with his tongue, and the examiner resists it from the outside.

DISCUSSION

The cranial nerves are examined thoroughly to detect the abnormalities of these nerves and to localise lesions at various levels of the brainstem. The lesions of the cranial nerve may occur either in the **supranuclear pathway** (in the corticonuclear fibres), **in the nucleus**, or in the **infranuclear pathway**, that is, in the cranial nerves. The nuclear and infranuclear palsies of the cranial nerves, whether unilateral or bilateral, manifest with definite clinical features. On the other hand, *unilateral supranuclear palsies* of most of the cranial nerves *do not manifest with physical signs* because of their **bilateral cortical representation**. Bilateral supranuclear lesions

of the cranial nerves manifest with specific features, especially lesions of the facial and hypoglossal nerves.

Olfactory Nerve

A lesion of the olfactory nerve manifests as various disorders of smell like **anosmia, parosmia, and olfactory hallucinations**. Disorders of smell have been described in detail in Chapter 48.

Anosmia: It is the *complete abolition of the sense of smell*. It can be **unilateral or bilateral**.

1. **Unilateral anosmia:** Seen in tumours of the olfactory bulb, tumours of the frontal lobe, and meningiomas pressing on the olfactory bulb or olfactory tract.
2. **Bilateral anosmia:** Seen in common cold, head injuries in which the cribriform plate of the ethmoid bone is fractured, and atrophic rhinitis.

Hyposmia: It refers to a *decreased sensation of smell*. The causes are the same as those for anosmia.

Parosmia: When the *sensation of smell is perverted*, it is known as parosmia. An offensive smell may seem like a pleasant odour or vice versa. This is also called **cacosmia**.

Causes: It could be a result of a mental disorder or occur as an aura in epilepsy; it is sometimes seen in cases of head injury.

Olfactory hallucination: When the sensation of smell is *perceived without the actual presence of any odour*, it is called an olfactory hallucination.

Causes: It is typically seen as an aura of temporal lobe epilepsy.

Optic Nerve

A lesion of the optic nerve results in defects in the acuity of vision, field of vision, and colour vision. The details of visual field defects, defects of visual acuity, and colour blindness are discussed separately under 'Perimetry', 'Acuity of Vision', and 'Colour Vision' (Chapters 44, 45, and 46, respectively).

Oculomotor Nerve

The lesion of the oculomotor nerve results in **ptosis, nystagmus, abnormal reaction of the pupil** to light and accommodation, **diplopia**, and **defects in eye movement**.

Ptosis

Definition: *Drooping of the eyelid* is called ptosis.

Causes:

1. Impairment of the functions of the third cranial nerve
2. Horner syndrome (sympathetic lesion)
3. Myasthenia gravis (disorder of neuromuscular junction)

The ptosis seen in **Horner syndrome** is always minimal. Therefore, the *presence of gross ptosis excludes sympathetic lesions*. In sympathetic lesions, the pupil of the affected side is smaller (constricted). In **third nerve palsy**, ptosis is complete, and the *pupil of the affected side is larger* (dilated). In **myasthenia**, ptosis is *usually bilateral*, and the pupil *remains unaffected*.

Nystagmus

Definition: This refers to involuntary, rhythmic, and jerky movements of the eyeball. Nystagmus may be **horizontal, vertical, or rotatory**.

Causes:
1. Vestibular lesion
2. Cerebellar lesion
3. Lesion of the third cranial nerve
4. Congenital

Nystagmus of visual origin is usually pendular and often rotatory on central fixation of the eyes.

Pupillary reactions

The pupils constrict in response to light (**light reflex**). The **pathways of direct and indirect light reflexes** are summarised in Fig. 56.22. In the *accommodation reflex*, there is *convergence of the eyeballs, constriction of the pupils, and increased convexity* of the lens. The **pathway of the accommodation reflex** is depicted in Fig. 56.23.

The **different abnormalities** in which pupillary reactions are altered are discussed here.

1. Argyll Robertson pupil (ARP)

Definition: It is characterised by the absence of the reaction of the pupils to light with **preservation of the reaction to accommodation;** the mnemonic **ARP** also stands for accommodation reflex present.

Causes: It is usually seen in **neurosyphilis**. Neurosyphilis has become rare since the advent of modern antibiotics.

2. Adie's pupil

Definition: It is characterised by *extremely decreased reactions* of the pupil *to light and darkness*. In light, the pupil constricts very slowly, and in darkness, it *dilates very slowly*. It also reacts sluggishly to accommodation.

Causes:
1. Holmes-Adie syndrome (decreased tendon reflexes)
2. Sometimes seen in young girls

3. Unilateral dilated and fixed pupil

Cause: Unilateral third nerve palsy. It is associated with ptosis and a laterally deviated eye.

4. Hippus

Definition: Alternating *rhythmic dilatation and constriction* of the pupil in response to light is called hippus.

Cause: It is usually seen in retrobulbar neuritis.

Abnormalities of ocular movement

Normally, the movement of the two eyes is symmetrical, so that the visual axes meet at the point at which the eyes are directed. This is called the **conjugate movement** of the eyes. In **third nerve palsy**, the ability of the eye to move medially, to move upward in the adducted position, and to move upward and downward in the abducted position is lost. The *eye deviates laterally* due to the unopposed

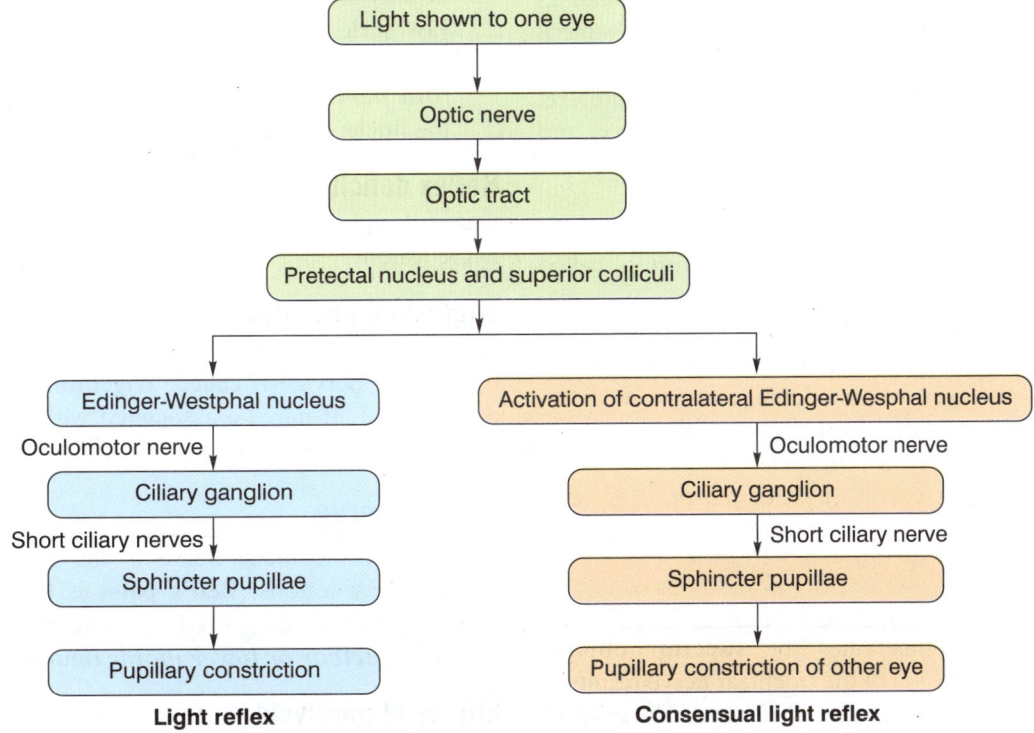

Fig. 56.22   Schematic diagram of the reflex pathway of direct and consensual light reflexes.

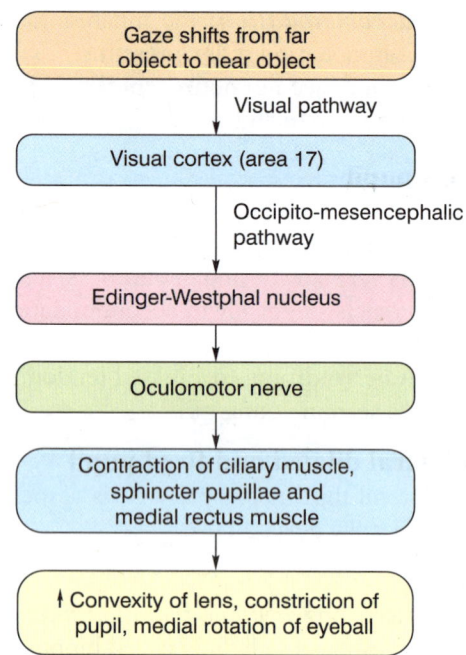

Fig. 56.23 Schematic diagram of the reflex pathway of the accommodation reflex.

action of the lateral rectus, which is supplied by the sixth cranial nerve.

Strabismus

Definition: *Deviation of the eyeball* is called strabismus or *squint*. The visual axes do not meet at the point of fixation.

There are **two types** of strabismus: paralytic and non-paralytic. *Paralytic strabismus* occurs due to weakness of the extraocular muscles. Paralytic strabismus causes *diplopia* (double vision) because the defective movement of one eye results in images formed by the two eyes falling upon non-identical points of the two retinas. Therefore, binocular fusion cannot occur in the visual cortex, and two separate images are perceived.

Diplopia

Definition: The occurrence of **double vision** is called diplopia.

Physiologic basis: Diplopia occurs only over that part of the field of vision *towards which the affected muscles move the eye*. If both the eyes are functional, and one deviates, **binocular diplopia** results. **Monocular diplopia** results from lens *opacities and astigmatism*.

Causes: Diplopia can occur in *third, fourth, and sixth nerve palsy*.

Trochlear Nerve

The trochlear nerve innervates the **superior oblique muscle**. Therefore, a lesion of the trochlear nerve results in *impaired downward movement of the eye*. The *eyeball rotates outward* by the unopposed action of the inferior rectus when the subject attempts to look downward.

Usually, there is *no squint, but diplopia may occur* below the horizontal plane.

Abducent Nerve

The abducent nerve innervates the **lateral rectus muscle**. Therefore, lesions of the sixth nerve result in the **inability to move the eye outwards**, and diplopia occurs when the *subject looks in that direction*. A *convergent squint* may occur because of the unopposed action of the medial rectus.

Trigeminal Nerve

A lesion of the trigeminal nerve results in **sensory and motor deficits**.

Sensory deficits

1. There is a loss of general sensation from different parts of the face depending on the division of the fifth nerve affected.
2. Though the fifth nerve **does not carry** the *taste sensation*, in a **suspected lesion** of the fifth nerve, the *sensation of taste should be examined* because the seventh nerve runs in close association with the fifth nerve in the brain.

Motor deficits

1. Paralysis of the fifth nerve of one side causes the muscles of *mastication on that side to fail to become prominent*. On opening the mouth, the **jaw deviates towards the paralysed side**, pushed over by the healthy lateral pterygoid muscle.
2. **Jaw jerk is diminished** in *infranuclear fifth nerve palsy*. The jaw jerk is **exaggerated in supranuclear fifth nerve palsy** (upper motor neuron lesion above the nucleus of the fifth nerve).

Reflex deficits

Corneal and conjunctival reflexes are abolished in fifth nerve lesions.

Trigeminal neuralgia

Neuralgia (nerve pain) of one or more branches of the trigeminal nerve is called **trigeminal neuralgia** (tic douloureux). It may be associated with sensory loss and muscle weakness in the area of its distribution.

Facial Nerve

A lesion of the facial nerve is the commonest of the cranial nerve lesions. **Bell's palsy** is the most common cranial nerve disorder. It is caused by the paralysis of the *infranuclear or lower motor neuron type*.

Effects of paralysis

Lesions that involve the facial motor nucleus or the infranuclear portion of the facial nerve result in *complete paralysis of all the facial muscles* on the ***ipsilateral side***.

1. The affected side of the face **loses its expression** (inability to frown; Fig. 56.24).
2. The *nasolabial fold* is **less pronounced**.
3. The eye on the affected side is *more widely open* than on the other side and **does not close completely** even during sleep.
4. The *mouth is drawn* to the healthy side.
5. *Food collects between* the lips and gum of the affected side.
6. *Fluid and saliva escape* from the affected angle of the mouth.
7. There is *loss of taste sensation* from the ***anterior two-thirds*** of the tongue. However, if the lesion is below the joining of the chorda tympani nerve that is distal to the stylomastoid foramen, taste will not be affected.

Types of paralysis

Facial nerve lesion may be **infranuclear or supranuclear**.

■ Infranuclear facial palsy

This is the commonest of all lesions of the cranial nerves. Idiopathic infranuclear facial palsy is called **Bell's palsy**. It usually occurs due to **viral infection,** or it may be **idiopathic**. The common features are:

1. *Both the upper and lower parts of the face* are **equally affected**.
2. *Taste sensation may be lost*, depending on the site of lesion.
3. There is ***no involvement of emotional components*** of facial expression.

■ Supranuclear facial palsy

Facial palsy due to a lesion above the nucleus, *involving the corticonuclear fibres*, is called supranuclear facial palsy. The common features are:

1. The ***lower part of the face is majorly affected,*** whereas the upper part of the face is either totally spared or affected minimally. This is because the frontal belly of the occipitofrontalis has bilateral cortical innervation.

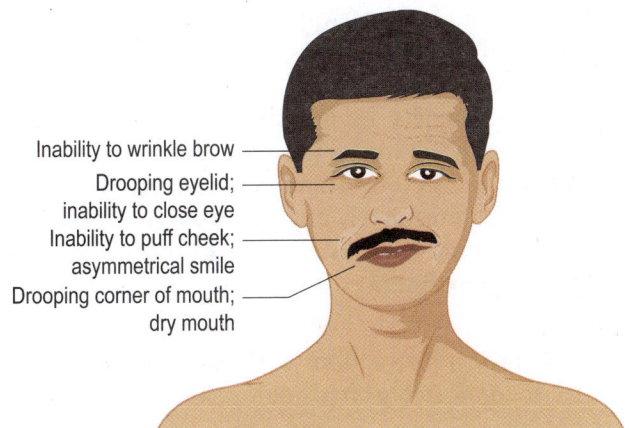

2. Taste sensation may not be altered.
3. The *muscles of the voluntary movement* of the face are ***paralysed***, but muscles involved in *emotional expressions* of the face, e.g., crying, remain ***intact or exaggerated (mimicking paralysis)***. This occurs because the emotional movements are not dependent on the same cortical innervation as voluntary movements.

Vestibulocochlear Nerve

The effect of **cochlear nerve lesions** is discussed separately in Chapter 47.

Effect of lesions of the vestibular nerve

1. The patient complains of *vertigo, dizziness, and giddiness*. **Vertigo** is the sensation of rotation in the absence of actual rotation (hallucination of movement).
2. The patient may vomit. **Nystagmus** may be present.
3. Orientation in space may be lost.

Glossopharyngeal Nerve

Effects of paralysis

1. Loss of **taste and general sensation from the posterior third** of the tongue.
2. **Absence of pharyngeal reflex** and *difficulty in swallowing*.
3. Decreased secretion of saliva.
4. *Orthostatic hypotension* may occur.

Vagus Nerve

Effects of paralysis

1. **Loss of the pharyngeal and palatal reflex**. Swallowing becomes difficult.
2. *Nasal regurgitation* of fluid may occur.
3. **Uvula deviates** to the *healthy side*.
4. *Paralysis of the vocal cord* causes **aphonia**.
5. **Paralysis of the larynx** (all the muscles of the larynx except the cricothyroid are supplied by the recurrent laryngeal nerve, a branch of the vagus nerve) results in hoarseness of the voice.
6. There is impairment of sensation from many organs.
7. Increase in heart rate and *impairment in the regulation of blood pressure*.

Accessory Nerve

A lesion of the accessory nerve results in the **inability to raise the shoulders** and **difficulty in turning the head**. There may be ***drooping of the shoulders***.

Hypoglossal Nerve

The features of hypoglossal nerve lesions depend on the **type of paralysis**.

Inability to wrinkle brow
Drooping eyelid;
inability to close eye
Inability to puff cheek;
asymmetrical smile
Drooping corner of mouth;
dry mouth

Fig. 56.24   Features of facial nerve palsy of the LMN type.

Lower motor neuron paralysis

■ Unilateral paralysis

The common features are:

1. **Tongue is pushed** to the *paralysed side*.
2. *Median raphe becomes concave* towards the paralysed side.
3. **Atrophy** (with flaccidity) of the tongue occurs on the affected side.
4. **Fasciculation** may be seen on the affected side.

■ Bilateral paralysis

The common features are:

1. Marked **wasting with fasciculation** *on both sides*.
2. Protrusion of the tongue becomes impossible.
3. **Dysarthria** and difficulty in pronouncing 'T' and 'D' may be seen.

Upper motor neuron paralysis

■ Unilateral paralysis

The common features are:

1. *Usually asymptomatic*.
2. Tongue may be pushed to the opposite side.

■ Bilateral paralysis

The common features are:

1. Tongue is **spastic**.
2. **Dysarthria** may be associated with *emotional disturbances*.
3. **Dysphagia** may be present. This is due to the inability to swallow because the tongue cannot manipulate food properly.

OSPE

I.   Check the acuity of vision of the subject by the confrontation test.

Steps

1. Give proper instructions to the subject.
2. Make the subject sit comfortably on a stool.
3. Sit at a distance of about 3 feet from the subject, taking care that your eye level remains at the eye level of the subject.
4. Ask the subject to fix his gaze at the tip of his nose and instruct him to say 'yes' when he sees the tip of his finger in the field of vision.
5. Ask the subject to close one of his eyes and close your opposite eye.
6. Move your finger midway between yourself and the subject from the periphery to the centre of the four quadrants to check the field of vision.
7. Compare the field of vision of the subject with your own field of vision.
8. Repeat the procedure with the other eye.

II.   Examine the III, IV, and VI cranial nerves of the subject and report your findings.

Steps

1. Instruct the subject to look at the tip of your finger and follow the movement of the finger.
2. Bring the tip of your index finger to the eye level of the subject, keeping a distance of 25 cm from the subject's eye.
3. Examine the functions of different extrinsic muscles of the eye by making appropriate movements with the finger.
4. Ask the subject to look straight at a distant object and then ask him to look immediately at the fingertip brought close to his eyes.
5. Examine the pupillary reflex (both direct and consensual) by focusing light to the eye of the subject. For this, focus the light by bringing it from the side of the head of the subject and by placing a piece of cardboard between the two eyes.

III.   Examine the VII cranial nerve of the subject and report your findings.

Steps

1. Give proper instructions to the subject.
2. Ask the subject to frown.
3. Ask the subject to shut his eyes against (examiner's) resistance.
4. Ask the subject to show his teeth, smile, and whistle.
5. Ask the subject to inflate his mouth and blow out his cheeks.
6. Ask the subject to clench his teeth. Look for the prominence of the platysma muscle.
7. Ask for testing taste sensations from the anterior two-thirds of the tongue (need not perform).

IV.   Examine the IX cranial nerve of the subject and report your findings.

Steps

1. Give proper instructions to the subject and ask him to sit comfortably on a stool.
2. Ask the subject to open his mouth wide, and with the help of a swab stick, tickle the back of the pharynx and observe the contraction of the posterior pharyngeal wall.
3. Ask the subject to lie down. Record his blood pressure in the supine position.
4. As the subject to stand and record the blood pressure immediately after the subject stands.

V.   Examine the XI cranial nerve of the subject and report your findings.

Steps

1. Give proper instructions to the subject and ask him to sit comfortably on a stool.

2. Stand behind the subject and place your hands on both the shoulders.
3. Ask the subject to elevate his shoulders and try to prevent this by applying counterpressure.
4. Ask the subject to move his chin to one side. Try to prevent it by opposing his chin movement and look for the prominence of the sternocleidomastoid muscle of the opposite side of the neck.
5. Repeat the procedure to check the action of the sternocleidomastoid muscle of the opposite side.

VI. Examine the XII cranial nerves of the subject and report your findings.

Steps

1. Give proper instructions to the subject.
2. Ask the subject to protrude his tongue and observe for the presence of fasciculation, tremor, or atrophy. Also check the position of the median raphe of the tongue.
3. Ask the subject to move his tongue to one side and to push the cheek of that side from inside. While the subject does this, try to assess the strength of the tongue by offering resistance from outside the cheek.
4. Repeat the procedure by asking the subject to push the cheek of the opposite side.

VIVA

1. *What parameters are tested to assess the higher functions?* (Ans. Refer to page 373, under the heading 'Higher Functions'.)
2. *What is the importance of testing speech in the examination of the nervous system?* (Ans. Refer to page 373, under the heading 'Speech Functions'.)
3. *Which cranial nerves are functionally sensory, motor, and mixed?* (Ans. Refer to page 374, under the heading 'Clinical Examination of the CN' and the subheading 'Introduction'.)
4. *What is the pathway for olfactory nerves?* (Ans. Refer to page 374, under the heading 'Olfactory nerve' and the subheading 'Anatomy'.)
5. *What are the precautions taken while examining the olfactory nerve.* (Ans. Refer to page 377, under the heading 'Examination of Olfactory nerve' and the subheading 'Precautions'.)
6. *What is meant by anosmia and parosmia? What are their causes?* (Ans. Refer to page 384, under the headings 'Anosmia' and 'Parosmia'.)
7. *Why should a distance of 3 feet be maintained between the subject and the examiner while performing the confrontation test and detecting acuity of vision?* (Ans. Refer to page 377, under the heading 'Assessment of the Optic Nerve' and the subheading 'Confrontation Test'.)
8. *Why should a distance of 25 cm be maintained between the subject's eye and the examiner's finger for assessing eye movements?* (Ans. Refer to page 377, See 'Assessment of the Optic Nerve' and the subheading 'Confrontation Test' and Fig. 56.4.)
9. *What are the effects of a lesion of the third cranial nerve?* (Ans. Refer to page 384, under the heading 'Oculomotor nerve'.)
10. *What is diplopia, and what are its causes?* (Ans. Refer to page 386, under the heading 'Oculomotor nerve' and the subheading 'Diplopia'.)
11. *What is ptosis, and what are its causes?* (Ans. Refer to page 384, under the heading 'Oculomotor nerve' and the subheading 'Ptosis'.)
12. *What is nystagmus?* (Ans. Refer to page 385, under the heading 'Oculomotor nerve' and the subheading 'Nystagmus'.)
13. *Describe Argyl Robertson pupil and Adie's pupil.* (Ans. Refer to page 385, under the heading 'Oculomotor nerve' and the subheadings 'Argyl Robertson pupil' and 'Adie's pupil'.)
14. *What are the causes of unilateral dilated and fixed pupil?* (Ans. Refer to page 386, under the heading 'Oculomotor nerve' and the subheading 'Unilateral dilated and fixed pupil'.)
15. *What are the divisions of the fifth cranial nerve, and what are their functions?* (Ans. Refer to page 375, under the heading 'Trigeminal nerve'.)
16. *How do you test for the motor function of the fifth cranial nerve?* (Ans. Refer to page 379, under the heading 'Assessment of the Trigeminal Nerve'.)
17. *Why is the fourth cranial nerve more liable to be affected by raised intracranial pressure?* (Ans. Refer to page 375, under the heading 'Trochlear nerve' and the subheading 'Anatomy'.)
18. *What is the course of the seventh cranial nerve?* (Ans. Refer to page 376, under the heading 'Facial nerve', Fig. 56.3.)
19. *How do you test the motor functions of the seventh cranial nerve?* (Ans. Refer to page 380, under the heading 'Assessment of the Facial Nerve'.)
20. *Why is the facial nerve more prone to injury in the facial canal?* (Ans. Refer to page 375, under the heading 'Facial nerve' and the subheading 'Sensory component'.)

21. *What is Bell's palsy?* (Ans. Refer to page 387, See 'Infranuclear Facial Palsy' and the subheading 'Bell's palsy'.)
22. *Differentiate between supranuclear and infranuclear palsy of the seventh nerve?* (Ans. Refer to page 387, under the headings 'Infranuclear Facial Palsy' and 'Supranuclear Facial Palsy'.)
23. *Why does the upper part of the face escape the effects of supranuclear seventh nerve palsy?* (Ans. Refer to page 387, under the heading 'Supranuclear Facial Palsy'.)
24. *How do you assess the functions of the vestibular division of the eight nerve?* (Ans. Refer to page 381, under the heading 'Assessment of the Vestibulocochlear Nerve'.)
25. *What are the functions of the ninth cranial nerve?* (Ans. Refer to page 376, under the heading 'Ninth Cranial Nerve' and the subheading 'Functions'.)
26. *What are the effects of a lesion of the ninth cranial nerve?* (Ans. Refer to page 387, under the heading 'Glossopharyngeal Nerve'.)
27. *What are the functions of the vagus nerve?* (Ans. Refer to page 376, under the heading 'Vagus Nerve' and the subheading 'Functions'.)
28. *What are the effects of a lesion of the vagus nerve?* (Ans. Refer to page 387, under the heading 'Vagus Nerve', and the subheading 'Effects of paralysis'.)
29. *How do you assess the functions of the eleventh cranial nerve?* (Ans. Refer to page 378, under the heading 'Accessory Nerve'.)
30. *What are the effects of a lesion of the eleventh cranial nerve?* (Ans. Refer to page 383, under the heading 'Accessory Nerve'.)
31. *How do you assess the functions of the twelfth cranial nerve?* (Ans. Refer to page 384, under the heading 'Hypoglossal Nerve'.)
32. *What are the effects of a lesion of the twelfth cranial nerve?* (Ans. Refer to page 388, under the heading 'Hypoglossal Nerve' and the subheading 'LMN and UMN paralysis'.)

57 | Clinical Examination of the Nervous System II (Sensory System)

Learning Objectives

After completing this practical, you will be able to (MUST KNOW):

1. Describe the importance of performing this practical in clinical physiology.
2. Classify different sensations and receptors.
3. Draw the sensory map of the body.
4. Elicit all the sensations.
5. List the precautions taken while eliciting sensations.
6. Trace the pathway of all sensations.
7. Name the common abnormalities of sensations.

You may also be able to (DESIRABLE TO KNOW):

1. Explain the abnormalities of sensations.
2. Correlate the clinical findings with abnormalities, if present.
3. Localise the diseases affecting different parts of the sensory system.
4. Explain the effects of lesions at various levels in the sensory pathways.

PY5.15: Demonstrate the correct clinical examination of the nervous system: higher functions, sensory system, motor system, reflexes, and cranial nerves in a normal volunteer or simulated environment.

CLINICAL EXAMINATION OF THE SENSORY SYSTEM

INTRODUCTION

Anatomical and Physiological Considerations

The sensory information conveyed to the central nervous system by the peripheral nerves originates in special structures distributed in the skin, subcutaneous tissues, muscles, tendons, and joints known as **receptors**. These are *modified nerve endings*. From the peripheral nerves, the sensations enter the spinal cord through the *posterior nerve roots*. In the spinal cord, the sensations ascend in **different sensory tracts** to finally reach the sensory cortex via the thalamus. *Some of the sensory inputs also reach the cerebellum*; these inputs are chiefly **unconscious proprioceptive** and **kinesthetic sensations,** which are involved in the modulation of motor activities.

Sensory Modalities

Sensations are broadly classified into **general sensations, special sensations, and visceral sensations.**

General sensations: The different types of general sensations are touch and pressure, warmth, cold, pain, vibration, and movement and position of joints (proprioception).

Special sensations: Sensations that originate in the special sensory receptors present in structures like the eye and ear are called special sensations. These are vision, hearing, smell, taste, and acceleration (rotational and linear). They have been discussed in Chapters 44 to 48.

Visceral sensations: Sensations that originate in visceral structures are referred to as visceral sensations. Some examples of visceral sensations are lung inflation, distension of the stomach, and changes in arterial blood pressure.

Receptors

Receptors are transducers that convert various forms of *energy in the environment into action potentials* in the neurons. They may be a part of the neuron or a specialised cell that generates action potential in the neurons. Very often, receptors are associated with **non-neural cells** that surround them to form a **sense organ.**

Types of receptors

Receptors are divided into **four categories:**

1. **Exteroceptors:** These receptors are concerned with **changes in the external environment** close to the body. Exteroceptors are distributed on the *surface of the body*, in the skin and subcutaneous tissues. These cutaneous sense organs are broadly divided into expanded endings and encapsulated endings.

   The **expanded endings** are:
   - Merkel's discs
   - Ruffini endings

   Merkel's discs and Ruffini endings are **slow-adapting touch receptors.**

The **encapsulated endings** are:
- Pacinian corpuscles
- Meissner's corpuscles
- Krause's end-bulbs

Meissner's and Pacinian corpuscles are **rapidly adapting touch receptors**. Most of these sensory endings are present ***around the hair follicles***. Therefore, the *slightest movement of hair* elicits the sensation of touch. Some of these endings, especially Ruffini endings and Pacinian corpuscles, are also found in deep fibrous tissues.

> **Note:** It appears that none of these endings is needed for the elicitation of sensations because sensory modalities can be elicited from areas that contain only free nerve endings.

2. **Interoceptors:** These are concerned with **changes in the internal environment** of the body, e.g., osmoreceptors respond to changes in the osmolality of body fluids.
3. **Proprioceptors:** These provide information about the **position of the body in space** at any given time. The conscious component of proprioception comes from the receptors in the joints and from cutaneous touch and pressure receptors.
4. **Teleceptors:** These are concerned with the events that occur at a distance from the body.

Sensory Pathways

Sensory pathways are divided into **two systems**. The pathways that ascend the posterior column of the spinal cord are frequently called the **lemniscal system**

(Fig. 57.1A) and the pathways that ascend the anterior and lateral quadrants of the spinal cord are referred to as the **anterolateral system** (Fig. 57.1B). The neurons in the sensory pathways are placed in sequential order and accordingly called *first, second, and third orders of neurons*.

1. The **first order of neurons** sends encoded information from the receptors to the spinal cord and medulla.
2. The **second order of neurons** transmits the impulse from the spinal cord and medulla to the thalamus, from where the **third order of neurons** conveys the information to the cortex.

Fine touch

Touch receptors are present in *large numbers in the skin of the fingers and lips* and in fewer numbers in the skin of the trunk.

1. The **first order of neurons** carrying fine touch sensation enters the spinal cord via the posterior root and then ascends the dorsal column of the spinal cord on the same side. They terminate in the **nucleus gracilis and cuneatus** of the medulla.
2. The **second order of neurons** arises from these nuclei, crosses to the opposite side in the medulla, and ascends the **contralateral medial lemniscus** to terminate in the **ventral posterior nucleus** and related *specific sensory nuclei* of the **thalamus**.
3. The **third order of neurons** arises from the thalamus and reaches the **sensory cortex via thalamic radiation**.

The **sensations that are carried in the posterior column** of the spinal cord are:

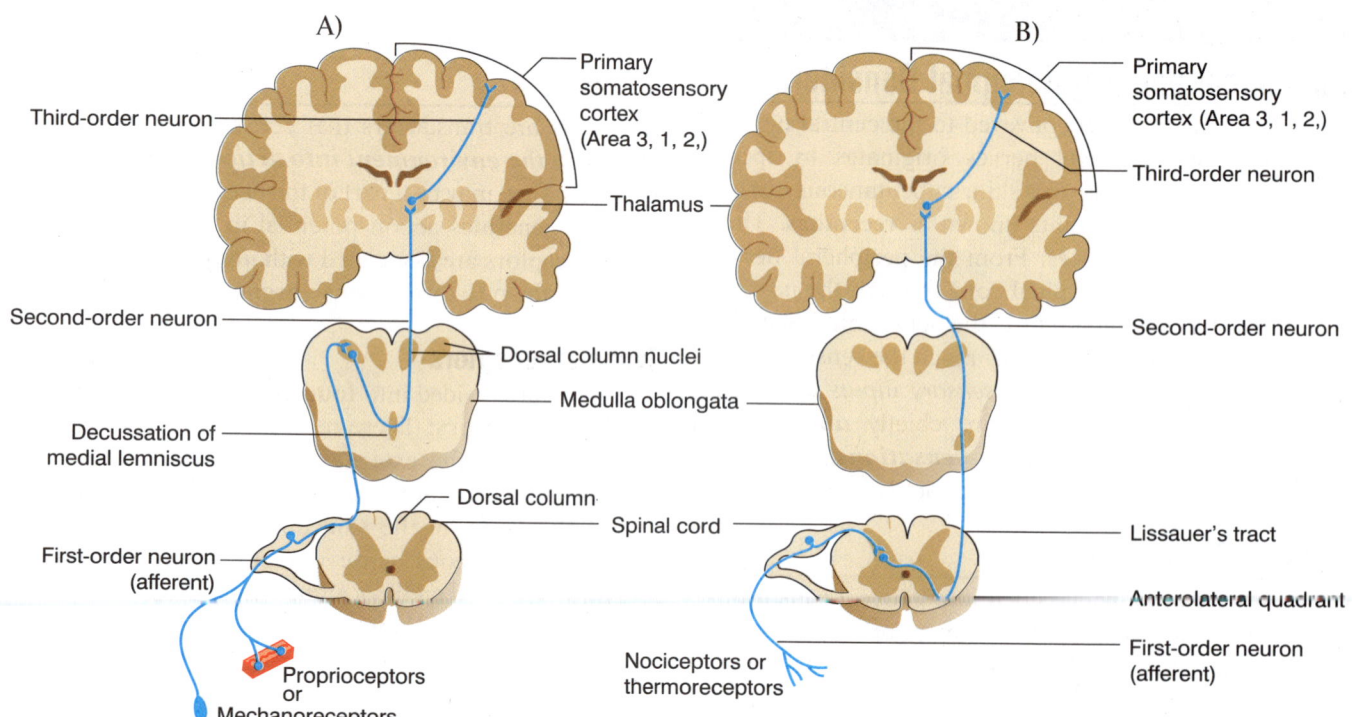

Fig. 57.1   Sensory pathways: **(A)** Dorsal column (lemniscal) pathway and **(B)** anterolateral (spinothalamic) pathway.

1. Fine touch
2. Proprioception (joint sensation and sense of position)
3. Sense of vibration
4. Tactile localisation
5. Two-point discrimination
6. Stereognosis

Crude touch

The *first order of neurons,* after entering the spinal cord, synapses on the *second order of neurons* in the dorsal horn of the cord. The second order of neurons crosses to *the opposite side* at that spinal segment and ascends up in the *contralateral ventral spinothalamic tract (anterolateral system)* to terminate in the *specific sensory relay nuclei* of the thalamus. The *third order of neurons* arises from the thalamus and terminates in the sensory cortex through thalamic radiation.

The **sensations that are carried in the anterolateral system** of the spinal cord are:

1. Crude touch
2. Pressure
3. Pain
4. Temperature (cold and warmth)

Sense of vibration

The pathway for the sense of vibration is the *same as that of fine touch.* The sensation of vibration is called **pallesthesia**. It is detected by mechanoreceptors, such as the Pacinian corpuscles, which respond to pressure and vibration. From the vibrating tuning fork, the vibration sensation is transmitted through the skin and bones to the mechanoreceptors in the tissues responsible for detecting vibration.

Pallhypesthesia: A diminished sense of vibration is known as pallhypesthesia. Loss or impairment of the vibration sensation may be associated with neurological disorders such as multiple sclerosis.

Proprioception

The pathway for proprioceptive inputs is the *same as that of fine touch.* A large part of proprioceptive input *goes to the cerebellum* in addition to its projection to the sensory cortex, which is involved in the modulation of motor activities.

Pain

The sense organs for pain are free nerve endings. The sensation of pain is transmitted to the central nervous system by a **two-fibre system**. The **Aδ fibres** carry fast pain whereas the **C fibres** carry slow pain.

1. The *Aδ fibres terminate mainly* on the neurons in **laminas I and V**, and the C fibres terminate on the neurons in **laminas I and II**.
2. The **second order of neurons** crosses to the opposite side of the spinal cord, at the same segmental level, and then ascends the *contralateral lateral spinothalamic* tract to terminate in the *specific sensory relay nuclei* in the thalamus.
3. From the thalamus, the **third order of neurons** arises and projects to the **sensory cortex**.

Many fibres activated by pain terminate in the reticular system, from where they project into the **midline and intralaminar** (*non-specific projection*) nuclei of the thalamus and from there, to *different parts of the cortex.* Many pain fibres also **terminate in the periaqueductal gray** in the midbrain.

Temperature

There are **two types of sense organs** for temperature sensation: one type for eliciting cold and the other one for eliciting warmth. The **afferents for cold are Aδ fibres and C fibres**, and **for warmth, only C fibres**.

1. The **first order of neurons** terminates at the same segmental level of the spinal cord.
2. The **second order of neurons** crosses to the opposite side and ascends the **contralateral lateral spinothalamic tract** to terminate in the thalamus from where the **third order of neurons** arises and terminates in the sensory cortex.

The **receptors and pathways** for various sensations are summarised in Table 57.1.

Table 57.1 Testing primary sensations.

Sensations	Testing method/object	Receptors	Afferent fibre size	Pathway
Pain	Pinprick	Cutaneous nociceptors	Small	Spinothalamic, also D
Temperature, heat	Warm metal object	Cutaneous thermoreceptors for heat	Small	Spinothalamic
Temperature, cold	Cold metal object	Cutaneous thermoreceptors for cold	Small	Spinothalamic
Touch	Cotton wisp, fine brush	Cutaneous mechanoreceptors, also naked endings	Large and small	Lemniscal (fine touch), also D and spinothalamic (crude touch)
Vibration	Tuning fork of 128 Hz	Mechanoreceptors, especially Pacinian corpuscles	Large	Lemniscal, also D
Joint position	Passive movement of specific joints	Joint capsule and tendon endings, muscle spindles	Large	Lemniscal, also D

D: diffuse ascending projections in ipsilateral and contralateral anterolateral columns; lemniscal: posterior column and lemniscal projection, ipsilateral; spinothalamic: spinothalamic projection, contralateral

Sensory Map

The spinal cord is made up of different segments. From each segment, a pair of motor and sensory nerve roots arise. The *sensory fibres from each segment* innervate a **specific dermatome of the body**. This **dermatomal innervation by sensory fibres constitutes the sensory map of the body** (Fig. 57.2). Sensations are elicited from the skin of different dermatomes to check the *intactness of a particular segment* of the spinal cord.

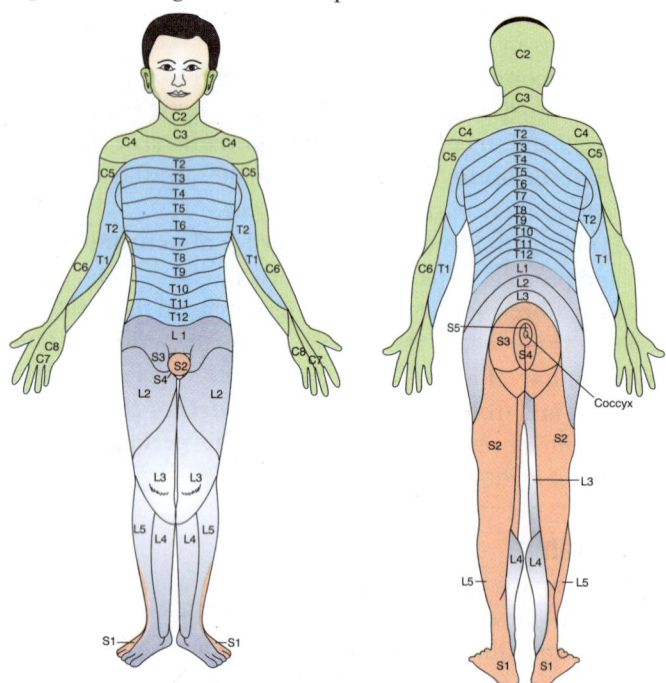

Fig. 57.2   Sensory map of the body.

METHODS OF EXAMINING THE SENSORY SYSTEM

Principle

Different sensory modalities are elicited from the different dermatomes of the two sides and compared.

Requirements

1. Cotton
2. Von Frey's hair aesthesiometer (Fig. 57.3)
3. Compass aesthesiometer (Fig. 57.4)
4. Tuning fork (128 Hz)
5. Pin
6. Algometer
7. Test tubes containing warm and cold water
8. Ballpoint pens

Procedure

The following different forms of sensation are tested.
1. **Tactile sensibility,** which includes:

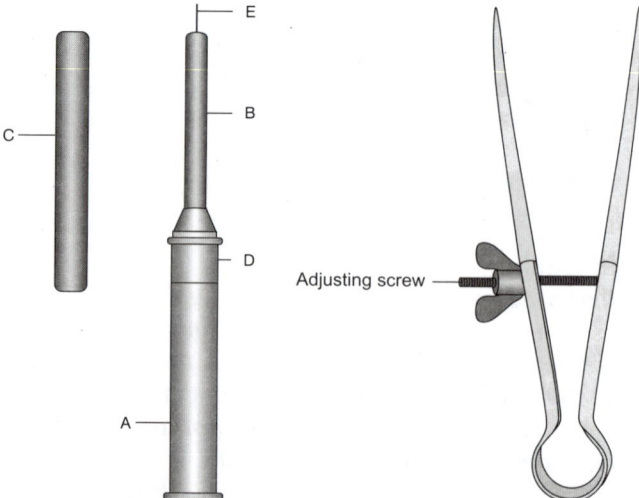

Fig. 57.3   Von Frey's hair aesthesiometer (A: body; B: sliding graduated tube; C: protective cap; D: body tube; E: protruding horsehair).

Fig. 57.4   Compass aesthesiometer.

- Fine touch
- Pressure (crude touch)
- *Tactile localisation* (ability to localise the point on the surface of the body that is being touched)
- *Two-point discrimination* (ability to discriminate between two points that are being touched simultaneously)
- *Stereognosis* (ability to feel and recognise familiar objects by their size, shape, and form)

2. **Position sense,** and the appreciation of passive movements (**proprioception**)
3. **Vibration**
4. **Pain**
5. **Temperature**

Fine touch
◼ Steps

1. Provide proper instructions to the subject (to raise his finger or say "Yes" when he feels the sensation of touch).
2. Ask the subject to close his eyes.
3. With the **help of cotton wool** (Fig. 57.5A) or **Von Frey's hair aesthesiometer** (Fig. 57.5B) lightly touch the skin on different parts of the subject's body.
4. If the subject raises his finger or says "Yes", **ask whether the sensation felt is normal or altered**. If the subject does not feel the sensation, compare carefully with the corresponding area on the opposite part of the body.
5. Elicit the sensation dermatome-wise on both sides of the body.

> **Note:** Areas of hypoasthesia, parasthesia, or hyperesthesia, if present, should be properly delineated.

6. Note down your observations.

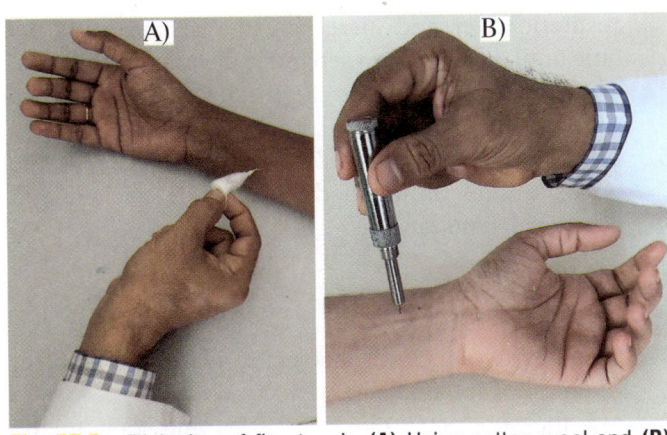

Fig. 57.5 Elicitation of fine touch: **(A)** Using cotton wool and **(B)** using a hair aesthesiometer.

Precautions

1. The subject should be properly instructed about the procedure to gain maximum cooperation.
2. The subject should keep his eyes closed throughout the procedure.
3. Sensations should be elicited according to the different dermatomes of the body.
4. Sensation of the corresponding area on the opposite side of the body should also be elicited simultaneously and compared.
5. If the sensation is altered in a particular part of the body, the area of altered sensation should be properly delineated.

Pressure (crude touch)
Steps

1. Provide proper instructions to the subject.
2. Ask the subject to close her eyes and look to the opposite side.
3. Elicit the pressure sensation by **pressing down with your fingertip** on the skin of different dermatomes (Fig. 57.6).

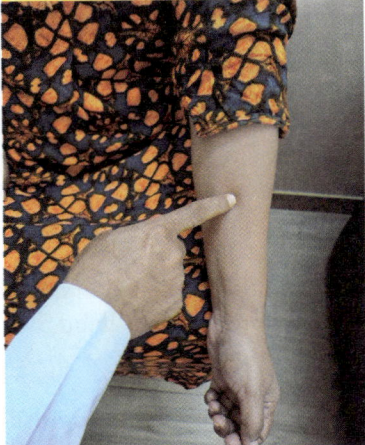

Fig. 57.6 Elicitation of crude touch.

4. Record your observations.

Precautions
Same as those described for 'Fine touch'.

Tactile localisation
Steps

1. Provide instructions to the subject to localise (with the help of a ballpoint pen) the part of the body that is being touched by the tip of the pen.
2. Ask the subject to **hold a pen and close her eyes** (Fig. 57.7A).
3. **Touch the skin of one area** of the patient's body with the help of a ball pen and ask the **subject to immediately localise** that point by touching it with the pen that he is holding.
4. **Measure the distance** between the two points (this is called the **localisation distance**) (Fig. 57.7B).

> **Note:** This distance varies greatly in different parts of the body. It corresponds to the **concentration of touch spots,** which are numerous on the tips of the fingers and palms and fewer on the back. The localisation distance is less if the concentration of touch spots is more.

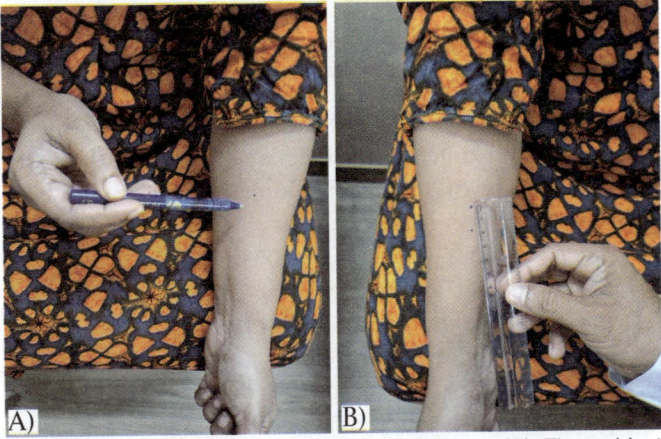

Fig. 57.7 Demonstration of tactile localisation: **(A)** The subject holding the pen and using it to touch the point being touched and **(B)** the distance between the two points (examiner's touch point and subject's touch point) is the localisation distance.

5. Likewise, determine the localisation distance on different parts of the body on both sides.

Precautions

1. The subject should be instructed properly regarding his role in the experiment.
2. The subject should keep his eyes closed throughout the procedure.
3. Sensations should be elicited according to different dermatomes of the body.

4. The localisation distance of the corresponding area on the opposite side of the body should be elicited simultaneously and compared.

Two-point discrimination

Steps

1. Instruct the subject to say whether she **feels the touch of one point or two points** when she is touched with a compass aesthesiometer. Use a *smaller aesthesiometer for the fingers* and hand, and a *big aesthesiometer for the forearm and trunk* of the body (Fig. 57.8A).
2. Ask the subject to close her eyes.

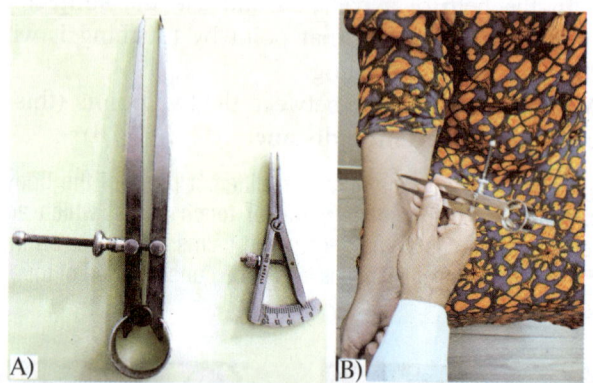

Fig. 57.8 **(A)** Big and small Weber's compass aesthesiometers and **(B)** procedure of testing for two-point discrimination.

3. Separate the two limbs of the compass aesthesiometer a little and touch the subject's skin **lightly with the two points of the aesthesiometer simultaneously.** Ask the subject to say whether she is being touched at one or two points (Fig. 57.8B).
4. If the subject appreciates only one point, *increase the distance between two points a little more* and keep *repeating the test till two separate points* are appreciated by the subject (the distance between two points when the subject feels it as two points is called the **minimum separable distance**).

Note: This distance varies greatly in different parts of the body according to the richness of the touch spots. Normally, it is about 2 mm on the fingertips, 5 mm on the hands, and more on other parts of the body.

5. Record the minimum separable distance on different parts of the body on both sides.

Precautions

1. Proper instruction should be given to the subject to gain maximum cooperation.
2. The subject should keep her eyes closed throughout the procedure.
3. The sensation should be elicited starting with the minimum distance between the two limbs of the

aesthesiometer and increasing the distance little by little until the minimum separable distance is obtained.

4. The two points of the aesthesiometer should be touched simultaneously.
5. The sensation of the corresponding part on the opposite side of the body should be elicited and compared simultaneously.

Stereognosis

Steps

1. Give instructions to the subject to **identify the object** when asked to handle it.
2. Ask the subject to close her eyes and look to the opposite side.
3. Place a **familiar object** in one hand of the subject and ask her to recognise it **by palpating the object** (Fig. 57.9A and B).
4. Repeat the procedure with *four or five familiar objects.*
5. Repeat the procedure with the opposite hand.

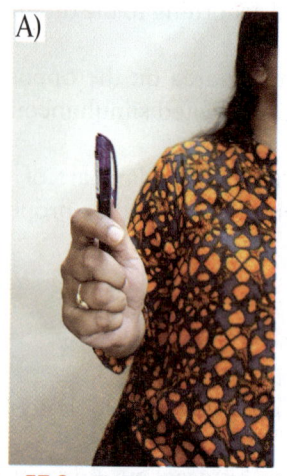
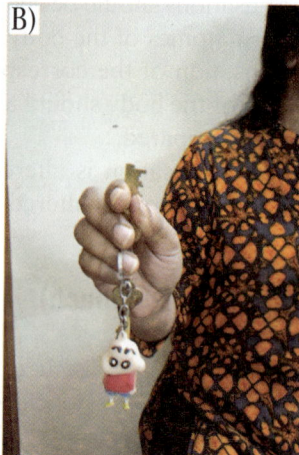

Fig. 57.9 Demonstration of the elicitation of stereognosis with **(A)** a pen and **(B)** a key chain.

Precautions

1. The subject should be instructed properly.
2. The subject should keep her eyes closed throughout the experiment.
3. The sensation should be elicited by giving the subject objects that are familiar to her.
4. The test should be repeated with at least three different objects.
5. The sensation should be elicited in one hand at a time and then repeated in the other hand.

Graphesthesia

Graphesthesia is the ability to **recognise writing on the skin through touch, without using vision.** It is a neurological function that involves the combined sensory and cortical processes of the somatosensory system.

Testing graphesthesia

Graphesthesia is typically tested by writing **numbers, letters, or shapes** on a patient's skin, usually the hand, while they have their eyes closed, and then asking them to identify what was drawn.

1. Ask the subject to close his eyes.
2. With an ink pen, write the number 7 (or any other number) on the subject's hand and ask him to identify the number (Fig. 57.10).

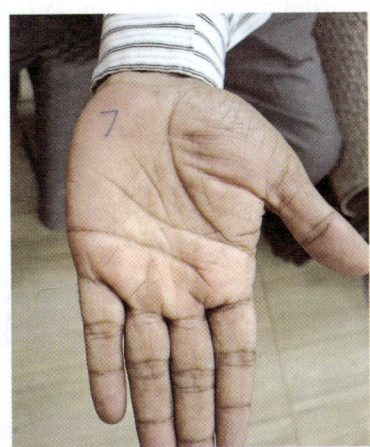

Fig. 57.10   Demonstration of eliciting graphesthesia. The number '7' is written on the hand, and the subject is asked to identify the number.

Physiological and clinical importance

Graphesthesia is a measure of fine tactile discrimination, the ability to distinguish between **different shapes and textures** on the skin.

Neurological Basis: It relies on intact sensory receptors in the skin, as well as the brain's ability to process and interpret those sensations.

Significance: Graphesthesia is a 'soft' neurological sign, meaning that it is not always present in every individual and can be affected by a variety of factors, including neurological conditions, learning disabilities, and even psychiatric disorders.

Loss of graphesthesia: The absence of graphesthesia—agraphesthesia—can be a sign of *damage to the parietal lobe, thalamus, or secondary somatosensory cortex* of the brain. It can also be associated with conditions such as multiple sclerosis, stroke, dementia, and brain injuries.

Sense of position and joint movement

This is tested by passively moving the subject's limbs to a specific position while his eyes are closed and asking him to recognise the position of the limb. The perception of movement is closely related to the sense of position; therefore, both senses are tested together.

Steps

1. Give proper instructions to the subject (to recognise the particular position of the limb when it is moved).
2. Ask him to close his eyes.
3. Move the subject's finger or hand up or down and ask him to identify the movement either by calling out the position of the finger/limb or by imitating the same movement with the other limb.
4. Repeat the procedure by changing the position of all limbs.
5. Make movements at all the joints (all small and big joints) and ask the subject to recognise the joint movement (Fig. 57.11A and B).

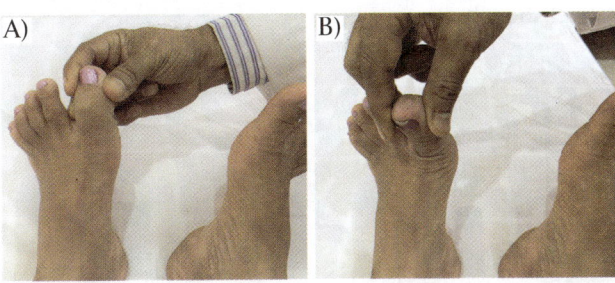

Fig. 57.11   Demonstration of joint movement by bending the great toe: **(A)** By forward bending and **(B)** by backward bending.

Note: Note the angle through which the limb was moved. If the sense of movement is decreased, this angle is greater than that in the normal limb. Movements of less than 10° are appreciated at all the normal joints.

6. Make a particular movement (flexion or extension at a joint) and ask the subject to recognise the direction of movement.

Note: The patient can sometimes recognise the occurrence of a movement but not its direction. The Romberg test for assessing body position is described in Chapter 58, under 'Coordination of Movement'.

Precautions

1. The subject should be properly instructed in order to get their full cooperation in the experiment.
2. The subject should keep his eyes closed during the experiment.
3. Movements at different joints and the position of different parts of the limbs should be performed.
4. Sensations should be elicited on both sides of the body and compared simultaneously.

Sense of vibration
Steps

1. Provide proper instructions to the subject.
2. Make the tuning fork vibrate by hitting the blades of the fork against the hypothenar eminence of the palm or the thigh.

3. Place the foot of the vibrating tuning fork on the surface of the subject's body, ideally **on a bony prominence** like the *lower end of the tibia, styloid process* of the ulnar (Fig. 57.12A), or the *medial or lateral malleolus* (Fig. 57.12B), and ask the subject whether he feels the vibration.

> **Note:** The vibrating tuning fork is placed on the surface of the body, especially *on a bony prominence* because **bones are good at transmitting vibration** to the receptors in the skin and deeper tissues. Bones per se do not contain vibration receptors; however, they are excellent conductors of vibration from the vibrating tuning fork to mechanoreceptors like the Pacinian corpuscles present in the tissues.

4. Ask the subject to raise his finger when he ceases to feel the vibration.

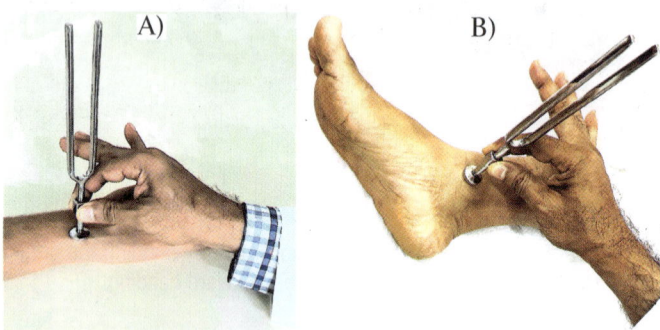

Fig. 57.12 Testing for sense of vibration: **(A)** In the upper limb (on styloid process of ulna) and **(B)** in the lower limb (on medial malleolus).

5. Immediately place the tuning fork on the corresponding bony prominence of your body and note whether you can still perceive the vibration.

> **Note:** If the examiner perceives the vibration after the subject ceases to perceive it, the subject's sense of vibration is impaired.

6. Elicit the vibration sense on all the bony prominences of the body.

▌Precautions

1. The subject should be instructed properly.
2. The tuning fork should be made to vibrate by hitting the blades of the fork against the hypothenar eminence of the palm or thigh, **not against a hard surface**.
3. The examiner should hold the tuning fork by the stem, close to the base, **without touching the blades**.
4. The vibrating fork should be placed only on the bony prominences.
5. After the subject ceases to feel the vibration, the examiner should immediately place the fork on the corresponding point on his own body to check whether the vibration has actually ceased.
6. The sensation should be elicited on the corresponding bony prominence on the opposite side of the body.

Pain
▌Superficial pain
Steps

1. Provide proper instructions to the subject.
2. Explain properly that you will be eliciting pain.
3. With the **help of a metallic pin** (Fig. 57.13A) or a **wooden pin** (Fig. 57.13B)—not a needle as it will cause bleeding—lightly **prick the skin** of different parts of the subject's body and ask him to indicate whether he feels pain.
4. Elicit pain from **all the dermatomes** on both sides of the body.
5. Delineate areas of analgesia, hypoalgesia, or hyperalgesia, if present.

Precautions

The precautions described for eliciting the fine touch sensation apply here.

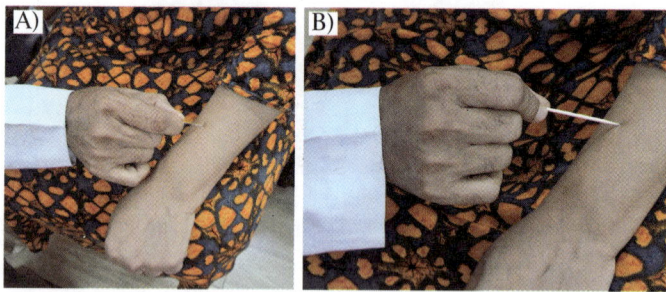

Fig. 57.13 Eliciting pain with **(A)** a metallic pin and **(B)** a wooden pin.

▌Pressure pain
Steps

1. Provide proper instructions to the subject.
2. With **an algometer** (Fig. 57.14), carefully press on the surface of the body and note the minimum pressure required to produce pain.
3. Repeat the procedure on the identical points of the body on the opposite side and compare the results.

> **Note:** Clinically, pressure pain is elicited by squeezing the muscle or tendon (Achilles tendon) till pain is produced.

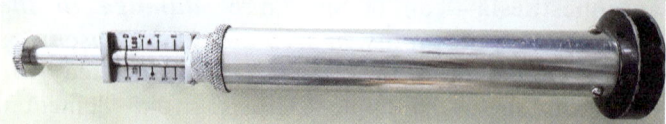

Fig. 57.14 Algometer for eliciting deep or pressure pain.

Temperature
▌Steps

1. Provide proper instructions to the subject—ask him to say whether he feels **cold** or **warm** when touched with different glass tubes.

2. Take two separate test tubes containing warm and cold water respectively (Fig. 57.15).
3. Place the test tubes on the subject's skin, each in turn or randomly, and ask the subject to report whether he feels warm or cold (Fig. 57.16A and B).
4. Examine warm and cold sensations on all the dermatomes on both sides of the body and note your observations.

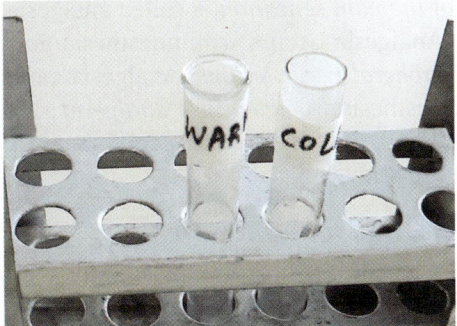

Fig. 57.15 Warm and cold solutions for eliciting the temperature sensation.

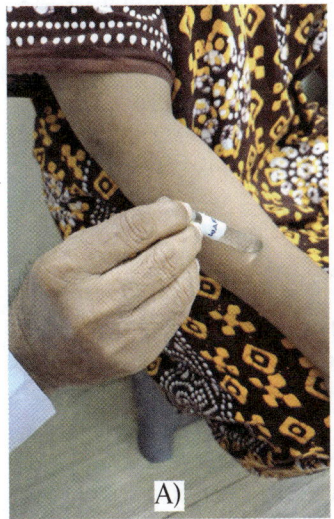
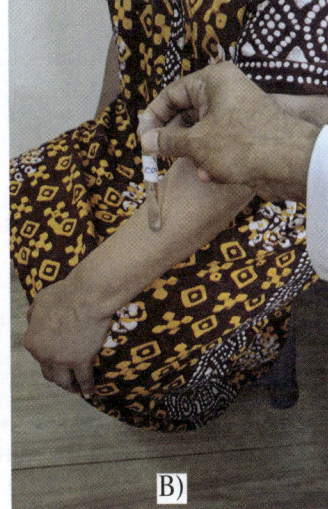

Fig. 57.16 Eliciting temperature sensation with **(A)** warm solution and **(B)** cold solution.

▌Precautions

The precautions described for eliciting the fine touch sensation apply here.

Observation and Results

1. Note your observations in a tabular format, dermatome-wise and on both sides, as given in the next column.
2. Analyse the results and report your findings with your comments on the functional integrity of the sensory system.

Parameters	Observation / Findings		
Patient's name, age, gender, height, and body weight.			
General examination			
i. Orientation and consciousness ii. Emotional state iii. Nutrition and pallor iv. Cyanosis v. Clubbing vi. Dyspnea vii. Vital signs			
Examination of sensory system			
Posterior column sensations	**Right side**	**Left side**	
i. Fine touch ii. Proprioception (sense of position and joint movement) iii. Vibration iv. Tactile localisation v. Two-point discrimination vi. Stereognosis vii. Graphesthesia			
Anterolateral system sensations	**Right side**	**Left side**	

i. Crude touch
ii. Pressure
iii. Temperature
  • Warm solution
  • Cold solution
iv. Pain
  • Fine pain (pin)
  • Deep pain (algometer)			

DISCUSSION

Abnormalities of Sensation

Tactile sensation

▌Anesthesia

Anesthesia refers to the **loss of all sensations**. Anesthesia is graded as **hypoesthesia** when the sensation is decreased or *complete anesthesia* when sensation is totally lost.

Causes of hypoesthesia: It is seen in **lesions of the central sensory structures**, such as the thalamus, internal capsule, or cortex. Usually, it affects the distal parts of the limbs more than the proximal parts.

Causes of complete anesthesia:

1. Usually occurs in **peripheral nerve lesions**. The common causes are leprosy and complicated diabetes mellitus.
2. Lesions of peripheral nerves result in anesthesia corresponding to the distribution of sensory fibres.
3. Complete anesthesia also occurs in **complete transection of the spinal cord** where anesthesia is seen in the limbs and trunk below the level of the lesion.

Dissociated anesthesia

When the **sensation of pain and temperature is lost with the preservation of the touch sensation**, the condition is known as dissociated anesthesia.

Physiological basis: Dissociated anesthesia occurs in conditions where the *grey matter of the spinal cord near the central canal* is damaged. The fibres carrying the touch sensation ascend the dorsal column of the spinal cord and, therefore, are spared. The **fibres carrying pain and temperature** cross to the opposite side of the spinal cord at the same segmental level of the cord. While crossing to the opposite side, these fibres *travel very close to the central canal*. Therefore, they are *damaged in disease processes* involving the grey matter of the spinal cord.

Causes:
1. Syringomyelia
2. Intramedullary tumours
3. Brainstem lesions (syringobulbia)
4. Thrombosis of the posterior inferior cerebellar artery

Hemianesthesia

This is a loss of sensation that affects the face, arm, and leg of one side (*usually the opposite side*) of the body.

Cause: Usually seen in lesions of the thalamus, internal capsule, or cortex.

Hyperesthesia

When the response to sensory stimulation is exaggerated, the condition is called hyperesthesia.

Cause: It is seen in cases of thalamic lesions.

Paraesthesia

When the touch **sensation is perverted** (touch may produce an unpleasant sensation almost amounting to pain), it is called paraesthesia. This consists of sensations like pricking, numbness, or band-like sensations around the trunk.

Causes:
1. *Nerve compression* is the commonest cause of paraesthesia. It occurs when peripheral nerves are stretched or subjected to pressure. The commonest example is paraesthesia (numbness and pricking) after sitting for a long time with the legs crossed.
2. Spinal tumours
3. Subacute combined degeneration of the spinal cord (vitamin B12 deficiency)
4. Disseminated sclerosis
5. Thalamic lesions

Proprioceptive sensation

The proprioceptive sensation is that of joint movement, the sense of the positions of different parts of the body, and the sense of vibration. The loss of proprioceptive sensation can occur without the loss of other sensations. It is characteristic of lesions of the posterior column or lesions of the fibres ascending in the posterior column to the medulla. The **Romberg test** to describe abnormalities of the sense of position is described in Chapter 57.

Loss of proprioception is seen in:
1. Tabes dorsalis
2. Subacute combined degeneration of the spinal cord

Pain

Analgesia

The *loss of the pain sensation* is called analgesia.

Causes: Analgesia occurs with anesthesia and is usually seen in *peripheral nerve lesions*. Analgesia can also occur without anesthesia. A *hereditary analgesia syndrome* has been described, in which pain receptors are completely absent in the body.

Hypoalgesia

Partial loss of pain sensibility is called hypoalgesia.

Cause: It occurs due to nerve compression.

Hyperalgesia

This is a condition of *exaggerated sensibility to pain*. In this condition, a mild stimulus, which ordinarily does not produce pain, causes severe pain. It may occur in response to a mild cutaneous stimulus or sometimes as an intractable spontaneous activity (without stimulus).

Causes:
1. Spinal cord disease, for example, tabes dorsalis
2. Thalamic lesions
3. Deep-seated lesions in the parietal lobe

Pain intensity scale

A pain intensity scale is a tool used to measure the **subjective level of pain** experienced by an individual. It is typically a **scale ranging from 0 to 10**, where *0 represents no pain* and *10 represents the most severe pain* imaginable.

Commonly used pain intensity scales:
1. **Numerical rating scale (NRS):** This is a widely used scale on which individuals rate their pain on a **scale from 0 to 10**, with 0 representing no pain and 10 representing the worst possible pain.
2. **Visual analogue scale (VAS):** This scale uses a horizontal line, with '**no pain**' at one end and '**worst pain imaginable**' at the other. Individuals mark the line to indicate their pain level.
3. **Verbal rating scale (VRS):** This scale uses descriptive words to represent different levels of pain intensity, such as '**none**', '**mild**', '**moderate**', '**severe**', and '**very severe**'.

Common Clinical Conditions

Peripheral nerve pain

This occurs due to *injury to the nerve, neuritis, and neuropathy*. It may be associated with *other sensory loss* with or without motor changes. Sometimes only nerve pain may occur without other sensory or motor loss. Then it is called **neuralgia**, for example, trigeminal neuralgia.

Root pain

Pain is seen in the area of **distribution of a particular root** that is affected. The most common examples are cervical and *lumbar root pain* distributed to the appropriate limb, as in *cervical spondylosis* or *lumbar disc prolapse*. It is characteristic of extramedullary cord compression.

Causalgia

This is an **abnormal burning sensation** that is usually seen after limb injuries. It occurs when the nerve injury is mild.

Visceral pain

This occurs due to diseases of the viscera. For example, *inflammation of the abdominal viscera* produces pain.

Visceral pain differs from somatic pain in the following ways:

1. **It is poorly localised** because the pain receptors in the viscera are relatively few.
2. **It is associated with autonomic changes** like hypotension, nausea, vomiting, and sweating. Autonomic changes occur due to the activation of visceral reflexes.
3. **It is associated with muscle guarding** (spasm of the abdominal wall). Muscle guarding occurs due to reflex contraction of the skeletal muscle in the abdominal wall. This is a protective reflex to prevent further injury to the viscera.
4. It often **radiates or is referred to other areas**. Usually, visceral pain is referred to a somatic structure that is developed from the same dermatome of the visceral structure in which the pain originates. The most common example is pain of myocardial infarction radiating to the ulnar border of the left hand or the pain of cholecystitis radiating to the tip of the shoulder.

Brown–Sequard syndrome

This occurs in a **hemisection of the spinal cord**. It is usually seen in injury to the spinal cord or in tumours that affect one half of the cord.

1. *On the side of the lesion, the dorsal column sensations* (the fine touch sensation, proprioceptive sensations, and tactile localisation and discrimination) **are lost.**
2. **On the opposite side** of the lesion *pain, temperature, and crude touch* sensations **are lost.**

This occurs because the sensation of fine touch, proprioception, and two-point discrimination *ascend the dorsal column of the same side*, whereas the sensation

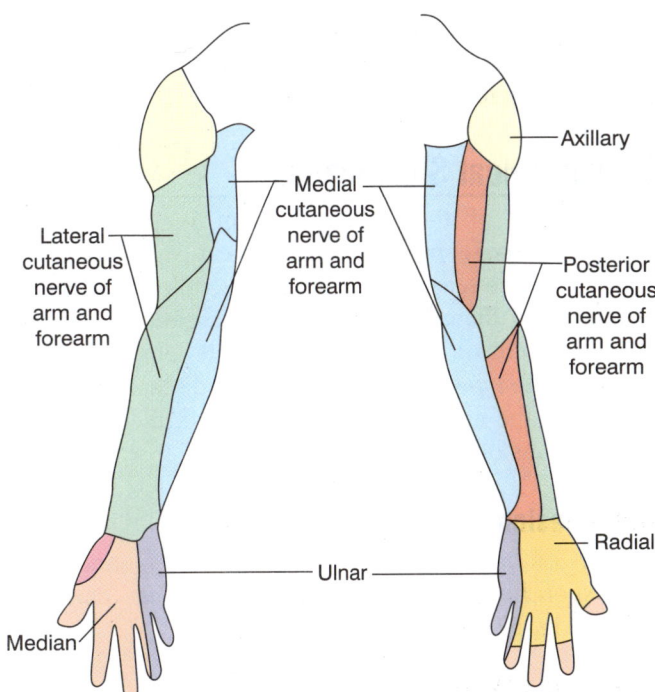

Fig. 57.17   Peripheral nerve lesions in the upper limbs.

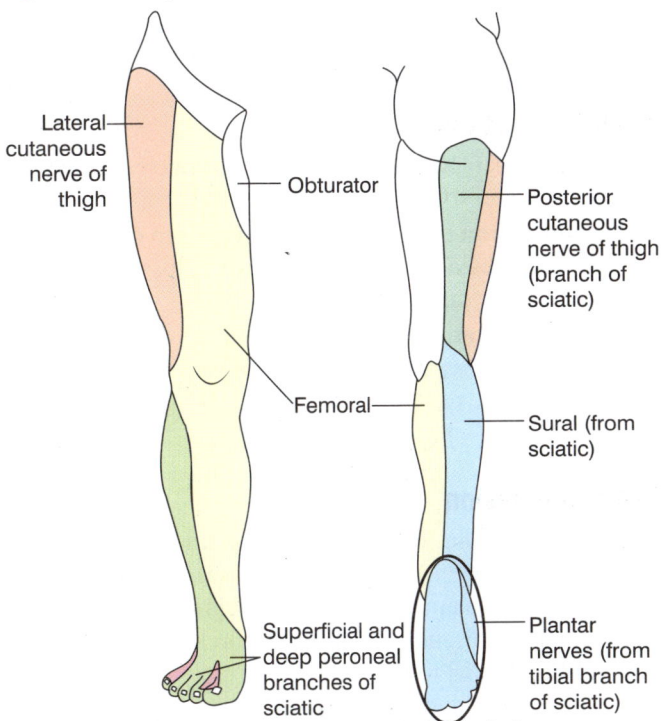

Fig. 57.18   Peripheral nerve lesions in the lower limbs.

of pain, temperature, and crude touch *ascend the anterolateral system of the opposite side* of the spinal cord.

Syringomyelia

In this condition, there is a lesion **around the central canal** of the spinal cord. The lesion interrupts the pain and temperature fibres passing to the opposite side of the spinal cord. Therefore, there is a **loss of the sensations of pain and temperature with preservation of touch** and **postural sensibility.**

Physiological Significance

Examination of the sensory system is performed to *localise disease processes* that affect any part of the neuraxis of the sensory system. This is called **localisation of lesions of the sensory system.** Localisation of a lesion partly depends on the distribution of the sensory loss and partly on the *type of sensory loss.* The disease may affect the nerve, the nerve root, the spinal cord, the brainstem, the thalamus or the cortex.

Nerve lesion

Lesion of a peripheral nerve results in anesthesia *corresponding to the distribution* of that particular nerve (Fig. 57.17 and 57.18).

Nerve root lesion

There is **segmental anesthesia** in root lesions corresponding to the *involvement of the segment* of the spinal cord from where the nerve root arises.

Spinal cord lesion

Complete transsection of the spinal cord causes anesthesia in the limbs and trunks below the level of lesion.

1. **Hemisection** of the spinal cord results in **dissociation of anesthesia** (dissociated sensory loss as seen in *Brown–Sequard syndrome*).
2. A lesion **around the central canal** of the spinal cord results *in loss of pain and temperature sensations on* both sides, below the level of the lesion with *preservation of other sensations.*

Brainstem lesion

Above the medulla, the spinothalamic tract (fibres of the anterolateral system) remains in close association with the trigeminothalamic tract in the tegmentum, whereas the medial lemniscus carrying the fibres of the posterior column lies medial to it.

1. A lesion of the **lateral part of the tegmentum** causes *hemianalgesia and thermoanesthesia* in the *opposite side* of the body without affecting other sensations (as the medial lemniscus is spared).
2. A deep-seated lesion in the **upper part of the brainstem** may involve the medial lemniscus without affecting the spinothalamic fibres. This results in *loss of posterior column sensations* with *preservation of pain and temperature sensations.*

Thalamic lesion

Severe and extensive lesions of the thalamus result in **gross impairment of sensory modalities** on the *opposite side* of the body. The threshold for pain may be raised, but a less painful stimulus may cause an exaggerated response (*hyperalgesia*). The touch sensation may induce an *unpleasant sensation* (paraesthesia). This is called the **thalamic syndrome,** which occurs in the lesions of the lateral and ventral nucleus.

Cortical lesion

The cortex is primarily involved in processing the **finer aspect of sensations,** especially the *spatial and discriminatory sensibility.* Tactile localisation, two-point discrimination, and stereognosis are therefore called cortical sensations. A cortical lesion results in the impairment of tactile localisation, two-point discrimination, and stereognosis. Other sensations may remain intact.

OSPE

I. **Elicit touch (fine touch) sensation of the anterior aspect of the forearms of the subject and report your findings.**

Steps
1. Provide proper instructions to the subject.
2. Ask the subject to close his eyes.
3. With cotton wool, lightly touch the skin of the anterior aspect of one forearm (according to the different dermatomes).
4. Elicit the touch sensation on the other forearm and compare the findings.
5. Report your findings.

II. **Elicit crude touch sensation of the anterior aspect of the forearms of the subject and report your findings.**

Steps
1. Provide proper instructions to the subject.
2. Ask the subject to close his eyes.
3. With the help of your fingertips, lightly press the skin of the anterior aspect of one forearm (according to the different dermatomes).
4. Elicit crude touch sensation on the other forearm and compare the findings.
5. Report your findings.

III. **Elicit two-point discrimination of the anterior aspect of the right forearm of the subject and report your findings.**

Steps
1. Provide proper instructions to the subject.
2. Ask him to close his eyes.

3. Separate the two limbs of the compass aesthesiometer a little and touch the subject's skin lightly with the two points of the aesthesiometer simultaneously. Ask the subject to say whether he is being touched at one or two points.

4. If the subject says one point, increase the distance between the two points a little more and repeat the test till the two separate points are appreciated by the subject as two points.

5. Repeat the procedure on the other forearm of the subject and compare.

6. Report your findings.

IV. Elicit pain sensation of the anterior aspect of the right forearm of the given subject and report your findings.

Steps

1. Provide proper instructions to the subject and explain properly that you will be eliciting pain.

2. With the help of a pin (not a needle) lightly prick the skin of the right forearm and ask the subject to say whether he feels pain.

3. Repeat the procedure on the opposite side of the body.

4. Delineate the area of analgesia, hypoalgesia, or hyperalgesia, if present.

5. Report your findings.

V. Perform tactile localisation on the anterior aspect of the forearms of the given subject and report your findings.

Steps

1. Provide proper instructions to the subject and ask him to hold a ballpen.

2. Ask the subject to close his eyes.

3. With the help of a pen, touch the right forearm at a particular point. Then, ask the subject to touch the same point with his pen.

4. Repeat the procedure on the other side of the body and compare.

5. Report your findings.

VI. Test the vibration sense in the upper limbs of the given subject and report your findings.

Steps

1. Select a tuning fork of 128 Hz or less.

2. Provide proper instructions to the subject.

3. Make the tuning fork vibrate by striking it against the hypothenar eminence of your hand or the thigh.

4. Hold the tuning fork by holding the stem of the fork close to the base without touching the blades.

5. Immediately place the vibrating tuning fork on the bony prominence of the upper limb and ask the subject to report when the vibration ceases.

6. When the subject gives indication of the cessation of vibration, immediately place the tuning fork on the same point on your body to determine whether the vibration has actually ceased.

7. Repeat on the other limb.

8. Report your findings.

VII. Test the sensation of joint movement and position in the lower limbs of the given subject and report your findings.

Steps

1. Give proper instructions to the subject (to recognise the particular position of the limb when it is moved).

2. Ask him to close his eyes.

3. Move the subject's toes or foot either up or down and ask the subject to recognise the movement by telling you the position of the toes/foot or ask him to imitate the same movement in his other limb.

4. Repeat the procedure by changing the position of the limb at different joints.

5. Make a particular movement (flexion or extension at a joint) and ask the subject to recognise the direction of the movement.

6. Repeat the procedure on the other limb.

7. Report your findings.

VIVA

1. *How do you classify sensations?* (Ans. Refer to page 391, under the heading 'Sensory Modalities'.)

2. *Define a receptor.* (Ans. Refer to page 391, under the heading 'Receptors'.)

3. *What are the types of receptors?* (Ans. Refer to page 391, under the heading 'Types of Receptors'.)

4. *What are the sensations carried in the dorsal column?* (Ans. Refer to page 392, under the heading 'Fine Touch'.)

5. *What are the sensations carried in the anterolateral system of the spinal cord?* (Ans. Refer to page 393, under the heading 'Crude Touch'.)

6. *Trace the pathway for fine touch.* (Ans. Refer to page 392, under the heading 'Fine Touch' and Fig. 57.1a.)

7. *Trace the pathway for proprioception.* (Ans. Refer to page 392, under the heading 'Proprioception' and Fig. 57.1a.)

8. *Trace the pathway for pain and temperature.* (Ans. Refer to page 393, under the heading 'Temperature', Fig. 57.1b.)

9. *What is a sensory map? What is its physiological significance?* (Ans. Refer to page 394, under the heading 'Sensory Map', Fig. 57.2.)

10. *What are the precautions to be observed during the elicitation of the fine touch sensation?* (Ans. Refer to page 395, under the heading 'Precautions'.)
11. *What are the precautions to be observed during the elicitation of tactile localisation and two-point discrimination?* (Ans. Refer to page 395, under the heading 'Precautions'.)
12. *Why is the tuning fork placed on the bony prominence to elicit the vibration sensation?* (Ans. Refer to page 397, under the heading 'Sense of Vibration' and the subheading 'Steps'.)
13. *What are the precautions to be taken during the elicitation of vibration sensation?* (Ans. Refer to page 398, under the heading 'Sense of Vibration' and the subheading 'Precautions'.)
14. *What is dissociated anesthesia?* (Ans. Refer to page 400, under the heading 'Dissociated Anesthesia'.)
15. *What are the causes of dissociated anesthesia? What is its physiological significance?* (Ans. Refer to page 402, under the heading 'Spinal Cord Lesion' and the subheading 'Hemisection'.)
16. *What is pallhypesthesia?* (Ans. Refer to page 393, under the heading 'Sense of Vibration'.)
17. *What is hyperesthesia? What are its causes?* (Ans. Refer to page 400, under the heading 'Hyperesthesia'.)
18. *Define paraesthesia. Name two causes of paraesthesia.* (Ans. Refer to page 400, under the heading 'Paresthesia'.)
19. *Trace the pathway for pain.* (Ans. Refer to page 393, under the heading 'Pain' and Fig. 57.1b.)
20. *What is hyperalgesia? What are its causes?* (Ans. Refer to page 400, under the heading 'Hyperalgesia'.)
21. *What is causalgia?* (Ans. Refer to page 401, under the heading 'Causalgia'.)
22. *How does visceral pain differ from somatic pain?* (Ans. Refer to page 400, under the heading 'Visceral Pain'.)
23. *What is the Brown–Sequard syndrome? What are its features?* (Ans. Refer to page 401, under the heading 'Brown Sequard Syndrome'.)
24. *What are the sensory changes seen in syringomyelia?* (Ans. Refer to page 401, under the heading 'Syringomyelia'.)
25. *What is the physiological significance of the examination of the sensory system?* (Ans. Refer to page 402, under the heading 'Physiological Significance'.)
26. *What are the sensory features of brainstem lesion?* (Ans. Refer to page 402, under the heading 'Brainstem Lesion'.)
27. *What is the effect of a lesion of the thalamus on sensory functions?* (Ans. Refer to page 402, under the heading 'Thalamic Lesion'.)
28. *What is the effect of a lesion of the cortex on sensory functions?* (Ans. Refer to page 402, under the heading 'Cortical Lesion'.)

58 | Clinical Examination of the Nervous System-III (Motor System)

Learning Objectives

After completing this practical, you will be able to (MUST KNOW):

1. Describe the importance of performing this practical in clinical physiology.
2. Measure the bulk of the muscles.
3. Estimate and grade the strength of various individual muscles and groups of muscles.
4. Assess the tone of flexors and extensors at various joints.
5. Elicit superficial and deep reflexes.
6. Test the coordination of movements in the upper and lower limbs.
7. Name the descending motor pathways.
8. Trace the pathway of corticospinal tracts.
9. List the differences between upper and lower motor neuron paralysis.

You may also be able to (DESIRABLE TO KNOW):

1. Trace the pathways of all descending motor tracts.
2. List the functions of the motor pathways, basal ganglia, cerebellum, and motor cortex.
3. Explain briefly the role of alpha and gamma motor neurons in the regulation of muscle tone.
4. Name the common conditions associated with alteration in bulk, tone, and strength of the muscles and reflexes.
5. Explain the changes in motor function in upper and lower motor neuron paralysis.
6. List the differences in coordination of movement in cerebellar, sensory, and corticospinal pathway disorders.
7. Describe the different types of abnormal gaits and involuntary movement.

PY5.15: Demonstrate the correct clinical examination of the nervous system: higher functions, sensory system, motor system, reflexes, and cranial nerves in a normal volunteer or simulated environment.

CLINICAL EXAMINATION OF THE MOTOR SYSTEM

INTRODUCTION

Anatomical and Physiological Considerations

The motor system consists of **motor areas in the brain, the upper motor neurons, the lower motor neurons, and the muscles**. The motor system deals with body functions related to the movement of different parts of the body and the regulation of posture and balance. Movement occurs due to the contraction and relaxation of the agonists and antagonists. **Agonists** are muscles that facilitate movement by their contraction, whereas **antagonists** facilitate movement by their relaxation. Movement depends on the maintenance of posture and balance. A balanced posture provides a stable background for movement.

Muscles

Muscles can be classified in various ways. However, to understand motor physiology, muscles are best classified as the **medial (proximal)** and **lateral (distal)** groups.

Proximal group of muscles

The proximal groups of muscles are the *muscles of the trunk, girdles, and proximal parts of the limbs*. These muscles are primarily involved in the **maintenance of posture** and equilibrium.

Distal group of muscles

The distal groups of muscles are the *intrinsic muscles of the digits and the muscles of the distal parts of the extremities*. They are not required for postural activities but are primarily involved in the **control of skilled voluntary movement**, i.e., manipulatory activities.

Lower Motor Neurons

The lower motor neurons are the *final common pathway for the output* of the motor system. The **cell bodies** of the lower motor neurons are present in the *anterior horn of the spinal cord*. The lower motor neurons consist of the **anterior horn cells and the homologous cells in the**

brainstem, their efferent nerve fibres that pass via the anterior spinal nerve roots and peripheral nerves to the muscles, and the **terminal axonal branches** that innervate the muscle fibres.

- In the ventral horn, the most **medially situated motor neurons** innervate the *proximal groups of muscles* (the axial muscles and the proximal limb muscles), and the most **laterally situated motor neurons** innervate the *distal groups of muscles* of the body.
- Therefore, the **medial groups of motor neurons are involved in postural control**, whereas the **lateral groups of motor neurons are involved in manipulatory (skilled) activities**.

Upper Motor Neurons

The upper motor neurons **originate in the motor cortex and other areas** in the brain that are involved in the regulation of motor activities and *terminate on the anterior horn cells*. The upper motor neurons are classically divided into **two types**: *pyramidal fibres* (corticospinal tract) and *extrapyramidal fibres*.

- The **pyramidal fibres** are motor neurons that *pass through the pyramid* in the medulla, regardless of their cells of origin. The **extrapyramidal fibres** are neurons that do not pass through the pyramid of the medulla.
- The **corticospinal tract** is synonymous with the *pyramidal tract* for all clinical purposes. The *extrapyramidal tracts* are the **rubrospinal, vestibulospinal, reticulospinal, and tectospinal** tracts.

Strictly speaking, some of the fibres of the pyramidal system do not pass through the pyramid, and some of the fibres of the extrapyramidal system pass through the pyramids. Therefore, from the physiological point of view, the upper motor neurons are better divided into the **medial system pathways** and **the lateral system pathways**.

Lateral system pathways

The upper motor neurons of the lateral system descend in the lateral funiculus of the spinal cord and terminate directly or indirectly on the laterally placed motor neurons in the anterior horns.

- This includes **two major pathways**: the **lateral corticospinal tract** and the **rubrospinal tract**.
- Since the lateral system fibres **terminate on the lateral group of motor neurons** (in the anterior horn) that innervate the distal group of muscles of the body, they are primarily involved in the **regulation of skilled voluntary activities**.

Medial system pathways

The upper motor neurons of the medial system descend the ventral funiculus of the spinal cord and terminate

mostly indirectly on the medially placed motor neurons in the anterior horns.

- This involves the **vestibulospinal** (lateral and medial), **reticulospinal** (medullary and pontine), **tectospinal**, and **interstitiospinal** tracts.
- Since the medial system fibres *terminate on the medial group of motor neurons* in the anterior horn cells that innervate the *proximal group of muscles* of the body, they are primarily involved in the **regulation of posture and equilibrium**.

Corticospinal tracts

Origin, course, and termination: The fibres of the corticospinal tract originate in the *fifth layer of the motor cortex*. Its fibres pass through the **posterior limb of the internal capsule** (Fig. 58.1), where all the fibres coming

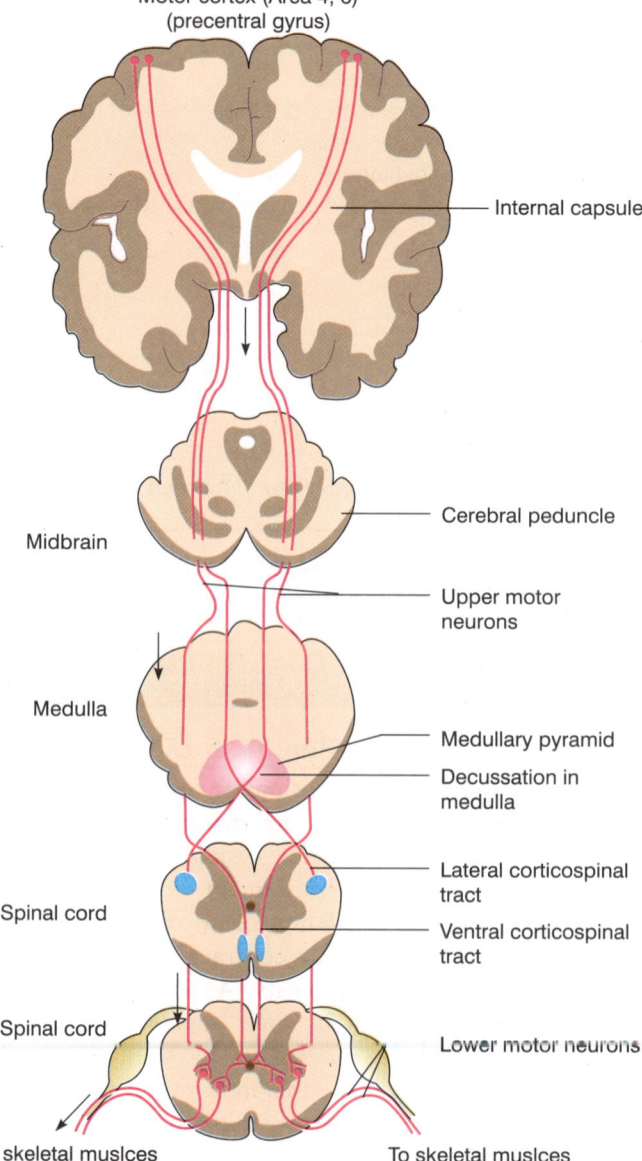

Fig. 58.1   Pyramidal (corticospinal) tract.

from different areas of the motor cortex converge into a narrow space (consequently, a *lesion in the internal capsule causes maximum motor deficit*). Then, the fibres descend down through the midbrain and pons into the medulla, where they form the pyramid.

- In the medulla, **80–90 per cent of the fibres,** after passing through the pyramid, **cross over (decussate) to the opposite side** and then enter the contralateral spinal cord to form the **lateral corticospinal tract.** These upper motor neurons enter the anterior grey horn of the spinal cord and project directly onto the lower motor neurons. Fibres of this tract have monosynaptic connections with the motor neurons that **innervate the distal groups of muscles.**

- The remaining *10–20 per cent of the fibres* in the medulla **do not cross over** to the opposite side. They *descend down ipsilaterally* on the same side of the spinal cord as the **anterior corticospinal tract** and **cross over to** *the opposite side* only at **the segmental level** (at the segments in the spinal cord where they innervate the muscles through the lower motor neurons). These fibres project onto the lower motor neurons (mostly indirectly) through interneurons that **supply the proximal groups of muscles.**

Functions:
- The **lateral corticospinal tract** conveys information from the motor cortex to the **distal group of skeletal muscles** on the opposite side of the body, which coordinates and regulates **skilled voluntary movement.**

- The **anterior corticospinal tract** conveys information from the motor cortex to the **proximal group of skeletal muscles** on the opposite side of the body, which coordinates and **regulates the movement of the axial skeleton** (that is involved in the **control of posture**).

Functions of other tracts

Rubrospinal tract: This tract conveys motor impulses from the red nucleus to the skeletal muscles on the opposite side of the body, which govern precise, discrete movements of the hands and feet (**skilled voluntary movements**).

Vestibulospinal tracts (VST): i) The **lateral VST** originates from Deiter's nucleus, which receives inputs from the utricles and saccules and traverses the length of the spinal cord. The tract is involved in the **adjustment of body posture in relation to linear acceleration**. ii) The **medial VST** originates from the medial and the descending vestibular nuclei, which receive inputs from the semicircular canals, and traverses up to the midthoracic level. This tract **adjusts body posture** (head, neck, and trunk movement) in relation to **angular or rotational acceleration**.

Reticulospinal tracts (RST): i) The **medullary reticulospinal tract** facilitates flexor reflexes, inhibits extensor reflexes, and decreases muscle tone. ii) The

pontine reticulospinal tract inhibits flexor reflexes, facilitates extensor reflexes, and increases the tone of antigravity muscles. Therefore, pontine *RST is the most important tract* involved in the **control of posture.**

Tectospinal tract: The tectospinal tract conveys impulses *from the superior colliculus* to the skeletal muscles on the opposite side of the body, which are involved in the movement of the head and neck in response to visual stimuli. Therefore, it controls **visually guided head movements.**

Motor Areas in the Brain

The motor areas in the brain include the **cortical motor areas** and the other areas that are involved in the regulation of motor activities. The other important motor areas in the brain are the **basal ganglia** and **cerebellum.**

Cortical motor areas

The cortical motor areas in the brain include the areas in the cortex that, **on stimulation, produce motor activities.**
- This includes the **primary motor cortex** (area 4), **premotor cortex** (lateral portion of area 6), the **supplementary motor cortex** (medial portion of area 6), the **somatosensory cortex** (areas 3, 1, and 2), and the **posterior parietal cortex** (areas 5 and 7).
- About **60 per cent of the fibres in the corticospinal tract** come from motor areas (primary motor cortex, premotor cortex, and supplementary motor cortex), whereas the remaining *40 per cent originate from the sensory areas* in the cortex.

Basal ganglia

The basal ganglia are subcortical structures that consist of several groups of nuclei in each cerebral hemisphere, including the **neostriatum** (caudate nucleus and putamen), **globus pallidus, subthalamic nucleus, and substantia nigra**.
1. The basal ganglia **receive inputs** from the *cortex and thalamus* and project back to the cortex via the thalamus.
2. They are involved in the **control of posture and movement**, especially in the **initiation, planning, programming, and smoothening** of movement.

Cerebellum

The cerebellum **receives inputs** from the *vestibular apparatus, the spinal cord, and the cortex*. It influences the lower motor neuron activities indirectly via its projection to the vestibular nuclei, the brainstem area, and the cortex.
1. The **vestibulocerebellum** (archicerebellum) is involved in the maintenance of equilibrium and balance.
2. The **spinocerebellum** (paleocerebellum) is involved in smoothening and coordination of movement.
3. The **corticocerebellum** (neocerebellum) is involved in the planning and programming of movement.

METHODS OF EXAMINING MOTOR FUNCTIONS

Principle

The integrity of the motor system is assessed by examining the size, tone, and strength of muscles, and by evaluating the reflex response of muscles to stretching and coordination of movement.

Requirements

1. Measuring tape (Fig. 58.2)
2. Knee hammer (Fig. 58.3)

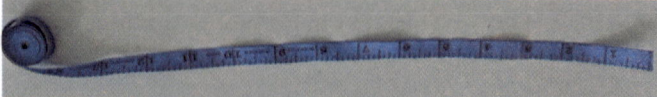

Fig. 58.2   Measuring tape.

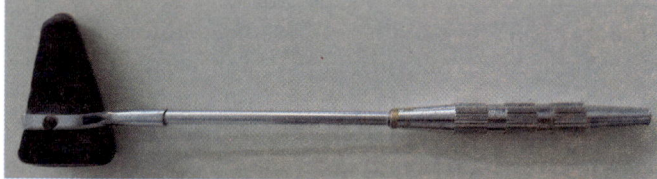

Fig. 58.3   Knee hammer.

Procedure

The following aspects of motor functions are assessed while examining the motor system:

1. Bulk of muscles
2. Tone of muscles
3. Strength of muscles
4. Reflexes
5. Coordination of movement
6. Gait
7. Involuntary movement (if present)

Bulk of muscles

The bulk of the muscles can be easily estimated by **inspection and palpation**.

1. Ask the subject to remove all his clothing (except the inner garments to cover the private parts) and sit comfortably on a stool or lie down on a couch.
2. **Inspect the muscle mass** of all parts of the body and note if *there is any wasting* (atrophy) *or hypertrophy* of any group of muscles.
3. **Palpate the muscles** to assess the consistency.

Note: Wasted or **atrophic muscles** are not only smaller but also softer and flabbier than normal muscles especially when they are contracted. **Hypertrophic muscles** are usually firm in consistency. If muscle wasting is associated with fibrosis, as seen in polymyositis, the muscles are hard to palpate and inelastic.

4. Compare the bulk of the muscles of both sides of the body.
5. Measure the **midarm** (Fig. 58.4A) and **midforearm** (Fig. 58.4B) circumferences in the upper limbs, and **midthigh** (Fig. 58.4C) and **midcalf** (Fig. 58.4D) circumferences in the lower limbs of both sides with a measuring tape.

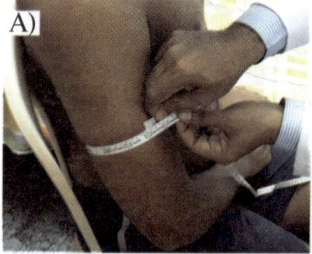 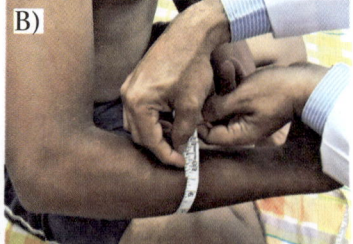

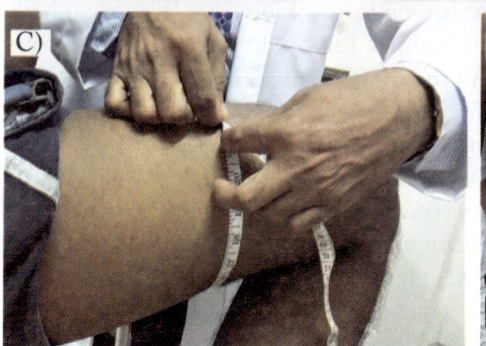 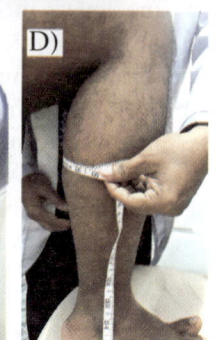

Fig. 58.4   Measurement of the circumference of the various parts of the limbs: **(A)** Midarm; **(B)** midforearm; **(C)** midthigh and **(D)** midcalf.

Note: Measurement of the girth of the muscles is the best way of estimating the bulk of the muscle.

Tone of muscles

Tone is a **state of partial contraction** of muscles. Clinically, tone means the **resistance of the muscle to passive stretching**. It is estimated by handling and passively moving various parts of the body.

1. Ask the subject to relax completely.
2. Passively move different parts of the body at various joints and try to feel the **degree of resistance encountered** during each passive movement (Fig. 58.5).

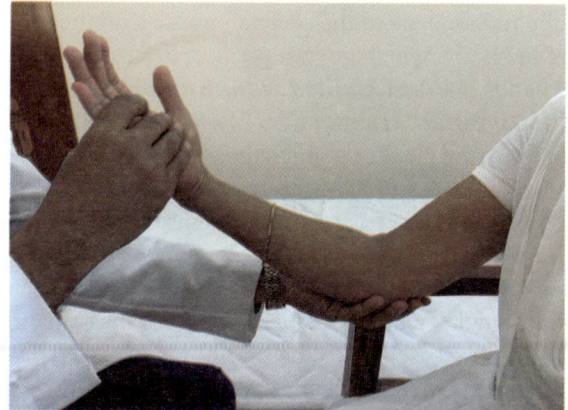

Fig. 58.5   Eliciting the tone of the biceps muscle by passively extending at the elbow joint. Note that the examiner appreciates the feeling of resistance offered to passive extension movement, not by actively palpating the muscle. The limb is supported to ensure and facilitate passive movement.

Note: The degree of resistance offered by the muscle during passive movement indicates the state of tone. This is perceived by **feeling the resistance to movement**, not by palpating the muscle. For example, passive flexion of the forearm stretches the triceps muscle, and passive extension of the forearm stretches the biceps muscle. Therefore, flexion assesses the tone of the triceps, and extension assesses the tone of the biceps muscle. The tone of a muscle may be normal, decreased (**hypotonia**), or increased (**hypertonia**). Do not palpate muscles while making passive flexion movements for eliciting tone because handling muscles could stimulate muscle sensory receptors and alter muscle tone due to interference.

3. Assess and compare the tone of the muscles on both sides of the body simultaneously.
4. Assess the tone of at least the extensors and flexors of the major joints (elbow and shoulder joints in the upper limb and knee and hip joints in the lower limb).

Strength of muscles

The strength of muscles is best assessed by eliciting **active movements against resistance**.

1. Ask the subject to **perform a movement** of any part of the body (say flexion of the forearm) and **you oppose the movement** actively (oppose flexion of the forearm by placing your palm on the subject's forearm and applying maximum resistance to stop flexion).

Note: The strength of the subject's muscle is assessed by comparing it with the strength of the examiner. The subject's age, sex, and build should be kept in mind while comparing the strength.

2. Compare the strength of the same group of muscles **on the other side** simultaneously.
3. Test the strength of the muscles of the lower limbs, upper limbs, and the trunk of the body.

Grading the strength of muscles

The strength or weakness of muscles is **graded into six degrees** by the Indian Medical Research Council Scale.

Grade 0: Complete paralysis (no contraction)
Grade 1: A flicker of contraction only (without any resultant movement of any limb or joint)
Grade 2: The muscle can make movements only when the opposing force of gravity is eliminated by appropriate positioning
Grade 3: The limb can be moved against the force of gravity, but not against the examiner's resistance
Grade 4: The muscle is able to make the full range of normal movement, but can be overcome (by resistance) to a variable extent
Grade 5: Normal power

Testing the strength of the muscles of the upper limbs

Interossei and lumbricals

First dorsal interosseous: Ask the subject to **abduct his index finger** against resistance; while doing so, the muscle becomes prominent, and the contraction of the muscle can be felt (Fig. 58.6).

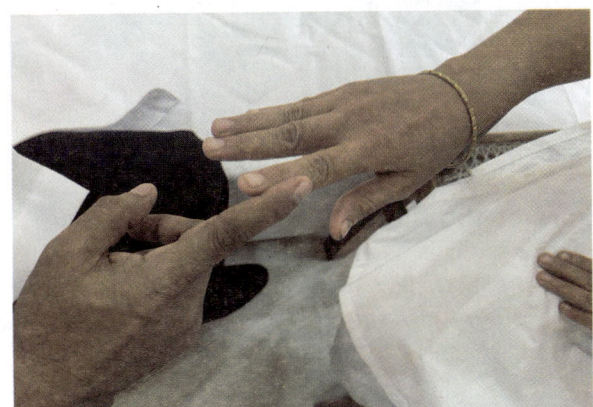

Fig. 58.6 Procedure of testing the strength of the first dorsal interosseous.

Dorsal interossei: These are the **abductors of the fingers**. Therefore, their power can be tested by asking the subject to *abduct the fingers* against resistance.

Palmar interossei: These are the **adductors of the fingers**. These are tested by placing a *paper or card between the subject's fingers* and trying to pull it out (Fig. 58.7).

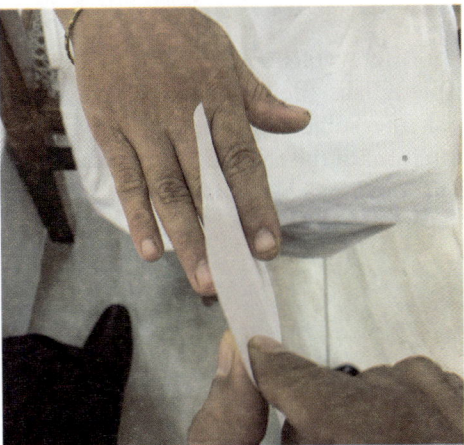

Fig. 58.7 Procedure of testing the strength of the palmar interossei.

Lumbricals: These are tested by asking the subject to **flex his metacarpophalangeal joints** and **extend his distal interphalangeal joints**. Ask the subject to **hold a pen**. While the terminal phalanx of the thumb is being apposed against the terminal phalanx of any other finger, the examiner tries to *dislodge the pen by force*. This is a **combined test for the opponens pollicis and lumbricals** (Fig. 58.8).

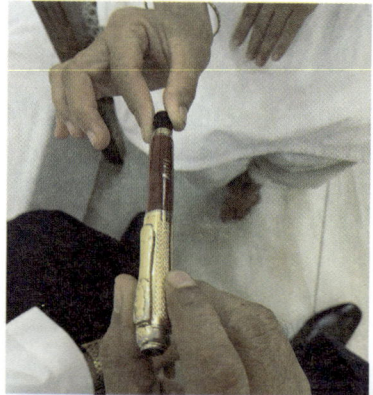

Fig. 58.8 Procedure of testing the strength of the lumbricals.

Flexors of the fingers: The flexors of the fingers are the flexor pollicis longus, flexor pollicis brevis, flexor digitorum superficialis, and flexor digitorum profundus. Ask the subject to *squeeze your index and middle fingers* (Fig. 58.9).

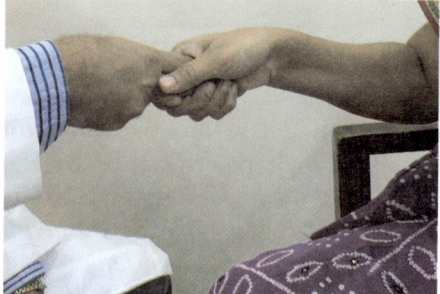

Fig. 58.9 Procedure of testing the strength of the flexors of the fingers.

Flexors of the wrist: The flexors of the wrist are the flexor carpi radialis, flexor pollicis brevis, and palmaris longus. Ask the subject to bring the tips of his fingers towards the front of the forearm so as to *touch the crease on the front of the wrist joint* (Fig. 58.10).

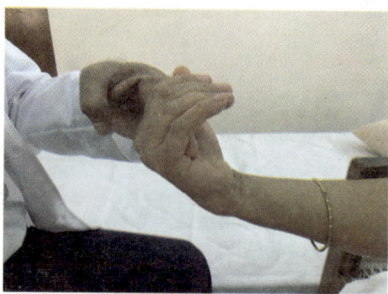

Fig. 58.10 Procedure of testing the strength of the flexors of the wrist.

Extensors of the wrist: These are extensor carpi radialis and extensor carpi ulnaris. Ask the subject to flex the fingers in the form of a fist and hold the hand with the palm facing downwards. Then, hold the wrist joint firmly and ask the subject to *extend the wrist joint against resistance* (Fig. 58.11).

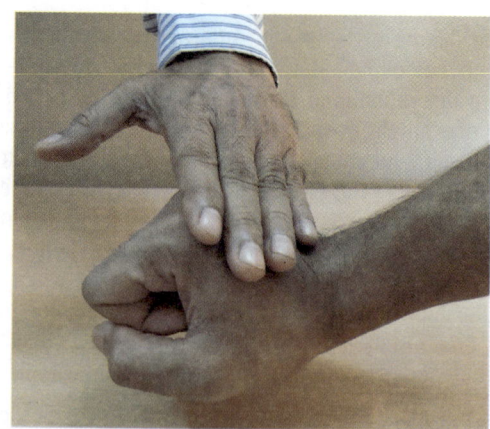

Fig. 58.11 Procedure of testing the strength of the extensors of the wrist.

Brachioradialis: Place the arm midway between the prone and the supine position. Then, ask the subject to *bend her forearm upwards. Oppose the movement* by *grasping the hand*. The brachioradialis becomes prominent (Fig. 58.12).

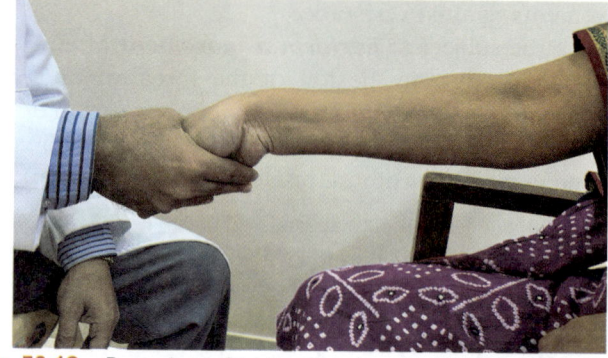

Fig. 58.12 Procedure of testing the strength of the brachioradialis. Note the prominence of the brachioradialis.

Biceps: Ask the subject to *lift up the forearm against resistance* offered by grasping the hand or wrist with the forearm in full supination. The biceps become prominent as they contract (Fig. 58.13).

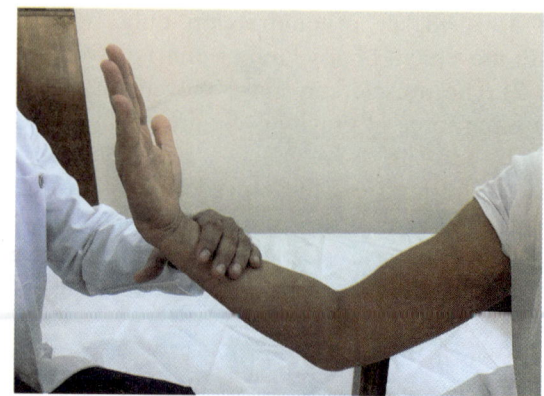

Fig. 58.13 Procedure of testing the strength of the biceps. Note the prominence of the biceps.

Triceps: Ask the subject to ***straighten out her forearm*** while *you try to keep it flexed* by applying passive resistance (Fig. 58.14).

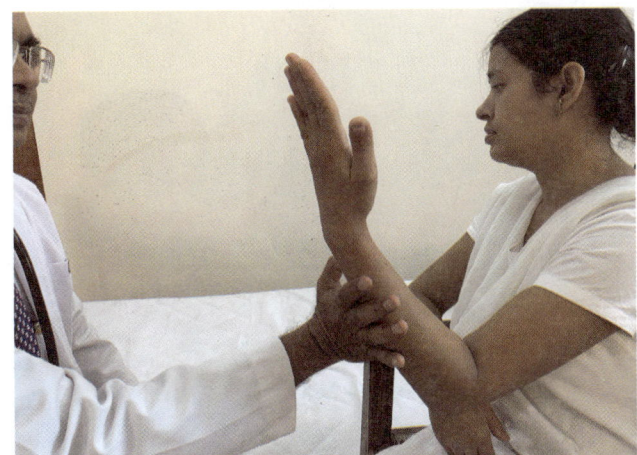

Fig. 58.14   Procedure of testing the strength of the triceps. Note the prominence of the triceps.

Supraspinatus: Ask the subject to keep her arms relaxed by the sides of her body. Then, instruct her to lift the arm straight outwards at a right angle to the body. The *first 30° angle of this movement* is primarily carried out by the **supraspinatus muscle** (Fig. 58.15). The remaining 60° angle is produced **by the deltoid**.

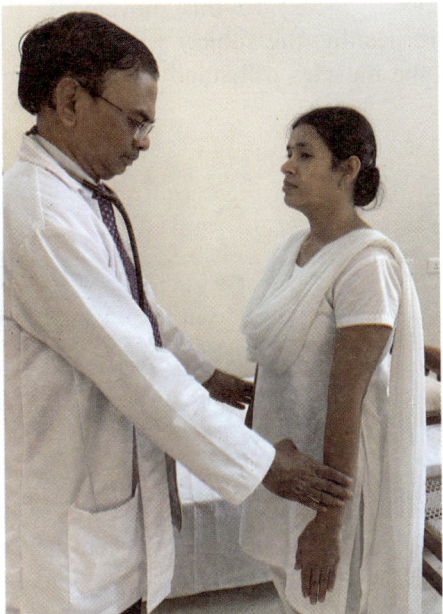

Fig. 58.15   Procedure of testing the strength of the supraspinatus.

Deltoid: It can be tested along with the supraspinatus. Ask the subject to make forward and backward movements of the abducted arm at *a 45° angle against resistance* (Fig. 58.16). The anterior and posterior fibres of the deltoid help to draw the abducted arm forward and backward, respectively.

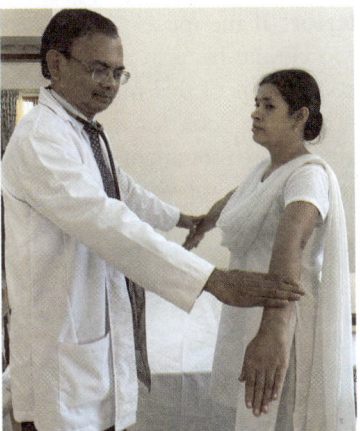

Fig. 58.16   Procedure of testing the strength of the deltoid. Note the prominence of the triceps. Note also that when arms are abducted at a 45° angle, resistance is applied against forward and backward movements as well as against lifting them.

Infraspinatus: Place the subject's elbow by her side with a forearm flexed to a right angle and then ask her to *rotate the limb outward against the resistance* applied to the middle of the outer aspect of the forearm (Fig. 58.17). The contraction of the muscle can be seen and felt.

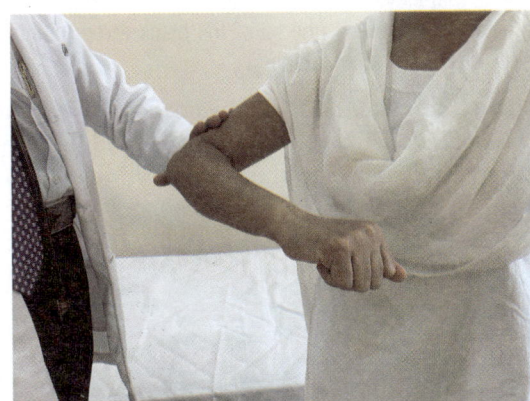

Fig. 58.17   Procedure of testing the strength of the infraspinatus.

Pectorals: Ask the subject to stretch her arms out in front of her and then **clap her hands while you attempt to hold them apart** (Fig. 58.18).

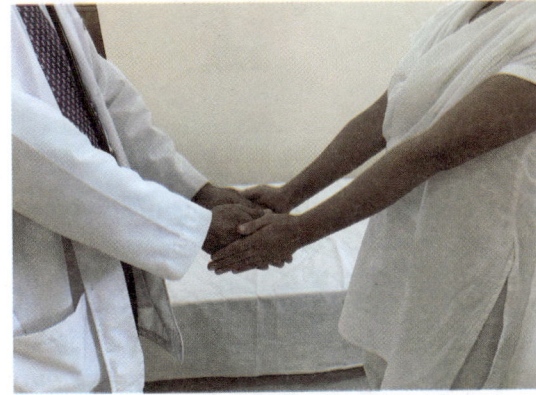

Fig. 58.18   Procedure of testing the strength of the pectorals.

Serratus anterior: If the muscle is paralysed, the subject will be unable to elevate his arm above a right angle when asked to do so. Paralysis of this muscle causes '**winging of the scapula**'. Therefore, look for a "winged scapula". The deformity becomes more prominent when the subject is asked to push forward against a wall with both hands (Fig. 58.19).

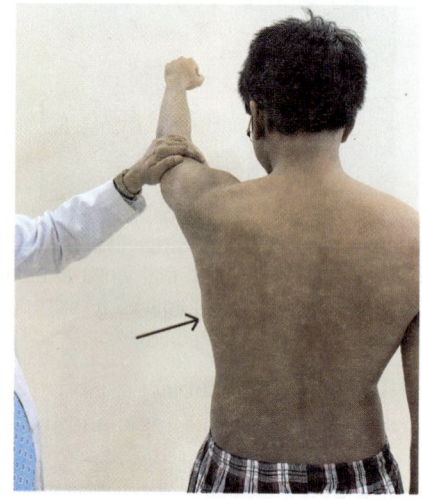

Fig. 58.19 Procedure of testing the strength of the serratus anterior. Note that elevating the arm above the right angle makes the serratus anterior prominent (the tip of the black arrow points to the prominence of the serratus anterior).

Latissimus dorsi: Ask the subject to **clap her hands behind her back** while you (standing behind the subject), offer passive resistance to the downward and backward movement (Fig. 58.20).

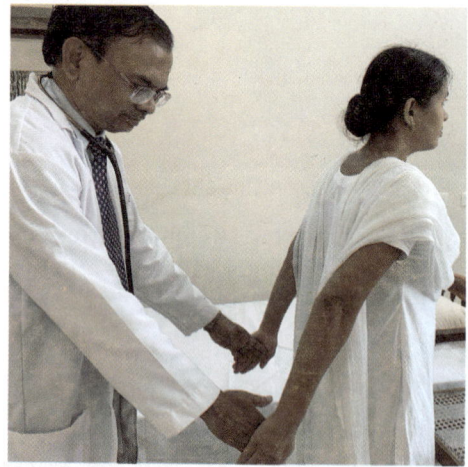

Fig. 58.20 Procedure of testing the strength of the latissimus dorsi.

■ **Testing the strength of muscles of the trunk**

Abdominal muscles: Weakness of the muscles of the abdomen is detected by observing the subject's *inability to raise herself in bed without the aid of her arms.* **Babinski's rising-up sign** is also elicited by asking the subject to lie on his back with her legs extended and *rise without using her hands* (Fig. 58.21).

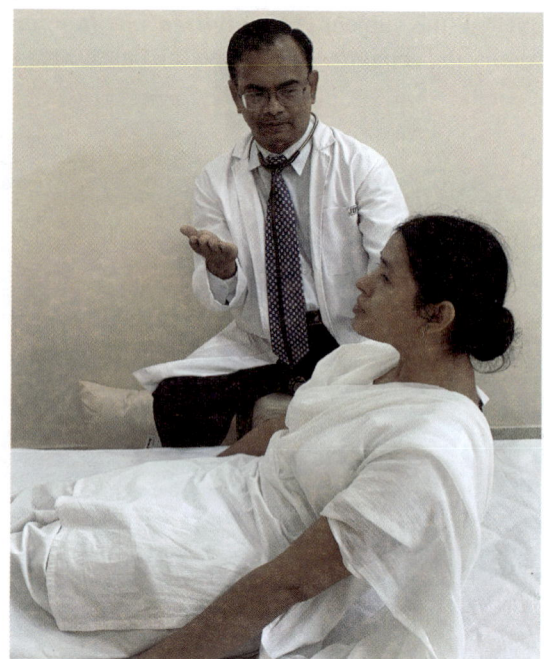

Fig. 58.21 Procedure of testing the strength of the abdominal muscles. Note that the subject rises without using her hands for support.

Erector spinae and muscles of the back: Ask the subject to *lie face down and try to raise her head from the bed* by extending the neck and back. *Provide passive resistance* (Fig. 58.22) to this movement. If the back muscles are healthy, the subject will be able to raise her head, and the muscles will stand out prominently during this effort.

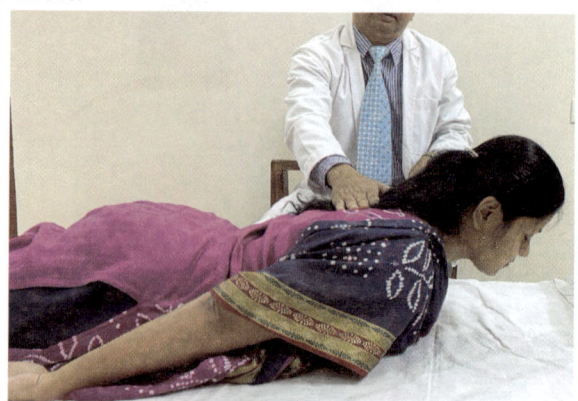

Fig. 58.22 Procedure of testing the strength of the erector spinae and muscles of the back.

■ **Testing the strength of the muscles of the lower limb**

Intrinsic muscles of the foot: It is difficult to examine the strength of the intrinsic muscles of the foot (lumbricals and interossei). If the interossei are weakened or paralyzed, claw-foot develops.

Dorsiflexor and plantar flexors of the feet and toes: The dorsiflexor is the peronei, and the plantar flexors are the tibialis posterior, gastrocnemius, and soleus. *Ask the subject to dorsiflex* (Fig. 58.23A) or *plantarflex* (Fig. 58.23B) *the part against resistance.* Try to fix the ankle or apply resistance against the subject's movement.

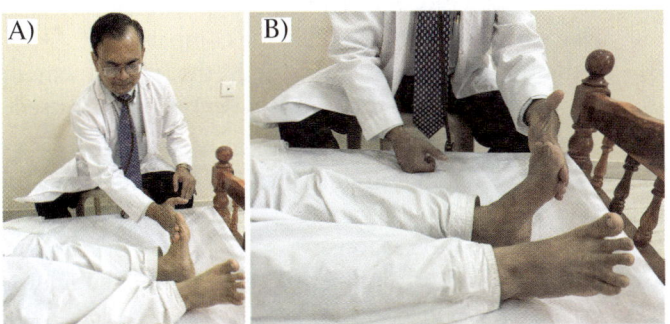

Fig. 58.23 Procedure of testing the strength of the muscles of the feet and toes: **(A)** Dorsiflexors and **(B)** plantar flexors.

Evertors and invertors of the foot: The evertors (Fig. 58.24A) are the peronei, and the invertors (Fig. 58.24B) are the tibialis anterior and tibialis posterior.

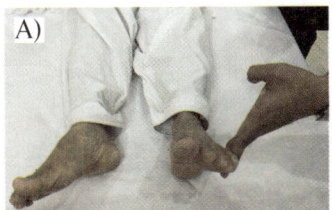 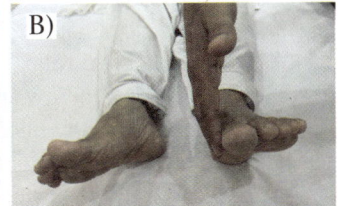

Fig. 58.24 Procedure of testing the strength of the muscles of the feet: **(A)** Evertors and **(B)** invertors.

Extensors of the knee: The quadriceps are the extensors of the knee. Bend the patient's knee, and then *pressing with your hand on the shin, ask him to straighten his limb* (Fig. 58.25).

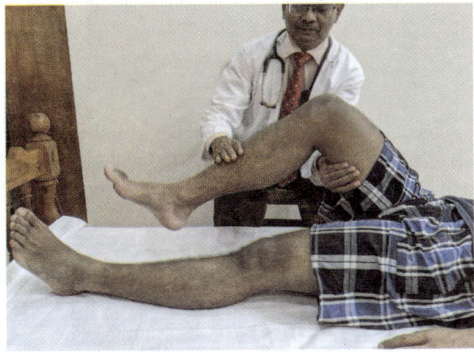

Fig. 58.25 Procedure of testing the strength of extensors of the knee. Note that the subject straightens their leg against resistance from the bent position of the knee.

Flexors of the knee: These are the biceps femoris, semitendinosus, and semimembranosus. Raise the straightened lower limb, supporting the thigh with your left hand and holding the ankle with your right hand. Then, *ask the subject to bend his knees against the resistance* (Fig. 58.26).

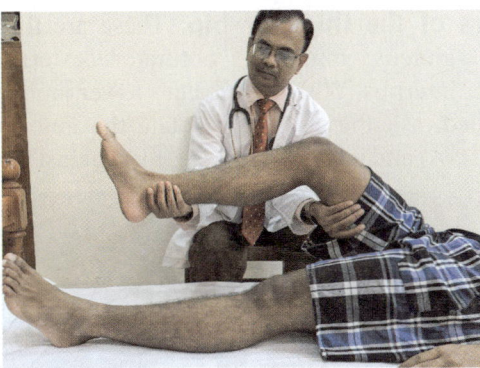

Fig. 58.26 Procedure of testing the strength of the flexors of the knee. Note that the subject bends the knees of the lifted and straightened limb against resistance applied at the ankle.

Extensors of the thigh: The gluteus maximus is the extensor of the thigh. Lift the subject's foot off the bed when the knee is extended and ask him to *depress the limb against resistance* (Fig. 58.27A).

Flexors of the thigh: These are the iliopsoas and the tensor fascia lata. In the extended leg, ask the subject to *raise his lower limb against resistance* without bending the limb at knee joints (Fig. 58.27B).

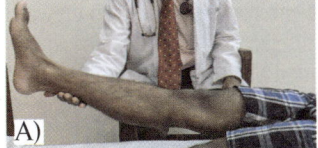 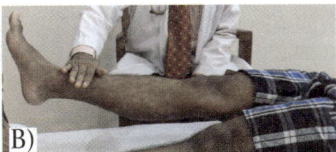

Fig. 58.27 Demonstration of the strength of extensors and flexors of the thigh: **(A)** For extensors of the thigh, the fully extended limb with extension at the knee joint is brought down from a small height by the subject against resistance given at the ankle from below by the examiner and **(B)** for flexors of the thigh, the fully extended limb is raised by the subject against resistance given at the ankle from above by the examiner.

Adductors of the thigh: These are the adductor longus, adductor brevis, adductor magnus, and gracilis. Abduct the lower limb and then ask the subject to bring it *back to the midline against resistance* (Fig. 58.28A).

Abductors of the thigh: These are the gluteus medius and gluteus minimus. Bring the lower limb to the midline and then ask the subject to move it *outward against resistance* (Fig. 58.28B).

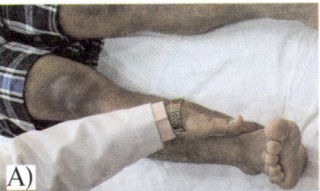 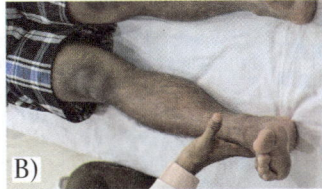

Fig. 58.28 **(A)** The demonstration of the strength of adductors and **(B)** demonstration of the strength of abductors of the thigh. Note that in the fully extended limb, the subject adducts and abducts the whole limb against resistance applied at the ankle from the side by the examiner.

Rotators of the thigh or hip: These are the gluteus medius, gluteus minimus, obturator externus, and obturator internus. With the subject's lower limb extended on the bed, ask the subject to rotate the limb outwards (Fig. 58.29A) and inwards (Fig. 58.29B) against resistance.

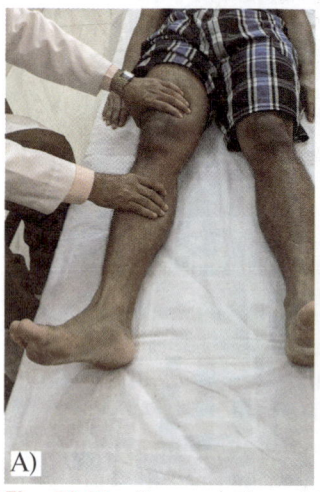 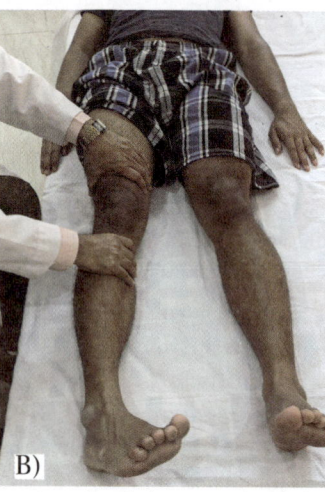

A)   B)

Fig. 58.29 Demonstration of the strength of the rotators of the thigh and hip. **(A)** For outward rotators, the subject rotates the entire limb in the outward direction in the fully extended position of the limb against resistance given by the examiner to prevent this outward rotation. **(B)** For inward rotators, the subject rotates the entire limb in the inward direction in the fully extended position of the limb against resistance applied by the examiner to prevent this inward rotation.

Reflexes

Clinically, reflexes are of **three types**: tendon or deep reflexes, superficial reflexes, and visceral or sphincteric reflexes.

▌ Tendon or deep reflexes

The **contraction of the muscle in response to a sudden stretch** produced by striking the tendon (with a knee hammer) is called a tendon reflex.

1. Tendon reflexes are **stretch reflexes** because they are elicited by stretching the muscle.
2. These stretch reflexes are **monosynaptic reflexes**.

The tendon reflexes assess the integrity of the afferent and efferent pathways and excitability of the anterior horn cells in the spinal segment of the stretched muscle.

The **following precautions** should be observed for eliciting tendon reflexes:

1. The subject should be completely relaxed.
2. Reassure the subject that the knee hammer is not a harmful instrument and will not cause pain while eliciting reflexes.
3. The subject's limb should be appropriately positioned.
4. Before striking the tendon, the muscle should be lightly stretched by positioning the limb.
5. The tendon should be stroked briskly with a knee hammer by making a sudden, jerky movement at the examiner's wrist.

6. The knee hammer should be appropriately held between the thumb and the index finger so that it swings freely in an arc, yet it is controlled in its direction.
7. The homologous reflex on the opposite side should always be tested immediately for comparison.
8. If the reflexes are not elicited, the reinforcement technique (**Jendrassik's maneuver**) should be used.

Grading of the tendon reflexes

Tendon reflexes can be graded into **five degrees** as given below.

Grade 0: Absent (no response)
Grade 1: Present but diminished (as a normal supinator jerk)
Grade 2: Brisk (as a normal knee jerk)
Grade 3: Very brisk (hyperactive)
Grade 4: Clonus

> **Note:** Normal supinator jerk is less than average and normal knee-jerk is brisker than average reflexes.

Biceps jerk (C5,6)

1. Ask the subject to relax.
2. Flex the subject's elbow and place his forearm in a semi-pronated position while supporting with your hand (Fig. 58.30), with the subject in the **sitting position** (Fig. 58.31), in the **supine position** (Fig. 58.32), or by placing his elbow on his abdomen, with the subject in the **lying down position** down on the bed (Fig. 58.33).

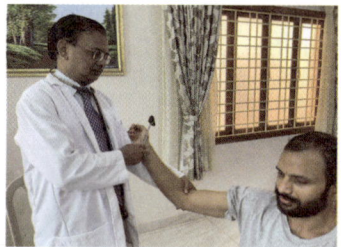

Fig. 58.30 Procedure to hold the forearm of the subject for eliciting biceps reflex. Note that the elbow of the subject has to be flexed and his forearm to be placed in a semi-pronated position while you support him with your hand. Ensure that the subject's upper limb is fully relaxed with your support.

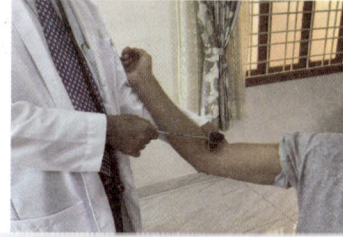

Fig. 58.31 Demonstration of biceps jerk in sitting or standing posture. Note that the subject rests his forearm on the examiner's forearm with the elbow joint flexed. The examiner strikes the biceps tendon by striking his own thumb (placed and pressed on the tendon) using the narrow end of the knee hammer.

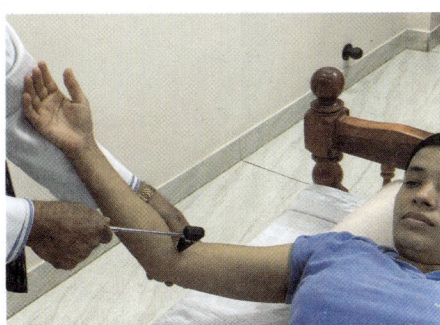

Fig. 58.32 Elicitation of biceps jerk in the supine position with the subject's limb outstretched and supported.

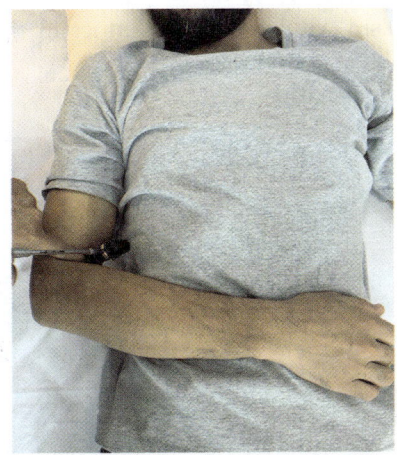

Fig. 58.33 Demonstration of biceps jerk in supine posture. Note that the subject rests his forearm on his abdomen with the elbow flexed at an angle of 90°. The examiner strikes the biceps tendon by striking his own thumb (placed and pressed on the tendon) with the narrow end of the knee hammer.

3. Place your thumb *firmly on the biceps tendon*.
4. *Strike your thumb* with the help of the pointed end of the knee hammer so that the biceps tendon stretches by striking the thumb.
5. Observe the **contraction of the biceps** muscle and the *flexion at the elbow*.
6. Elicit the biceps jerk on the other limb (Fig. 58.34) and compare.

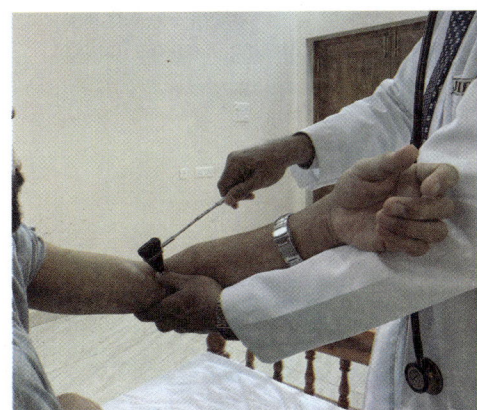

Fig. 58.34 Elicitation of biceps reflex of the opposite side (left side).

Triceps jerk (C6,7)
1. Flex the subject's arm at the elbow and allow the forearm to rest on her abdomen (Fig. 58.35) or be supported by your hand (Fig. 58.36).
2. Tap the triceps tendon directly above the olecranon.

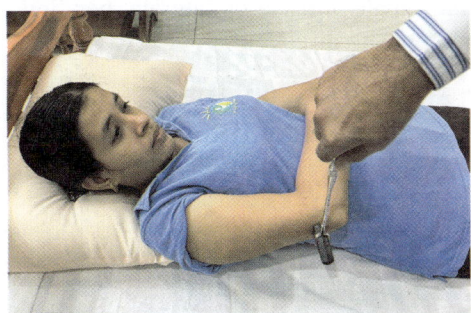

Fig. 58.35 Demonstration of triceps jerk in the supine posture. Note that the subject rests her forearm on her abdomen with the elbow flexed at an angle of 90°. The examiner strikes the triceps tendon using the broad end of the knee hammer.

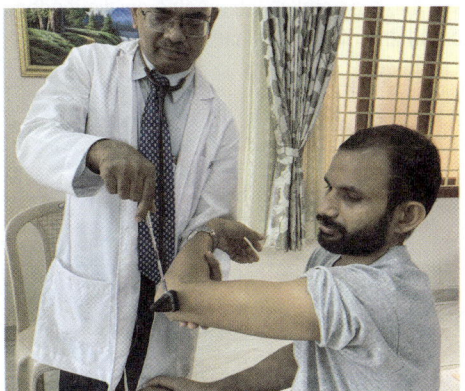

Fig. 58.36 Demonstration of triceps jerk in sitting or standing posture. Note that the subject's forearm rests on the examiner's forearm with his elbow joint flexed at 90°. The examiner strikes the triceps tendon using the broad end of the knee hammer.

Note: Take care not to strike the belly of the triceps muscle.

3. Observe the **contraction of the triceps muscle** and extension at the elbow.
4. Elicit the triceps jerk of the other side and compare (Fig. 58.37).

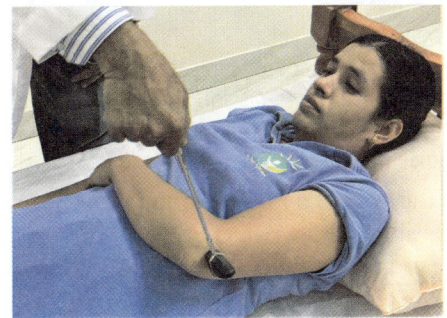

Fig. 58.37 Elicitation of triceps jerk of the opposite side (left side of the subject).

Supinator or brachioradialis jerk (C5,6)

1. Hold the subject's hand in the *sitting position* (Fig. 58.38) or *supine position* (Fig. 58.39) or allow the subject's forearm *to rest on his abdomen* in the supine position (Fig. 58.40) and slightly stretch the brachioradialis muscle by laterally bending the hand in the opposite direction.

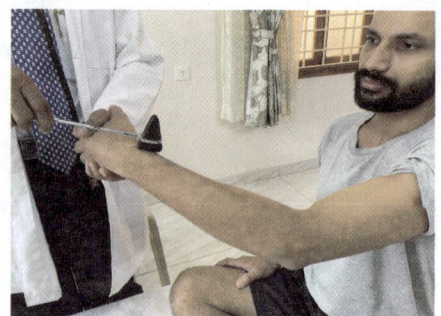

Fig. 58.38   Demonstration of supinator jerk in the sitting or standing posture. Note that the examiner holds the subject's hand, slightly dorsiflexes it, and then strikes the brachioradialis tendon at the wrist using the broad end of the knee hammer.

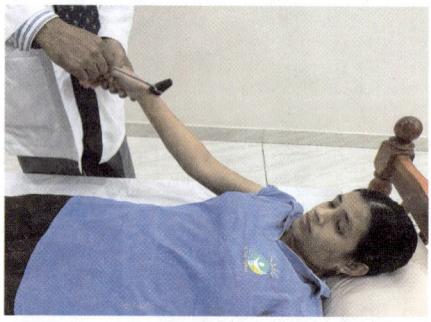

Fig. 58.39   Elicitation of supinator jerk with the subject in the supine position.

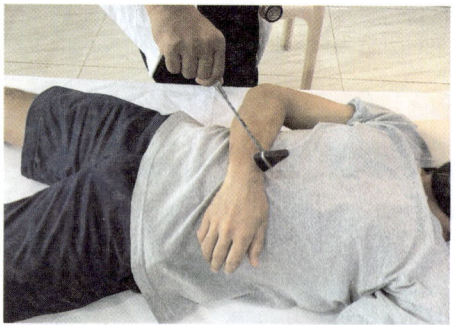

Fig. 58.40   Demonstration of supinator jerk in the supine posture. Note that the subject rests his forearm on his abdomen, and the examiner strikes the brachioradialis tendon at the wrist with the broad end of the knee hammer.

2. With the help of a knee hammer, strike the radius 1–2 inches above the wrist, over its styloid process.
3. Observe the flexion at the elbow and supination of the forearm.
4. Elicit the supinator jerk of the other side (Fig. 58.41) and compare.

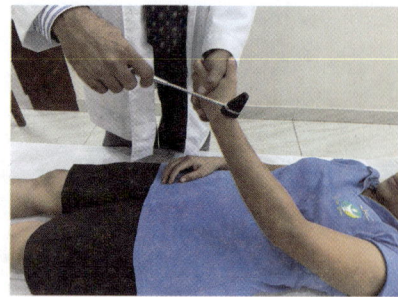

Fig. 58.41   Elicitation of supinator jerk of the opposite side (left side of the subject).

■ Knee jerk (L2, 3, 4)

It can be tested with the subject either in the supine or sitting position.

In the supine position (Fig. 58.42, 58.43, and 58.44):

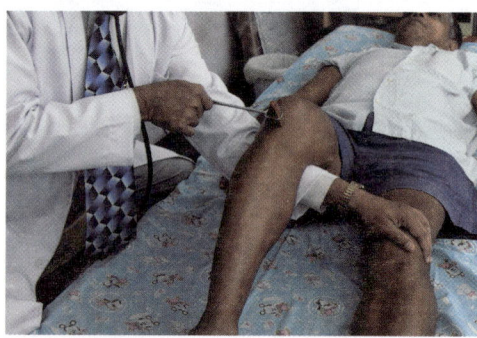

Fig. 58.42   Demonstration of knee jerk in the supine position. Note that the examiner supports the leg to be examined by placing his hand below the leg in such a way that he lifts it with the help of the other leg.

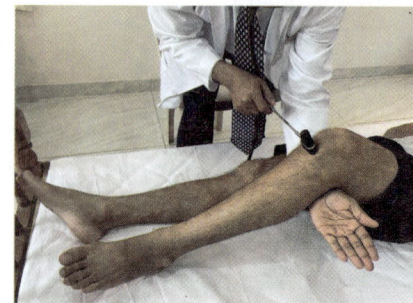

Fig. 58.43   Elicitation of knee jerk of the left side, in the supine position, the examiner lifting the leg using his forearm.

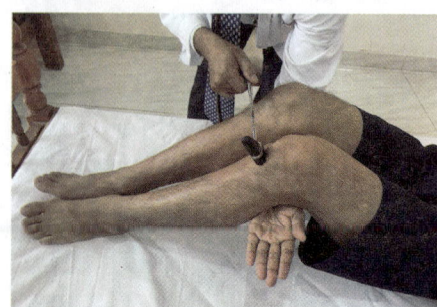

Fig. 58.44   Elicitation of knee jerk of both sides with a single lift in the supine position.

1. Expose the leg up to the upper thigh.
2. Pass your forearm under the knee to be tested and place your hand on the opposite knee (the knee to be tested should rest on the dorsum of your wrist and forearm).
3. Semiflex the knee and lift your hand slightly so that the weight of the knee rests on your hand.
4. Strike the patellar tendon directly with the help of a knee hammer (using the narrow end of the hammer).
5. Observe the **contraction of the quadriceps** and the brief extension at the knee.
6. Elicit the knee jerk of the opposite side and compare.

In the sitting position (Fig. 58.45 and 58.46):

1. Ask the subject to sit at the edge of the bed or on a stool in such a way that his legs dangle freely from the edge. Alternately, ask the subject to keep one knee (the knee to be tested) on the other knee.
2. Ask him to relax completely.
3. Strike the patellar tendon.
4. Observe the contraction of the quadriceps and the extension at the knee joint.

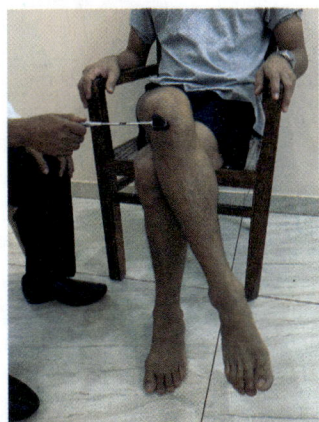

Fig. 58.45 Demonstration of knee jerk in the sitting position. Note that the subject sits on a stool or chair crossing the leg to be examined over the other leg. The examiner strikes the patellar tendon. The subject's legs should hang freely (should not touch the ground).

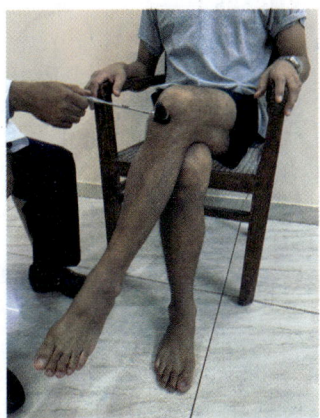

Fig. 58.46 Elicitation of knee jerk on the opposite side (left side of the subject) in the sitting position.

Ankle jerk (S1,2)

The ankle jerk can be tested with the subject in the supine, kneeling, or prone position.

In the supine position:

1. Place the subject's lower limb (to be examined) on the bed in such a way that it is everted and slightly flexed.
2. With one hand, slightly dorsiflex the foot so as to stretch the Achilles tendon (Fig. 58.47).
3. With the other hand, strike the tendon on its posterior surface (using the broad end of the knee hammer).
4. Observe for any **contraction of calf muscles** and *plantar flexion* of the foot.
5. Elicit the ankle jerk of the other side (Fig. 58.48) and compare.

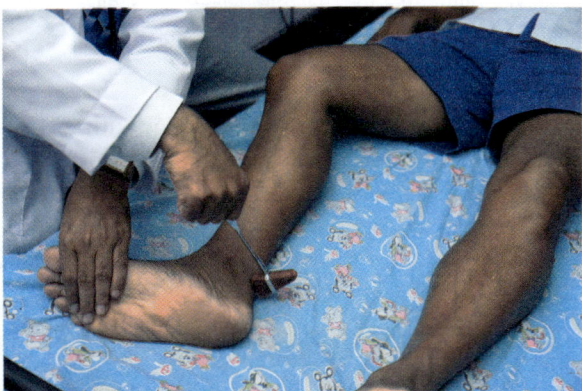

Fig. 58.47 Demonstration of elicitation of ankle jerk in the supine posture. Note that the examiner strikes the Achilles tendon after slightly dorsiflexing the foot. Also note that the knee of the examined leg is flexed to an angle of 120°.

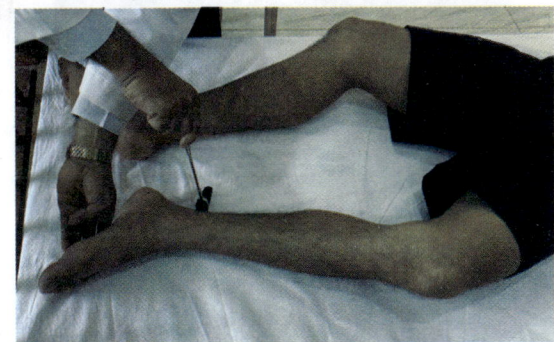

Fig. 58.48 Elicitation of ankle jerk on the opposite side (left side of the subject) in the supine position.

In the kneeling and prone position:

1. Ask the subject to kneel on a chair with his feet projecting outwards (Fig. 58.49A).
2. With the subject in the prone position, keep the ankle at a right angle and slightly dorsiflex the foot (Fig. 57.49B).
3. Strike the Achilles tendon.
4. Observe for **contraction of the calf muscles** and *plantar flexion* of the foot.

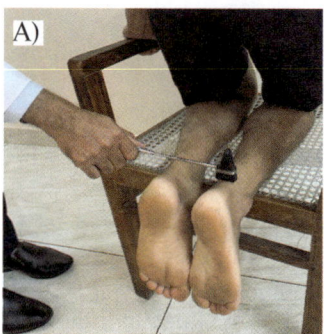
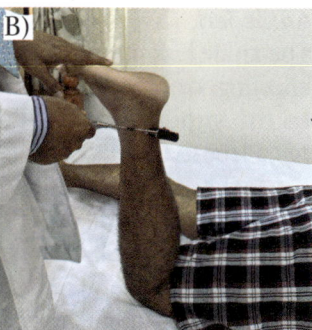

Fig. 58.49 Demonstration of ankle jerk: **(A)** in the kneeling posture and **(B)** in the prone posture. Note that the subject kneels on a chair or lies down on the bed in a prone posture with his knee bent at a right angle while the examiner strikes the Achilles tendon. Slight dorsiflexion of the foot may be needed if the ankle is not at a right angle.

Jaw jerk

1. Ask the subject to partially open his mouth.
2. Place a finger firmly on his chin (Fig. 58.50).
3. Strike the finger with the narrow end of a knee hammer.
4. Observe for immediate closure of the mouth (due to the contraction of the elevators of the jaw).

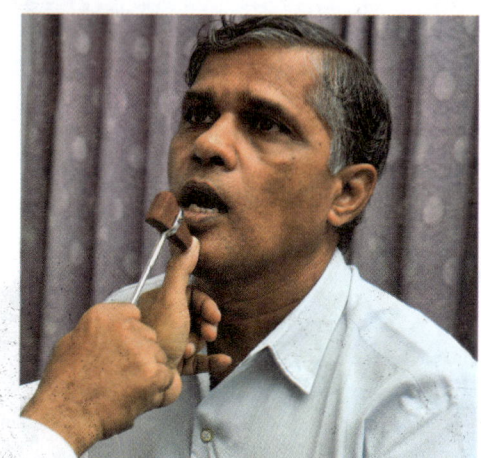

Fig. 58.50 Demonstration of jaw jerk. Note that the examiner strikes his own thumb placed on the subject's chin (the subject partially opens his mouth).

Jendrassik's maneuver

This is performed after asking the subject to make a strong voluntary muscular effort using the following methods:

1. While testing the **reflexes of the lower limb**, ask the subject to hook the fingers of two hands together and then pull them apart (against one another) as hard as possible (Fig. 58.51).
2. While testing the **reflexes of the upper limb**, ask the subject to clench his teeth or make a fist with the other hand (Fig. 58.52).

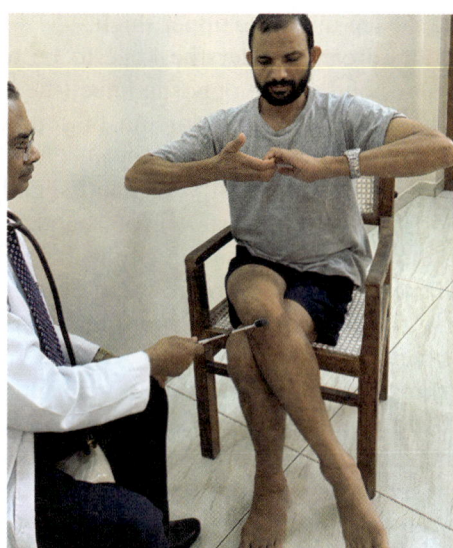

Fig. 58.51 Demonstration of Jendrassik's maneuver. Note that the subject pulls apart the fingers of the two hands hooked against each other, during which time, the examiner elicits the jerk.

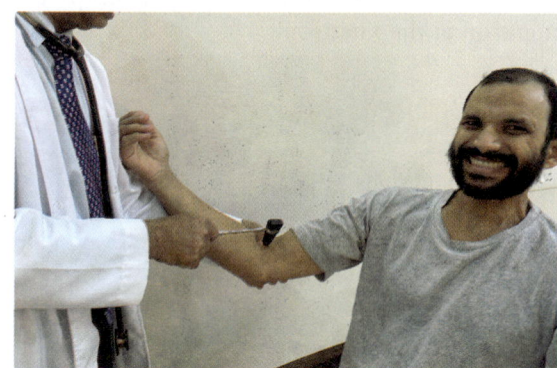

Fig. 58.52 Jendrassik's maneuver for upper limbs. Note that the subject clenches his teeth firmly while the examiner elicits the reflex.

Note: Jendrassik's maneuver works by increasing the excitability of the anterior horn cells and the sensitivity of the muscle spindle primary sensory endings to stretch by increasing the gamma fusimotor discharge.

Superficial reflexes

Superficial reflexes are elicited by **stimulating the cutaneous receptors**. The stimulation of an area of the skin by scratching results in the contraction of certain muscles supplied by the same spinal segment. These reflexes are polysynaptic reflexes. Superficial reflexes are of two types, spinally mediated and cranially mediated (Table 58.1).

The **chief superficial reflexes of spinal origin** are:

1. Plantar reflex
2. Cremasteric reflex
3. Bulbocavernosus reflex
4. Anal reflex
5. Abdominal reflex
6. Scapular reflex

Superficial reflexes of cranial origin are:
1. Conjunctival reflex (refer to Fig. 56.9A)
2. Corneal reflex (refer to Fig. 56.9B)
3. Pupillary reflexes (light and accommodation reflex)
4. Palatal reflex (described under '10th Cranial Nerve' and Fig. 56.7 and 56.8 in Chapter 56)

Plantar reflex (L5,S1)
1. Ask the subject to lie down on a couch.
2. Partially flex the lower limb and rotate it externally.
3. With one (left) hand, grasp the leg just above the ankle joint.
4. Ask the subject to relax completely.
5. With the other hand, using *a pointed object* (the pointed, metallic part of the knee hammer or a pointed key), **gently scratch the outer edge of the sole** of the foot, from the heel towards the little toe, and then medially across the metatarsus towards the ball of the great toe (Fig. 58.53).
6. Observe for the *plantar response* (as described below in 'Note').

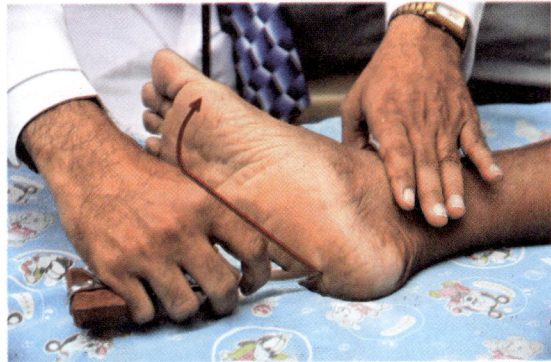

Fig. 58.53 Demonstration of plantar reflex. Note that a pointed object is used to stroke or scratch on the lateral aspect of the sole in the direction of the arrow depicted in the figure.

Note: The **plantar response** may be a flexor plantar response or an extensor plantar response. The **flexor plantar response** is characterised by inversion and dorsiflexion of the ankle with flexion of all the toes at the metatarsus. This is normally present in healthy subjects. The **extensor plantar response** is characterised by dorsiflexion of the great toe and abduction or fanning of the other toes with dorsiflexion of the ankle. It is found in patients with corticospinal tract lesions and is a pathognomonic feature of upper motor neuron paralysis. This abnormal response is also called **Babinski sign** as it was first described by Joseph Babinski. It is also normally seen in newborns and infants.

Other methods of eliciting plantar reflex: In addition to *Babinski sign* as described above, several alternative methods are considered for eliciting the plantar reflex, including the *Chaddock, Gonda, Oppenheim, and Gordon signs*.

Chaddock sign: This involves stroking the lateral malleolus.
Gonda sign: This method involves flexing and suddenly releasing the fourth toe.
Oppenheim sign: This involves applying pressure to the medial side of the tibia.
Gordon sign: This involves squeezing the calf muscle.

Cremasteric reflex (L1,2)
This is elicited only in male subjects.
1. Expose the part (genitalia and upper thigh).
2. Lightly scratch the inner aspect of the upper part of the thigh.
3. Observe the **elevation of the testicle** on that side and the **contraction of the dartos muscle** as evidenced by an increase in the wrinkling of the skin of the scrotum.
4. Elicit the cremasteric reflex on the opposite side.

Abdominal reflex (T8–12)
1. Ask the subject to lie down on the bed.
2. Expose the abdomen fully.
3. Ask him to relax completely
4. *Stroke lightly but briskly each side of the abdomen above and below the umbilicus, with a key, pencil, or the pointed, metallic end of a knee hammer* (Fig. 58.54), *from the outer aspect towards the midline* (Fig. 58.55).
5. Observe the contraction of the abdominal muscles after every stroke as evidenced by the **deviation of the umbilicus** towards the stimulus.
6. The reflex elicited in the upper part of the abdomen (above the umbilicus) is called the **upper abdominal reflex** (T8–10) and in the lower part of the abdomen (below the umbilicus) is called the **lower abdominal reflex** (T10–12).

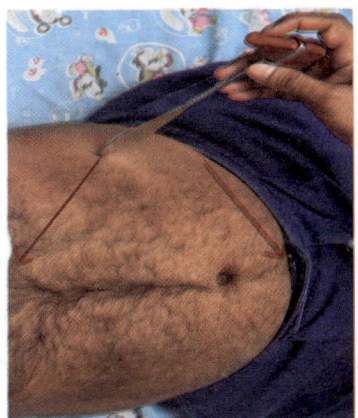

Fig. 58.54 Note that with the pointed, metallic end of the knee hammer, the surface of the abdomen is scratched from the outer aspect towards the midline in the direction of the arrow.

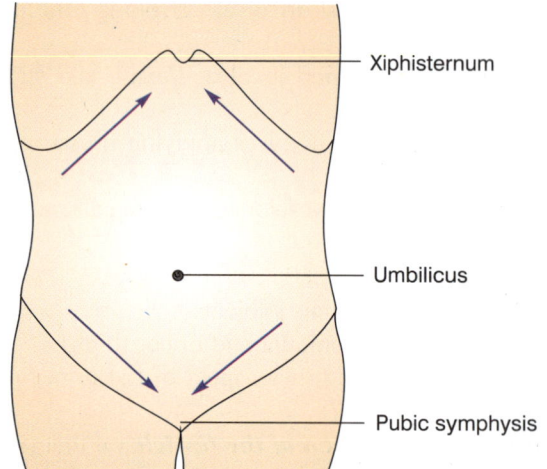

Fig. 58.55 Site and direction of stimulation for elicitation of the upper and lower abdominal reflex.

> **Note:** It is often impossible to elicit abdominal reflexes in obese, elderly, and anxious patients and in multiparous women.

Bulbocavernosus reflex (S3,4)

This is elicited only in male subjects.
1. Expose the part (external genitalia).
2. Pinch the dorsum of the glans penis.
3. Observe the contraction of the bulbocavernosus muscle.

Anal reflex (S3,4)

1. Expose the anal region.
2. Ask the subject to relax completely.
3. Stroke or scratch the skin near the anus.
4. Observe the contraction of the anal sphincter.

Scapular reflex (C5–8, T1)

1. Expose the upper portion of the back.
2. Stroke the skin in the interscapular region.
3. Observe the contraction of the scapular muscles.

All deep and superficial reflexes are summarised in Table 58.1.

Sphincteric reflexes

These reflexes are concerned with **swallowing, defecation, and micturition**. They depend on complex muscular movements excited by increased tension in the wall of the viscera concerned.

Swallowing: Ask the subject whether he has any *difficulty in swallowing* (dysphagia). Also ask whether there is any *regurgitation of food* through the nose. If dysphagia is present, ascertain whether it is *predominantly for liquids or solids or both*.

Defecation: Ask the subject if he experiences *any problems while passing stools*. The subject should also be questioned about the presence of normal or abnormal anorectal sensations while defecating.

Micturition: The subject should always be asked about his bladder habits and whether he has *any problem in controlling or initiating micturition*. **Retention of urine, incontinence, or urgency** of micturition should be noted.

Coordination of movement

Coordination of movement means smooth recruitment, interaction and cooperation of muscles or groups of muscles to carry out *a precise and definite motor act*. Coordination of movement should be tested both in the upper and lower limbs.

In the upper limbs

Finger–nose test
1. Properly instruct the subject about the procedure and the steps involved.
2. Ask the subject to touch the tip of her nose with the tip of her index finger from the maximally outstretched hand (Fig. 58.56A), rapidly and repeatedly, first with the eyes open (Fig. 58.56B) and then with the eyes closed (Fig. 58.56C).
3. Observe whether the subject is able to touch her nose every time, especially when the speed increases.
4. Ask the subject to repeat the test with the other hand (Fig. 58.56D and 58.56E).

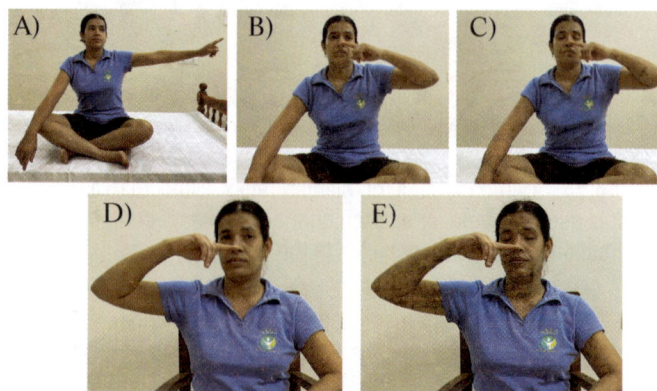

Fig. 58.56 Procedure for the finger–nose test. **(A)** The subject is asked to touch the tip of her nose with the tip of her index finger with her maximally outstretched hand; **(B)** then, she repeats the same rapidly, first with the eyes open and **(C)** repeats the same with the eyes closed; **(D and E)** then, she repeats the entire procedure with the other hand.

Finger–finger–nose test: In addition to the procedure of the finger-nose test, the subject, with the outstretched hand (Fig. 58.57A), first touches the finger of the examiner (Fig. 58.57B) and then the tip of her nose (Fig. 58.5C), and does it rapidly and repeatedly. Then, she repeats the procedure with the other hand (Fig. 58.57D).

Table 58.1   Summary of tendon and superficial reflexes

Name of reflex	Root value (Centre of integral)	How the reflex is elicited	Normal response
A. Deep or tendon reflexes			
Biceps jerk	C5,6	Striking the thumb placed on the biceps tendon	Contraction of biceps and flexion of the elbow
Triceps jerk	C6,7	Striking the triceps tendon directly above the olecranon	Contraction of the triceps and extension of the elbow
Supinator (brachioradialis) jerk	C5,6	Striking the radius 1–2 inches above the wrist, over its styloid process	Flexion at elbow and supination of the forearm
Knee jerk	L2,3,4	Striking the patellar tendon directly	Contraction of quadriceps and brief extension at the knee
Ankle jerk	S1,2	Striking the Achilles tendon on its posterior surface	Contraction of the calf muscle and plantar flexion of the foot
Jaw jerk (masseter reflex)	Mesencephalic trigeminal nucleus in the midbrain	Striking the finger placed firmly on the subject's chin with the mouth partially open	Closure of mouth due to contraction of the elevators of the jaw
B. Superficial reflexes			
Plantar reflex	L5,S1	Gently scratching the outer edge of the sole of the foot from the heel towards the ball of the great toe	Flexor plantar response: Inversion and dorsiflexion of ankle with flexion of all toes
Cremasteric reflex	L1,2	Lightly scratching the inner aspect of the upper part of the thigh	Elevation of the testicle and contraction of the dartos muscle of that side
Abdominal reflex i) Upper abdominal reflex ii) Lower abdominal reflex	T8–12 i) (T8,9,10) ii) (T10,11,12)	Stroking lightly but briskly on each side of the abdomen above and below the umbilicus	Contraction of the abdominal muscle and deviation of the umbilicus towards the stimulus
Bulbocavernosus reflex	S3,4	Lightly pinching the dorsum of the glans penis	Contraction of the bulbocavernosus muscle
Anal reflex	S3,4	Stroking or scratching the skin near the anus	Contraction of the anal sphincter
Scapular reflex	C5–8, T1	Stroking the skin of interscapular region	Contraction of the scapular muscle
Conjunctival reflex	Trigeminal (spinal) nucleus in pons and brainstem facial motor nuclei	Touching the conjunctiva with a piece of cotton wool	Blinking of the eye and tear production (**Afferent** by the ophthalmic branch of the 5th CN, and **efferent** by the 7th CN to the orbicularis oculi muscle for the blinking response)
Corneal reflex	i) Chief sensory nucleus of the 5th CN in rostral pons ii) Brainstem facial motor nucleus	Touching the sclerocorneal junction (limbus) with a piece of cotton wool	Blinking of the eye (**Afferent** by the ophthalmic branch of the 5th CN, and **efferent** by the temporal and zygomatic branches of the 7th CN to the orbicularis oculi muscle for the blinking response
Light reflex (pupillary reaction to light)	Midbrain nuclei: i) Pretectal nucleus and superior colliculi ii) Edinger–Westphal nucleus	Focusing light with a pencil torch on the corresponding eye	Constriction of the pupil of the eye on the same side (**direct light reflex**) and pupillary constriction of the opposite eye (**consensual or indirect light reflex**)
Accommodation reflex	i) Edinger Westphal nucleus ii) Visual cortex iii) Oculomotor nucleus	Making the subject quickly look at the tip of the examiner's finger placed close to his eyes after being allowed to look at a faraway object for some time	i) Constriction of the pupils ii) Medial rotation (convergence) of the eyeball iii) Increased convexity of the lens

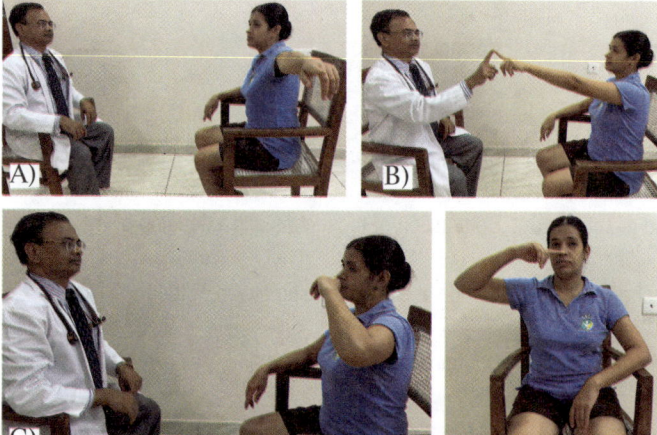

Fig. 58.57   Procedure for the finger–finger–nose test. **(A)** The subject stretches out her hand; **(B)** with outstretched hand, she touches the finger of the examiner; **(C)** she then touches the tip of her nose. She repeats these steps in quick succession with her eyes open. **(D)** Then, she repeats the procedure using the other hand.

Making a circle

1. Properly instruct the subject about the procedure and the steps involved.
2. Ask the subject to draw a circle in the air with his forefinger.
3. Observe whether the subject is able to draw a circle.
4. Ask him to repeat the test with the other hand.

Dysdiadokokinesis

Dysdiadokokinesia is the inability to **execute rapidly repeated alternate movements**. Diadokokinesis is tested by the following methods:

1. Ask the subject to flex his elbow to a right angle and then ask him to **perform supination and pronation of his forearm as rapidly** as possible.
2. Ask the subject to *tap his palm with the tips of his fingers* as fast as possible in an arhythmic manner.
3. Ask the subject to clap on the dorsum of one hand with the palm of the other hand as quickly as possible. He may be asked to perform this movement alternately on either hand.

Romberg test: This test is used to assess the **body's sense of positioning and proprioception**, which requires **intactness of the dorsal column**. It is also used to *investigate the cause of loss of motor coordination* (ataxia). It is performed to *differentiate between* **cerebellar disease and sensory system disease.**

*   The patient is asked to *stand fully erect with both the feet close together* and then *instructed to close her eyes* (**Fig. 58.58**).
*   If the patient has *loss of balance after closing her eyes*, the **Romberg test is positive**, which indicates that **ataxia is due to sensory deficit** (loss of proprioception and sense of body position).

*   If the **Romberg test is not positive** (the subject does not lose her balance after closing her eyes), but the subject *loses balance as soon as she is made to stand with her eyes open*, the **ataxia is cerebellar in nature**.
    Romberg test is performed mainly for assessing coordination of the trunk of the body including the neck and head.

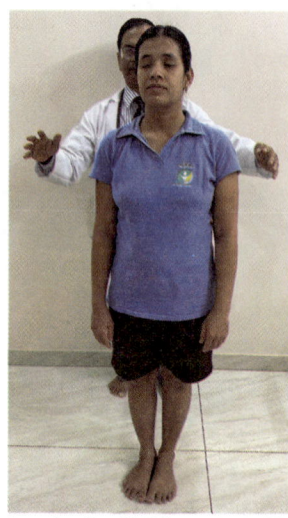

Fig. 58.58   Procedure for the Romberg test. The patient is asked to stand with her feet close together and close her eyes. If the patient has a loss of balance after closing her eyes, the Romberg test is positive.

■ In the lower limbs

Knee–heel test

1. Ask the subject to lie down in the supine position.
2. With the eyes open, ask her to place the heel of one foot (**Fig. 58.59A**) on the opposite knee and then slide the heel down the shin of the leg towards the ankle (**Fig. 58.59B**).
3. Ask the subject to repeat the procedure in quick succession.
4. Observe whether she performs the action properly.
5. Ask the subject to repeat the procedure with the other limb.

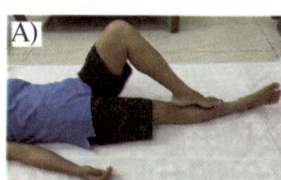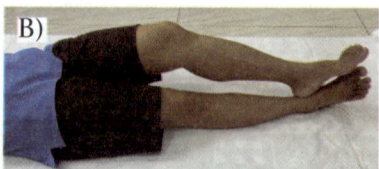

Fig. 58.59   Procedure for the knee–heel test. **(A)** With the eyes open, the subject is asked to place one heel on the opposite knee and **(B)** slide the heel down the shin of the leg towards the ankle. The subject is asked to repeat this step in quick succession and then perform it with the other limb.

Making a circle

1. Ask the subject to draw a circle in the air with his toes.
2. Observe whether he is able to draw a circle.

Walking
1. Ask the subject to walk in a straight line.
2. Observe whether he is able to walk in a straight line.

Gait
Gait refers to the **attitude of walking**. Ask the subject to walk **barefoot along a straight line**. Ask him to walk a certain distance and then to turn round and come back. While the subject is walking, observe the following points:
1. Whether the subject can walk at all.
2. If he walks, whether *he walks in a straight line* or if he tends to deviate to one side.
3. If he *tends to fall*, what direction he falls towards.

Involuntary movements

Involuntary movements are not seen normally. In some diseases of the nervous system, there are involuntary, unintended movements. Observe whether there is any *involuntary movement of any part of the body*. If involuntary movements are present, note the **type of movement,** such as, fibrillation, fasciculation, tremor, myoclonus, tonic or clonic spasm, dystonia, ballism, chorea, or athetosis.

Observation and Results

1. Note your observations, as recorded on both sides of the body, in a tabular format as given below.

Parameters	Observation / Findings	
Patient's name, age, gender, height, and body weight.		
General examination		
i. Orientation and consciousness ii. Emotional state iii. Nutrition and pallor iv. Cyanosis v. Clubbing vi. Dyspnea vii. Vital signs		
Examination of motor system		

Bulk of the muscles	Right side	Left side

i. In the forelimb
  • Midarm
  • Midforearm
ii. In the lower limb
  • Midthigh
  • Midcalf		

Tone of the muscles	Right side	Left side
i. Flexors of elbow joint ii. Extensors of elbow joint iii. Flexors of shoulder joint iv. Extensors of shoulder joint v. Flexors of knee joint vi. Extensors of knee joint vii. Flexors of hip joint viii.Extensors of hip joint		

Strength of the muscle		

i. Muscle of the upper limb
  • Interossei and lumbricals
  • Flexors of fingers
  • Flexors of wrist
  • Extensors of wrist
  • Brachioradialis
  • Biceps
  • Triceps
  • Supraspinatus
  • Infraspinatus
  • Deltoid
  • Pectoralis
  • Serratus anterior
  • Latissimus dorsi
ii. Muscles of the trunk
  • Abdominal muscles
  • Erector spinae and muscles of the back		

iii. Muscles of the lower limb
  • Intrinsic muscles of foot
  • Dorsiflexor and plantar
  • flexors of the feet and
  • toes
  • Evertors and invertors of
  • foot
  • Extensors of knee
  • Flexors of knee
  • Extensors of thigh
  • Flexors of thigh
  • Adductors of thigh
  • Abductors of thigh
  • Rotators of thigh or hip		

Reflexes
i. Tendon or deep reflexes
  • Biceps jerk
  • Triceps jerk
  • Supinator jerk
  • Knee jerk
  • Ankle jerk
  • Jaw jerk
ii. Superficial reflexes
a. Superficial reflexes of spinal origin:
  • Plantar reflex
  • Cremasteric reflex
  • Bulbocavernosus reflex
  • Anal reflex
  • Abdominal reflex
  • Scapular reflex
b. Superficial reflexes of cranial origin:
  • Conjunctival reflex
  • Corneal reflex
  • Pupillary reflexes
  • Light reflex
  • Accommodation reflex
  • Palatal reflex
iii. Sphincteric reflexes
  (swallowing, defecation, micturition)		

Coordination of movement
i.   In the upper limb
  • Finger–nose test
  • Finger–finger–nose test
  • Finger–finger test
  • Making a circle
  • Dysdiadokokinesis
  • Romberg test
ii.   In the lower limb
  • Knee–heel test
  • Making a circle
  • Walking		

Gait
  • Attitude of walking
  • Walking in a straight line
  • Swinging or falling		

Involuntary movements, if any
  • Fibrillation
  • Fasciculation
  • Tremor
  • Myoclonus
  • Tonic/clonic spasm
  • Dystonia
  • Ballism
  • Chorea
  • Athetosis		

2. Compare the findings of both sides, analyse the results, and report your findings with your comments on the functional integrity of the motor system.

DISCUSSION

Bulk of the Muscle

The bulk of the muscle may be **normal, decreased** (atrophy), or **increased** (hypertrophy).

Muscle atrophy

Muscle atrophy is seen in neurological disorders, especially in **lower motor neuron disease**. *Generalised wasting* of the muscle occurs in non-neurological conditions like malignancy, diabetes, thyrotoxicosis, and tuberculosis. *Localised wasting* is seen in arthritis or myopathy.

Muscle hypertrophy

Hypertrophy occurs due to the *excessive use of muscles,* as seen in athletes and gymnasts. It can also occur in some *myotonic disorders*.

Tone of the Muscle

The tone of the muscle is the **state of partial contraction** of the muscle. Healthy muscles always exhibit certain degrees of tone. In some diseases, the *tone of the muscles increases* (hypertonia), and in others, the *tone of the muscles decreases* (hypotonia).

Hypertonia

Hypertonia is a feature of **upper motor neuron lesions**. It manifests as **spasticity or rigidity**.

■ Spasticity

Spasticity is a term used to describe a state of *increased tone of muscle* of the 'clasp-knife' type.
•   The tone is much **more increased in the antigravity muscles**, i.e., in the *flexors of the upper limbs and the extensors and adductors of the lower limbs*.
•   Clasp-knife rigidity is seen in **pyramidal tract lesions**.

■ Rigidity

Rigidity is **seen in all muscles** *without any relation to gravity*. It is seen in **lesions of the extrapyramidal tracts**. There are **two types of rigidity**: lead pipe and cogwheel.
Lead pipe rigidity: The resistance to passive movement is **uniform throughout the range of movement**. It is seen in catatonic states, dementia, and Parkinsonism.
Cogwheel rigidity: The resistance to passive movement is seen alternately, i.e., there is *alternate resistance and relaxation*. This is typically seen in diseases of the basal ganglia, particularly in the involvement of the substantia nigra.

Strength of Muscles

If muscle strength is decreased, there is **paresis**; if there is no strength, there is **paralysis**. **Hemiplegia** refers to paralysis of one side of the body, especially of the arms and legs. **Paraplegia** refers to paralysis of both legs; **monoplegia** means paralysis of one limb; and **quadriplegia** means paralysis of all four limbs.
•   **Hemiplegia** is usually seen in lesions of the *corticospinal tract at the level of the internal capsule*.
•   **Paraplegia** is seen in spinal cord lesions below the midthoracic level, and **quadriplegia** is seen in spinal cord lesions above the upper thoracic level.
•   **Monoplegia** usually occurs due to lesions of a nerve plexus.
•   **Crossed paralysis** refers to paralysis of the ipsilateral cranial musculature with contralateral hemiplegia. It is usually seen in brainstem disease.
  Weakness of the muscle may occur in the absence of paralysis. It occurs due to *myasthenia gravis, myopathies, and myotonic dystrophy*.

Reflexes
Tendon reflexes

Tendon reflexes are stretch reflexes that are activated in response to a **sudden stretch of the muscle**. These are **monosynaptic reflexes** that are activated by stretching of the muscle spindle, which conveys information via **Ia fibres** directly to the motor neurons in the spinal cord

(Fig. 58.60). Stimulation of the α motor neuron causes the contraction of the muscle that was stretched.

- The presence of the tendon reflexes indicates the **integrity of the afferent and efferent pathways** and of the **excitability of the anterior horn cells** in the spinal segment of the stretched muscles.
- Tendon reflexes are continuously affected by the activities in the *descending (from the supraspinal centres)* pathways. The higher centres **usually inhibit** the spinal reflexes. Therefore, the tendon reflexes are *exaggerated in upper motor neuron lesions*.
- Tendon reflexes are **diminished or absent in lower motor neuron lesions** because there is disruption in the final common pathway.

Role of γ motor neurons: The γ motor neurons *increase the sensitivity of the muscle spindle to stretch*. Therefore, *increased γ motor neuron discharge increases the reflex activity*. The γ motor neurons are usually under the *inhibitory influence* of supraspinal inputs. Therefore, *a lesion of the upper motor neurons* results in the *exaggeration of deep reflexes*.

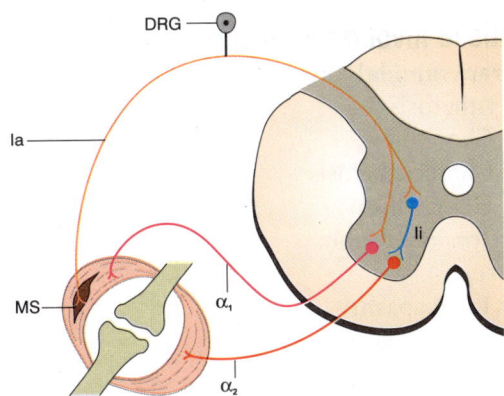

Fig. 58.60 The stretch reflex (DRG: dorsal root ganglion; MS: muscle spindle; Ii: inhibitory interneuron; α₁ and α₂: motor neurons to agonist and antagonist muscle respectively; and Ia: Ia afferents).

Superficial reflexes

The superficial reflexes are **polysynaptic** and involve many centres in the neuraxis. These are elicited by stimulating the cutaneous receptors that carry information to *higher centres by sensory pathways*. The higher centres then convey information to the concerned muscles by *motor pathways*. Therefore, superficial reflexes **are lost in both upper and lower motor neuron paralysis**.

Coordination of Movement

Normal movement is dependent on the ability of the *agonist muscles to contract* to the degree needed and the simultaneous relaxation of the antagonist muscles. *Impairment in these abilities* produces incoordination of movement. This incoordination may be due to a disease of the *cerebellum, the corticospinal tract, or the sensory system*. The lack of proper coordination is known as **ataxia**.

Cerebellar disease

In **cerebellar ataxia**, the errors of movement tend to occur at *right angles to the intended direction* of movement. A *useful sign* of cerebellar ataxia is *dysdiadokokinesia*, which is the impaired ability to execute rapidly repeated alternate movements. *All the aspects of movement* (initiation, rate, range, direction, and termination) are affected.

Corticospinal tract disease

The incoordination is characterised by **slowness and clumsiness of the finger movements**. This is tested by asking the patient to rapidly approximate each finger to the thumb. Corticospinal tract disease *does not cause incoordination of movement* at the more proximal joints, i.e., the knee, hip, elbow, and so on; it *also does not cause incoordination of movement in the leg*. However, if it is associated with muscle weakness, *impairment in walking* occurs.

Sensory system disease

Incoordination of movement can be produced in the arms or legs by *impaired sensation*. This is called **sensory ataxia**. It is tested by the *Romberg sign*. The patient is asked to stand with his feet close together, and if he can do so, he is asked to continue with his eyes closed. If the subject *sways or falls*, the **Romberg sign is positive**. It is an important physical sign of **impaired position and joint sense in the lower limb**.

Gait

Gait is the **posture of the subject while walking**. The *character of the gait* is often important in the diagnosis of neurological diseases. Normally, when a person walks, he partially flexes the hip and knee joint of one lower limb and dorsiflexes his foot. As he does so, his foot lifts up from the ground while the other lower limb supports the whole weight of the body. As the first lower limb moves forward and takes up the weight, the other lower limb flexes, and the entire cycle is repeated. If the smooth manner in which the whole movement is performed is disturbed, the gait becomes abnormal. The common **abnormal gaits** are: spastic gait, ataxic gait, festinant gait, waddling gait, high-stepping gait, and limping gait.

Spastic gait

This is probably the commonest abnormal type. The person **walks on a narrow base**, has difficulty in bending his knees, and drags his feet along *as if they are glued to the ground*.

- The movement is slow, and *the flexion of the knee and hip joints is either absent or imperfectly performed.* The affected leg tends *to remain adducted.*
- The foot is raised from the ground *by tilting the pelvis* and then *swinging the leg forward* so that the foot tends to describe an arc (circumduction) with the *toe scraping along the floor.*

It is characteristically seen in **corticospinal tract lesions**. There are two types of spastic gaits: (i) hemiplegic and (ii) scissor.

Hemiplegic gait: In this type of gait, *only one leg is affected.* It is ***seen in hemiplegia***.

Scissor gait: The *spasticity is present on both sides.* The person walks in a typical *criss-cross fashion.* It is typically seen in ***congenital spastic paraplegia***.

Ataxic gait

This occurs due to ataxia. Ataxic gaits are of **two types**, stamping and drunken.

Stamping gait: It is a **high-stepping ataxic gait** in which the movements in the lower limbs are not coordinated. The person *raises his feet suddenly and often to an abnormally high level* and then jerks them forward, *bringing them to the ground again with a stomp,* often, heel first. The degree of ataxia tends to increase in the darkness or if the person's eyes are closed. It is best seen in **tabes dorsalis** and **severe peripheral neuritis**.

Drunken gait: The patient walks on a **broad and irregular base** with the feet planted widely apart. The degree of ataxia is equally severe whether the eyes are opened or closed. It is typically seen in **cerebellar disorders**.

Festinant gait

The patient walks with an *attitude of generalised flexion* (bent forward) so that the centre of gravity of the body lies outside, in front of him. To bring the centre of gravity to its proper place, the patient takes **rapid, short, and shuffling steps**. However, the centre of gravity moves forward and continues to elude him. Thus, he **attempts to catch the centre of gravity**. *His arms do not swing.* It is typically seen in **Parkinsonism**.

Waddling gait

This is like the **gait of a duck**. The patient sways from side to side, the body is tilted backwards with an increase of *lumbar lordosis and a protuberant abdomen.* The feet are planted widely apart, and the heels and toes tend to be brought down simultaneously. It occurs in **proximal muscular weakness**, which is seen in **myopathies and muscular dystrophies**. It is also seen in **advanced pregnancy**.

High-stepping gait

The patient walks by **taking high steps**. It is typically seen in **foot drop**, as seen in **peripheral neuritis and preseason muscular dystrophy**.

Limping gait

The person **limps with short steps**, keeping the painful limb semiflexed, and dropping the pelvis towards the painful side. It is seen in *tuberculosis of the knee* and hip joints and in sciatica.

Involuntary Movements

Involuntary movements can occur either at rest or during voluntary movement. They are classified into two types, localised and generalised.

Localised involuntary movement

1. Fibrillation
2. Fasciculation
3. Myoclonus
4. Tremor

Generalised involuntary movement

1. **Extrapyramidal abnormalities**
   - Athetosis
   - Chorea
   - Choreoathetosis
   - Hemiballism
   - Torsion dystonia
2. **Spasms**
   - Tonic spasm
   - Clonic spasm

▌Fibrillation

This occurs due to the *contraction of a single muscle fibre.* It cannot usually be seen. Clinically, fibrillation, if present, can be observed *in the tongue,* but it can be recorded electromyographically.

▌Fasciculation

This occurs due to the contraction of *a bundle of muscle fibres.* It can be seen as well as recorded electromyographically. It occurs due to **irritation of the anterior horn cells** or **nerve roots** during inflammation or degeneration.

Causes:
- Motor neuron disease
- Cervical spondylosis
- Syringomyelia
- Peroneal muscular dystrophy

Myoclonus

A sudden, *shock-like contraction of a single muscle or group of muscles* is called myoclonus. It is involuntary and arrhythmic. There are different types of myoclonus: when it occurs in the face, it is called **facial myoclonus;** when it occurs during muscular activity, it is called **action myoclonus**; and when it occurs in different parts of the body and disappears during sleep, it is called **myoclonus simplex.**

Tremor

Tremor is a *regular, rhythmic, purposeless, to-and-fro movement* of a part of the body (usually limbs) due to the contraction of a group of muscles and their antagonists. *It usually involves the distal parts of the limbs, tongue,* and rarely, the trunk. It is divided into **resting and static tremors** (when it occurs at rest) and **intention and kinetic tremors** (when it occurs during a purposeful movement of the limbs).

- **Resting tremor** is typically seen in *Parkinsonism* and **intention tremor** in *cerebellar disorder.*
- Tremor is also divided into *fine and coarse tremors.* **Fine tremor** is seen in anxiety and hyperthyroidism. **Coarse tremor** is seen in Parkinsonism (pin-rolling tremor).

Causes of tremor:

I. **Physiological**
   1. Anxiety
   2. Exposure to cold
   3. Old age (senile tremor)
   4. Congenital
II. **Pathological**
   A. *Neurological*
   1. Parkinsonism
   2. Cerebellar disorder
   3. Disseminated sclerosis
   4. Benign essential tremor
   B. *Metabolic*
   1. Thyrotoxicosis
   2. Hypoglycemia
   3. Hepatic coma
   4. Uremia
   C. *Toxic*
   1. Alcoholism
   2. Barbiturate poisoning
   3. Opium poisoning
   4. Heavy metal poisoning

Chorea

This is a *rapid, involuntary, dancing* type of movement. It occurs in *lesions of the caudate nucleus.* It is seen in Huntington's disease (**Huntington's chorea**) and chronic rheumatic disease (**Sydenham's chorea**).

Athetosis

This is characterised by continuous, *slow or writhing movements.* It occurs due to a *lesion in the globus pallidus.*

Choreoathetosis

When *chorea and athetosis are present together*, the condition is called choreoathetosis.

Ballism

This is an involuntary movement that is *sudden, flailing, intense, and violent.* It occurs in *lesions of the subthalamic nucleus.* When it occurs in one side of the body, it is called **hemiballism.**

Torsion dystonia

The torsion of the limbs and vertebral column results in a *distorted posture of the limbs and trunk.* A persistent increase in muscle tone occurs. This dystonia *disappears during sleep.*

Tonic spasm

Tonic spasm of the muscle is seen in *tetanus and strychnine poisoning.*

Clonic spasm

Clonic spasm of the muscle is *seen in epilepsy.*

Tics

These are *sudden rapid, repeated, coordinated,* and *purposeless* movements that usually occur in the same region intermittently. Generally, tics occur in the form of *blinking of the eyes* or *wriggling of the shoulders.*

Upper Motor Neuron (UMN) Paralysis

Features

1. Muscles are **affected in groups** (individual muscles are never affected)
2. **No muscle atrophy** (disuse atrophy may occur in chronic patients)
3. **Spasticity** (hypertonia)
4. **Exaggeration of tendon reflexes**
5. **Loss of superficial reflexes**
6. Positive Babinski sign (**extensor plantar response**)
7. No fascicular twitches
8. No denervation potential in EMG
9. Normal nerve conduction studies

Causes

The corticospinal pathways can be interrupted by *lesions at any level*, starting from the cerebral cortex, subcortical white matter, internal capsule, brainstem, to the spinal cord.

- The ***most common site of lesion*** of the corticospinal tract is the **internal capsule,** which is usually involved in cerebral hemorrhage due to ***damage to Charcot's artery*** (the **artery of cerebral hemorrhage**), a branch of the middle cerebral artery.
- Corticothalamic, corticostriate, corticorubral, corticopontaine, cortico-olivary, and corticoreticular fibres also *pass through the internal capsule.* Therefore, a lesion in the internal capsule not only affects the pyramidal (corticospinal) tract, ***but also the extrapyramidal and other fibres.*** Therefore, the resulting paralysis is called ***upper motor neuron paralysis***, instead of pyramidal paralysis.

The **extrapyramidal motor system** includes the *basal ganglia and the cerebellum.* These two structures influence the extrapyramidal tracts by projecting directly or indirectly to the brainstem. ***Extrapyramidal lesions do not cause paralysis*** (Table 58.2).

Table 58.2   Differences between pyramidal (corticospinal) and extrapyramidal lesions

	Pyramidal	**Extrapyramidal**
Muscle tone	Spasticity (clasp-knife rigidity)	Plastic (cogwheel rigidity)
Distribution of hypertonus	Flexors of arm and extensors of leg	Generalised
Shortening and lengthening reaction	Present	Absent
Involuntary movement	Absent	Present
Tendon reflexes	Exaggerated	Normal
Babinski sign	Positive	Negative
Paralysis	Of voluntary movement	No paralysis

Physiological basis

In upper motor neuron (UMN) paralysis, in addition to **lesions of the corticospinal tract** (the so-called pyramidal tract), a few extrapyramidal fibres (especially ***corticoreticular fibres*** that project onto the reticulospinal tract) are also disrupted. This occurs in UMN paralysis due to a **lesion at the internal capsule** (the commonest site of UMN lesion).

- The **pontine reticulospinal tract** is *excitatory to the muscles involved in postural control,* i.e., the **antigravity muscle**. This reticulospinal tract is under the inhibitory control of corticoreticular fibres. In UMN lesions, the *disruption of corticoreticular fibres* facilitates the excitatory output of the pontine reticulospinal pathway. Therefore, ***hypertonia and spasticity*** occur in a UMN lesion.

- Deep reflexes are exaggerated because of the ***increased discharge and sensitivity of the gamma motor neurons***. Excitability of the gamma motor neurons regulates spinal reflex activity. Gamma motor neurons are usually inhibited by many supraspinal influences. In UMN lesions, the ***loss of inhibitory influence*** increases gamma motor neuron discharge and thereby ***increases the reflex activity***.
- The corticospinal tract *excites the flexor motor neurons and inhibits the extensor motor neurons* of the digits of the limbs. Therefore, normally stroking the sole elicits plantar flexion. In UMN paralysis, disruption of corticospinal influence on the lumbosacral motor neurons causes *dorsiflexion of the big toe and fanning of other toes* (***Babinski sign or extensor plantar response***).

Lower Motor Neuron (LMN) Paralysis

The lower motor neurons may be injured or diseased in the *cranial nerve nuclei* or *spinal anterior horn cells*, in the *anterior nerve roots*, or in the nerves themselves.

- The **anterior horn cell** lesions may be *acute or chronic*. The most common *acute lesion of the anterior horn cell* is **poliomyelitis**. The *chronic degeneration* of anterior horn cells occurs in **motor neuron disease** (progressive muscular atrophy).
- The **anterior nerve roots** may be damaged by *trauma*, especially in association with cervical spondylosis or by an *inflammatory or neoplastic lesion*.
- The **peripheral nerves** are chiefly affected by *injury, inflammation*, and *toxic or metabolic disorders* (neuropathies). As the nerves carry both motor and sensory information, pure motor deficits *rarely occur*. Usually, muscular paralysis is *associated with sensory changes*.

Features

1. Usually, **individual muscles** are affected
2. **Muscle atrophy** is pronounced (Table 58.3)
3. **Flaccidity**
4. **Hypotonia** is seen in the affected muscles
5. Tendon reflexes and superficial **reflexes are diminished or absent**
6. *Babinski sign* is **negative** (plantar flexion)
7. **Fascicular twitches** may be present
8. Denervation potentials (**fibrillation, fasciculation, positive sharp waves**) are observed in the EMG
9. *Nerve conduction studies* reveal **abnormalities**

Table 58.3 Comparison of upper motor neuron and lower motor neuron paralyses

	UMN paralysis	LMN paralysis
Muscles affected	Muscles are affected in groups	Individual muscles are affected
Size of the muscles	Atrophy not seen (slight atrophy may occur due to disuse)	Pronounced atrophy (may be up to 80 per cent of the total bulk) of muscles
Type of paralysis	Spastic paralysis	Flaccid paralysis
Tone of the muscles	Hypertonia	Hypotonia
Power of the muscles	Paralysis occurs (no voluntary movement)	Paralysis occurs
Tendon reflexes	Exaggerated	Diminished or absent
Superficial reflexes	Absent	Absent
Plantar reflex	Extensor plantar response (Babinski sign positive)	Flexor plantar reflex (Babinski sign negative)
Involuntary movement	Absent	Fascicular twitches may be present
EMG changes	No denervation potentials seen in EMG	Denervation potentials (fibrillations, fasciculations, and sharp waves) are seen in EMG
Nerve conduction	No abnormalities in nerve conduction	Abnormal nerve conduction (decreased studies conduction)

OSPE

I. Measure the bulk of the muscles of the right arm of the subject.

Steps
1. Provide proper instructions to the subject.
2. Detect the midpoint of the subject's right arm by measuring (with the help of a measuring tape) the distance between the median olecranon process and the tip of the humerus.
3. Ask him to relax completely.
4. Measure the midarm circumference with a measuring tape.
5. Measure the midarm circumference of the other (left) side and compare.

II. Assess the tone of the flexors and extensors of the right elbow of the subject.

Steps
1. Provide proper instructions to the subject.
2. Ask him to relax completely.
3. Make passive movements (flexion and extension) of the forearm at the elbow joint.
4. Feel (can also palpate the muscles) the tone of the extensors and flexors.
5. Repeat the procedure on the other elbow joint and compare.

III. Assess the strength of the biceps muscle of the right side of the subject.

Steps
1. Properly instruct the subject on the steps of the procedure.
2. Ask the subject to bend his right forearm against resistance (the examiner prevents the flexion of the forearm by applying resistance).
3. Look for the prominence of the biceps muscle and assess the strength (in terms of grade) of the biceps.
4. Repeat the procedure on the opposite side and compare.

IV. Elicit biceps jerk of the right side of the subject.

Steps
1. Provide proper instructions to the subject.
2. Flex the subject's right elbow and make the forearm semipronated by resting it on the subject's abdomen or on your (examiner's) left forearm.
3. Expose the front of the arm.
4. Ask the subject to relax completely.
5. Place your thumb on the biceps tendon firmly to stretch the muscle.
6. Strike with the narrow end of a knee hammer on his thumb.
7. Observe the contraction of the biceps and flexion of the forearm.
8. Elicit the biceps jerk on the opposite side and compare.

V. Elicit triceps jerk on the right side of the subject.

Steps
1. Provide proper instructions to the subject.
2. Flex the subject's right elbow and rest the forearm on his (the subject's) chest or on your own (examiner's) forearm.
3. Expose the back of the arm.
4. Ask the subject to relax completely.
5. Tap the triceps tendon with the broad end of the hammer with movements at the wrist joint.
6. Look for contraction of the triceps and extension of the forearm.
7. Elicit the triceps jerk on the opposite side and compare.

VI. Elicit right side supinator jerk of the subject.

Steps

1. Provide proper instructions to the subject.
2. Slightly flex the subject's right forearm and support the forearm by holding the subject's hand.
3. Ask the subject to relax completely.
4. Tap the radius about 1–2 inches above the wrist over its styloid process.
5. Look for flexion at the elbow and supination of the forearm.
6. Elicit supinator jerks on the opposite side and compare.

VII. Elicit knee jerk of the right side of the subject in the supine position.

Steps

1. Provide proper instructions to the subject.
2. Pass your hand under the knee to be tested and place it on the opposite knee in such a way that the tested knee rests on the dorsum of your wrist.
3. Ask the subject to relax completely.
4. Strike the patellar tendon with the broad end of the hammer with movement at the wrist joint.
5. Observe the contraction of the quadriceps and extension at the knee joint.
6. Elicit the knee jerk on the opposite side and compare.

VIII. Elicit ankle jerk of the right side of the subject in the supine position.

Steps

1. Provide proper instructions to the subject.
2. Place the subject's right lower limb on the bed so that it lies everted and slightly flexed.
3. Slightly dorsiflex the foot so as to stretch the Achilles tendon.
4. Strike the tendon on its posterior surface with the broad end of the hammer with movement at the wrist joint.
5. Observe the contraction of the calf muscles and plantar flexion at the ankle joint.
6. Elicit ankle jerk on the other side and compare.

IX. Elicit plantar reflex of the subject.

Steps

1. Properly instruct the subject on the steps of the procedure. Ask the subject to lie down in the supine position.
2. Fix the foot by placing the left hand on the medial malleolus.
3. Ask the subject to relax completely.

4. Gently scratch with a key or the pointed, metallic end of a knee hammer on the outer edge of the sole of the foot, from the heel towards the little toe, and then medially across the metatarsus.
5. Observe the response.
6. Elicit the plantar reflex on the opposite side and compare.

X. Elicit the abdominal reflex of the subject in the supine position.

Steps

1. Provide proper instructions to the subject.
2. Expose the abdomen.
3. With the help of a key or the pointed, metallic end of a knee hammer, scratch lightly but briskly from the outer aspect of the abdomen towards the midline in all four quadrants.
4. Look for contraction of the muscle and deviation of the umbilicus.

XI. Elicit the cremasteric reflex of the subject.

Steps

1. Provide proper instructions to the subject.
2. Expose the external genitalia and upper portion of the thigh.
3. With the help of a key, scratch the upper and inner aspect of the thigh lightly and briskly.
4. Look for the contraction of the dartus muscle and lifting of the testicle.
5. Elicit the cremasteric reflex of the other side and compare the findings.

XII. Perform the finger–nose test on the subject.

Steps

1. Provide proper instructions to the subject.
2. Ask the subject to touch the tip of his nose with the tip of one of his index fingers rapidly and repeatedly, first with the eyes open and then with the eyes closed.
3. Ask him to repeat the same with the opposite index finger; compare the findings.

XIII. Perform the knee-heel test on the subject in the supine position.

Steps

1. Provide proper instructions to the subject.
2. Ask the subject to place one of his heels on the opposite knee and then to slide the heel down his shin towards the ankle.
3. Ask him to repeat the same rapidly 4–5 times.
4. Ask him to do the same on the other side; compare the findings.

VIVA

1. *What are the different aspects of motor functions that are assessed while examining the motor system?* (**Ans.** Refer to page 408, under the heading 'Procedure'.)
2. *How do you measure the bulk of the muscles in the upper and lower limbs?* (**Ans.** Refer to page 408, under the heading 'Procedure' and the subheading 'Bulk of muscles'.)
3. *What is muscle tone and how is it assessed clinically?* (**Ans.** Refer to page 408, under the heading 'Tone of Muscles'.)
4. *How do you grade the strength of muscles?* (**Ans.** Refer to page 409, under the heading 'Grading the Strength of Muscles'.)
5. *How do you estimate the strength of the intrinsic muscles of the hands?* (**Ans.** Refer to page 409, under the heading 'Testing strength of muscles of the upper limb' and the subheading 'Interossei and lumbricals'.)
6. *How do you assess the strength of the flexors and extensors of the wrist?* (**Ans.** Refer to page 410, under the heading 'Testing strength of muscles of the upper limb' and the subheading 'Flexors of the wrist'.)
7. *How do you assess the strength of the biceps, triceps, and brachioradialis?* (**Ans.** Refer to page 410-411, under the heading 'Testing strength of muscles of the upper limb' and the subheadings for biceps, triceps, and brachioradialis'.)
8. *How do you assess the strength of the abdominal muscles?* (**Ans.** Refer to page 412, under the heading 'Testing strength of muscles of muscles of the trunk'.)
9. *How do you assess the strength of the intrinsic muscles of the foot?* (**Ans.** Refer to page 412-413, under the heading 'Testing strength of muscles of the lower limb'.)
10. *How do you assess the strength of the extensors and flexors of the knee and those of the thigh?* (**Ans.** Refer to page 413, under the heading 'Testing strength of muscles of the lower limb'.)
11. *What are the precautions observed for eliciting deep reflexes?* (**Ans.** Refer to page 414, under the heading 'Reflexes' and the subheading 'Precautions. . .'.)
12. *How do you grade tendon reflexes?* (**Ans.** Refer to page 414, under the heading 'Grading of Tendon Reflexes'.)
13. *What is the root value of different important tendon jerks?* (**Ans.** Refer to page 421, see Table 58.1.)
14. *Name the superficial reflexes.* (**Ans.** Refer to page 418, under the heading 'Superficial Reflexes'.)
15. *What are the tests for coordination of movement in the upper and lower limbs?* (**Ans.** Refer to page 420, under the heading 'Coordination of Movements' and the subheading 'In the upper limbs'.)
16. *What is dysdiadokokinesis?* (**Ans.** Refer to page 422, under the heading 'Dysdiadokokinesis'.)
17. *Define gait, and name the parameters observed for assessing gait.* (**Ans.** Refer to page 423, under the heading 'Gait'.)
18. *In what conditions are atrophy and hypertrophy of muscles observed? Why?* (**Ans.** Refer to page 424, under the heading 'Discussion' and the subheadings for atrophy and hypertrophy.)
19. *What is the cause of spasticity in upper motor neuron paralysis?* (**Ans.** Refer to page 424, under the heading 'UMN Paralysis' and the subheading 'Physiological basis'.)
20. *Why are deep tendon reflexes exaggerated in UMN paralysis?* (**Ans.** Refer to page 428, under the heading 'UMN Paralysis' and the subheading 'Physiological basis'.)
21. *What is the role of gamma motor neurons on maintaining muscle tone?* (**Ans.** Refer to page 424, under the heading 'Tendon Reflexes'.)
22. *In addition to Babinski sign, what other methods are followed for eliciting the plantar reflex?* (**Ans.** Refer to page 419, under the heading 'Plantar Reflex'.)
23. *What are the receptors, afferents, efferents of the stretch reflex?* (**Ans.** Refer to page 425, under the heading 'Tendon reflexes'.)
24. *What is the cause of flaccidity in lower motor neuron paralysis?*
    (**Ans.** In LMN paralysis, the motor neurons supplying the muscles are diseased. Normally, discharge of motor neurons keeps the muscle in a state of partial contraction and maintains the muscle excitability. As motor neurons (LMN.) are damaged, the discharge to the muscle is decreased or absent. Hence, the muscle becomes flaccid.)
25. *What are the differences between pyramidal and extrapyramidal tract lesions?* (**Ans.** Refer to page 428, see Table 58.2.)
26. *What are the differences between upper motor neuron and lower motor neuron paralysis?* (**Ans.** Refer to page 429, see Table 58.3.)
27. *How do you classify muscles clinically?* (**Ans.** Refer to page 405, under the heading 'Muscles'.)
28. *What do you mean by lower and upper motor neurons? Give examples.* (**Ans.** Refer to page 405-406, under the headings 'Lower Motor Neuron' and 'Upper Motor Neuron'.)
29. *What are the descending motor tracts?* (**Ans.** Refer to page 406, under the headings 'Lateral System' and 'Medial System'.)
30. *Name the extrapyramidal systems.* (**Ans.** Refer to page 406, under the heading 'Upper Motor Neuron' and the subheading 'Extrapyramidal tracts'.)

31. *Trace the pathway of corticospinal tracts.* (Ans. Refer to page 405, under the heading 'Corticospinal Tract' and see Fig. 57.1.)
32. *What are the functions of the corticospinal tracts?* (Ans. Refer to page 406, under the heading 'Corticospinal Tract' and the subheading 'Functions'.)
33. *What are the functions of extrapyramidal systems?* (Ans. Refer to page 407, under the heading 'Functions of Other Tracts'.)
34. *What are the areas in the brain that are involved in the regulation of motor activities?* (Ans. Refer to page 407, under the heading 'Motor Areas in the Brain'.)
35. *What are the functions of the motor cortex?* (Ans. Refer to page 407, under the heading 'Cortical Motor Areas'.)
36. *What are the ataxic gaits, and in what conditions are they seen?* (Ans. Refer to page 426, under the heading 'Ataxic Gait'.)
37. *What gait is seen in Parkinsonism and how do you describe it?* (Ans. Refer to page 426, under the heading 'Festinant Gait'.)
38. *What are the functions of the basal ganglia?* (Ans. Refer to page 407, under the heading 'Basal ganglia'.)
39. *What are the types of alterations in the tone of muscles observed in Parkinsonism?* (Ans. Refer to page 424, under the heading 'Rigidity'.)
40. *What are the functions of the cerebellum?* (Ans. Refer to page 407, under the heading 'Cerebellum'.)

59 | Introduction to Animal Experiments and Appliances

Learning Objectives

After completing this practical, you will be able to:

1. Identify and describe the uses of the appliances used in experimental physiology.
2. List the advantages of using an electrical stimulus.
3. List the advantages of using frog and gastrocnemius-sciatic preparations.
4. State the basic principle of the apparatus used in amphibian practicals.
5. List the factors that affect the strength of induced current.
6. List the precautions taken for amphibian practicals.
7. Make primary and secondary circuits.
8. Smoke the paper pasted on the drum.
9. Varnish (fix) the recording.

INTRODUCTION TO ANIMAL EXPERIMENTS

A student of physiology should be familiar with the apparatus used in experimental physiology. He should know the basic working principles of various instruments, the uses of the apparatus, and the instructions for the safe use of the apparatus. Since electric current is used as the stimulus for most experiments, proper earthing (grounding) and insulation of the wires must be ensured before starting an experiment.

In most experimental work, especially the kind dealing with the study of the response of tissues to various stimuli, **four components are needed:** (i) a source of stimulation, (ii) a stimulating device, (iii) tissue preparation, and (iv) a recording device.

Source of Stimulation

The stimulus may be mechanical, chemical, thermal, or electrical. In most experimental procedures, the **electrical stimulus is usually preferred** because of its *many advantages:*

1. The electrical stimulus is easy to deliver and can be handled conveniently by most operators.
2. The apparatus for delivering the stimulus is compact.
3. The stimulus is easily controlled by the break or make of a key.
4. It is possible to stimulate the tissue with the desired strength, frequency, and duration, accurately and easily.
5. The stimulus can be accurately localised on the tissue.
6. The stimulus can be remotely controlled from a distance.
7. This is the least injurious type of stimulus to tissues.

Stimulating Device

The stimulating device is the inductorium, which is described in detail later in this chapter.

Tissue Preparation

For amphibian nerve muscle experiments, the **sciatic nerve and the gastrocnemius muscles** of frogs are usually used.

Advantages of using frogs

1. They are easily available.
2. They are easy to handle.
3. They are harmless.
4. They are not expensive to procure.
5. To maintain a tissue preparation of frogs, no extra supply of oxygen is needed because their muscles can directly imbibe oxygen from the environment.
6. The tissue preparation of a frog can be maintained for a long time, if handled properly.
7. It is easy to dissect frogs.

Note: Frogs are **no longer used** in academic or research-based experimental studies, as they are now classified as *endangered species*. The above information is intended solely for *computer-assisted learning purposes.*

Advantages of the gastrocnemius-sciatic preparation

1. The sciatic nerve and gastrocnemius muscle are easy to locate and dissect.
2. The sciatic nerve is the longest nerve and, therefore, is easy to place on electrodes that are kept a short distance away from the muscle.
3. The gastrocnemius muscle is a big muscle (with a larger cross-sectional area), and therefore, on contraction, produces more force to lift the lever and yields a good magnitude of contraction.
4. The gastrocnemius muscle is not easily fatigued.

Recording Device

Muscle contractions are recorded using a **writing lever** that inscribes on the smoked surface of a rotating drum fitted to a **kymograph**.

DESCRIPTION AND USES OF APPLIANCES

Source of Current

Electrical stimulation can be provided either with a **direct current** (DC) source and a pair of stimulating electrodes (**galvanic current**) or by using an induction coil with electrodes (**faradic current** or **induced current**). In most experiments, direct current is used.

Direct current (6 volts) is available at the battery terminals of all experimental tables. To obtain an induced current, a constant current (galvanic) of low voltage is fed into the primary coil of the inductorium. To supply low-voltage direct current, a central low-voltage unit is installed in most laboratories. The output terminals feed a direct current of 3–15 volts to all the working seats at a table. This direct current is a rectified current, which comes from the central eliminator. Direct current can also be obtained from dry cells connected in series.

Wires

Generally, **copper or aluminium wires** are used in laboratories to carry electric current. A single, thick wire is used to supply direct current. The wires are insulated by cotton, silk, or enamel. While connecting the wires to supply current, the insulation from the tip of the wires is removed and polished with the help of fine sandpaper to ensure sufficient contact. The wire should not be damaged or cracked. The wires are usually rolled on glass rods into spirals.

Keys

The key is a device used for completing or interrupting a circuit. Two types of keys are used, the simple or tap key and the short-circuiting key.

The tap key: This key (Fig. 59.1A) is connected in the primary circuit in series with the DC source. The key is pressed gently and released to make and break the circuit.

The short-circuiting key: This key (Fig 59.1B) is connected in the secondary circuit in parallel to prevent accidental leakage of current into the tissue. This also prevents unipolar induction. The key is kept closed to check unnecessary stimulation of the tissue, and when stimulation is required, it is left open. Different types of short-circuiting keys are available, but the **Du Bois-Reymond key** (Fig. 59.1C) is usually used in the laboratory.

The reversing key: This key (Fig. 59.1D) is also used in the laboratory when two electrodes are required for shunting the current from one electrode to the other.

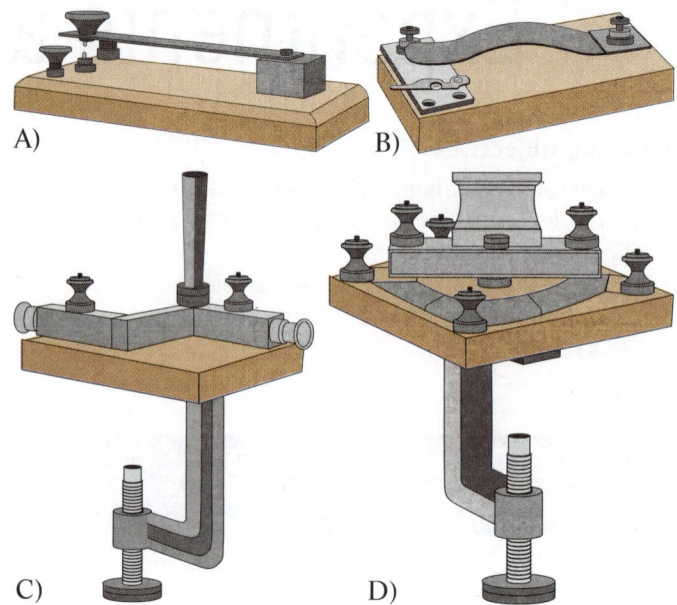

Fig. 59.1   Keys: **(A)** Tap key; **(B)** short-circuiting key; **(C)** Du Bois key; and **(D)** reversing key.

Inductorium

The inductorium (induction coil) (Fig. 59.2) is a device from which a faradic (alternate) current is obtained by feeding a galvanic current. The most commonly used inductorium is the **Du Bois-Reymond inductorium**, named after its inventor who introduced it in 1849. This is a simple device used for transforming direct current into induced current. It basically functions as a step-up transformer to obtain a high-voltage stimulus from a low-voltage direct current source using the principle of Faraday's electromagnetic induction. It consists of **two separate coils:** *the primary coil* and *the secondary coil*. The **primary coil** is fixed on a frame. The **secondary coil** is a movable one that covers the primary coil but has no connection with it.

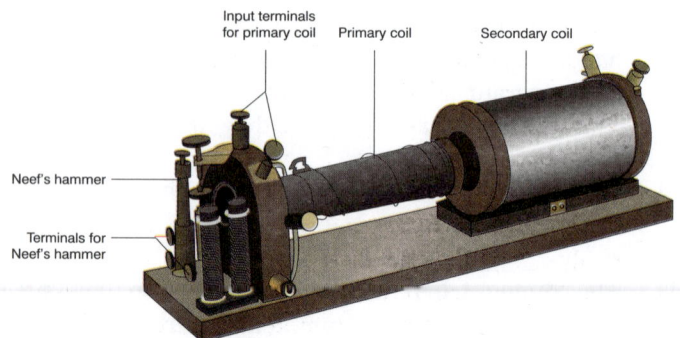

Fig. 59.2   Du Bois-Reymond inductorium.

The primary coil: The primary coil consists of 300 turns of insulated, thick copper wire wound around a soft iron core. The primary coil, the direct current source, and the tap key are connected in a series; this constitutes the primary circuit.

The secondary coil: The secondary coil is made of 5000 turns of very fine copper wire. It is designed to slide along **two horizontal metal slide rods**, one of which is marked with a **centimetre scale** to measure the distance between the two coils. The two terminals of the secondary coil are connected to **stimulating electrodes**. The secondary coil and the stimulating electrodes form the secondary circuit.

A current is induced in the secondary coil only when there is a change in the strength of the magnetic field of the primary coil. When the strength of the current passing through the primary coil is constant, changes in the strength of the magnetic field occur only at the commencement (**make**) and termination (**break**) of the current. Therefore, a current is induced in the secondary coil at 'make' or 'break' of the current in the primary coil. No current is induced in the secondary coil when the current passing through the primary coil is constant. The induced current is **brief** and **transient**.

The time taken by the current in the primary circuit at 'make' to develop from zero to maximum voltage is longer than that taken by it to fall from maximum to zero at 'break'. This is due to the development of Faraday's extra current at 'make'. Therefore, the ***induced current in the secondary coil is stronger at 'break' than at 'make'.*** *The break stimulus is always stronger than the make stimulus.* The strength of the stimulating current can be increased or decreased by changing the distance or the angle between the primary and secondary coils. Other factors also determine the strength of the induced current.

The inductorium also has a built-in interruptor (**Neef's hammer**) which works on the same principle as that of an electric bell. When Neef's hammer is introduced in the primary circuit, the alternate make and break stimuli are rapidly repeated (40/s); this produces repeated induced current in the secondary circuit.

Factors that affect the strength of induced current

1. **The distance between the two coils**—when the distance between the two coils increases, the strength of the stimulating current decreases, and when the distance decreases, the strength of the current increases.
2. **The angle between the coils**—when the two coils are placed in a line, the strength of the current is maximum. The strength of the current is reduced by turning the secondary coil away from the primary coil. When the secondary coil is placed at right angles to the primary coil, there is no induction of current.
3. **Number of turns in the coils**—usually fixed.
4. The **strength of the direct current** fed into the primary coil.

Stimulating Electrodes

Electrodes used in biological experiments differ depending on their manufacture and use. They are designed to *provide low resistance* between the preparation and the amplifier input. Stimulating electrodes (Fig. 59.3) are used to deliver electrical stimuli to the tissues. A stimulating electrode consists of two copper wires held together by a piece of perspex.

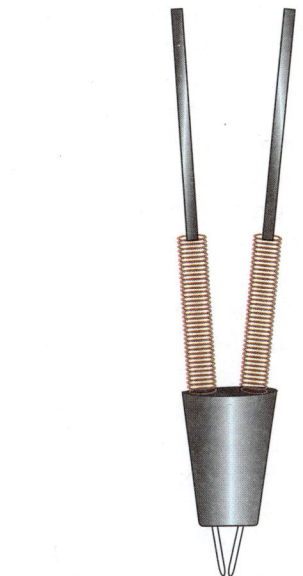

Fig. 59.3   Stimulating (simple) electrode.

Signal Marker

It is always better to indicate the point of application of the stimulus below the tracing. A **signal marker** (Fig. 59.4A) marks the exact moment of stimulation below the recording of the muscle contractions. It has two electromagnets and a writing lever. The lever marks the point of stimulation on the smoked paper. It is always included in the primary circuit.

This simple time marker (Fig. 59.4B) with a single magnet can also be used for this purpose.

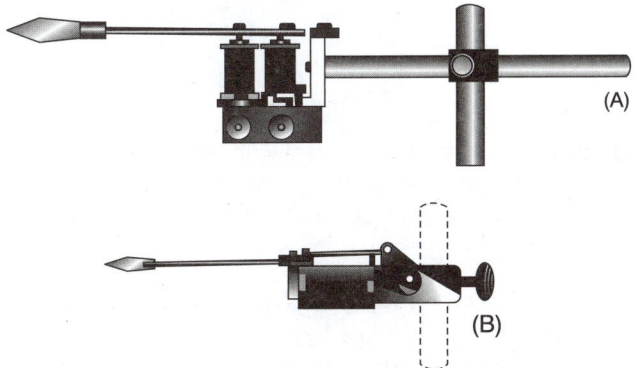

Fig. 59.4   **(A)** Signal marker and **(B)** simple time marker.

Power Shaft and Pulleys

A horizontal power shaft driven by an electric motor is provided on the table. Cone pulleys with four grooves are fixed to the power shaft at each seat.

Kymograph

Kymograph (Fig. 59.5) is the name given to any instrument that records movements on a moving surface. It consists of a **metal gearbox** to which a *vertical rotating shaft* is connected. The shaft is powered by a horizontal axis running through the metal case. To one side of this axis, a *series of pulleys* is attached. A belt connects one of these pulleys to one of the pulleys in the power shaft. A cylinder (6″×6″) called the **drum** is fixed to the shaft. The *drum rotates with the shaft*. A gear switch on the left side of the kymograph provides high and low gear. In each gear, the drum can be made to turn at different speeds by connecting different-sized pulleys and the power shaft. The drum can be started or stopped by turning a clutch on the left side of the metal gearbox.

There are two horizontal **contact arms** that project from the lower end of the vertical shaft. These contact arms can be separated and fixed with various angles between them. When the tips of the arms revolve, they make contact with a spring at the top of the kymograph. The insulated carrier of the spring is adjustable and is clamped by a screw.

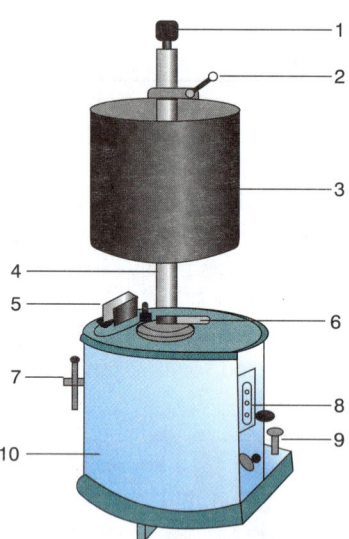

Fig. 59.5   The kymograph (1: screw lift for cylinder; 2: cylinder fixing lever; 3: cylinder; 4: spindle; 5: contact block; 6: contact arm; 7: clutch lever; 8: speed regulator; 9: levelling screw; 10: body of kymograph).

There are *two terminals for electrical connection:* one is attached to the insulated spring and the other to the metal case of the gearbox. By means of these connecting terminals, the insulated carrier along with the spring can be made to act as a key in the primary circuit. The circuit is 'made' or 'broken' when the tip of the contact arm makes and breaks contact with the insulated spring.

Muscle Trough

The muscle trough (Fig. 59.6) is a perspex or plastic chamber used to keep the muscle moist and viable in Ringer's solution. A block carrying the stimulating electrodes is fixed on one side of the wall of the trough. The writing lever is fixed on the other side. From the base of the muscle trough, a drainage pipe is attached, with a clamp that helps to drain the Ringer's solution from the trough whenever required.

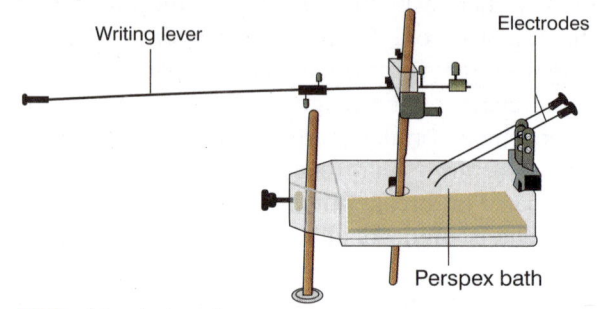

Fig. 59.6   Muscle trough.

Levers

Different types of levers are used in experimental physiology for various purposes. The commonly used levers are the **writing simple lever, the starling heart lever, the isometric lever, the afterload lever** (Fig. 59.7), and the **frontal lever** (Fig. 59.8).

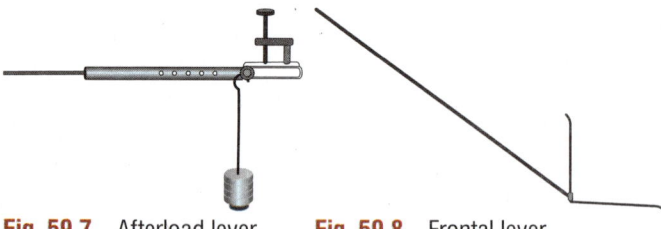

Fig. 59.7   Afterload lever.   **Fig. 59.8**   Frontal lever.

Writing lever

This is used to magnify and record the muscle contraction on the drum. The lever consists of a horizontal arm that bears holes and notches for hanging the weights (Fig. 59.9). The lever is fixed to the side wall of the muscle trough. The writing point of the lever is made up of a triangular piece of photographic film.

An ink writing stylus can be fitted into the writing lever, which can write on white glazed paper instead of a smoked drum. There is a screw (afterload screw) near the fulcrum of the lever, which limits its downward movement.

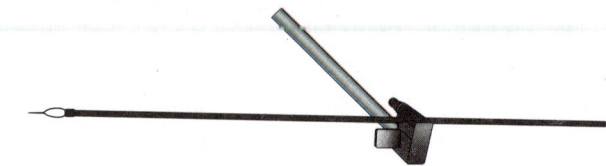

Fig. 59.9   Simple lever.

The Starling heart lever

This is used for recording the cardiogram of a frog's heart. This lever is more sensitive than the writing lever because it records the contractions of the heart, which are weaker than the contractions of the gastrocnemius muscle. It consists of a frame with a light steel lever, with holes and notches, supported by a fine, adjustable nickel–silver spring (Fig. 59.10).

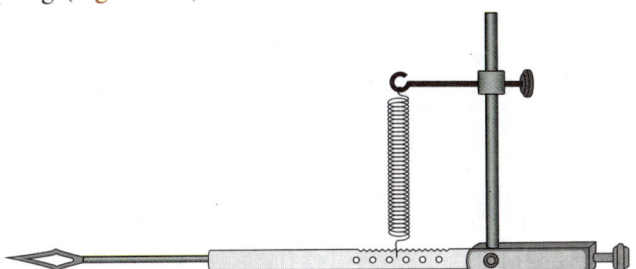

Fig. 59.10   Starling heart lever.

Isometric Lever

This consists of a holder that carries a steel tension spring and a flat writing lever (Fig. 59.11). It is used for recording isometric contractions.

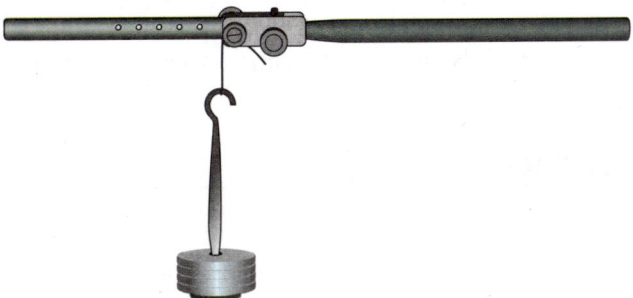

Fig. 59.11   Isometric lever.

Myograph Stand

This is a vertical rod fixed to a heavy and triangular base (Fig. 59.12). The muscle trough can be fitted to the rod and

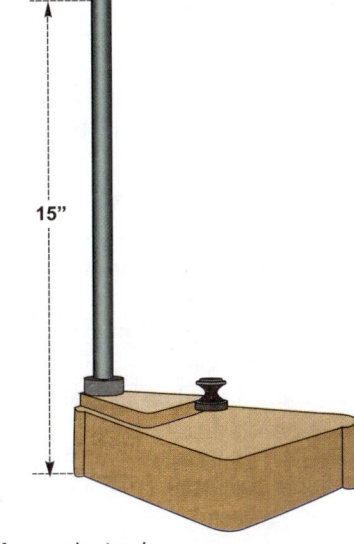

15"

Fig. 59.12   Myograph stand.

can be moved up and down with the help of a fitted screw. The rod can be turned on its axis so that the writing point of the muscle lever can be made to touch or be removed from the drum without disturbing other adjustments.

Tuning Fork

A tuning fork (Fig. 59.13) with a frequency of 100 vibrations per second (100 Hz) is used for **measuring different time intervals**. To the end of one arm of the tuning fork, a **writing point** is attached. The tuning fork is set to vibrate and is then made to write on the fast-rotating drum to obtain a tracing. This tracing consists of different waves, each measuring (from crest to crest) 0.01 seconds (10 ms).

Fig. 59.13   Tuning fork.

Pohl's Commutator

This is used to change the direction of the current. It consists of a vulcanite base with a rocking metallic cradle mounted on top (Fig. 59.14). There are six mercury-filled cup-like depressions, connected to six terminals. Two narrow copper strips connect the diagonally opposite corner cups.

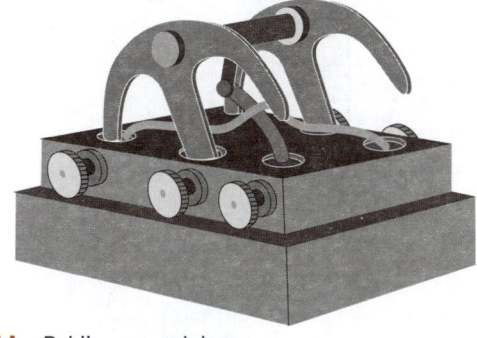

Fig. 59.14   Pohl's commutator.

Student's Stimulator

This is an electronic stimulator with **a DC output of 0–15 volts**. The strength (volts), frequency, and duration of the stimulus are indicated on the apparatus. More advanced stimulators, which are required for special experiments and research, are also available.

EXERCISES

Making Electrical Connections

Make the **primary and secondary circuits** as depicted in Fig. 59.15A and B. Check whether the primary and secondary circuits are made correctly.

1. To check the primary circuit, connect a short piece of wire to one of the low-volt terminals and strike the

other terminal with the free end of the wire. A spark indicates the presence of a current. Check the simple key and the contact block on the kymograph. Each time the striker makes contact, a spark is produced.

2. To check the secondary circuit, place the tissue on the wires connected to the secondary coil terminals. If twitching occurs in the tissue with each revolution of the spindle, the connection is correct. If the muscle does not contract, place electrodes directly on the muscle. If the muscle contracts due to direct stimulation, check whether the nerve is damaged from the dissection.

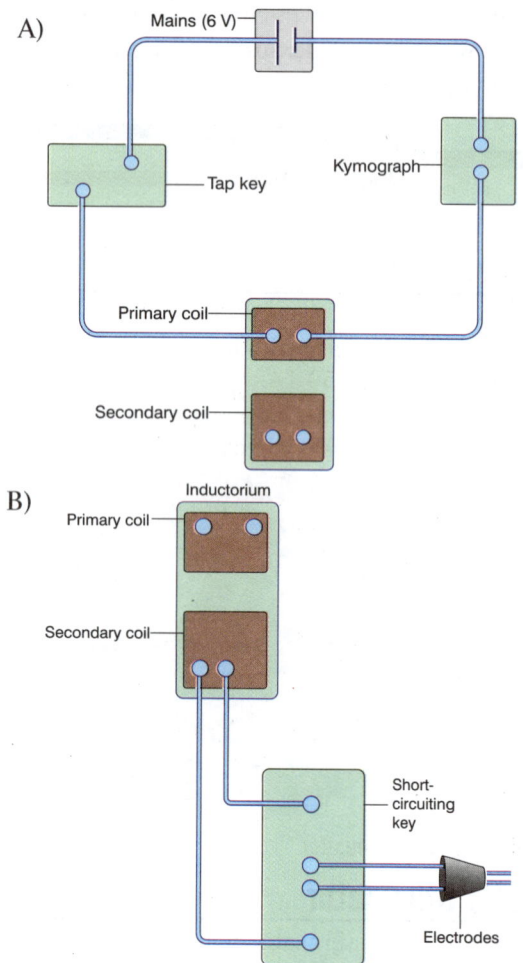

Fig. 59.15   **(A)** Primary circuit and **(B)** secondary circuit.

Smoking

Before smoking, paste a sheet of glazed paper onto the drum. Turn on the burner, place the drum on the smoking stand (Fig. 59.16), and rotate it manually over a flame to produce a thin and uniform black coating.

Note: Smoking **is no longer practised** for experimental purposes due to the harmful effects of smoke. Modern setups use **ink writers** on **white, glazed paper** instead. Instead, **ink-writer on white paper wrapped over the drum** is used these days.

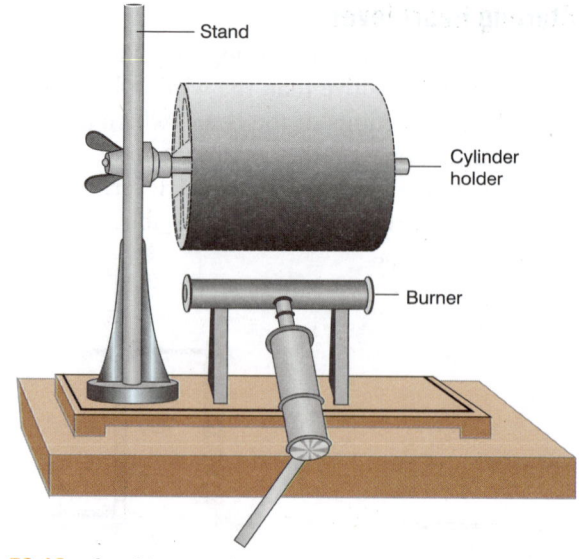

Fig. 59.16   Smoking stand.

Varnishing

Varnishing is performed to fix the recording on the smoked paper.

Label the recording before removing the paper. Cut the sheet at the joint and remove it from the drum. Dip it in a 2% resin or methylated spirit solution. Clip and hang until completely dry.

Precautions

1. The primary and secondary circuits should be made perfectly.
2. Loose connections in the circuits should be detected and fixed.
3. The wires used for making the circuit should be as short as possible. Long wires can be shortened by winding them around a glass rod or a pencil.
4. The kymograph should be properly levelled using the levelling screws at its base.
5. The drum should be tightly fixed to the vertical shaft.
6. The drum should always be rotated clockwise.
7. The writing lever should always be arranged on the right side of the drum.
8. The writing lever should be tangential to the recording surface.
9. The tip of the writing lever should touch the smoked surface evenly and lightly.
10. The initial and resting positions of the writing lever should always be horizontal.
11. The tracing should be taken at least one inch above the lower edge of the drum.
12. The contact arm should be tightly fixed.

VIVA

1. *What are the different types of stimuli, and why is the electrical stimulus usually preferred?* (**Ans.** Refer to page 433, under the heading 'Source of Stimulation'.)
2. *Why are frogs used for amphibian practicals?* (**Ans.** Refer to page 433, under the heading 'Tissue preparation' and the subheading 'Advantages of using frogs'.)
3. *What are the advantages of using the gastrocnemius-sciatic preparation?* (**Ans.** Refer to page 433, under the heading 'Tissue preparation' and the subheading 'Advantages of using the gastrocnemius-sciatic preparation'.)
4. *What are the types of keys used in amphibian experiments, and what are their uses?* (**Ans.** Refer to page 434, under the heading 'Keys'.)
5. *What is the working principle of the inductorium?* (**Ans.** Refer to page 434, under the heading 'Inductorium'.)
6. *What are the factors that determine the strength of induced current?* (**Ans.** Refer to page 435, under the heading 'Inductorium' and the subheading 'Factors that determine the strength of induced current'.)
7. *Why is the 'break' stimulus stronger than the 'make' stimulus?* (**Ans.** Refer to page 435, under the heading 'Inductorium'.)
8. *What is the use of the short-circuiting key?* (**Ans.** See page 434, under the heading 'Keys'.)
9. *What is the use of a signal marker?* (**Ans.** Refer to page 435, under the heading 'Signal Marker'.)
10. *What is the working principle of a kymograph?* (**Ans.** Refer to page 436, under the heading 'Kymograph'.)
11. *How is the speed of the kymograph regulated?* (**Ans.** Refer to page 436, under the heading 'Kymograph'.)
12. *What is the use of the contact arm of the kymograph?* (**Ans.** Refer to page 436, under the heading 'Kymograph'.)
13. *How is the time tracing obtained in the recording?* (**Ans.** See Page 437, under the heading 'Tuning Fork'.)
14. *What are the precautions taken for making electrical circuits?* (**Ans.** Refer to page 438, under the heading 'Precautions'.)
15. *How are the recordings fixed?* (**Ans.** Refer to page 438, under the heading 'Varnishing'.)

60 | Nerve–Muscle Preparation

Learning Objectives

After completing this practical, you will be able to:

1. Hold a living albino rat.
2. Anesthetise the rat.
3. Dissect the rat to isolate the sciatic nerve and gastrocnemius muscle.
4. List the precautions taken during the nerve–muscle preparation.
5. List the reasons why the gastrocnemius muscle and sciatic nerve are preferred for amphibian nerve–muscle experiments.
6. State the composition of the modified Krebs–Henseleit buffer (MKHB) solution.
7. Understand, via computer-assisted learning, the preparation of amphibian nerve–muscle.

PY3.18: Observe with computer-assisted learning: (i) amphibian nerve–muscle preparation and (ii) amphibian cardiac experiment.

INTRODUCTION

For any nerve–muscle experiment, the **sciatic nerve and the gastrocnemius muscle are used for the following reasons**:

1. The sciatic nerve is a long nerve and, therefore, easy to mount in the muscle trough.
2. The gastrocnemius muscle is a bulky muscle, producing strong contractions upon stimulation. It cannot be fatigued easily.

Discontinuation of the use of frogs: In the past, frogs were routinely used for academic experimental purposes for the students, and the preparation was called the amphibian nerve muscle preparation. Recently, however, the government has declared the *frog to be an endangered species*. Consequently, its use for any kind of experiment **has been banned**. Therefore, frogs can no longer be used for teaching and training purposes. The best alternative is to *use albino rats* (preferably of the Wistar strain, which is easy to breed and handle). This preparation is called *mammalian nerve–muscle preparation*. However, *amphibian nerve–muscle experiments* are demonstrated by **computer-assisted learning** (described below).

Rat Nerve-Muscle Preparation

The most ideal laboratory animal for the mammalian nerve–muscle experiment is the albino rat. The procedure typically involves a dual-chamber nerve bath filled with a **physiological salt solution**. This solution, typically a **modified Krebs–Henseleit buffer (MKHB)**, provides a stable environment for the nerve and muscle tissue. The bath is designed to maintain the nerve's integrity, ensuring that it remains free from kinks, twists, or excessive stretching.

Physiological salt solution: This solution is crucial for maintaining the physiological environment of the nerve and muscle tissue. MKHB, a common choice, contains essential **electrolytes** like sodium, potassium, calcium, magnesium, and chloride, along with **glucose** for energy. The pH and osmolality of the solution are also carefully controlled.

Dual-chamber nerve bath: A dual-chamber bath, sometimes referred to as a *modified Krebs–Henseleit buffer (MKHB) chamber,* provides separate compartments for the nerve and the muscle. This arrangement allows for independent manipulation of the nerve and muscle and also facilitates the attachment of electrodes.

Oxygenation and temperature control: The solution is typically gassed with a mixture of oxygen and carbon dioxide to ensure adequate oxygenation. The bath is also maintained at a controlled temperature, usually around 37°C, to mimic in vivo conditions.

METHOD FOR NERVE–MUSCLE PREPARATION

Principle

An anesthetised albino rat is dissected to isolate the intact sciatic nerve and gastrocnemius muscle. This nerve–muscle preparation is mounted in the dual-chamber nerve bath to perform various experiments.

Requirements

1. Albino rat
2. Dissecting set: Dissection board, a pair of scissors with blunt ends (8″), a pair of scissors with sharp ends (6″), a pair of pointed forceps, AND a glass rod
3. Anesthetic agent: Ketamine (100mh/kg bw) and xylazine (10 mg/kg bw)
4. MKHB solution

Procedure

There are two broad stages in nerve–muscle preparation: anesthetising the rat and dissecting it to make the nerve–muscle preparation.

Anesthetising the rat

After obtaining permission from the IAEC to use an albino rat for the academic training of medical students, a normal Wistar albino rat (body weight of 200–300 g) may be procured from an authorised vendor. The rat is kept in a cage in an air-conditioned animal lab for the purpose, with food and water available *ad lib*. Once in the lab, the animal is anesthetised with an i.p. injection of ketamine (100 mg/kg bw) and xylazine 10 mg/kg bw) by an experienced technician posted in the animal lab, following all the steps of the procedure. Once the rat is anesthetised, the dissection is performed as described below.

Dissection

1. Cut the skin of the rat around the middle of the trunk and strip off the skin from the trunk and hind limbs.
2. On the rat board, place the rat on its abdomen.
3. Dissect from the thigh side, taking care not to injure the underlying sciatic nerve.
4. Identify the sciatic plexus.
5. Isolate a 2 cm long piece of vertebral column from where the sciatic plexus originates by cutting the vertebral column above and below the exit of the sciatic nerve with scissors.
6. Bisect the vertebral column vertically into two halves with the help of bone-cutting scissors.
7. Expose the sciatic nerve in the thigh between the muscle mass posteriorly by separating the muscle with the help of the blunt glass probe (Fig. 60.1).
8. Clean the nerve of its surrounding fascial attachments.

> **Note:** Do not pull the nerve or touch it with a metal object. Only use a glass rod to handle the nerve.

9. Identify, separate, and cut the gastrocnemius tendon from its attachment and tie a long thread around the tendon.
10. Free the muscle from the tibia and cut the tibia close to the knee joint. Then, cut the femur close to the knee joint. The knee joint should be kept intact.
11. Remove all redundant muscles (other than the gastrocnemius).
12. Lift the nerve–muscle preparation (Fig. 60.2) carefully and transfer it to a container filled with MKHB solution.
13. Keep the nerve–muscle preparation immersed in MKHB solution until it is used for the experiment.

> **Note:** If required, a nerve–muscle preparation from the other side can also be obtained.

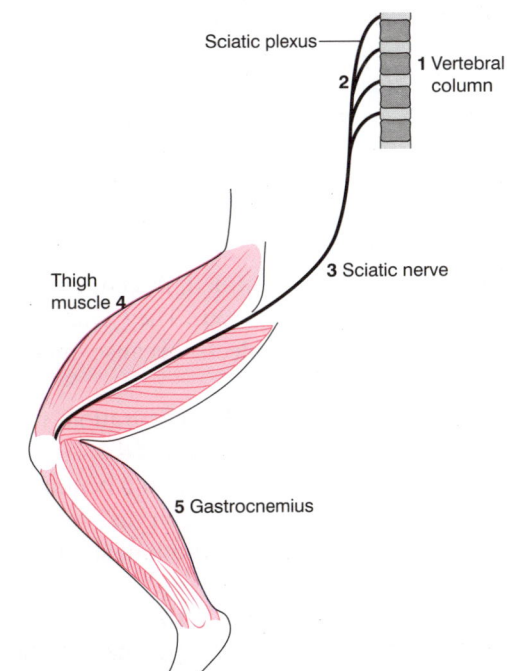

Fig. 60.1 Anatomical position of the sciatic nerve and gastrocnemius muscle of rats.

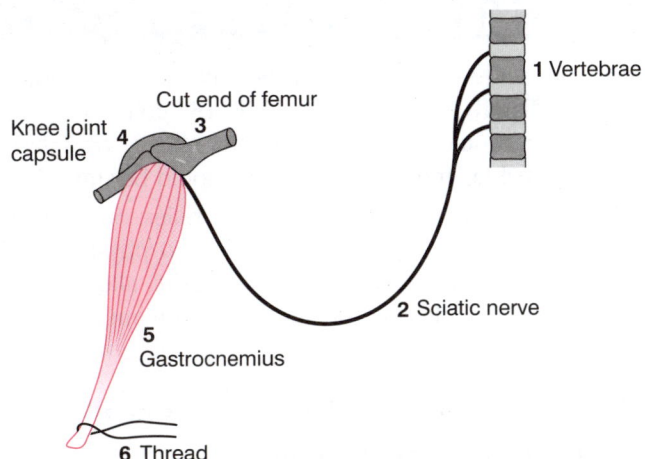

Fig. 60.2 The sciatic–gastrocnemius preparation. Note that a thread is tied to the tip of the tendon and that a portion of the vertebral column is kept intact with the nerve.

Precautions

1. The rat should be kept in a cage in the animal house under appropriate ethical and hygienic conditions.
2. While administering anesthesia, **proper dosage** and procedure should be followed to minimise discomfort to the animal.
3. Care should be taken not to injure the sciatic nerve plexus while performing the dissection.

4. The knee joint should be kept intact with the preparation because it is easier to fix the muscle through the knee joint in the muscle trough.

5. A piece of the vertebral column should be kept intact with the nerve (the nerve should not be cut from its origin). It becomes easy to place the nerve on the electrodes if the vertebral column is intact along with the nerve.

6. The nerves should be identified, traced, and exposed with the help of a glass rod. They should not be handled with metallic objects because metals may stimulate nerves.

7. While dissecting to obtain the preparation, the nerve and the muscle should not be strained.

8. The nerve–muscle preparation should be immediately transferred into MKHB solution as soon as the dissection is over. The preparation should not be allowed to dry.

9. Once the preparation is ready, it should be mounted in the muscle trough to start the experiment. Otherwise, the muscle may become fatigued.

DISCUSSION

Once the nerve–muscle preparation is made, it should be immediately immersed in MKHB solution. The preparation should be mounted in the muscle trough as early as possible, and the experiment should be started.

The rat nerve–muscle preparation relies on a well-defined solution that provides a stable and physiological environment for the nerve and muscle tissue, allowing for accurate and reliable experimental measurements.

Computer-assisted Demo of Amphibian Nerve-muscle Preparation

The procedure for amphibian nerve–muscle preparation may be demonstrated to students through computer-assisted learning. The procedure is broadly the same as that for the rat but with three major differences: i) instead of the first step of anesthetisation, **pithing of the frog** is demonstrated; ii) the preparation is immersed in **Ringer's solution**, and iii) a muscle trough is used for mounting the preparation. Thus, there are **two broad steps** in nerve–muscle preparation: *pithing of the frog* and *dissection* to make the nerve–muscle preparation.

Pithing of the frog

1. Hold the frog gently but firmly with a piece of cloth or cotton.

Note: The skin of the frog is slippery. Therefore, the animal should be held with a dry cloth or cotton.

2. Strike a blow to the **head** to induce unconsciousness.

Note: This procedure is called stunning.

3. Hold the unconscious frog in your hand and ventroflex its head.

4. Feel the depression at the junction of the skull and vertebral column.

Note: This corresponds to a point in the middle of the line joining the posterior borders of the tympanic membranes.

5. At this junction, insert a pithing needle firmly through the skin, muscle, and bone tissue into the spinal cord.

6. Manipulate the needle anteriorly into the skull and rotate it to destroy the brain.

7. Withdraw the needle and direct it backwards into the spinal cord and rotate the needle to destroy the cord.

Note: Immediately after the needle is directed into the spinal cord, the muscles of the lower limb and trunk become spastic. They become flaccid after the destruction of the spinal cord. This procedure is called pithing. After pithing, the animal loses its voluntary and reflex movements but is still alive and can be used for experiments.

Dissection

1. Cut the skin of the frog around the middle of the trunk and strip off the skin from the trunk and hind limbs.

2. Place the frog on the frog board on its abdomen.

3. Pick up the tip of the urostyle with the forceps and lift it carefully. Cut the pelvic girdle on its sides, taking care not to injure the underlying sciatic nerve.

Continue with dissection steps similar to those performed for the rat. The preparation is kept in Ringer's solution.

Composition of Ringer's solution

1. NaCl: 0.6% (isotonic with frog plasma)
2. KCl: 0.014% (maintains membrane potential)
3. $CaCl_2$: 0.012% (maintains muscle excitability)
4. $NaHCO_3$: 0.02% (maintains pH)
5. NaH_2PO_4: 0.001% (maintains pH)
6. Dextrose: 0.1% (provides nutrition)

VIVA

1.   Why are the gastrocnemius muscle and sciatic nerve selected for nerve–muscle experiments? (**Ans.** Refer to page 440, under the heading 'Introduction'.)

2. *How is the anesthetization done?* (Ans. Refer to page 441, under the heading 'Procedure' and the subheading 'Anesthetising the rat.')
3. *What are the precautions to be followed during dissection for the nerve–muscle preparation?* (Ans. Refer to page 441, under the heading 'Procedure' and the subheading 'Dissection.')
4. *Why is the knee joint kept intact with the muscle for making the preparation?* (Ans. Refer to page 441-442, under the heading 'Precautions.')
5. *Why is the nerve not handled with metallic objects?* (Ans. Refer to page 441-442, under the heading 'Precautions.')
6. *Why is the preparation immersed in MKHB solution immediately after dissection?* (Ans. Refer to page 442, under the heading 'Precautions.')
7. *What is the composition of MKHB solution?* (Ans. Refer to page 440, under the heading 'Rat Nerve–Muscle Preparation.')
8. *What is the composition of Ringer's solution, and what are its uses?*

61 | Simple Muscle Twitch

Learning Objectives

After completing this practical, you will be able to:

1. Dissect and make a sciatic nerve and gastrocnemius muscle preparation.
2. Make primary and secondary circuits.
3. Record the response of the muscle to a single electrical stimulus to the nerve.
4. Record the time-tracing below the simple muscle curve.
5. Calculate the latent period, contraction period, and relaxation period from the recording.

PY3.18: Observe with computer-assisted learning: (i) amphibian nerve–muscle preparation and (ii) amphibian cardiac experiments.

INTRODUCTION

When a muscle is stimulated with a single induction shock, it exhibits a momentary twitch like a contraction. This momentary contraction of the muscle in response to electrical stimulation is called a **simple muscle twitch**. The contraction recorded on a moving kymograph is known as a **simple muscle curve**. The simple muscle curve is recorded to study the latent period, contraction period, and relaxation period of skeletal muscles (Fig. 61.1).

The latent period is the period from the point of the stimulus to the point of onset of the contraction. The **contraction period** is the period between the point of onset of contraction and the point that corresponds to the peak of the contraction. The relaxation period is the period from the peak of a contraction to the end of relaxation.

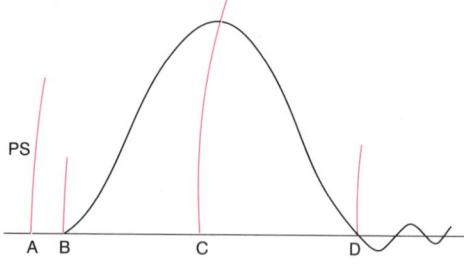

Fig. 61.1 Simple muscle twitch with time-trace below the curve (PS: point of stimulation; AB: latent period; BC: contraction period; CD: relaxation period).

METHOD TO STUDY SIMPLE MUSCLE TWITCH

Principle

When a muscle is stimulated with a single induction shock, the muscle contracts. This lifts the lever to record a curve on a revolving smoked drum.

Requirements

1. Dissection instruments
2. Kymograph
3. Muscle trough
4. Inductorium
5. Short-circuiting key
6. Tap key
7. Ringer's solution
8. Smoked drum
9. Low-resistance wires
10. Electrodes
11. Tuning fork (100 Hz)
12. Thread
13. Hook and weights (Fig. 61.2)

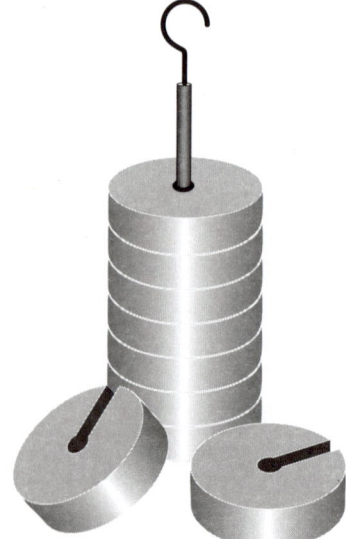

Fig. 61.2 Hook with weights.

Procedure

1. Arrange the primary and secondary circuits for recording a muscle twitch (see Fig. 59.15).
2. Include the kymograph in the primary circuit.
3. Select the fastest speed of the kymograph (first gear; pulleys 4:1).

4. Dissect a frog to obtain a sciatic nerve–gastrocnemius preparation.
5. Fix the nerve–muscle preparation in the muscle trough.
6. Pour Ringer's solution into the trough.
7. Hang a 10 g weight from the writing lever and keep the muscle in the after-loaded position.
8. Adjust the writing lever in such a way that it touches the drum lightly in the horizontal position.
9. Adjust the secondary coil to obtain a contraction at the 'break' stimulus only.
10. Set the drum in motion, and record a baseline.
11. Press the tap key and release it as soon as you record the first contraction.
12. Make the tuning fork vibrate by striking it against the thigh or the hypothenar eminence of the hand and record a time-tracing below the simple muscle curve.
13. Stop the drum and close the short-circuiting key.
14. Rotate the drum manually so that the contact arms touch the kymograph key.

Note: This marks the instant when the primary circuit becomes complete upon closing the tap key, thereby inducing a stimulus in the secondary coil.

15. Mark the point of stimulation by moving the writing lever over the smoked drum.
16. Mark the beginning of the contraction, the peak of the contraction, and the end of relaxation by moving the lever vertically on the drum manually on the corresponding points in the curve.
17. Calculate and record the duration of the latent period (LP), contraction period (CP), and relaxation period (RP).

Precautions

In addition to the measures described for 'nerve–muscle preparation' in Chapter 59, the following precautions should be observed.

1. The stimulus should be brief and limited to a single induction shock.
2. The point of the stimulus should be accurately marked.
3. While marking the latent period, contraction period, and relaxation period, the lever should be placed exactly on the points.
4. The time-tracing should be recorded just below the muscle contraction curve for easy correlation.

Observations and Results

Observe and study the simple muscle curve (Fig. 61.1). Express the duration of LP, CP, and RP in ms. Calculate the CP and RP as a percentage of the total muscle curve (CP + RP) duration.

DISCUSSION

The latent period, contraction period, and relaxation period vary according to the type of muscle. **The latent period** is due to the following:

- Time taken for the stimulus to travel along the nerve to the neuromuscular junction.
- Time taken for the impulse to cross the neuromuscular junction to stimulate the muscle.
- Time taken for the excitation–contraction coupling to occur.
- Time taken by the lever to overcome the inertia of rest.
- Time taken to overcome the viscous resistance of the muscle.

The latent period is normally about 10 ms. The contraction period represents the duration of mechanical contraction. It normally ranges between 20 and 40 ms. The relaxation period represents the time taken by the muscles to relax. It is normally more than the contraction period and ranges between 30 and 50 ms.

VIVA

1. *What are the causes of the latent period?* (**Ans.** Refer to page 445, under the heading 'Discussion'.)
2. *What is the normal duration of the contraction and relaxation periods of the frog skeletal muscle and what do they represent?* (**Ans.** Refer to page 445, under the heading 'Discussion'.)
3. *Can the duration of LP, CP, and RP be determined without obtaining the time-tracing below the curve?* (**Ans.** Yes, it can be derived from the speed of the drum.)
4. *Why is induced current used for recording a simple muscle twitch?* (**Ans.** Induced current is preferred because it proved a brief stimulus of the desired intensity.)
5. *Why is a 10 g weight placed on the lever?* (**Ans.** The weight placed on the lever checks the amplitude of the contraction, overcomes the inertia of the lever, and keeps the lever horizontal.)

62 | Effect of Temperature on Simple Muscle Twitch

Learning Objectives

After completing this practical, you WILL be able to:

1. Demonstrate the effect of temperature on muscle contraction.
2. State the precautions taken for recording the effects of temperature on muscle contraction.
3. Explain the effects of temperature on muscle contraction.

PY3.18: Observe with computer-assisted learning: (i) amphibian nerve–muscle preparation and (ii) amphibian cardiac experiments.

INTRODUCTION

A change in the temperature of Ringer's solution causes a change in muscle contraction. With a change in temperature, there is a change in amplitude and the duration of different periods of contraction (latent, contraction, and relaxation periods). These changes are mainly due to changes in the rate of conduction velocity in the nerve, enzymatic and chemical activities in the muscle, and a change in the viscosity of the muscle.

METHOD TO STUDY THE EFFECT OF TEMPERATURE ON MUSCLE CONTRACTION

Principle

A change in the temperature of the environment affects muscle contraction. The effects of temperature on muscle contraction are studied by changing the temperature of Ringer's solution. The effects are studied on the same point of stimulus and the same baseline. The change in amplitude of contraction, the duration of the latent period, contraction period, and relaxation period are noted.

Requirements

1. Same as those for 'simple muscle twitch'
2. Cold Ringer's solution (10°C)
3. Warm Ringer's solution (40°C)
4. Centigrade thermometer

Procedure

1. Pith and dissect the frog to make the nerve–muscle preparation.

2. Set up the nerve–muscle preparation for recording the simple muscle curve.
3. Record a simple muscle curve on the revolving drum with Ringer's solution in the muscle trough at room temperature.
4. Drain the Ringer's solution from the muscle trough and replace it with warm Ringer's solution. Wait for 1–3 minutes to allow the muscle to warm up.
5. Using the same baseline, same point of stimulation, and same strength of stimulus, record the effect of warm Ringer's solution on the simple muscle curve.
6. Note the temperature of the Ringer's solution and then drain the solution from the muscle trough.
7. Refill the trough with room-temperature Ringer's solution and wait for some time for the preparation to come back to normal temperature. Then replace it with cold Ringer's solution and wait 2–5 minutes to cool the muscle.
8. Using the same baseline, point of stimulation, and strength of stimulus, record the effect of the solution on muscle contraction.
9. Record a time-tracing below the muscle curve with the help of a tuning fork.
10. Calculate the latent period, contraction period, and relaxation period of the muscle contraction with different temperatures.
11. Record your observations in a tabular form (Table 62.1).

Table 62.1 Tabulation of experimental recordings.

Temperature of Ringer's soln.	L P (ms)	C P (ms)	R P (ms)	Height of contraction (cm)
Normal (25°C)				
Warm (40°C)				
Cold (10°C)				

Observations

Compare the recordings of the **three muscle curves** at the three different temperatures of Ringer's solution. Study the *height and slope* of contraction, and the *duration of the latent period, contraction period,* and *relaxation period* of each curve (Fig. 62.1).

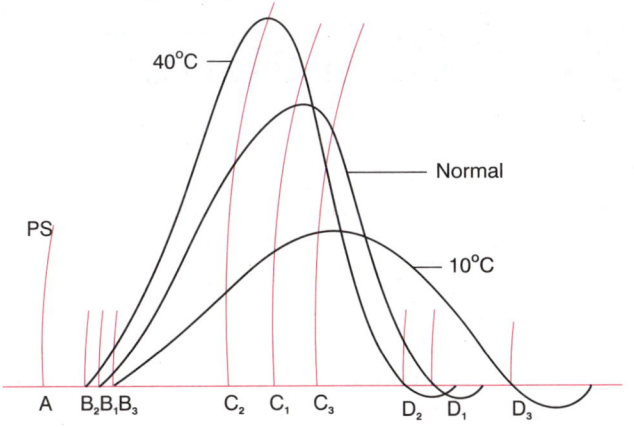

Fig. 62.1   Effect of temperature on simple muscle twitch. AB_1, AB_2, and AB_3 are the latent periods; B_1C_1, $B2C_2$, and $B3C_3$ are the contraction periods; C_1D_1, C_2D_2, and C_3D_3 are the relaxation periods of normal, high (40°C), and low (10°C) temperatures respectively.

Precautions

The precautions are the same as those taken while eliciting the simple muscle twitch. In addition, the following precautions are also to be kept in mind:

1. The point of stimulation, the baseline, and the strength of stimulation should be kept constant for all the recordings.
2. The temperature of the Ringer's solution **should not exceed 42°C.**

> **Note:** When the temperature of the solution is 43°C or more, the muscle proteins are denatured and consequently remain in a state of sustained contraction. This phenomenon is known as heat rigor.

3. The temperature of the cold solution **should not be less than 4°C.**

> **Note:** When the temperature of the solution is very low, the muscle proteins are coagulated. This prevents muscle contraction.

4. The temperature of the solution should be recorded just before or immediately after muscle contraction.

5. The effects of the warm solution should be recorded before recording the effects of cold Ringer's because cold Ringer's inhibits all enzymatic and metabolic activities of the muscle. It may be difficult to revive muscle activities from these effects.

DISCUSSION

When muscle contraction is recorded with **a higher temperature of** Ringer's solution, *the latent period, contraction period, and relaxation period decrease,* and *the height of contraction increases.* The decrease in the latent period is due to the following factors:

1. Increase in the conduction velocity of the nerve
2. Increased rate of neuromuscular transmission
3. Inertia of the lever being overcome faster

The shortening of the contraction and relaxation periods is due to faster contraction and relaxation. This occurs due to the **activation of myosin ATPase activity** and **decreased resistance** of the muscle to contractions as the viscosity of the muscle decreases with increased temperature. The amplitude of contractions increases due to *increased enzymatic and chemical activities* in the muscle.

When muscle contraction is recorded with **a lower temperature of** Ringer's solution, *the opposite effects* are observed. This is attributed to the **decreased rate of conduction** of impulses in the nerve and through the neuromuscular junction, **increased viscosity of the muscle, and decreased enzymatic and chemical activities** in the muscle.

Changes in the muscular activities of **human beings** due to changes in environmental temperature, though similar, may be different from these experimental observations. This is because physical efficiency depends on various factors like **training, motivation, state of nutrition,** environmental temperature, humidity, and so on. Normally, the body temperature never rises to the extent of causing heat rigor. However, if a person is exposed to a high temperature for a long time, a phenomenon akin to heat rigor occurs; if a person is exposed to very low temperatures, muscle contraction is inhibited.

VIVA

1. *What are the precautions taken when recording the effects of temperature on muscle contraction?* (Ans. Refer to page 447, under the heading 'Precautions'.)
2. *What changes in muscle contraction occur in response to warm Ringer's solution? What are the causes of these changes?* (Ans. Refer to page 447, under the heading 'Discussion'.)
3. *What changes in muscle contraction occur in response to cold Ringer's solution? What are the causes of these changes?* (Ans. Refer to page 447, under the heading 'Discussion'.)
4. *What is heat rigor?* (Ans. Refer to page 447, under the heading 'Discussion'.)
5. *Why is the effect of warm Ringer's recorded before recording the effect of cold Ringer's?* (Ans. Refer to page 447, under the heading 'Precautions', point no. 5.)
6. *What is the effect of temperature on performance in human beings?* (Ans. Refer to page 447, under the heading 'Discussion'.)

63 Effect of Increasing Strength of Stimuli on Muscle Contraction

Learning Objectives

After completing this practical, you will be able to:
1. Define subthreshold, threshold, and supramaximal stimuli.
2. Differentiate between 'make' and 'break' stimuli.
3. Demonstrate the effect of an increase in the strength of stimuli on muscle contraction.
4. Explain the physiological basis of these changes.

PY3.18: Observe with computer-assisted learning: (i) amphibian nerve-muscle preparation and (ii) amphibian cardiac experiments.

INTRODUCTION

The amplitude of contraction increases with increases in the strength of the stimuli. There are different types of stimuli:
1. A **subminimal stimulus** or subthreshold stimulus is a stimulus that does not evoke a response.
2. A **threshold stimulus** is the minimum strength of a stimulus that is just enough to evoke a response. This is also called minimal or liminal stimulus.
3. A **maximal stimulus** produces the maximum response.
4. A **supramaximal stimulus** is stronger than a maximal stimulus but does not change the magnitude of the contraction after reaching the peak level.

When a muscle is stimulated with increasing strengths of stimuli, **more and more motor units are recruited**. This results in an *increase in the amplitude of the contraction*.

A *motor unit* is defined as a single motor neuron (together with its branches) and the muscle fibres that it supplies.

Factors that affect the magnitude of contraction:
1. Number of motor units activated by the stimulus
2. The strength of the stimulus
3. The frequency of the stimulus

METHOD TO STUDY EFFECTS OF STRENGTH OF STIMULI ON MUSCLE CONTRACTION

Principle

The amplitude of muscle contraction increases with increase in the strength of the stimulus. In this experiment, single 'make' and 'break' stimuli of increasing intensity are applied to the nerve supplying the muscle, starting from subthreshold levels and progressing to supramaximal levels. The resulting muscle contractions are recorded on a stationary drum.

Requirements

1. Electrical connections for single induction stimulus (with a spring key in the primary circuit and a short-circuiting key in the secondary circuit)
2. Kymograph
3. Muscle trough and lever
4. Nerve–muscle preparation (freshly dissected)

Procedure

1. Set up the myograph and the nerve–muscle preparation for recording a simple muscle twitch.
2. Exclude the drum from the primary circuit and engage the gear in the neutral position.
3. Move the secondary coil of the inductorium far away from the primary coil.
4. Keep the writing point of the lever away from the drum and press and release the spring key. Observe the muscle for the contraction at 'make' and 'break'.
5. If there is no contraction, move the secondary coil 1 cm closer to the primary coil and press and release the key. Again, look for a contraction at 'make' and 'break'.
6. Repeat the procedure till the break shock yields a contraction. Record the contraction on the smoked drum. Measure and note the distance (in cm) between the primary and secondary coils.
7. Move the secondary coil 1 cm closer to the primary coil, rotate the drum manually and record the contraction at **both 'make' and 'break'**. Record each pair of 'make' and 'break' contractions close to each other, as shown in Fig. 63.1.
8. Repeat this procedure by moving the secondary coil closer to the primary coil until there is no further increase in the amplitude of contraction on increasing

the intensity of the stimulus. Measure the distance between the primary and secondary coils for each stimulus.

9. Label the response as **M for the 'make'** stimulus and **B for the 'break'** stimulus below each pair of recordings.

Summation of subminimal stimuli

1. Set up the apparatus for a simple muscle twitch with a spring key in the primary circuit.
2. Reduce the strength of the induction shock to just below the minimum.
3. Deliver a single induction shock and observe that no contraction occurs.
4. Repeatedly stimulate the muscle by rapidly and repeatedly tapping the key; a contraction typically appears after the fifth or sixth stimulus due to the summation of subminimal stimuli.

Observations

Observe and study the recording (Fig. 63.1). Note that **no contraction is produced at the subminimal stimulus** and that a contraction is recorded only with the break stimulus at minimal strength. As stimulus strength increases, contractions occur with both 'make' and 'break' stimuli and the amplitude of contractions increases in a graded manner.

1. In all recordings, the height of the *contractions of the 'break' stimuli is more than the height of the contractions of the make stimuli*, when the stimuli were submaximal.

2. **At maximal stimulus**, *the height of the contraction is maximum*, but there is no difference between the recordings of the 'make' and 'break' stimuli.

3. After reaching the maximal level, there is *no further increase in the height of contractions* following the application of supramaximal stimuli. In the case of supramaximal stimuli, the heights of the contractions at 'make' and 'break' stimuli also remain the same.

Precautions

1. The drum should be excluded from the primary circuit.
2. Contractions of both 'make' and 'break' stimuli should be recorded.
3. The recording should start from the subminimal level and progress to the supramaximal stimuli.
4. Each pair of recordings should be labelled to indicate the 'make' and 'break' stimuli.
5. The writing point should be brought in contact with the drum with the same friction for all the recordings.
6. A minimum of 15 seconds should be allowed between the application of the 'make' and 'break' stimuli to avoid any beneficial effects on muscle contraction.

DISCUSSION

At subminimal (subthreshold) stimulus strength, *the muscle does not contract* because the current supplied does not have enough strength to excite muscle fibres to result in a muscle contraction. A **threshold stimulus** excites

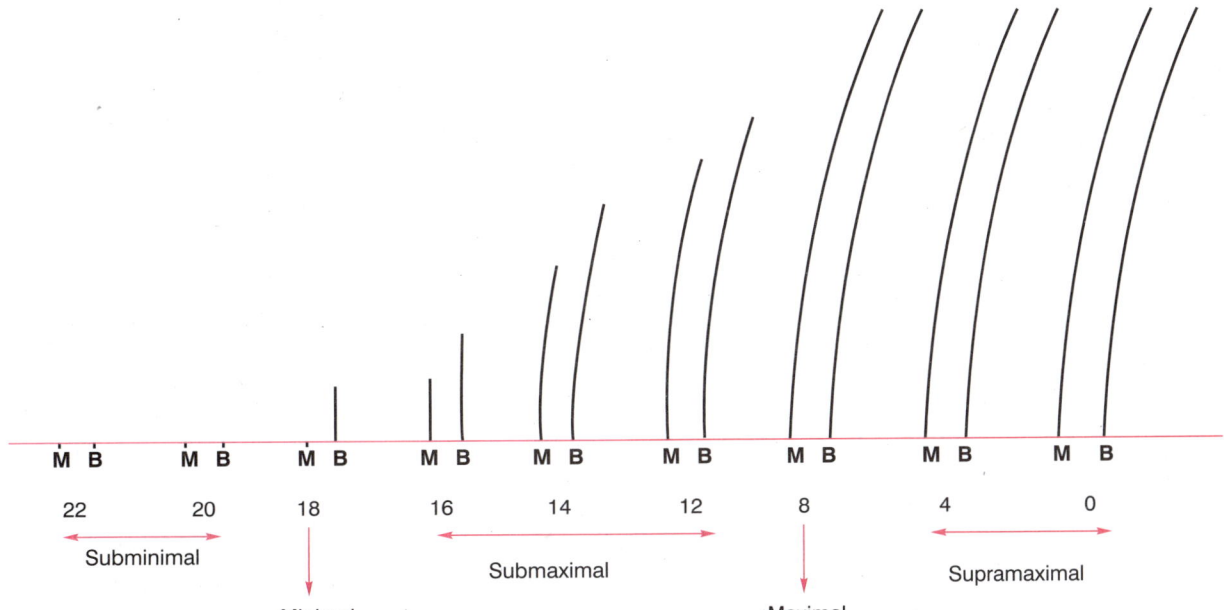

M B	M B	M B	M B	M B	M B	M B	M B	M B
22	20	18	16	14	12	8	4	0

Subminimal ← → | Minimal | Submaximal ← → | Maximal | Supramaximal ← →

Fig. 63.1   Effect of the strength of stimuli on muscle contractions (M: 'make' stimulus; B: 'break' stimulus). The numbers below the stimuli indicate the distance (in cm) between the primary and secondary coils.

a few motor units and produces a *weak contraction*. At minimal stimulus strength, a contraction is recorded only with the 'break' stimulus because the break stimulus is stronger than the make stimulus.

As the **strength of stimuli increases**, ***more and more motor units are recruited***, which results in a *greater magnitude of contraction*. When the strength of the stimulus reaches maximal level, there is no increase in the magnitude of contraction with further increase in the strength of stimuli (**supramaximal stimuli**) because the *maximum number of motor units have already been utilised*.

VIVA

1. *Define subminimal, threshold, and supra-maximal stimuli.* (Ans. Refer to page 448, under the heading 'Introduction'.)
2. *Why does the contraction occur only with the 'break' stimulus at the threshold level?* (Ans. Refer to page 449, under the heading 'Discussion'.)
3. *Why does the magnitude of contraction increase with increase in the strength of stimuli?* (Ans. Refer to page 449–450, under the heading 'Discussion'.)
4. *Why is no change observed in the magnitude of the contraction with an increase in the strength of the contraction after reaching the maximal level?* (Ans. Refer to page 449–450, under the heading 'Discussion'.)
5. *Define a motor unit.* (Ans. Refer to page 448, under the heading 'Introduction'.)
6. *Why does only the 'break' stimulus evoke a response with the application of the minimal stimulus?* (Ans. Refer to page 449, under the heading 'Discussion'.)
7. *Why are 15 seconds allowed between the application of the 'make' and 'break' stimuli?* (Ans. Refer to page 449, under the heading 'Discussion'.)

64 | Effect of Two Successive Stimuli on Muscle Contraction

Learning Objectives

After completing this practical, you will be able to:
1. Define absolute and relative refractory periods.
2. Describe the physiological basis of the beneficial effect.
3. Demonstrate the effect of two successive stimuli on muscle contraction.
4. Explain the mechanisms of these effects.

PY3.18: Observe with computer-assisted learning: (i) amphibian nerve-muscle preparation and (ii) amphibian cardiac experiment.

INTRODUCTION

When two successive stimuli are paired, the response of the muscle to the paired stimulus depends **on the timing of the second stimulus**. If the second stimulus is applied in *the absolute refractory period* of the previous stimulation, *it does not evoke* any response. If it falls in the **relative refractory period**, a response may be obtained. The muscle and nerve are unresponsive during the refractory period of the action potential. However, the *mechanical response (the contractile machinery) has no refractoriness*. Therefore, the two successive stimuli *can be added up*.

Absolute Refractory Period

This is the period during which a second stimulus **does not produce any response**, no matter how strong the stimulus is or the duration of the application of the stimulus.

Relative Refractory Period

This is the period during which a **strong stimulus may evoke a response**.

Beneficial Effect

When a muscle is stimulated by two successive stimuli, the *magnitude of the contraction of the second stimulus* is **greater than the first**. This occurs because the **first stimulus becomes beneficial for the second one**.
1. The **calcium ions released** from the terminal cisterns during muscle contraction are pumped back into the cisterns during relaxation. Therefore, when the second stimulus falls in the relaxation period or immediately following the relaxation period of the first one, **some amount of calcium is left** in the sarcoplasm due to incomplete relaxation. This *increases the calcium*

concentration for the second stimulus, as it adds to the calcium that has been left in the sarcoplasm from the first stimulus. Therefore, the height of the contraction increases with the second stimulus.
2. The **increase in temperature and the decrease in viscosity** of the muscle by the first contraction also contribute to the beneficial effect.

METHOD TO STUDY EFFECT OF TWO SUCCESSIVE STIMULI ON MUSCLE CONTRACTION

Principle

When two successive stimuli are paired and applied to the muscle, the magnitude of contraction changes depending on the timing of the second stimulus. This is recorded by separating the contact arms of the kymograph and recording the contractions at different angles between the arms.

Requirements

The requirements are the same as those for eliciting the simple muscle twitch.

Procedure

1. Set up the nerve–muscle preparation for recording a simple muscle twitch.
2. Arrange the induction coil to obtain maximal or supramaximal stimuli.
3. Separate the two contact arms attached to the spindle of the drum by an angle such that the second twitch immediately follows the first twitch.
4. Stimulate the nerve, and record the muscle contraction. Mark the two points of stimulation.
5. Reduce the angle between the two contact arms to such an extent that the second stimulus falls during the relaxation period of the first twitch. Record the contraction and mark the point of stimulation.

6. Continue recording while gradually reducing the angle between the two arms so that the second stimulus falls during the contraction phase, as well as during the first and second halves of the latent period of the first contraction.

Observations

Study your observations.
1. Note that there is **no effect of the second stimulus** on muscle contraction if the stimulus *falls in the first half of the latent period* of the first muscle twitch.
2. However, if the second stimulus *falls in the second half of the latent period* or in the contraction period, the **magnitude of the contraction increases**.
3. When the second stimulus *falls in the relaxation period of the first contraction*, a **conjoint second contraction** (two peaks of the contraction) appears, which obscures the relaxation period of the first contraction. The **second peak is bigger** than the first one.
4. When the second stimulus *falls immediately after the relaxation period* of the first contraction, the **second contraction is bigger** than the first one (Fig. 64.1).

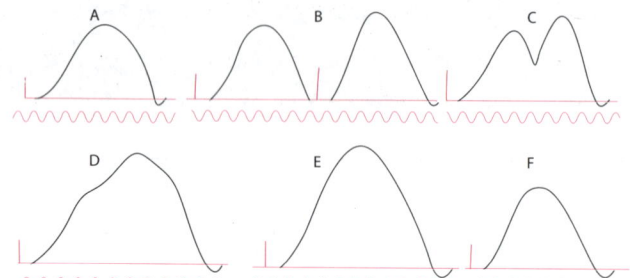

Fig. 64.1   Effect of two successive stimuli on muscle contraction. **(A)** Simple muscle twitch; **(B)** Second stimulus given immediately following the relaxation period of the first one; **(C)** Second stimulus applied during the relaxation period of the first one; **(D)** Second stimulus applied during the contraction of the first one; **(E)** Second stimulus applied during the second half of the latent period of the first stimulus; **(F)** Second stimulus applied in the first half of the latent period of the first stimulus.

Precautions

1. The distance between the contact arms should be gradually decreased to apply the second stimulus on different phases of contraction elicited by the first stimulus.
2. The point of stimulus of both the twitches should be marked.
3. The beneficial effect should be demonstrated.
4. The stimuli should be of maximal or supramaximal strength as these stimuli activate all motor units and yield the maximum response.

DISCUSSION

When the second stimulus falls in the **first half of the latent period** of the first contraction, it *does not evoke any response* because it falls in the absolute refractory period of the first stimulus.

1. When the second stimulus falls in the **second half of the latent period or in the contraction period**, there is a *summation of contraction*, and *the magnitude of the contraction increases*.
2. When the second stimulus **falls in the relaxation period** of the first, the *relaxation is arrested, and the second contraction occurs*. In this case, the height of the second contraction is more than the first one because of the beneficial effect.
3. When the second stimulus falls **immediately following the relaxation** of the first contraction, a *second twitch is recorded, which is of higher magnitude than the first one*. The increase in magnitude of the second twitch is also due to the beneficial effect. The increased magnitude of contraction is *due to the summation of the responses* (contractions) rather than the summation of stimuli.

VIVA

1. *Why is the supramaximal stimulus used in this experiment?* (**Ans.** Refer to page 452, under the heading 'Precautions'.)
2. *What is the beneficial effect, and what is its physiological basis?* (**Ans.** Refer to page 451, under the heading 'Beneficial Effect'.)
3. *Define absolute and relative refractory periods.* (**Ans.** Refer to page 451, under the headings 'Absolute refractory period and 'Relative refractory period'.)
4. *Explain why the second stimulus does not evoke any response if it falls in the first half of the latent period of the first twitch.* (**Ans.** Refer to page 452, under the heading 'Discussion'.)
5. *Why is the magnitude of a contraction more when the second stimulus falls in the second half of the latent period or the contraction period of the first twitch?* (**Ans.** Refer to page 452, under the heading 'Discussion'.)
6. *Why is the magnitude of a contraction of the second stimulus more than the first one when the second stimulus falls in or following the relaxation period of the first one?* (**Ans.** Refer to page 452, under the heading 'Discussion'.)

65 | Genesis of Tetanus

Learning Objectives

After completing this practical, you will be able to:
1. Define treppe, clonus, and tetanus.
2. Demonstrate the effects of increasing the frequency of stimulation on muscle contraction.
3. List the precautions taken during the genesis of tetanus in this experiment.
4. Calculate the minimal tetanisable frequency (MTF).
5. List the factors that affect MTF.
6. Explain the physiological basis of treppe, clonus, and tetanus.
7. Differentiate between experimental and clinical tetanus.
8. List the causes, features, and prevention of tetanus (the disease).

PY3.18: Observe with computer-assisted learning: (i) amphibian nerve–muscle preparation and (ii) amphibian cardiac experiment.

INTRODUCTION

Tetanus refers to a **state of sustained tonic contraction** of the muscle (without relaxation) due to *rapidly repeated stimulation*. It does not occur if the muscle is stimulated at a low rate (lower frequency). If *the rate of stimulation* increases (higher frequency), tetanus ensues. When the muscle is *stimulated below the tetanising frequency*, **incomplete tetanus (clonus)** occurs.

METHOD TO STUDY GENESIS OF TETANUS

Principle

If a muscle is stimulated at high frequencies, *there is sustained tonic contraction of the muscle* (tetanus). In this experiment, the nerve–muscle preparation is stimulated at different frequencies using a vibrating interrupter till tetanus ensues.

Requirements

1. The apparatus used to elicit a simple muscle twitch
2. Vibrating variable interrupter (Fig. 65.1): The reed is calibrated to vibrate at a frequency of 5, 7, 10, 20, 30, and 40 vibrations per sec. This is achieved by sliding the clamping plate along the metal guides fixed to the base board.
3. Signal marker

Procedure

1. Arrange an electrical circuit for single induced shocks, including the vibrating interrupter and signal marker in the primary circuit. Exclude the kymograph from the circuit.
2. Set up the kymograph and nerve–muscle preparation as done for the recording of the simple muscle curve.
3. Adjust the inductorium for weak 'break' shocks.
4. Adjust the length of the vibrating reed of the interrupter to provide five interruptions (stimuli) per second.
5. Start the kymograph using slow speed (fast gear; pulley 1:4) and set the reed vibrating. Open the short-circuiting key to stimulate the muscle and close it after recording 5–7 contractions on the drum.
6. Now increase the rate of interruptions (stimulation) to 10, 15, 20, 30, and 40 per second and record each stimulation on a fresh space on the smoked paper. Avoid unnecessary stimulation.

Note: If a high frequency is not available for obtaining tetanus, use Neef's hammer by including it in the primary circuit.

7. Note the frequency of stimulation that produced complete tetanus in your experiment.
8. Above each set of recordings, indicate the rate of stimulation as shown in the figure.
9. Fix the smoked paper recording by varnishing the paper.

Observations

Observe and study the graph (Fig. 65.2). Observe the **staircase phenomenon (treppe)** of the first initial stimuli. At the low frequency of stimulation, single contractions occur; with increasing frequency, first clonus (partial tetanus) and then tetanus occur.

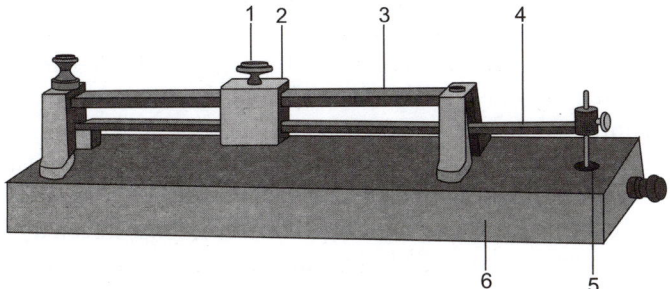

Fig. 65.1 Vibrating reed (1: clamping plate; 2: thumb screw; 3: vibration scale; 4: metal guide; 5: mercury cup; 6: base board).

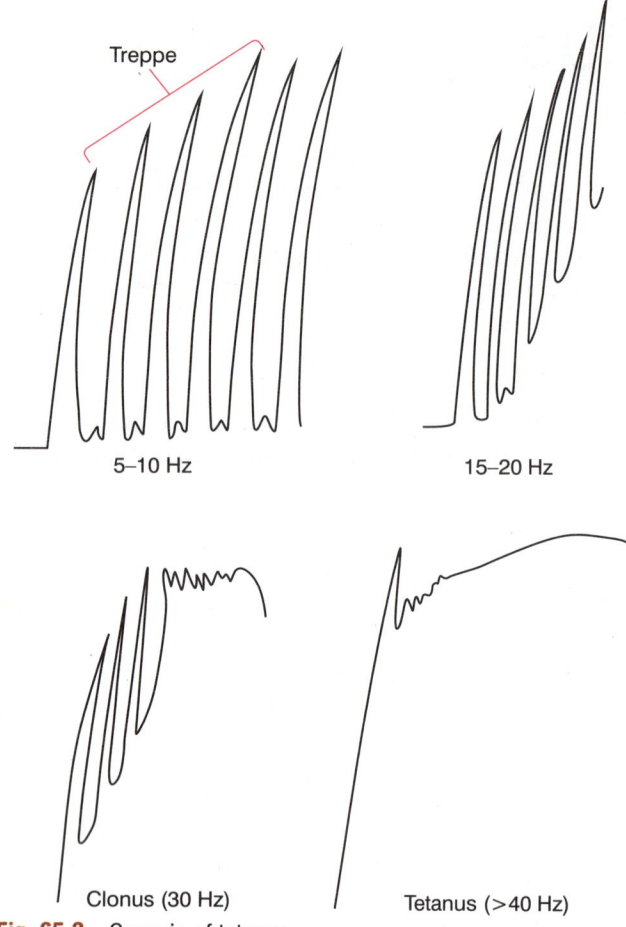

Fig. 65.2   Genesis of tetanus.

Precautions

1. The kymograph should be excluded from the circuit.
2. The inductorium should be adjusted for weak 'break' shocks.
3. The preparation should be stimulated from lower frequencies to higher frequencies.
4. Unnecessary stimulation should be avoided.
5. If the tetanising frequency is not obtained, Neef's hammer should be included in the primary circuit.

DISCUSSION

Minimal Tetanisable Frequency

The minimal tetanisable frequency (MTF) of a muscle can be calculated from the simple muscle curve (measuring the contraction period) by using the following formula:

$$MTF = \frac{1}{\text{Contraction period}}$$

For example, if the contraction period is 0.04 seconds, the MTF = 1/0.04 = 25 Hz.

Factors That Affect MTF

1. **Type of muscle:** In **slow muscles**, the *MTF is low* because the muscles produce slow, sustained contractions (longer contraction period). In **fast muscles**, the *MTF is greater* because the contraction period is less. An example of a slow muscle is the soleus, and examples of fast muscles are the muscles of the eye.
2. **Temperature of the environment:** The tetanisable frequency *is lower in a hot environment* and *higher in a cold environment*.
3. **Load acting on the muscle:** If the *load acting on the muscle is greater*, the tetanisable *frequency decreases*.

Treppe

Treppe is also known as the **staircase phenomenon**; it is the *progressive increase in the force of contractions for the first two to three contractions* when a muscle is stimulated repeatedly. This occurs due to the **accumulation of calcium** in the sarcoplasm due to the application of repeated stimuli. Treppe *is also seen in cardiac muscles*. However, the **cardiac muscle cannot be tetanised** because it has a *longer refractory period*.

Clonus

Clonus is a state of **partial tetanus** observed in experimental conditions (*experimental clonus*). This should not be confused with the *clinical clonus*, e.g., *ankle clonus*, seen in upper motor neuron type of paralysis. In experimental clonus, relaxation is incomplete.

Tetanus

Tetanus is a **state of sustained contraction**. The muscle remains in a **state of tonic contraction without relaxation**. This occurs when a nerve-muscle preparation is stimulated at a higher frequency. Rapid and repeated stimulation causes the stimuli to fall during the contraction phase so that the **contractile processes are repeatedly activated**. The muscle does not get time to relax. Therefore, with each stimulation, the *muscle contracts without relaxation*. *Individual responses fuse* to give a state of sustained contraction (tetanus). The muscles of the body that are involved in the maintenance of posture exhibit *tetanic contraction* (sustained contraction). An erect posture is maintained due to sustained contraction of the antigravity muscles. Tetanic contraction of the skeletal muscles is also observed during an isometric exercise.

Tetanus is also seen clinically when a person is infected by a group of bacteria called *Clostridium tetani*. Tetanus usually occurs *following an injury* (cut or wound) through which the bacteria enter the body. The **tetanus toxin** released by the bacteria *stimulates the motor neurons repeatedly* at a high frequency and results in tetanus. The *facial muscles* are commonly affected. In severe cases, all the skeletal muscles of the body may be affected. The disease can be **prevented by** prior *immunisation with the tetanus vaccine* or administering the vaccine *within twelve hours of injury*.

VIVA

1. *Define treppe, clonus, and tetanus.* (Ans. Refer to page 455, under the heading 'Discussion'.)
2. *What is the mechanism of the staircase phenomenon?* (Ans. Refer to page 455, under the heading 'Discussion' and the subheading 'Treppe'.)
3. *How is tetanus produced experimentally?* (Ans. Refer to page 454, under the heading 'Procedure'.)
4. *What is the minimal tetanisable frequency (MTF)? How is the MTF calculated, and what are the factors that affect MTF?* (Ans. Refer to page 456, under the heading 'Discussion' and the subheading 'Minimal tetanisable frequency'.)
5. *Explain why the cardiac muscle cannot be tetanised.* (Ans. Refer to page 455, under the heading 'Discussion' and the subheading 'Treppe'.)
6. *Give an example of tetanic contractions in our body.* (Ans. Refer to page 454-455, under the heading 'Discussion'.)
7. *Why is the tension developed by a tetanically contracting muscle more than the tension developed by the muscle during a single twitch?*
   (Ans. During a single contraction of the muscle, any calcium released into the sarcoplasm is quickly taken back into the cisterns during relaxation. But if the muscle is stimulated repeatedly, there is an accumulation of calcium in the sarcoplasm because calcium cannot be pumped back fully into the cisterns. This increases the tension in the muscle.)
8. *What is the cause of tetanus (disease)? How is the disease prevented?* (Ans. Refer to page 454, under the heading 'Discussion'.)
9. *What is tetany?*
   (Ans. Tetany occurs due to hypocalcemia, for example, in hypoparathyroidism. It does not bear any connection to tetanus.)

66 | Genesis of Fatigue

Learning Objectives

After completing this practical, you will be able to:
1. Define fatigue.
2. Demonstrate the site of fatigue in the nerve–muscle preparation.
3. List the precautions taken during the recording of the genesis of fatigue.
4. Name the site of fatigue in isolated and intact preparations.
5. Explain the causes of fatigue in isolated preparations.
6. Explain how recovery can be expedited.

PY3.18: Observe with computer-assisted learning: (i) amphibian nerve–muscle preparation and (ii) amphibian cardiac experiment.

INTRODUCTION

Fatigue is defined as a *decrease in performance due to continuous and prolonged activity*. It can occur in the whole organism or in isolated preparations. The mechanism of fatigue is different in an intact organism and in an isolated preparation. Fatigue is a **reversible phenomenon** in which there is no permanent functional or structural damage to the tissues. **In humans**, fatigue first occurs **in the central nervous system**, whereas **in isolated preparations**, the *neuromuscular junction* is the first site of fatigue.

METHOD TO STUDY THE GENESIS OF FATIGUE

Principle

A muscle is fatigued when it is stimulated repeatedly and continuously. The phenomenon of fatigue is recorded by stimulating the preparation without changing the baseline, the point of stimulation, and the strength of the stimulus.

Requirements

The requirements are the same as those for 'simple muscle twitch'.

Procedure

1. Dissect the frog to prepare the nerve–muscle preparation.
2. Mount the preparation in the muscle trough and set it up for recording a simple muscle curve. Mark the point of stimulation.
3. *Repeatedly stimulate* the nerve and **record the first, second, and third contractions** on a fast-moving drum without changing the point of stimulation. Note the beneficial effect.
4. Move the writing lever away from the drum.
5. Without changing the point of stimulation, **stimulate the nerve repeatedly** by keeping the tap key pressed and *record every tenth contraction* by applying the writing lever to the drum.

> **Note:** The drum rotates without recording the muscle contraction. Only the tenth contraction is recorded on the drum. This is done to avoid overlapping recordings. Recordings can be made with each stimulation, but overlapping of the recordings will make it difficult to study the graph.

6. Continue to *record every tenth contraction* until the contractions are too feeble to be recorded.
7. Change the point of the stimulus to record a muscle contraction at a different place adjacent to the fatigue curve and on the same baseline.
8. **Stimulate the muscle directly** and record the contraction on the changed point of stimulus.
9. Drain the Ringer's solution and replace it with fresh solution.
10. Allow the nerve–muscle preparation to **rest for five minutes**.
11. Again, change the point of stimulus on the same baseline in such a way that the next recording will be adjacent to the previous recording.
12. **Stimulate the nerve** to record the muscle contractions.

Observation

Record the **amplitude and duration** of the phases of the first three contractions and the subsequent contractions. Note that with the onset of fatigue, the relaxation period of the muscle twitches is prolonged, and the baseline goes up (Fig. 66.1A). Muscle contraction occurs by direct stimulation of the muscle (Fig. 66.1B) following fatigue. Muscle contraction also occurs in response to nerve stimulation following recovery (Fig. 66.1C).

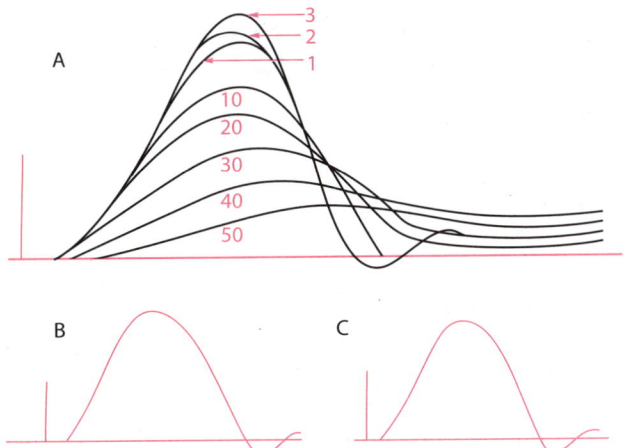

Fig. 66.1   Demonstration of the phenomenon and site of fatigue. **(A)** Genesis of fatigue following repeated stimulation of the nerve. Numbers depicted with the curves indicate the number of stimuli. Note the beneficial effects of the first three contractions. Also, note the decrease in amplitude, prolongation of the relaxation period, and rise in baseline with the onset of fatigue; **(B)** recording of the curve by directly stimulating the muscle immediately following the onset of fatigue; **(C)** recording of the curve by stimulating the nerve following recovery.

Precautions

1. All the precautions described for the recording of simple muscle twitch should be taken (Chapter 61).
2. All the contractions should be recorded on the same point of the stimulus and on the same baseline for the fatigue curve (fatigue produced by the stimulation of the nerve).
3. The muscle should be directly stimulated immediately after recording the fatigue by stimulating the nerve, and the contraction should be recorded on a different point of the stimulus but on the same baseline.
4. The preparation should be allowed a minimum of five minutes for recovery before stimulating the nerve to record the effect of recovery.

5. To facilitate recovery, the old Ringer's solution should be removed and replaced with fresh solution.

DISCUSSION

In isolated preparations, fatigue can occur at **three sites**: *the muscle, the neuromuscular junction, and the nerve.* The *nerve is theoretically unfatiguable*, and therefore, the possible sites of fatigue are either the muscle or the neuromuscular junction. However, the muscle contraction recorded by directly stimulating the muscle following the genesis of fatigue indicates that the muscle is not fatigued. Therefore, it can be inferred that the *first site of fatigue is the neuromuscular junction.*

The *cause of this fatigue is the depletion of acetylcholine*, the neurotransmitter from the myoneural junction. If the preparation is allowed to rest for some time and fresh Ringer's solution is supplied to the preparation, the muscle contracts in response to the stimulation of the nerve (following the period of recovery). This again proves that the site of fatigue is the neuromuscular junction because recovery allows for the re-synthesis of neurotransmitters at the nerve endings. The Ringer's solution supplies nutrition and facilitates recovery.

If the *muscle is directly stimulated continuously*, it can also be *fatigued due to the exhaustion of glycogen storage*. However, in this condition, there will be no recovery, as the utilised glycogen cannot be replaced.

An **early sign of fatigue** is the *prolongation of the relaxation period*. When a muscle is fatigued, the relaxation becomes incomplete, and it remains in a state of partial contraction. This is called **contraction remainder**. It occurs due to a decrease in the ATP content and accumulation of the metabolites in the muscle. The baseline increases due to contraction remainder.

In **human beings**, the *first site of fatigue could be the CNS*, not the neuromuscular junction.

VIVA

1. *Define fatigue.* (**Ans.** Refer to page 456, under the heading 'Introduction'.)
2. *What is the difference between the fatigue of an intact animal and that of an isolated preparation?* (**Ans.** Refer to page 456, under the heading 'Introduction'.)
3. *What is the site of fatigue in an isolated preparation and how do you demonstrate it?* (**Ans.** Refer to page 456, under the heading 'Procedure'.)
4. *What is the mechanism of fatigue in an isolated preparation?* (**Ans.** Refer to page 457, under the heading 'Discussion'.)
5. *How can recovery be facilitated?* (**Ans.** Refer to page 457, under the heading 'Discussion'.)
6. *What is contraction remainder?*
    (**Ans.** When a muscle is fatigued, the relaxation becomes incomplete, and it remains in a state of partial contraction. This is called **contraction remainder**. It occurs due to a decrease in the ATP content and accumulation of the metabolites in the muscle.)
7. *What is the early sign of fatigue in an isolated preparation?* (**Ans.** Refer to page 457, under the heading 'Discussion'.)

67 | Conduction Velocity of Nerves in Frogs

Learning Objectives

After completing this practical, you will be able to:
1. State the importance of determining nerve conduction in clinical physiology.
2. Demonstrate the recording of the conduction velocity of the nerves of a frog.
3. List the factors that affect nerve conduction velocity.

PY3.18: Observe with computer-assisted learning: (i) amphibian nerve–muscle preparation and (ii) amphibian cardiac experiment.

INTRODUCTION

The detection of the velocity of nerve conduction is one of the most important tests in clinical neurophysiology. In human beings, the velocity of conduction is determined by using nerve conduction apparatus (see Chapter 31). Recording the conduction velocity in frogs, however, is a simple experiment. Conduction velocity chiefly depends on the **diameter and myelination** of the nerve.

METHODS TO DETERMINE THE CONDUCTION VELOCITY OF NERVES IN FROGS

Principle

The velocity of conduction is determined by dividing the distance between the two points of stimuli (proximal and distal) by the difference in the latent period of the two recordings.

Requirements

1. Same as those for simple muscle twitch
2. Scale

Procedure

1. Prepare a gastrocnemius–sciatic nerve preparation and the setup to record a simple muscle twitch.
2. **Stimulate the vertebral end** of the sciatic nerve and record a simple muscle twitch. Mark the point of placement of the electrodes on the nerve.
3. Mark the point of stimulus and the point of onset of the contraction to **record the latent period**.
4. **Stimulate the muscular end** of the sciatic nerve and record a simple muscle twitch on the same baseline and on the same point of the stimulus and calculate the latent period. Mark the point of placement of the electrodes on the nerve.
5. **Deduct the latent period** of the second recording (recording of the stimulation at the muscular end) from the latent period of the first recording (recording of the stimulation at the vertebral end).
6. **Measure the distance between the points of stimulation** of the vertebral end and the muscular end of the nerve in centimetres.
7. Calculate the **conduction velocity** by dividing the distance by time, i.e., D/T, where D: length in cm between two points of stimuli and T: time difference (in ms) between the latent periods of the two recordings.

Note: The distance is the length of the nerve (in cm) between the two points of stimuli. The 'time' is the difference in the latent periods of the two recordings (in ms).

Observations

Observe the difference in the latent period of the two recordings (Fig. 67.1) and calculate the conduction velocity from the given recordings. Express the result in m/s.

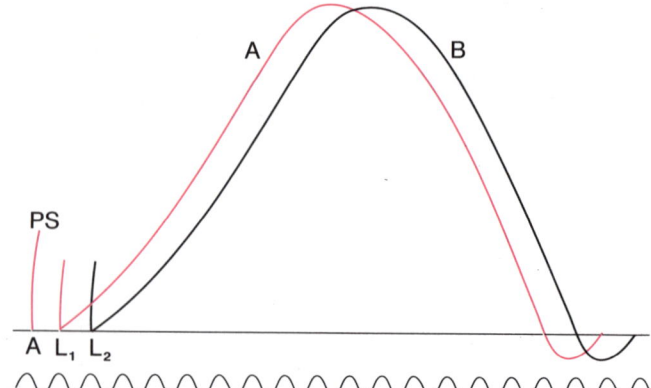

Fig. 67.1 Determination of nerve conduction velocity in frog. (A: Simple muscle curve following the stimulation of the nerve close to the muscle; B: simple muscle curve following stimulation of the nerve close to the vertebra; PS: point of stimulation; AL_1: latent period of the curve A; AL_2: latent period of the curve B).

Note: The normal value of conduction velocity of the sciatic nerve of a frog is **40–60 m/s.**

Precautions

1. The point of stimulus at both ends of the sciatic nerve should be marked at the time of stimulation.
2. The distance between the two points should be accurately measured.
3. The difference between the latent periods should be accurately measured.

DISCUSSION

The sciatic nerve is a **thick, mixed nerve** composed of both motor and sensory fibres.

The conduction velocity of a nerve is mainly determined by the *fibre diameter and the degree of myelination* of the nerve. As the fibre diameter increases, the velocity of conduction increases. The velocity of conduction is higher in myelinated than in unmyelinated fibres. The velocity of conduction of a somatic nerve (like the sciatic nerve) with a fibre diameter of 12–20 μm ranges between **60 and 120 m/s.** A decrease in conduction velocity indicates injury to the nerve or some defect in the nerve.

Other factors that affect nerve conduction are **temperature, height of action potential, and stimulating and recording systems.**

VIVA

1. *What is the clinical significance of determining the conduction velocity of nerves?* (Ans. Refer to page 459, under the heading 'Discussion'.)
2. *What is the normal velocity of conduction of the sciatic nerve of the frog?* (Ans. Refer to page 458, under the heading 'Observation.)
3. *What are the factors that affect the velocity of conduction in the nerve?* (Ans. Refer to page 459, under the heading 'Discussion'.)
4. *In which condition does the velocity of conduction decrease?* (Ans. Refer to page 459, under the heading 'Discussion'.)

68 | Normal Cardiogram of a Frog

Learning Objectives

After completing this practical, you will be able to:

1. Dissect and open the thorax and the pericardium of a frog, pin the apex of the heart, and fix the heart to the lever.
2. Identify the different parts of the heart.
3. Record a normal cardiogram.
4. Explain the different waves in the cardiogram.
5. List the properties of the heart demonstrated in this experiment.
6. List the differences between amphibian and mammalian hearts.

PY3.18: Observe with computer-assisted learning: (i) amphibian nerve–muscle preparation and (ii) amphibian cardiac experiment.

INTRODUCTION

A normal frog cardiogram is a recording of the mechanical activity of the frog's heart on a smoked drum. Since a cardiogram is a **recording of the mechanical activities of the heart**, it records the systole and diastole of the different chambers of the heart.

In a frog, the atria are called **auricles**, the **ventricles are single-chambered**, and the electrical rhythm for generating an impulse is located in the **sinus venosus** instead of the SA node as seen in the mammalian heart (Table 68.1). Therefore, in an ideal tracing, the mechanical activities of the sinus venosus, auricles, and ventricles are recorded. A **white crescentic line** is present between the auricles and the sinus venosus (Fig. 68.1). The normal heart rate of a frog is **40–50 beats** per minute.

METHOD OF RECORDING A NORMAL CARDIOGRAM OF A FROG

Principle

The mechanical activities of the amphibian heart are directly recorded by connecting the heart to the writing lever with a thread, which transmits the waves of contraction and relaxation from the heart to the lever. The cardiac activities are recorded on a moving drum.

Requirements

1. Kymograph with Sherrington–Starling drum
2. Frog board
3. Myograph stand
4. Starling's heart lever or simple heart lever
5. Frog's Ringer's solution
6. Pins (also one hooked pin)
7. Thread

Procedure

1. Pith the frog (destroy only the spinal cord).
2. Lay the pithed frog on its back on the frog board.
3. Make a median incision through the skin over the sternum.
4. Raise the xiphisternum with blunt forceps and separate it from the underlying tissue using a pair of blunt scissors, taking care not to injure the heart.
5. Insert one of the blades of the scissors under the pectoral girdle and cut on both sides so that the anterior wall of the thorax can be removed.
6. Pull the forelimbs laterally and fix them on the board with pins so as to keep the chest wide open.
7. Identify the heart, beating inside the thin membrane (pericardium).
8. Observe that at the apex of the heart, there is a small, clear space between the heart and pericardial membrane. With the help of forceps, pinch and lift the pericardium at the apex in this clear space, taking care not to touch the heart.
9. Make a slit in the pericardium with a pair of fine scissors and then cut the pericardium up to the base of the heart, taking care not to injure the heart.
10. Study the different parts of the heart (Fig. 68.1A and B).

Note: On the ventral aspect of the heart, the initial dilated portion of the aorta, which is known as the bulbus arteriosus, divides into two aortae. On the dorsal aspect (lift the ventricle), identify the sinus venosus separated from the auricles by a white crescentic line. Note that two superior vena cavae and the inferior vena cava enter the sinus venosus. Observe the change in the colour of the chambers during systole (contraction) and diastole (relaxation).

11. Fix the pericardium through the base of the heart to the frog board with a pin.
12. Hook a bent pin through the apex of the heart, taking care not to puncture the chambers of the ventricle.
13. Tie one end of the thread to the pin and lift the ventricle by the thread. Tie the other end of the thread to the heart lever.

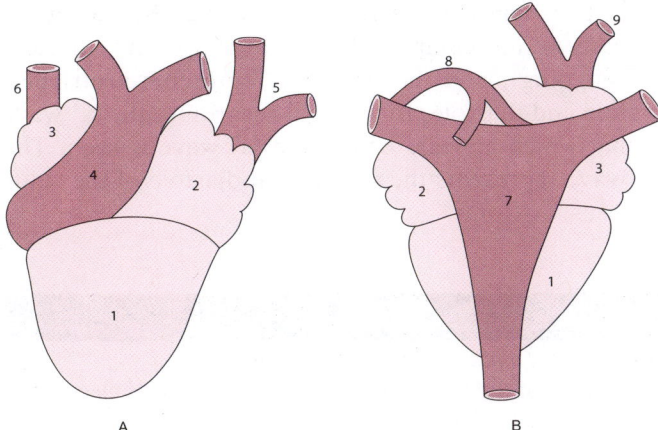

Fig. 68.1 Frog's heart: **(A)** Dorsal view and **(B)** ventral view (1: ventricle; 2: left auricle; 3: right auricle; 4: truncus arteriosus; 5: left anterior caval vein; 6: right anterior caval vein; 7: sinus venosus; 8: pulmonary vein; 9: right systemic arch; 10: posterior caval vein).

> **Note:** Keep the thread vertical and taut enough to transmit the contraction of the heart to the writing point of the lever.

14. Keep the writing arm of the lever horizontal.
15. Touch the writing point of the heart lever lightly to the smoked paper on the drum in the lower third (about 5 cm from the lower margin) of the drum.
16. Set the drum to rotate at a slow speed (1.2 mm/s) and record the cardiogram starting from just after the joint of the paper on the drum.
17. Take a time-tracing below the recording.
18. Repeat the recording of the cardiogram at a higher speed (2.5 mm/s).

> **Note:** Recording at a faster speed will clearly show the different components of the cardiogram.

Observation

Identify the different components of the cardiogram recorded at slow and fast speeds as shown in Fig. 68.2A, B, and C. Observe the rhythmicity (whether regular or irregular) and calculate the heart rate.

Precautions

1. While making a median incision on the sternum of the frog, care should be taken not to damage the heart.
2. The heart should be exposed by cutting the pericardium.
3. While cutting the pericardium, care should be taken not to damage the heart.
4. The hooked pin should be introduced at the apex of the heart, through the wall of the ventricle. While introducing the hooked pin, care should be taken not to puncture the ventricle (the pin should not enter the ventricular cavity).

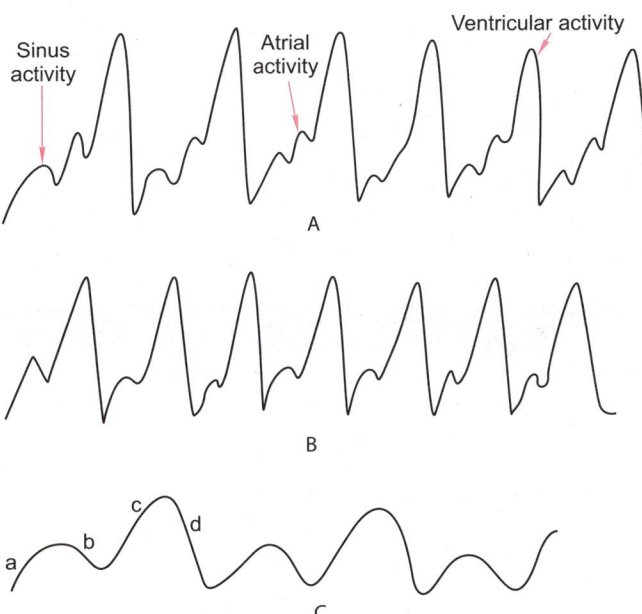

Fig. 68.2 Normal cardiogram of frog. **(A)** Ideal recording (at slow speed; 1.2 mm/s); **(B)** usual recording (at slow speed; 1.2 mm/s); **(C)** usual recording at fast speed (a: atrial systole; b: atrial relaxation; c: ventricular contraction; d: ventricular relaxation).

5. The thread connecting the heart and the lever should be placed vertically.
6. The lever should be placed horizontally.
7. The base of the heart should be fixed. This increases the amplitude of the recording because the force of contractions is directly transmitted to the lever due to the pulling of the apex towards the fixed base during each systole.
8. Frog Ringer's solution should be poured on the heart at regular intervals to prevent it from drying.

DISCUSSION

The properties of the heart that are studied in this experiment are **automaticity, rhythmicity, conductivity, and contractility**. Automaticity is studied by observing the automatic beating of the heart, which occurs due to the impulse generated automatically in the heart; rhythmicity is studied by the rhythmical beating of the heart; conductivity is studied by the conduction of impulses from the sinus venosus to the ventricles (*better demonstrated by **Stannius ligatures***); and contractility is recorded by observing the contraction of the heart and recording the systole and diastole in the tracings.

In the heart of a frog, the cardiac impulse is generated in the sinus venosus. Impulse is transmitted from the sinus venosus to the auricles and then to the ventricles. A slight pause is seen between auricular and ventricular contractions and this is due to the delay (partial conduction block) in the conduction of the impulse from the auricles to the ventricles. In a frog, the rate of impulse generation is maximum in the sinus venosus. Therefore, the *sinus venosus is the natural pacemaker* of the heart.

The Cardiogram

Different waves in the cardiogram represent the activities of different chambers of the heart. Usually, only two **types of waves** are seen. The **'a' wave** represents auricular systole (upgoing) and diastole (downgoing), and the **'v' wave** represents ventricular systole and diastole. In an ideal recording, the **'s' wave** is that which appears before the **'a' wave** is seen. The **'s' wave** represents the systole and diastole of the sinus venosus.

VIVA

1.   *What is the difference between a cardiogram (recorded in this experiment) and an electrocardiogram?*
     (**Ans.** A cardiogram is a recording of mechanical activities (contractions) of the heart. An ECG is the recording of electrical activities of the heart.)
2.   *What is the normal heart rate in a frog?* (**Ans.** Refer to page 460, under the heading 'Introduction'.)
3.   *What are the properties of the cardiac muscle? What properties of the cardiac muscle are demonstrated in this experiment?* (**Ans.** Refer to page 461, under the heading 'Discussion'.)
4.   *What are the differences between the amphibian and mammalian hearts?* (**Ans.** Refer to page 460, under the heading 'Introduction'.)
5.   *Where is the pacemaker of a frog's heart situated?* (**Ans.** Refer to page 461, under the heading 'Discussion'.)
6.   *What does the crescentic line represent?* (**Ans.** Refer to page 460-461, under the heading 'Procedure', see the Note under point no. 10.)
7.   *What are the different waves recorded in a normal cardiogram of a frog's heart? How are these waves produced?* (**Ans.** Refer to page 461, under the heading 'Discussion' and the subheading 'The cardiogram'.)
8.   *What are the precautions taken during dissection to expose the heart?* (**Ans.** Refer to page 461, under the heading 'Precautions'.)
9.   *Why is the base of the heart fixed?*
     (**Ans.** The base of the heart should be fixed, because this increases the amplitude of the recording because the force of contractions is directly transmitted to the lever due to the pulling of the apex towards the fixed base during each systole.)
10. *Why should only the spinal cord be destroyed during pithing?*
     (**Ans.** Cardiovascular centres are present in the brain. Therefore, if the brain is destroyed with pithing, there may be an alteration in heart function.)

69 | Effect of Temperature on Frog's Heart

Learning Objectives

After completing this practical, you will be able to:
1. State the physiological importance of performing this practical.
2. Demonstrate the effect of cold and warm Ringer's solution on the sinus venosus and the ventricle.
3. List the precautions taken for studying the effect of cold and warm Ringer's solution on the sinus venosus and the ventricle.
4. Explain the changes in cardiac activities following the application of cold and warm Ringer's solution on the sinus venosus and the ventricle.

PY3.18: Observe with computer-assisted learning: (i) amphibian nerve–muscle preparation and (ii) amphibian cardiac experiment.

INTRODUCTION

The application of cold and warm Ringer's solution on the sinus venosus changes the heart rate by changing the pacemaker activity, which is present in the sinus venosus in frogs. The application of cold and warm Ringer's solution on the ventricle changes the force of contraction by directly affecting the contractile machinery of the myocardium.

This experiment is carried out to study the effect of temperature on the sinus venosus and the ventricle, and to know the site of impulse generation in the frog's heart.

METHOD TO STUDY THE EFFECT OF TEMPERATURE ON FROG'S HEART

Principle

The application of cold and warm Ringer's solution on the sinus venosus changes the heart rate and that on the ventricle changes the force of contraction. These changes are observed by applying cold and warm Ringer's solution separately on the sinus venosus and on the ventricle and recording the effects on a moving drum.

Requirements

1. The same as those mentioned in Chapter 68
2. Cold Ringer's solution (15°C)
3. Warm Ringer's solution (35°C)
4. Dropper
5. Blotting paper

Procedure

Expose the heart of a pithed frog and record a normal cardiogram as described in Chapter 68. Then carry out the experiment separately on the sinus venosus and on the ventricle as described below.

On the sinus venosus

1. Record a normal cardiogram (about 10 beats).
2. Apply cold (15°C) Ringer's solution to the sinus venosus with the help of a dropper and record its effect on the cardiogram (about 10 beats).
3. Apply Ringer's solution at normal room temperature and record a normal cardiogram (about 10 beats).
4. Apply warm Ringer's (35°C) to the sinus venosus with the help of a dropper and record its effect on the cardiogram (about 10 beats).
5. Apply Ringer's solution at normal room temperature and record a normal cardiogram (about 10 beats).

On the ventricle

1. Record a normal cardiogram (about 10 beats) at room temperature.
2. Apply cold (15°C) Ringer's solution to the ventricle with a piece of blotting paper and record its effect on the ventricle.

Note: A small piece of blotting paper is soaked in cold Ringer's solution and placed on the ventricle with the help of forceps, taking care not to allow the solution to trickle down to the sinus venosus.

3. Apply Ringer's solution at normal room temperature and record a normal cardiogram (about 10 beats).
4. Apply warm Ringer's (35°C) to the ventricle with blotting paper and record its effect on the ventricle.

Note: The blotting paper is soaked in warm Ringer's solution and then placed on the ventricle with forceps, taking care not to allow the solution to trickle down to the sinus venosus.

5. Apply Ringer's solution at normal room temperature and record a normal cardiogram (about 10 beats).

   Tabulate the effects of temperature on the sinus venosus and on the ventricle with reference to heart rate and force of contraction.

Observation

Study the effect of temperature on the sinus venosus and the ventricle. Note that cold Ringer's decreases the heart rate but increases the force of contraction, and warm Ringer's increases the heart rate but decreases the amplitude of contraction when applied to the sinus venosus. Cold Ringer's decreases the amplitude of contraction without changing the heart rate and warm Ringer's increases the amplitude of contraction without changing the heart rate when applied to the ventricle (Fig. 69.1).

Precautions

1. The normal cardiogram should be recorded before recording the effects of cold and warm Ringer's solution on the sinus venosus and the ventricle.
2. The temperature of cold Ringer's should be 15°C, and the temperature of warm Ringer's should be 35°C. If the solution is very cold or very hot, it may damage the heart.
3. The temperature of the solutions should be recorded just before their application.
4. Care should be taken to apply the solution only on the sinus venosus when the effect of cold and warm Ringer's solution is being elicited.
5. Care must be taken to prevent the trickling down of the solution to the sinus venosus from the ventricle when the effect of cold and warm Ringer's is being elicited. While recording the cardiogram, the ventricle should be placed above the sinus venosus, and a blotting paper (not the dropper) should be used to pour cold

and warm Ringer's solution on the ventricle so that the solution does not trickle down to the sinus venosus.
6. The heart should be moistened with normal Ringer's solution frequently to prevent drying.
7. When not recording, the lever of the heart should be lowered to prevent deterioration of the function of the heart.

DISCUSSION

Cold Ringer's on the Sinus Venosus

The application of cold Ringer's solution on the sinus venosus *decreases the heart rate and increases the amplitude of contractions*. The heart rate decreases because cold Ringer's directly inhibits the pacemaker activity of the heart. This is the **primary effect**. The increase in the amplitude of contractions is *due to the Frank–Starling law*—when the heart rate decreases, the ventricular end diastolic volume increases because the ventricle gets more time to fill up. The increased ventricular filling increases the length of the ventricular muscle fibre before the onset of systole. Therefore, the force of the contraction increases. This is **the secondary effect**.

Warm Ringer's on the Sinus Venosus

The application of warm Ringer's solution on the sinus venosus *increases the heart rate and decreases the force of contraction*. The **increase in heart rate** is the **primary effect** and the ***decrease in the force of contractions is the secondary effect.*** The heart rate increases due to the stimulation of the pacemaker activity in the sinus venosus by the warm solution. The force of contractions decreases due to decreased filling of the heart (decreased end diastolic volume) as the heart gets less time to fill up.

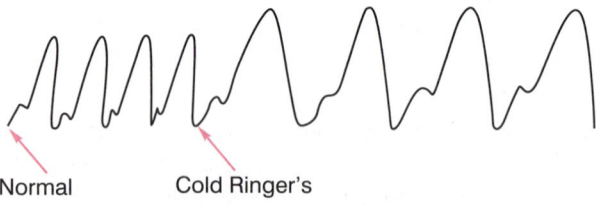

Normal   Cold Ringer's

A. On sinus venosus

Normal   Warm Ringer's

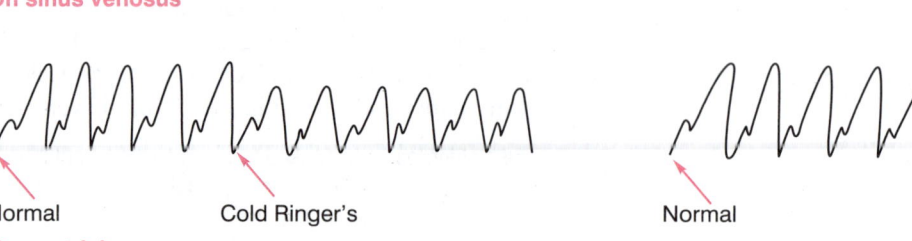

Normal   Cold Ringer's

B. On ventricle

Normal   Warm Ringer's

Fig. 69.1   Effect of temperature on frog's heart.

Cold Ringer's on the Ventricle

The application of cold Ringer's solution to the ventricle **decreases the force of contraction** due to the *inhibition of myocardial contractility* by the cold solution. The heart rate does not change because the pacemaker of the heart is present in the sinus venosus, which remains unaffected in this experiment. The myocardial activity is depressed by the cold Ringer's solution because at the low temperature, the *enzymatic activity of the myocardium decreases*, and *the viscosity of the myocardial tissue increases*.

Warm Ringer's on the Ventricle

The application of warm Ringer's solution to the ventricle *increases the force of contraction* due to the accentuation of myocardial activity by the direct action of warm solution on it. The heart rate remains unchanged because the pacemaker is present in the sinus venosus. Warm Ringer's stimulates myocardial contractility by **increasing the *enzymatic activity and decreasing the viscosity*** of the myocardial tissue.

These experiments prove that the **sinus venosus is the pacemaker** of the frog heart.

VIVA

1. *What is the effect of cold Ringer's on the sinus venosus and the ventricle? What is the physiological basis?* (Ans. Refer to page 464, under the heading 'Observation'.)
2. *What is the Frank–Starling law of the heart?* (Ans. Refer to page 464, under the heading 'Discussion'.)
3. *What is the effect of warm Ringer's solution on the sinus venosus and the ventricle? What is the physiological basis?* (Ans. Refer to page 464, under the heading 'Observation'.)
4. *What are the precautions taken for demonstrating the effect of cold and warm Ringer's on the sinus venosus and the ventricle?* (Ans. Refer to page 464, under the heading 'Precautions'.)
5. *What is the physiological basis of the difference between the effect of cold and warm Ringer's on the sinus venosus and the ventricle?* (Ans. Refer to page 464, under the heading 'Observation'.)

70 | Effect of Stannius Ligatures on Frog's Heart

Learning Objectives

After completing this practical, you will be able to:
1. Explain the clinical implication of this practical.
2. Demonstrate the effect of Stannius ligature on the frog heart.
3. Explain the effect of Stannius ligatures.
4. State the rate of discharge of different potential pacemakers of the heart.
5. Classify heart blocks.

PY3.18: Observe with computer-assisted learning: (i) amphibian nerve–muscle preparation and (ii) amphibian cardiac experiment.

INTRODUCTION

In humans, the cardiac impulse is generated in the SA node and conducted to all parts of the heart. Therefore, the SA node is the pacemaker of the heart. In a **frog's heart**, the **pacemaker is present in the sinus venosus**. The cardiac muscle has the property of automaticity, that is, it has the power to generate its own impulses. Though normally an impulse is generated in the SA node (primary pacemaker), automaticity is not limited to the SA node alone. When the SA node is diseased, the other potential pacemakers of the heart take over the responsibility of generating the impulse. The first to take over the work of the SA node is the AV node. The next in the hierarchy are the bundle of His, the Purkinje system, and the ventricular muscle. In humans, *the rate of discharge is maximum in the SA node because it is the natural pacemaker of the heart*. The rate of discharge *gradually decreases in the hierarchy of the pacemakers*.

In humans, the **rates of discharge of the different pacemakers** are as follows:
SA node: 60–100/min
AV node: 50–70/min
His bundle: 40–60/min
Purkinje system: 30–50/min
Ventricular muscle: 15–40/min

This practical demonstrates the hierarchy of the pacemaking activity of the different tissues of the heart.

METHOD TO STUDY THE EFFECT OF STANNIUS LIGATURES ON FROG'S HEART

Principle

The rate of discharge of impulses is different in different potential pacemakers of the heart. Their rhythms are demonstrated by separating (appropriately placing ligatures) them from each other.

Requirements

1. Same as those listed in Chapter 68
2. Aneurysm needle
3. Thread

Procedure

1. Set up the experiment as done for recording a normal cardiogram.
2. Pass a threaded aneurysm needle between the truncus arteriosus and the atria.
3. Hook up the heart and record the normal cardiogram on a slow-moving drum.
4. Bring forward the thread under the truncus arteriosus and tie it at the junction of the sinus venosus and the atria (on the white crescentic line).

Note: This is the first Stannius ligature (Fig. 70.1). It records the atrial rhythm.

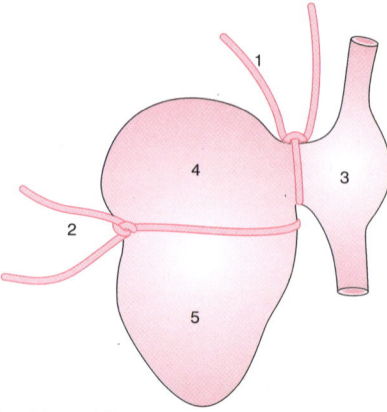

Fig. 70.1 Position of Stannius ligatures as seen in the side view of the heart (1: first Stannius ligature; 2: second Stannius ligature; 3: sinus venosus; 4: auricles; 5: ventricle).

5. Record the effect of ligation on the cardiogram.
6. Apply the ligature at the atrioventricular junction and record the effect of ligation on the cardiogram.

Note: This is the second Stannius ligature. It records the ventricular rhythm. Note that the ventricle starts beating after a pause, and at a much slower rate (idioventricular rhythm).

Observation

Note that the frequency of the heart beat after placing the first Stannius ligature is significantly less than the normal rhythm. The frequency of the heart beat is much lower after placing the second Stannius ligature (Fig. 70.2).

Precautions

1. The first Stannius ligature should be tied between the truncus arteriosus and the atria.
2. The second Stannius ligature should be tied between the atria and ventricle.
3. The recording should be taken immediately after placing the ligatures.

DISCUSSION

The **sinus venosus (SA node in humans)** is the **primary pacemaker** of the heart. Therefore, the **first Stannius ligature**, which prevents the transmission of impulses from the sinus venosus to the atria, decreases the heart rate as the impulse is now generated by the atria (**atrial rhythm**). After placing the **second Stannius ligature**, which prevents transmission of impulses from the atria to the ventricle, the heart rate decreases further because the impulse is now generated by the ventricle (**ventricular rhythm**). This indicates that the primary pacemaker in the frog heart is present in the sinus venosus.

Clinical Significance

Heart blocks

As discussed, the SA node normally controls the heart rate. Interruption of impulse transmission from the atria to the ventricle is called heart block. There are three degrees of heart blocks: first, second, and third. In **first and second degree heart blocks**, impulse transmission between the atria and the ventricle is not completely interrupted; therefore, these are called **incomplete heart blocks**. In **third-degree heart blocks**, impulse transmission between the atria and the ventricle is completely blocked, and therefore, these are called **complete heart blocks**.

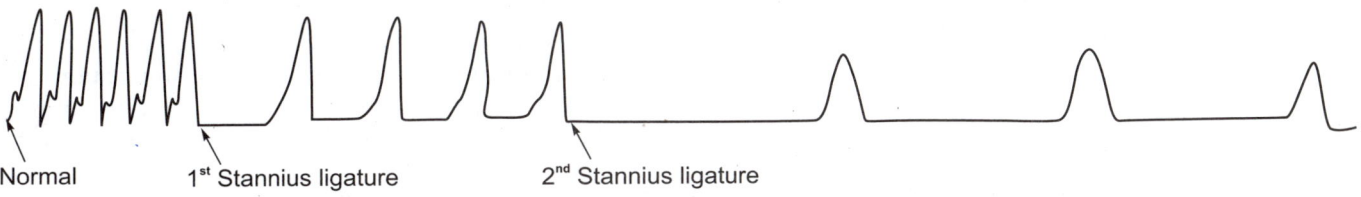

Normal   1ˢᵗ Stannius ligature   2ⁿᵈ Stannius ligature

Fig. 70.2 Recording of the effects of the Stannius ligature on a frog's heart.

VIVA

1. *What is the effect of the first Stannius ligature on the heart?* (**Ans.** Refer to page 467, under the heading 'Discussion'.)
2. *What is the effect of the second Stannius ligature on the heart?* (**Ans.** Refer to page 467, under the heading 'Discussion'.)
3. *What are the rates of discharge of the different potential pacemakers of the heart?* (**Ans.** Refer to page 466, under the heading 'Introduction'.)
4. *What is a heart block? What are the different types of heart blocks?* (**Ans.** Refer to page 467, under the heading 'Discussion'.)

71 | Properties of the Cardiac Muscle

Learning Objectives

After completing this practical, you will be able to:
1. Explain the importance of studying the properties of the cardiac muscle.
2. List the properties of the cardiac muscle.
3. Define extrasystole, compensatory pause, refractory period, all-or-none law, and the staircase phenomenon.
4. Elaborate on the physiological basis of the different properties of the cardiac muscle.
5. Explain why the cardiac muscle cannot be tetanised.
6. Explain the physiological basis of the staircase phenomenon.

PY3.18: Observe with computer-assisted learning: (i) amphibian nerve–muscle preparation and (ii) amphibian cardiac experiment.

INTRODUCTION

The properties of the cardiac muscle can be divided into two groups: properties that can be studied in a **beating heart** and those studied in a **quiescent heart**.

Properties that can be studied in a beating heart:
1. Automaticity
2. Rhythmicity
3. Contractility
4. Conductivity
5. Excitability
6. Long refractory period
7. Extrasystole and compensatory pause

Properties that can be studied in a quiescent heart:
1. All-or-none law
2. The staircase phenomenon
3. Length–tension relationship
4. Summation of subminimal stimuli

In this practical, the properties that you will study are extrasystole, compensatory pause, refractory period, all-or-none law, the staircase phenomenon, and the summation of subminimal stimuli. The last three properties can be studied in a quiescent heart.

METHOD TO STUDY PROPERTIES OF THE CARDIAC MUSCLE

Principle

The properties of the cardiac muscle are studied in a beating heart and in a quiescent heart.

Requirements

1. The same as those for recording a normal cardiogram
2. Electrical circuit for cardiac stimulation
3. Signal marker
4. Aneurysm needle

Procedure

Recording of extrasystole, compensatory pause, and refractory period

I. In a beating heart
1. Set up the experiment as you would for recording a normal cardiogram.
2. Apply electrodes to the base of the ventricle to stimulate it with single induction shocks.
3. Adjust a signal marker close to the heart lever to record the movement induced by the stimulation.
4. Record normal heartbeats on a slow-moving drum.
5. Stimulate the ventricle during different phases of the cardiac cycle.

> **Note:** While stimulating the ventricle, it is important to observe that the stimuli applied during the systole are ineffective, whereas the stimuli applied during diastole elicit a premature contraction (extrasystole), which is followed by a compensatory pause. The contraction following the compensatory pause is of a greater magnitude than the previous one (Fig. 71.1A).

6. Label your record to show the systole and diastole in a normal heartbeat, point of application of the extra stimulus, extrasystole, and compensatory pause.

II. In a quiescent heart
1. Make electrical connections for delivering single induced shocks with a drum in the circuit.
2. Apply the first Stannius ligature by tying the heart with a thread at the white crescentic line to make the heart quiescent.
3. Place the electrodes at the base of the ventricle.
4. Stimulate the ventricle by adjusting the angle between the contact arms so that the stimuli fall during different phases of the cardiac cycle.
5. Record the effect of the stimuli on the drum running at medium speed.

6. Mark the point of stimulation for each graph before changing the angle of the contact arms and the position of the cylinder.
7. Obtain at least **three sets of graphs** as mentioned below:
   i. The second stimulus is applied when the **ventricle is completely relaxed** after the first contraction.
   ii. The second stimulus is applied **during the diastole of the first heartbeat** (relative refractory period).
   iii. The second stimulus is applied **during the systole of the first heartbeat** (absolute refractory period).

III. All-or-none law

1. Make electrical connections to stimulate the ventricle with single induced shocks.
2. Apply the first Stannius ligature to make the heart quiescent.
3. Apply electrodes to the base of the ventricle.
4. Adjust the writing lever to record on a stationary drum.
5. Stimulate the ventricle with subthreshold stimuli and observe the effect.
6. Increase the strength of the stimulus till a contraction is recorded.
7. Increase the strength of the stimulus every thirty seconds; rotate the drum through 1 cm each time and record the contraction.

> **Note:** Observe that the **height of the contraction remains the same** irrespective of the strength of the stimulus, that is, the amplitude of contraction of the threshold stimulus is the same as the amplitude of contraction recorded with the stimuli of higher strength. No recording occurs with subthreshold stimuli (Fig. 71.1B).

IV. Staircase phenomenon

1. Adjust the inductorium for a single effective shock.
2. Make the heart quiescent by applying the first Stannius ligature.
3. Stimulate the ventricle repeatedly at intervals of two seconds and record each contraction at 1 cm intervals on a stationary drum.

> **Note:** Observe that the first few contractions show a successive increase in amplitude, which is known as the staircase phenomenon (Fig. 71.1C).

V. Summation of subminimal stimuli

1. Make the heart quiescent by placing the first Stannius ligature.
2. By adjusting the position of the inductorium, find a stimulus that only just fails to produce a contraction.

> **Note:** This is a subthreshold stimulus.

3. Repeatedly stimulate the ventricle at intervals of one second till the ventricle produces a full contraction.

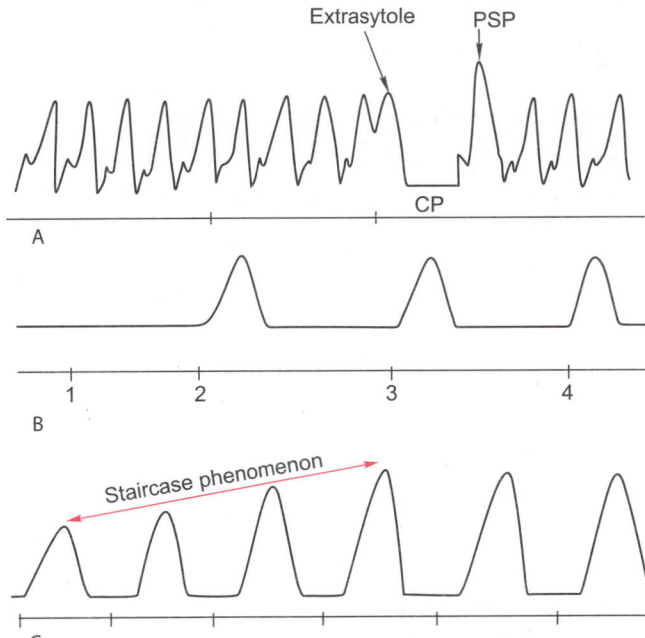

Fig. 71.1   Demonstration of the properties of the cardiac muscle. **(A)** Extrasystole (1: stimulus applied during systole produces no extrasystole; 2: stimulus applied during diastole produces an extrasystole which is followed by a compensatory pause; PSP: postextrasystolic potentiation); **(B)** all-or-none law (1: subthreshold stimulus; 2: threshold stimulus; 3 and 4: suprathreshold stimuli); **(C)** staircase phenomenon (stimuli applied every 2 seconds).

> **Note:** Usually between the tenth and twentieth stimulus, the ventricle contracts.

Observation

Observe and study the properties of the cardiac muscle recorded in a beating heart and in a quiescent heart.

Precautions

1. For recording the extrasystole and compensatory pause, the stimulus should be applied in the diastole of the heart.
2. To study the refractory period, one stimulus should be applied in the systole and another in the diastole of the heart.
3. The all-or-none law, staircase phenomenon, and summation of subminimal stimuli should be studied in a quiescent heart.
4. To study the all-or-none law, stimuli should be delivered in different strengths starting from the subthreshold to the suprathreshold level.
5. To study the staircase phenomenon, the ventricle should be stimulated repeatedly at intervals of 2 seconds.
6. To study the effect of the summation of subminimal stimuli, the subthreshold (that just fails to evoke a

response) stimuli should be delivered repeatedly at intervals of 0.5–1 second.

DISCUSSION

Extrasystole and Compensatory Pause

When the ventricle is **stimulated in the relaxation period** (relative refractory period), the heart muscle may contract. This **contraction comes earlier** than the normally expected contraction. Therefore, it is called an **extrasystole**. The next impulse arrives in the refractory period of the extrasystole, hence fails to evoke a response. This results in **a pause (silence)** following the extrasystole, which is known as a **compensatory pause**. The response following the compensatory pause is greater than the previous one due to the accumulation of calcium ions during the pause.

Refractory Period

The cardiac muscle has a **long refractory period**. The **absolute refractory period** is about 250 ms and the **relative refractory period** is around 50 ms (Fig. 71.2). During the absolute refractory period, a stimulus cannot re-excite the tissue, no matter how strong the stimulus is. The duration of the action potential of the cardiac muscle is almost the same as the duration of the mechanical activity. A fresh action potential should be accompanied by a mechanical response. The mechanical responses of the cardiac muscle cannot be merged. Therefore, contraction and relaxation of the cardiac muscle to a stimulus must be over before the muscle responds to another stimulus. Therefore, the **cardiac muscle cannot be tetanized.**

All-or-None Law

The **threshold stimulus** is the weakest stimulus that evokes a response. If the heart muscle is stimulated with subthreshold stimuli, no response is seen. The **amplitude of contractions** in response to the suprathreshold stimuli remains the same as that of the threshold stimuli. This is known as the all-or-none law. This is due to **two reasons:** (a) the heart muscle, being an excitable tissue, follows the all-or-none law and (b) the heart muscle behaves as the functional syncytium, and therefore, the whole heart contracts with the same force.

Staircase Phenomenon

If the heart is stimulated repeatedly with the interval between the consecutive stimuli not less than 10 seconds,

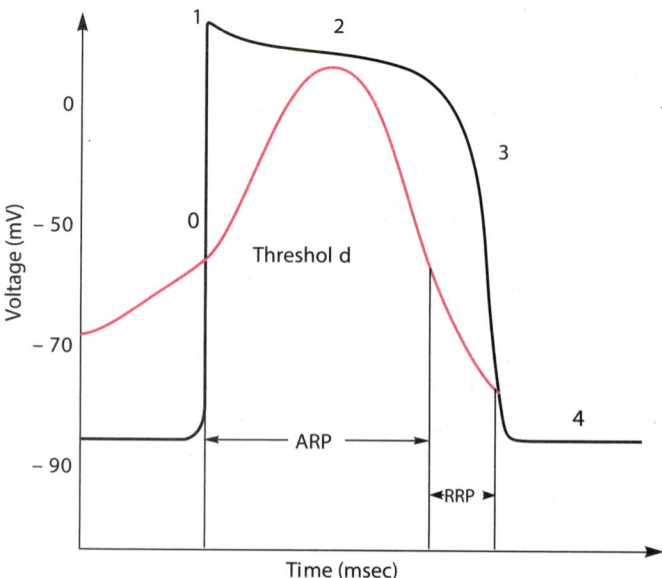

Slow fibres, present in the SA and   AV nodes. Resting membrane potential is −50 to −70 mV and the conduction velocity is 2–10 cm/sec. Note the spontaneous diastolic depolarisation in phase 4 and slow phase 0.

Fast fibres (atrial and ventricular myocardial cells and cells in specialised conduction tissues). Resting membrane potential is −90 mV and the conduction velocity 30–100 cm/sec.

ARP : absolute refractory period, i.e., an interval in which no stimulus. however strong, can initiate an action potential

RRP : relative refractory period, i.e., an interval during which   a supranormal stimulus can initiate an action potential

Fig. 71.2 Action potential of cardiac muscle showing five phases.

the **first 2–5 contractions progressively increase in amplitude**. This is called the **staircase phenomenon**. This is due to the accumulation of calcium ions in the sarcoplasm. With each stimulus, calcium ions are released into the sarcoplasm; if the next stimulus is delivered within 10 seconds, the calcium ions may not be totally pumped back into the sarcotubular system. Therefore, the next contraction is accentuated due to the **increase in the concentration of calcium ions** (calcium released by the stimulus plus the extra calcium from the previous stimulus). The staircase phenomenon also occurs due to the **increase in the temperature** of the muscle during the previous contraction.

Summation of Subminimal Stimuli

When subminimal stimuli are applied repeatedly, with the interval between the consecutive stimuli being less than one second, the stimuli summate and produce a response.

VIVA

1. *What is extrasystole? Why is extrasystole followed by a compensatory pause?* (Ans. Refer to page 470, under the heading 'Discussion' and the subheading 'Extrasystole and compensatory pause'.)

2. *Explain why the cardiac muscle cannot be tetanised.* (Ans. Refer to page 470, under the heading 'Discussion' and the subheading 'Refractory period'.)

3. *Define and explain the absolute and relative refractory periods.* (Ans. Refer to page 470, under the heading 'Discussion' and the subheading 'Refractory period'.)

4. *What is the all-or-none law? Why does the cardiac muscle exhibit this phenomenon?* (Ans. Refer to page 470, under the heading 'Discussion' and the subheading 'All-or-none law'.)

5. *Why should the intervals between the stimuli be less than 10 ms to demonstrate the all or none law?* (Ans. Refer to page 470, under the heading 'Discussion' and the subheading 'Staircase phenomenon'.)

6. *What is the staircase phenomenon? What is its physiological basis?* (Ans. Refer to page 470, under the heading 'Discussion' and the subheading 'Staircase potential'.)

7. *What is the mechanism of summation of the subminimal effects?* (Ans. Refer to page 470, under the heading 'Discussion' and the subheading 'Summation of subminimal stimuli'.)

72 Effect of Stimulation of Vagosympathetic Trunk on Frog's Heart

Learning Objectives

After completing this practical, you will be able to:

1. Explain the clinical implications of performing this practical.
2. Explain the differences between vagal and sympathetic innervation of the frog and human hearts.
3. Identify the vagosympathetic trunk in the frog.
4. Demonstrate the effect of vagal stimulation on the heart.
5. Understand the phenomenon of vagal inhibition and vagal escape.
6. Explain the physiological basis of vagal inhibition and vagal escape.
7. Explain the effect of vagal stimulation in human beings.

PY3.18: Observe with computer-assisted learning: (i) amphibian nerve–muscle preparation and (ii) amphibian cardiac experimen

INTRODUCTION

The vagal and sympathetic fibres to the frog's heart cannot be stimulated separately because these fibres are mixed to form a single nerve, the vagosympathetic trunk (VST). **Stimulation of VST results in cardiac inhibition** because the vagal effect is dominant over the sympathetic effect. However, if VST is stimulated for a long time, the facilitatory effect of the sympathetic may become dominant. The **white crescentic line** is the parasympathetic ganglion (**Remak's ganglion**) in the frog's heart; its stimulation causes cardiac inhibition.

The postganglionic parasympathetic neurons that are embedded in the heart muscle at the junction of atria and ventricle form the white crescentic line.

METHODS TO STUDY EFFECTS OF STIMULATION OF THE VAGOSYMPATHETIC TRUNK OF THE FROG'S HEART

Principle

Stimulation of the vagosympathetic trunk results in cardiac inhibition. However, if the stimulation continues, the heart recovers from this inhibitory effect. This is demonstrated by the effect of vagosympathetic stimulation of the heart recorded on a moving drum.

Requirements

1. Same as those for recording a normal cardiogram
2. Electrical circuit for stimulating the heart
3. Frog

Procedure

1. Pith the frog.
2. Expose the chest of the frog by making an incision on the sternum.
3. Extend the incision upwards to the lower jaw.
4. Cut the platysma.
5. Remove the tissue running from the angle of the jaw to expose the petrohyoid muscle (a thin muscle that runs from the base of the skull to the posterior corner of the hyoid bone).

Note: The petrohyoid muscle is identified by its shining colour. The glossopharyngeal and the hypoglossal nerves are seen superficial to the petrohyoid. Along the lower border of the petrohyoid, a neurovascular bundle is seen. This neurovascular bundle is formed by the laryngeal nerve, the carotid artery and the vagosympathetic trunk. The vagosympathetic trunk is identified by its close association with the artery (Fig. 72.1).

6. Isolate the vagosympathetic trunk carefully with a thin glass rod and pass a thread below the nerve.
7. Confirm the vagosympathetic trunk by observing the cardiac inhibition (slowing of the heart) by stimulating the nerve.
8. Record a normal cardiogram.
9. Stimulate the vagosympathetic trunk with a stimulus of lower strength and record the effect of stimulation.
10. Repeat the procedure by gradually increasing the strength of the stimuli till the heart stops.

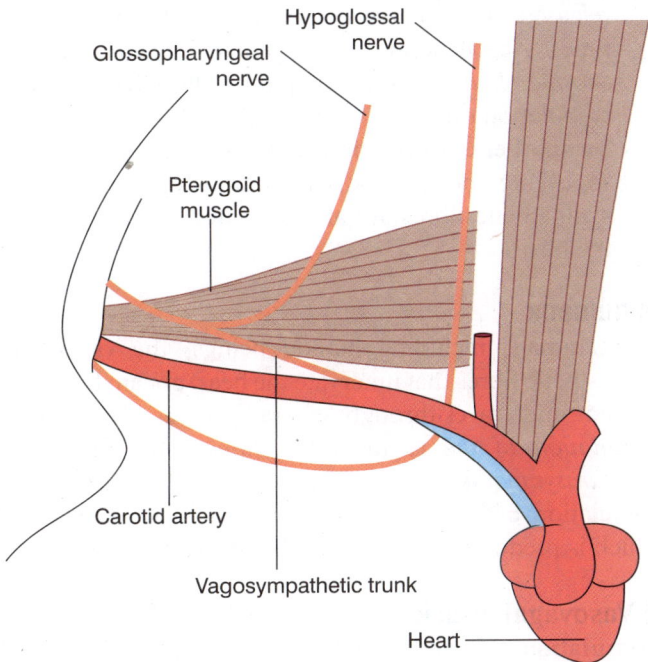

Hypoglossal nerve

Glossopharyngeal nerve

Pterygoid muscle

Carotid artery

Vagosympathetic trunk

Heart

Fig. 72.1   Anatomy of the vagosympathetic trunk.

Note: For studying the effect of different strengths of stimuli, record the cardiogram before, during, and after the stimulation of the vagosympathetic trunk. The slowing and final stopping of the heart due to vagosympathetic stimulation is known as vagal inhibition.

11. After the heart stops, continue stimulating the vagosympathetic trunk till the heart starts beating.

Note: The recovery of the heart from the inhibitory influence of the vagus when the vagosympathetic trunk is stimulated for a longer duration is known as vagal escape.

12. Indicate the beginning and termination of vagal stimulation on the recording and label the vagal inhibition and vagal escape.

Observation

Study the effect of stimulation (of different strengths) of the vagosympathetic trunk on the cardiac activities (Fig. 72.2). Note that at a lower strength of stimulation, there is a slowing down of the heart, but the heart stops with a higher strength of stimulus. Also note that the *heartbeat reappears when stimulation is continued* for a long time. The *heart rate of the vagal escape is significantly less* than the heart rate prior to the vagal stimulation (normal heart rate).

Precautions

1. The vagosympathetic trunk should be identified by its anatomical landmark.
2. Before carrying out the experiment, the vagosympathetic trunk should be confirmed by stimulating the trunk and observing the slowness of the heart.
3. The effect of vagal stimulation on the heart should be studied from a stimulus of lower strength to one of higher strength.
4. After recording vagal inhibition, the stimulation should be continued to study the phenomenon of vagal escape.
5. The cardiogram should be recorded before, during, and after the stimulation of the vagosympathetic trunk.
6. The recording should be labelled properly to mark the start and termination of the stimulation.

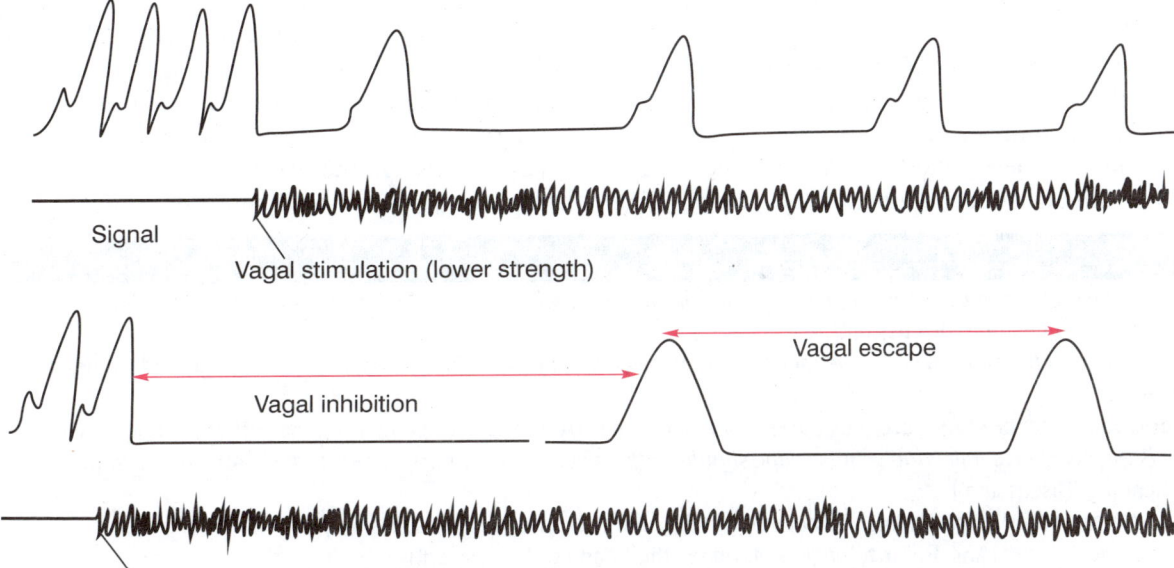

Signal

Vagal stimulation (lower strength)

Vagal inhibition

Vagal escape

Vagal stimulation (higher strength)

Fig. 72.2   Effect of vagal (vagosympathetic trunk) stimulation on a frog's heart.

DISCUSSION

Effect of Stimulation of the Vagus Nerve

In frogs

■ Vagal inhibition

When the vagus nerve (vagosympathetic trunk) is stimulated in a frog, the heart is inhibited. As a result, the *heart rate* and *the force of contraction decrease*. This is called vagal inhibition. If the stimulus is strong, the heart stops. **Cardiac inhibition** occurs due to the ***release of acetylcholine*** at the nerve endings. This increases the potassium conductance in the nodal tissues by *opening a special set of potassium channels*. Acetylcholine also *decreases the concentration of cyclic AMP* in the cells. The decrease in cyclic AMP *slows the opening of the calcium* channels, which decreases the firing rate. A decrease in calcium concentration in the myocardial cells *decreases the force of contraction*.

■ Vagal escape

A **strong vagal stimulation** may abolish the spontaneous discharge of the heart for some time, and the heart stops temporarily. However, the ***heart recovers automatically*** even after the continuation of vagal stimulation. This is called **vagal escape**. The heart rate following vagal escape is *significantly lower* than the normal heart rate because the escape rhythm is the ventricular rhythm.

Causes of vagal escape:

1. **Idioventricular rhythm:** When the heart stops due to vagal stimulation, the *ventricle starts generating an impulse*, which is known as idioventricular rhythm. It is so named because the cardiac rhythm is due to the pacemaker activity of the ventricular muscle, and the exact cause of the ventricular pacemaking activity is not known (idiopathic). As the ***discharge rate of the ventricle is much lower***, the idioventricular rhythm is significantly lower than the normal heart rate.
2. **Depletion of acetylcholine:** When the vagus nerve is stimulated continuously, the acetylcholine released at the nerve ending is depleted after some time. Acetylcholine is *degraded rapidly by the enzyme cholinesterase*. Therefore, the effect of vagal stimulation on the heart is temporary.

3. **Sympathetic stimulation:** It is assumed that when the vagosympathetic trunk is continuously stimulated, the sympathetic fibres are also activated; these stimulate the heart.

In humans

In mammals, including human beings, the vagal and sympathetic fibres that innervate the heart are anatomically distinct and travel through separate nerves. As a result, *stimulation of the vagus nerve shows only the effects of parasympathetic activation*. However, continuous stimulation of the vagus nerve results in **vagal escape**, which is predominantly due to ***idioventricular rhythm***.

■ Vasovagal attack

Stimulation of the vagus nerve causes sudden and transient loss of consciousness. This is known as **vasovagal syncope** or vasovagal attack. It occurs due to inadequate cerebral blood flow, which results from abrupt vasodilation and decreased cardiac output.

■ Vagal tone

The normal heart rate in humans is about 70/mm (the range is 60–100), which is significantly lower than the **intrinsic heart rate** (100–120/mm). Intrinsic heart rate is the heart rate when the heart is denervated (devoid of parasympathetic and sympathetic innervation). This reduced heart rate (in comparison to the intrinsic heart rate) is **due to vagal tone**. Therefore, vagal tone is the tonic inhibitory influence of the vagus nerve on the heart. There is also the **sympathetic tone**, which stimulates the heart. However, normally, the **vagal tone is dominant over the sympathetic tone**. This is the reason why the heart rate is normally lower than the intrinsic rate. The balance between the vagal and sympathetic drives is known as **sympathovagal balance**.

VIVA

1. *What is the difference between vagal and sympathetic innervation of the heart in frogs and humans?* (**Ans.** Refer to page 474, under the heading 'Discussion'.)
2. *What is vagal inhibition? What is the mechanism involved in vagal inhibition?* (**Ans.** Refer to page 474, under the heading 'Discussion'.)
3. *What is vagal escape? What are the causes of vagal escape?* (**Ans.** Refer to page 474, under the heading 'Discussion'.)
4. *Why is the heart rate following vagal escape significantly lower than the normal heart rate?* (**Ans.** Refer to page 474, under the heading 'Discussion'.)
5. *What is a vasovagal attack?* (**Ans.** Refer to page 474, under the heading 'Discussion'.)
6. *What is vagal tone?* (**Ans.** Refer to page 474, under the heading 'Discussion'.)

73 | Perfusion of Frog's Heart and Effect of Drugs and Ions

Learning Objectives

After completing this practical, you will be able to:
1. Explain the importance of performing this practical in cardiovascular physiology.
2. List the effects of drugs and chemicals on the normal cardiogram.
3. Explain the effect of various chemicals on the heart.

PY3.18: Observe with computer-assisted learning (i) amphibian nerve–muscle preparation and (ii) amphibian cardiac experiment.

INTRODUCTION

The activity of the heart primarily depends on the concentration of intracellular and extracellular ions. Various drugs and chemicals change cardiac function by changing the ionic concentration of the nodal tissues and myocardial cells by either acting directly on the ion channels or by acting on different receptors that affect the ion channels. Usually, chemicals **alter heart function by changing the cyclic AMP and calcium** concentration in the cardiac cells. Many of the drugs used in clinical practice for cardiac ailments act by modulating the ionic concentration of cardiac cells.

METHOD TO STUDY PERFUSION OF A FROG'S HEART AND EFFECT OF DRUGS AND IONS

Principle

Various drugs and ions change the rate and force of contraction of the heart. The effects of these chemicals are observed on the cardiogram of a frog and recorded on a moving drum.

Requirements

1. Same as those for recording a normal cardiogram
2. Different chemicals (1% $CaCl_2$, 1% KCl, 1% NaCl, 1 in 100,000 adrenaline, and 1 in 10,00,000 acetylcholine)
3. Perfusion set for frog's heart, which include Syme's cannula, Mariotte's bottle (Fig. 73.1)

Procedure

1. Pith the frog.
2. Expose the thorax of the frog.
3. Remove the pericardium.
4. Pass a fine thread around the sinus venosus.
5. With a pair of sharp scissors, make a small slit in the sinus venosus and introduce Syme's cannula.
6. Tie the thread around the neck of the cannula and cut the heart out of the frog.
7. Connect the cannula with Mariotte's perfusion bottle containing frog's Ringer's solution.
8. Perfuse the heart with Ringer's solution and record the heartbeat on a slow-moving drum (Fig. 73.1).
9. Record the effect of the following drugs and ions by applying each chemical separately with the help of separate droppers:
   i.   1 ml of 1% $CaCl_2$
   ii. 1 ml of 1% KCl
   iii. 2 ml of 1% NaCl
   iv. 0.5 ml of 1 in 100,000 solution of adrenaline hydrochloride
   v.   0.5 ml of 1 in 10,00,000 acetylcholine

Note: A normal cardiogram should be recorded before and after recording the effect of each chemical.

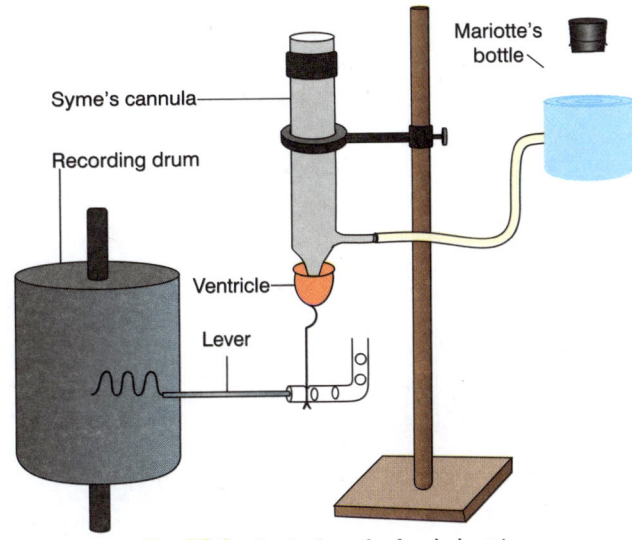

Fig. 73.1 Perfusion of a frog's heart.

Observation

Observe the changes in the cardiogram following the application of different chemicals. Note that *calcium chloride and adrenaline stimulate the heart*, whereas *potassium chloride and acetylcholine depress the heart*. Sodium chloride *increases the heart rate but decreases the force of contraction* (Fig. 73.2).

Observe the effect of different chemicals on the recording (Fig. 73.2).

Precautions

1. The precautions taken while recording a cardiogram also apply to this experiment.
2. While introducing the cannula into the sinus venosus, care should be taken not to puncture the other heart chambers.
3. The thread should be tied tightly so that it does not loosen during the experiment.
4. The concentration and amount of the chemicals should be appropriate.
5. Separate droppers should be used for applying different chemicals.
6. A normal cardiogram should be recorded before applying the chemicals.
7. The heart should be washed with frog's Ringer's solution before the application of each chemical.

8. The effect of stimulatory chemicals should be recorded before the recording of inhibitory chemicals.

DISCUSSION

Adrenaline

Adrenaline **increases the inotropic, chronotropic, dromotropic,** and **bathmotropic** actions of the heart. It exerts its effect on the heart by acting **on β_2 adrenergic receptors** that *increase intracellular cyclic AMP* concentration. Increased intracellular cyclic AMP in the nodal cells facilitates the *opening of longstanding calcium channels*, which increases the depolarization phase of the impulse, thereby **increasing the heart rate**. Adrenaline also increases intracellular calcium in the myocardial cells by **acting on β_1 receptors** present on the cardiac muscles and thereby increases the *force of contraction*.

Acetylcholine

Acetylcholine **decreases the heart rate and the force of contraction**. The heart rate decreases because the membrane becomes hyperpolarized, and the slope of prepotentials is decreased due to the action of acetylcholine on **muscarinic receptors and K^+ channels**. Acetylcholine increases the K^+ conductance in the nodal tissue by directly opening the

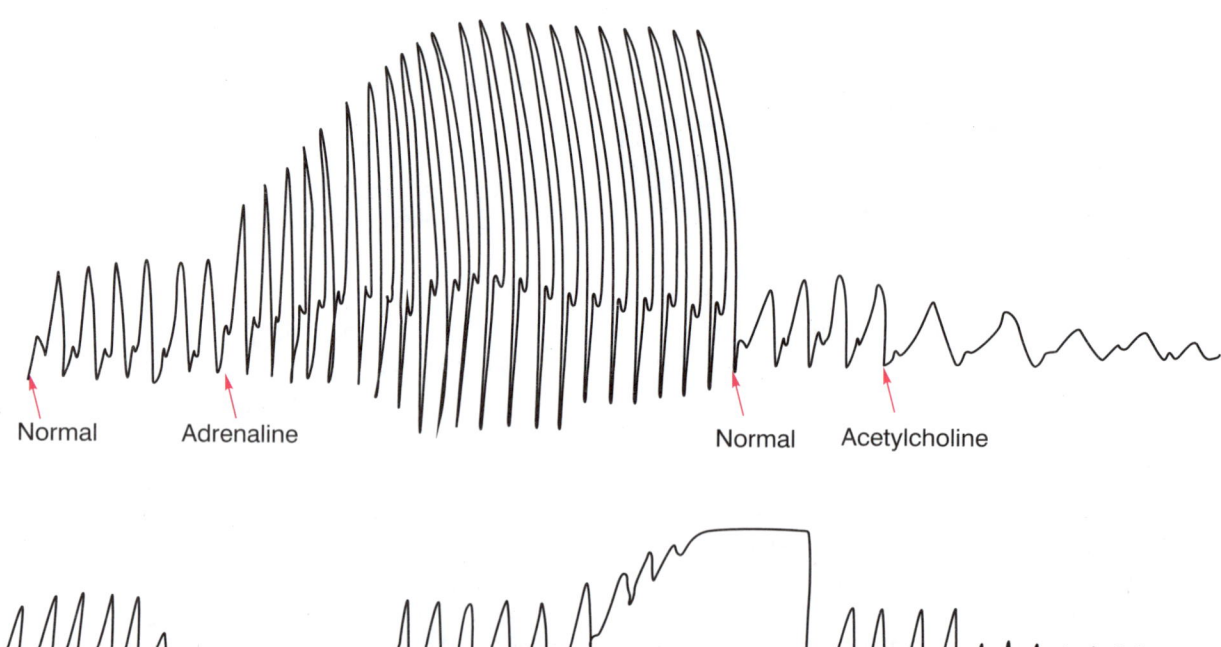

Fig. 73.2   Recording of the effects of drugs and ions on the frog's heart.

K$^+$ channels. By acting on **M$_2$ receptors** on the nodal cells, acetylcholine *decreases the concentration of intracellular cyclic AMP*, which slows down the opening of calcium channels. This *decreases the firing rate* of the nodal tissue. Therefore, the heart rate decreases. Acetylcholine *also decreases cyclic AMP in* the myocardial cells, and therefore, *decreases the magnitude of contraction*.

Potassium Chloride

Potassium chloride **decreases the resting membrane potential**. Therefore, the fibres become inexcitable. The heart stops in diastole.

Calcium Chloride

Calcium chloride **increases the force of contraction and decreases the relaxation time**. Therefore, the heart stops in systole (tonic contraction). This is called **calcium rigor**. It may not affect the heart rate.

Sodium Chloride

Sodium chloride **facilitates depolarization** and hence **increases the heart rate**. However, it competes with calcium ions and therefore decreases the force of contraction.

VIVA

1. *What are the effects of various drugs and chemicals on the heart? State the physiological basis for each.* (Ans. Refer to page 476–477 under the heading 'Discussion'.)
2. *What is calcium rigor?* (Ans. Refer to page 477, under the heading 'Discussion' and the subheading 'Calcium chloride'.)

74 | Effect of Drugs and Ions on Isolated Mammalian Intestine

Learning Objectives

After completing this practical, you will be able to:
1. Classify smooth muscles.
2. List the properties of smooth muscles.
3. Name the steps of contraction of smooth muscles.
4. Describe the effect of various drugs and chemicals on intestinal movement.
5. Explain the mechanism of action of these drugs and chemicals.

PY3.18: Observe with computer-assisted learning: (i) amphibian nerve–muscle preparation and (ii) amphibian cardiac experiment.

INTRODUCTION

Intestinal movements are possible due to the activities of smooth muscles present in the walls of the intestine, which generate their own impulses.

Smooth Muscles

Smooth muscles are broadly classified into **two types**: (a) visceral or single-unit smooth muscles and (b) multiunit smooth muscles. **Visceral smooth muscles** are found in the stomach, intestines, uterus, urinary bladder, and the walls of the small arteries and veins. **Multiunit smooth muscles** are found in the walls of the large arteries, in the large airways (bronchioles), in the erector pili (muscles in the hair follicles), and radial and circular muscles of the eye.

Properties of visceral smooth muscles

1. They are **involuntary** and innervated by **autonomic fibres**.
2. They exhibit continuous, irregular contractions independent of their nerve supply. This enables them to maintain a state of partial sustained contraction called **tonus or tone**. This sustained contraction occurs due to the **latch-bridge mechanism** in which dephosphorylated myosin cross-bridges remain attached to the actin for some time after the cytoplasmic calcium concentration falls.
3. Visceral smooth muscle is unique in that it **contracts in response to a stretch** in the absence of any extrinsic innervation. The stretch causes a decline in membrane potential, increased spike frequency, and increased tone.
4. There is **no true resting membrane potential**. During periods of quiescence, the RMP is about −50 mV.
5. Spikes (slow **sine wave-like fluctuations**) of a few millivolts appear on the resting potential.
6. They exhibit **autorhythmicity**. Pacemaker potentials appear at multiple foci.
7. The **excitation contraction coupling is very slow**. The muscle contracts about 200 ms after the start of the spikes and 150 ms after the spike is over. The peak contraction is reached about 500 ms after the spike.
8. The thick and thin filaments **are not arranged in an orderly fashion**. Therefore, there are no A and I bands. As a result, smooth muscles do not exhibit cross striations, hence their name. They also contain intermediate filaments.
9. They **lack transverse tubules and contain very few sarcoplasmic reticula** for the storage of calcium. For contraction, they receive calcium chiefly from ECF.
10. Intermediate filaments attached to the **dense bodies** play a role during contraction. During contraction, intermediate filaments pull the dense bodies attached to the sarcolemma, which causes lengthwise shortening of the muscle fibre.
11. Muscles exhibit **plasticity**, which is the variability of the tension that it exerts at any given length. This allows the smooth muscle to undergo great changes in length while retaining the ability to contract effectively.
12. **Calmodulin** and myosin light chain kinase are the regulator proteins for contraction.

Major steps in the contraction of visceral smooth muscle

1. Acetylcholine binds to the muscarinic receptors.
2. Calcium influx of the cell increases.
3. Calcium binds with calmodulin-dependent myosin kinase.
4. Phosphorylation of myosin occurs.
5. Myosin binds with actin, which increases myosin ATPase activity.
6. This causes contraction of the muscle.

7. Dephosphorylation of myosin occurs by various phosphatases.
8. Sustained contraction or relaxation occurs due to the latch-bridge mechanism.

METHOD TO STUDY EFFECTS OF DRUGS AND IONS ON ISOLATED MAMMALIAN INTESTINE

Principle

Segments of the small intestine continue to contract and respond to various stimuli if they are kept in a suitable medium at optimum temperature with the provision for oxygen supply.

Requirements

1. **Dale's apparatus:** This consists of a large perspex rectangular bath meant for keeping water at an appropriate temperature (37°C) with the help of a heating element and thermostat. There is a central organ bath of 20 ml capacity, which is provided with an outlet. There is a hollow bent glass tube curved at the lower end for fixing the intestine and other tissues. This tube can be inserted into the centre of the organ bath and is also used for supplying oxygen through the solution. A frontal lever can be attached to the assembly for recording movements on a moving kymograph (Fig. 74.1).
2. **Tyrode's solution:** The composition of Tyrode's solution (for preparing 10 litres of stock solution) is as follows:

- NaCl: 80 g
- KCl (10%): 20 ml
- MgSO$_4$ (10%): 26 ml
- NaH$_2$PO$_4$ (5%): 13 ml
- Glucose: 10 g
- NaHCO$_3$: 10 g
- CaCl$_2$ (molar): 18 ml
- Aerating gas: Oxygen or air

3. Petri dish
4. Thread and needle
5. Oxygen supply
6. Frontal lever
7. Kymograph and smoked drum
8. Pipette/syringe
9. A living rabbit
10. Drugs and chemicals

Procedure

1. Keep the rabbit fasting overnight to ensure active spontaneous intestinal contractions.

Note: The intestine of a fasting rabbit exhibits strong contractions.

2. Fill the organ bath with Tyrode's solution and the outer bath with water.
3. Heat the water of the outer bath to maintain the temperature at about 37°C.
4. Keep the petri dish containing Tyrode's solution ready.
5. After stunning the rabbit, open up its abdomen.
6. Take out a small part (about 5 cm) of the jejunum close to the duodenum, and place the intestine in a petri dish containing Tyrode's solution.
7. Rinse the intestinal lumen with Tyrode's solution with the help of a pipette or by pushing the solution gently through the lumen with the help of a syringe.
8. Pass the threaded needle through the wall of one of the cut ends of the segment and make a loop with the thread.
9. To the other end of the intestinal segment, tie a long thread to attach the tissue to the lever.
10. Mount the segment in the organ bath filled with Tyrode's solution by securing the threaded loop to the curved end of the glass tube.
11. Allow oxygen to pass through the solution at a rate of 2–3 bubbles per second.
12. Maintain the temperature of the water bath at 37°C. Check the temperature frequently.
13. Attach the intestine to the frontal lever.
14. Record the normal movements of the intestine on a slow-moving drum.

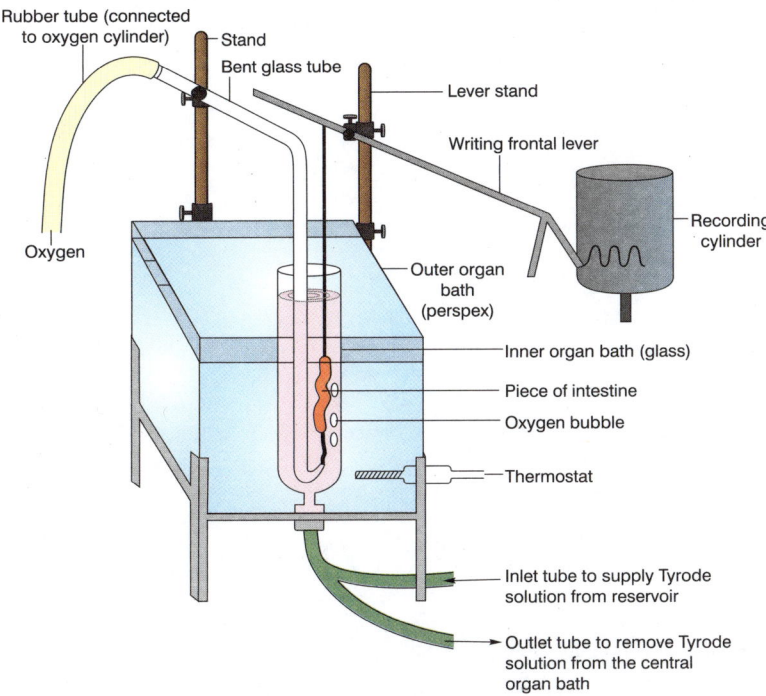

Rubber tube (connected to oxygen cylinder)
Stand
Bent glass tube
Lever stand
Writing frontal lever
Oxygen
Recording cylinder
Outer organ bath (perspex)
Inner organ bath (glass)
Piece of intestine
Oxygen bubble
Thermostat
Inlet tube to supply Tyrode solution from reservoir
Outlet tube to remove Tyrode solution from the central organ bath

Fig. 74.1 Dale's apparatus.

15. Study the effect of the following drugs/chemicals by adding 1 ml of each test solution to the central organ bath using pipettes.
    - Acetylcholine: 1 in 10,00,000
    - Adrenaline: 1 in 1,00,000
    - Atropine: 0.01%
    - Histamine: 50 mg
    - KCl solution: 1%
    - CaCl$_2$ solution: 1%
    - Barium chloride: 2%

Note: After recording the effect of each drug, the Tyrode's solution should be drained and replaced with fresh Tyrode's solution. The effect of the next drug should be recorded only after the intestine exhibits the normal movement.

16. By placing arrow marks below the recordings, indicate the drugs used for the recordings.

Observation

Observe the rate and amplitude of movement of intestinal contractions following the application of each chemical (Fig. 74.2).

Precautions

1. The animal must not be fed the previous night to ensure good intestinal contractions.

2. The temperature of the outer organ bath should be maintained at 37°C throughout the experiment.
3. All the required apparatus should be kept ready before killing the animal and dissecting the intestine.
4. The lumen of the intestine should be rinsed quickly and placed in Tyrode's solution immediately after separating it from the GI tract of the animal.
5. Oxygen should be supplied throughout the experiment.
6. Separate pipettes should be used to add chemicals to the organ bath. If reusing a single pipette, it must be thoroughly cleaned before taking the next chemical.
7. Between applications of chemicals into the organ bath, Tyrode's solution should be replaced with fresh solution every time.
8. Normal recordings should be taken before and after the recording of the effect of each chemical.
9. The effect of acetylcholine should be studied before the application of atropine.
10. The effect of acetylcholine should also be studied immediately after the application of atropine.

DISCUSSION
Adrenaline

When adrenaline is added to the preparation, the membrane potential becomes larger, **the frequency of**

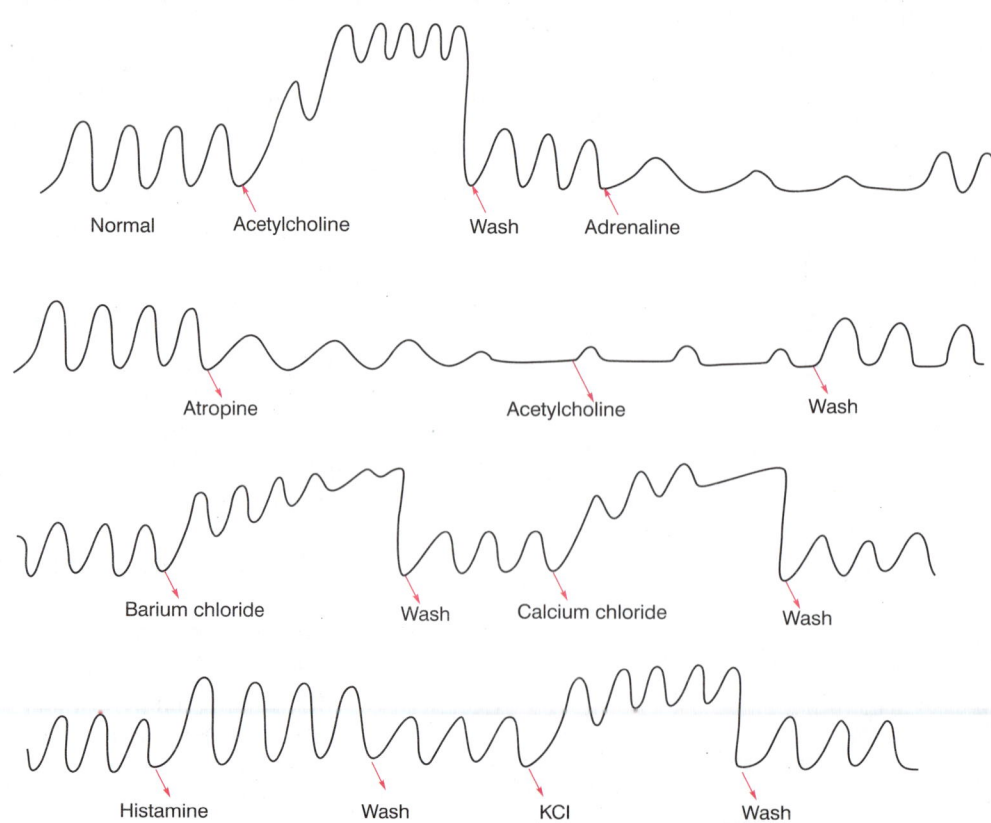

Fig. 74.2   Recording of the effects of drugs and ions on rabbit intestine.

contraction decreases, the muscle relaxes, and the amplitude of contraction decreases. Adrenaline exerts its inhibitory effect by acting on both α and β receptors present on the muscle. The *action on the β receptor* is mediated by a **decrease in cyclic AMP** in the cells and increased intracellular binding of calcium so that less calcium is available in the cell. This decreases the muscle tension in response to excitation. The action *on the α receptor* is mediated by **increased calcium efflux** from the cells so that *less calcium is available* in the cell. This also decreases the magnitude of contractions.

Acetylcholine

Acetylcholine decreases the membrane potential, and the muscle becomes more active. The **rate and height of contraction increase.** There is an increase in tonic tension in the muscle. Acetylcholine exerts its effect by **activating the phospholipase C**, which in turn, forms ionositol triphosphate (IP3). *IP3 increases the intracellular calcium* concentration by mobilising calcium from the intracellular stores and facilitating calcium entry into the cell. This increases the activity of the muscle.

Atropine

Atropine is a cholinergic **muscarinic blocker**. It prevents the action of acetylcholine on the smooth muscle of the intestine. It *decreases muscle activity*. If acetylcholine is applied to the preparation following the application of atropine, the effect of acetylcholine is abolished.

Histamine

Histamine *increases the tone* of the smooth muscle. It increases the amplitude of contractions. It acts by activating the H_1 and H_2 receptors. By acting on H_1 **receptors**, it *activates phospholipase C*, which in turn *increases intracellular calcium concentration* and by acting on H_2 receptors, increases cyclic AMP concentration in the cells.

Potassium Chloride

Just like acetylcholine, potassium chloride **stimulates** intestinal movements.

Calcium Chloride

$CaCl_2$ increases calcium entry into the cell and **stimulates the contraction** of the intestine. Calcium causes tonic contraction of the muscle.

Barium Chloride

Barium chloride **mimics the action of acetylcholine**. The intestine *contracts strongly* due to the direct action of barium ions on the intestinal smooth muscle.

VIVA

1. *What are the types of intestinal movement?*
   (Ans. The major intestinal movements are peristalsis, segmentation, mass peristalsis, and reverse peristalsis.)
2. *What are the types of smooth muscles?* (Ans. Refer to page 478, under the heading 'Smooth Muscles'.)
3. *What are the special properties of smooth muscles?* (Ans. Refer to page 478, under the heading 'Smooth Muscles'.)
4. *What are the steps of contraction of smooth muscles?* (Ans. Refer to page 478, under the heading 'Smooth Muscles'.)
5. *What are the effects of different chemicals on intestinal movement? What are their mechanisms of action?* (Ans. Refer to page 480-481 under the heading 'Discussion'.)

75 Effect of Drugs on Mammalian Uterine Contraction

Learning Objectives

After completing this practical, you will be able to:
1. Describe the physiological and clinical significance of performing this practical.
2. Name the hormones that affect uterine activity.
3. List the effects of different hormones on uterine contraction.
4. Describe the mechanism of their action.

> **PY3.18:** Observe with computer-assisted learning: (i) amphibian nerve–muscle preparation and (ii) amphibian cardiac experiment.

INTRODUCTION

The **myometrium** of the uterus is made up of **smooth muscles**. Uterine smooth muscles respond to various hormones in different phases of the menstrual cycle and pregnancy. The ovarian hormones, especially **estrogen, progesterone and relaxin, and oxytocin** secreted from the posterior pituitary, modify the activities of the uterus by acting on the myometrial and epithelial cells. These hormones alter the activities of the myometrial cells of the uterus in different phases of gestation to facilitate smooth continuation and termination of pregnancy. This practical is designed to study the effect of some of these drugs on uterine contraction.

METHOD TO STUDY EFFECT OF DRUGS ON MAMMALIAN UTERINE CONTRACTION

Principle

An estrogen-primed uterus is sensitive to various drugs. The effect of different drugs is studied on an isolated uterus using Dale's apparatus.

Requirements

1. Dale's apparatus (a detailed description is given in Chapter 74)
2. Dale's solution
3. Gas mixture (95% O_2 and 5% CO_2)
4. Frontal lever
5. Petri dish
6. Needle and thread
7. Kymograph with smoked drum
8. Live adult female rat primed with estrogen
9. Drugs: oxytocin, estrogen, progesterone, acetylcholine, and adrenaline

Procedure

1. Select a female rat in the estrous phase or prime a female rat with estrogen.

> **Note:** Estrogen-priming is done by injecting estrogen into the animal 24 hours before starting the experiment. The primed uterus increases the sensitivity of the uterine tissue to different drugs.

2. Stun (kill) the animal and open up its abdomen.
3. Locate the two cornu (horns) of the uterus.
4. Cut the upper end of each horn to separate it from the ovary and the surrounding fat.
5. Split the lower end of the uterus and separate each horn.
6. Divide each horn into two pieces so that four segments are available from each rat.
7. With the help of the needle, loop the thread around one cut end and attach a long piece of thread to the other end.
8. Mount the segment in Dale's solution by placing the hook in the curved glass rod in Dale's organ bath, and connect the other end to the frontal lever.
9. Maintain the temperature of the solution at 37°C.
10. Allow bubbles of the gas mixture to pass through the solution continuously.
11. Record the normal contraction of the uterus.
12. Study the effect of oxytocin, estrogen, progesterone, acetylcholine, and adrenaline on uterine contraction. Wash the tissue with fresh Dale's solution before and after the application of each drug. Record normal uterine contractions before studying the effect of each drug.
13. Indicate on the recording by placing arrow marks below the points of application of drugs.

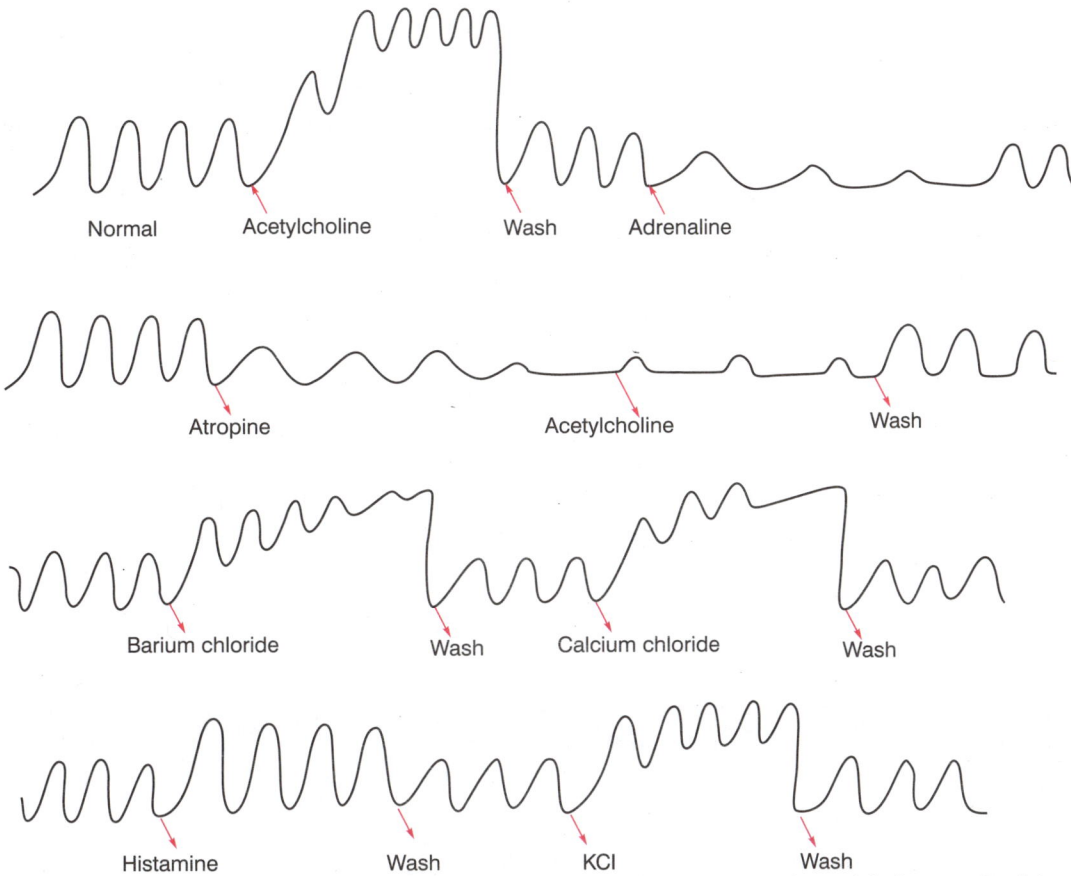

Fig. 75.1   Effect of drugs on uterine contraction. Note that oxytocin, estrogen, and acetylcholine are stimulatory, whereas progesterone and adrenaline are inhibitory. Oxytocin and acetylcholine increase the tone of the uterine muscle.

Observation

Observe the normal uterine contraction and the effect of different drugs on uterine contraction (Fig. 75.1).

Precautions

1. The animal should be in the estrous phase or should be primed with estrogen.
2. Each uterus should be cut into two separate segments.
3. The temperature of the organ bath should be maintained at about 37°C.
4. The tissue should be washed with fresh Dale's solution before recording the effect of each drug.
5. Normal uterine contraction should be recorded before recording the effect of each drug.

DISCUSSION

Effect of Different Drugs

Oxytocin

Oxytocin *increases the frequency and amplitude of uterine contraction* and **the tone of the muscle**. It acts on the receptors present on the myometrium. It *increases intracellular calcium concentration* and thereby stimulates contraction.

Estrogen

Estrogen **stimulates uterine contraction** by acting on the receptors in the myometrial cells. It combines with the intracellular protein receptors, and the hormone receptor complex binds to the DNA; this ***promotes the formation of mRNA***, which in turn, regulates the formation of new proteins that facilitate cell function.

Progesterone

Progesterone **inhibits uterine contraction and decreases the tone** of the muscle. It inhibits myometrial cells, *decreases the excitability of the myometrium*, and *decreases the sensitivity* of the myometrium to oxytocin. It also *decreases the number of estrogen receptors* in the myometrial cells. Progesterone works by acting on the receptors inside the cell, which regulates DNA, which in turn controls new mRNA synthesis.

Acetylcholine

Acetylcholine **increases the tone, frequency, and amplitude** of the uterine contraction, probably by similar mechanisms as those occurring in intestinal smooth muscle.

Adrenaline

Adrenaline **decreases uterine contraction**, probably by similar mechanisms as those occurring in intestinal smooth muscle.

Clinical Significance

Oxytocin

The number of *oxytocin receptors* in the myometrium *increases 100 times in the later part of pregnancy* and reaches a peak at term. *Estrogen increases the number of oxytocin receptors* on the myometrial cells. At term, the distension of the uterus and dilatation of the cervix gives **feedback information** to the posterior pituitary to release more oxytocin. It also increases the sensitivity of the myometrium to the normal oxytocin concentration in the blood. Oxytocin facilitates uterine contraction, which finally leads to **parturition**.

Estrogen

Estrogen *increases uterine muscle mass* and its *content of contractile proteins*. The myometrial cells become more excitable and active. The **estrogen-dominated uterus is more sensitive to oxytocin**. During the early part of pregnancy, the estrogen concentration in plasma is low. Therefore, there are no uterine contractions; this prevents abortion. Close to term, the estrogen concentration increases in plasma, which along with oxytocin, facilitates parturition.

Progesterone

Progesterone has antiestrogenic activity. It **decreases uterine excitability and contraction**, decreases the estrogen receptors on the myometrial cells, and decreases the sensitivity of the uterus to estrogen. Progesterone concentration increases during pregnancy; it is the main hormone that **maintains pregnancy**.

VIVA

1. *What are the hormones produced by the ovary that act on the uterine myometrium?* (Ans. Refer to page 483, under the heading 'Discussion'.)
2. *What are the actions of oxytocin, estrogen, progesterone, acetylcholine and adrenaline on uterine contraction? What is their mechanism of action?* (Ans. Refer to page 483, under the heading 'Discussion'.)
3. *What is the mechanism of initiation of labour?* (Ans. Refer to Page 484, see under the heading 'Clinical Significance' and the subheading 'Oxytocin'.)
4. *What is the role of oxytocin in parturition?* (Ans. Refer to page 483, under the heading 'Discussion'.)
5. *What is the role of estrogen in parturition?* (Ans. Refer to page 483, under the heading 'Discussion'.)
6. *What is the role of progesterone in pregnancy?* (Ans. Refer to page 483-484, under the heading 'Discussion'.)

76 | Estrus Cycle in Rat

Learning Objectives

After completing this practical, you will be able to:
1. Describe the different phases of the estrus cycle in rats.
2. Identify different phases by performing microscopic examination of vaginal smears.
3. Correlate these changes with the phases of the menstrual cycle in humans.

PY3.18: Observe with computer-assisted learning: (i) amphibian nerve–muscle preparation and (ii) amphibian cardiac experiment.

INTRODUCTION

Under the influence of hormones, cyclical changes occur in the reproductive organs of females during their reproductive life. The regular cyclic changes in females are meant for their preparation for fertilisation and pregnancy. In primates, the cycle is referred to as menstrual cycle, and periodic vaginal bleeding (menstruation) is an important feature of the cycle. In **non-primate mammals** like rats that do not menstruate, sexual cycles are referred to as **estrus cycles**. The cyclical changes in vaginal smears in rats are relatively well-marked, whereas similar vaginal changes in humans and other species, though present, are not so specific. In humans, specific changes occur in the uterus and the ovaries during the cycles, but it is not easy to study the changes in these organs.

METHOD TO STUDY THE ESTRUS CYCLE IN RATS

Principle

The vaginal epithelium undergoes cyclical changes during the estrus cycle under the influence of ovarian hormones. These changes are identified by examining the vaginal smears under the microscope.

Requirements

1. Microscope
2. Pipette
3. Methylene blue
4. Slides and coverslips
5. Adult non-pregnant female rats

Procedure

1. Place a drop of methylene blue stain on a slide.
2. With the help of a pipette, aspirate vaginal fluid from the rat.
3. Mix the vaginal fluid with the stain and place a coverslip on the mixture.
4. Make similar smears from five different rats (in different phases of the cycle).
5. Observe the cellular pattern under the high-power microscope.

Observations

The presence of vaginal cells and leucocytes helps in the identification of different phases of the cycle (Fig. 76.1).

1. **Proestrus:** Predominance of vesicular (nucleated) cells

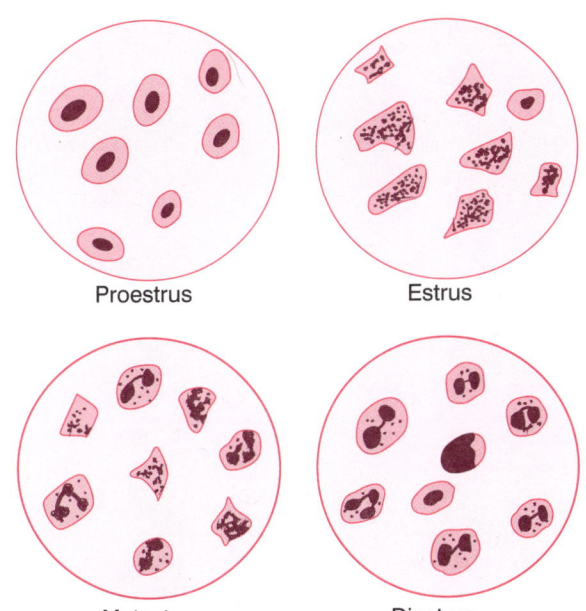

Fig. 76.1 Microscopic appearance of vaginal smears of different phases of the estrus cycle in rats.

2. **Estrus:** Predominance of non-nucleated, cornified or keratinised cells
3. **Metestrus:** Presence of leucocytes and cornified cells
4. **Diestrus:** Primarily leucocytes and a few other cells

Precautions

1. Adult non-pregnant female rats should be used for the experiment.
2. Smears should be prepared by collecting vaginal fluid from different rats.
3. Vaginal fluid should be collected by introducing the tip of the pipette into the vagina and then by aspirating the fluid.
4. Vaginal smears should be examined under the high-power microscope.

DISCUSSION

The *estrus cycle in rats is 4–5 days long*. The **proestrus phase** lasts *only for a few hours*. The *estrus phase* is the heat phase, which marks the ***first day*** of the cycle and *denotes ovulation in rats*. The **estrus phase** corresponds to the **ovulation phase** in humans.

In humans, the menstrual cycle is divided into *two phases*, **proliferative, and secretory.** In the first half of the cycle (proliferative or follicular phase), the ovarian follicle matures. In the middle of the cycle, ovulation occurs, which is followed by the secretory or luteal phase, the second half of the cycle. Menstrual bleeding occurs at the end of the secretory phase.

VIVA

1. *Why are non-pregnant adult female rats selected for this experiment?*
   (**Ans.** Pregnant rats will have effects of hormones of pregnancy on the vaginal smear.)
2. *What are the different phases of the estrus cycle in rats? How do you identify these phases by studying the vaginal smear?*
   (**Ans.** Refer to page 485, under the heading 'Observations'.)
3. *In which phase of the estrus cycle does ovulation occur in rats?* (**Ans.** Refer to page 486, under the heading 'Discussion'.)
4. *What are the phases of the menstrual cycle in humans?* (**Ans.** Refer to page 486, under the heading 'Discussion'.)
5. *What are the uterine changes observed in different phases of the menstrual cycle?* (**Ans.** Refer to page 486, under the heading 'Discussion'.)
6. *What is the mechanism of ovulation? What are the indicators of ovulation?*
   (**Ans.** In rats, indicators of ovulation are the changes in the vaginal smear in the estrous phase.)
7. *Why is it important to know the date of ovulation?*
   (**Ans.** It is highly essential to know ovulation for both conception [pregnancy to occur] and contraception [to prevent pregnancy].)

77 | Charts, Graphs, Spotters and Derived Questions

Spotter, Chart–Graph 1

The following schematic diagram represents an activity happening across the cell membrane. Answer the following questions related to the diagram.

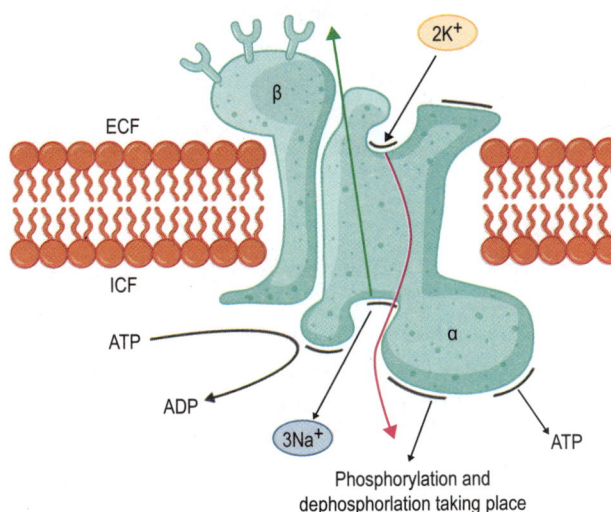

Phosphorylation and dephosphorlation taking place

Questions

i. Identify the physiological process illustrated in the picture.
ii. What is the structure represented by the symbol alpha? What is its function?
iii. Briefly outline the principle of operation of this process.
iv. Mention two important functions served by the process.
v. Name one important blocker of the process and its clinical use.

Answers

i. The process represents the **mechanism of action of Na⁺–K⁺ ATPase**.
ii. The structure represented by the symbol alpha is the α **subunit of Na⁺–K⁺ ATPase**. On its cytoplasmic side, it has **ATPase activity** and the binding sites for 3 Na⁺, ATP, and phosphate, and at the extracellular side, the α subunit has the binding sites for 2 K⁺ and ouabain.
iii. On activation, Na⁺–K⁺ ATPase pumps **three Na⁺ ions out of the cell and two K⁺ into the cell**. The Na⁺–K⁺ pump catalyses the hydrolysis of ATP to ADP

and uses the energy released to pump three Na⁺ out of the cell and two K⁺ into the cell for each mole of ATP hydrolysed. Therefore, the Na⁺–K⁺ pump is an **electrogenic pump.**

iv. The two important functions served by the pump are:
  a. **Cytosolic ion concentration: The** Na⁺–K⁺ pump prevents Na⁺ from accumulating in the cell and K⁺ from exiting from the cell along their respective concentration gradients. Thus, Na⁺–K⁺ pump maintains a high concentration of K⁺ and low concentration of Na⁺ in the cell.
  b. **Cell volume:** By maintaining the ion concentration on both sides of the cell, the Na⁺–K⁺ pump regulates water movement across the cell membrane. This maintains the intracellular water content and therefore, the cell volume.

v. The cardiac glycosides **digoxin and digitoxin** are the most commonly used Na⁺–K⁺ pump blockers. They are used in the **treatment of congestive heart failure**.

Spotter, Chart–Graph 2

The following schematic diagram is a graphic representation of a specific membrane transport process. Answer the questions related to this diagram.

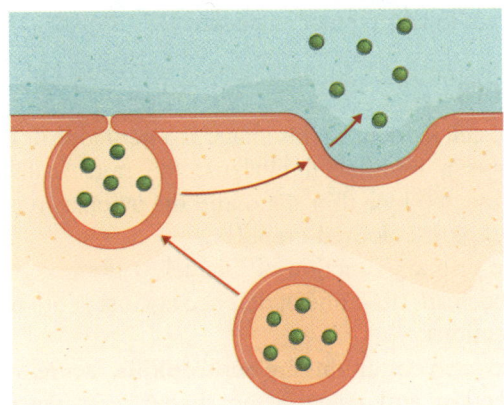

Questions

i. Identify the type of transport illustrated in the picture.
ii. Name two categories of substances that use this transport process.
iii. Name the ion required in this process.
iv. Does this process require energy?
v. Name the types of this process.

Answers

i. Exocytosis
ii. Hormones and neurotransmitters
iii. Calcium ion
iv. Yes, this process requires energy
v. Constitutive exocytosis and regulated exocytosis

Spotter, Chart–Graph 3

Observe the cells in the microscopic field prepared for a differential leucocyte count (DLC), and answer the following questions:

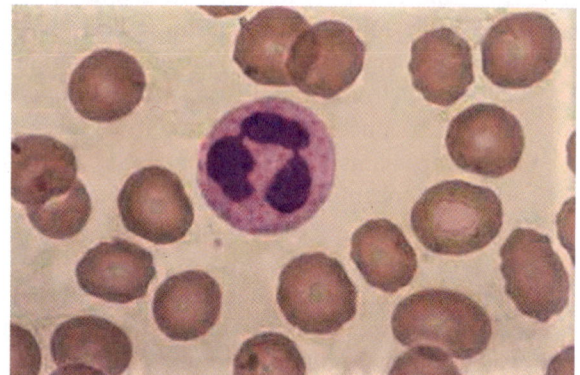

Questions

i. Identify the cell in the microscopic field and mention two important identifying features of this cell.
ii. Mention the primary function of this cell.
iii. Name two pathological conditions in which there is increase and decrease of this cell count.
iv. Mention the precursor for this cell in the bone marrow.
v. Name two common conditions in which there is a defect in this type of leucocyte.

Answers

i. The cell in focus in this image is a **neutrophil**. Usually, it has a multilobed nucleus; the nuclear lobes are connected by a thin stand and the cytoplasm contains fine, pink-coloured granules.
ii. The primary function of this cell is the **phagocytosis** of bacteria (first line of defence against acute bacterial infection).
iii. Two such conditions are **neutrophilia** (acute pyogenic infection and acute hemorrhage) and **neutropenia** (typhoid and malaria).
iv. The precursor cells are: myeloblast, promyelocyte, myelocyte, and metamyelocyte.
v. a. **Chediac–Higashi syndrome** (autosomal recessive, granule defects, poor chemotaxis)
   b. **Pelger–Huet anomaly** (autosomal dominant, lack of nuclear segmentation, nucleus has a bilobed, spectacular shape)

Spotter, Chart–Graph 4

Observe the cells in the microscopic field prepared for a differential leucocyte count (DLC), and answer the following questions:

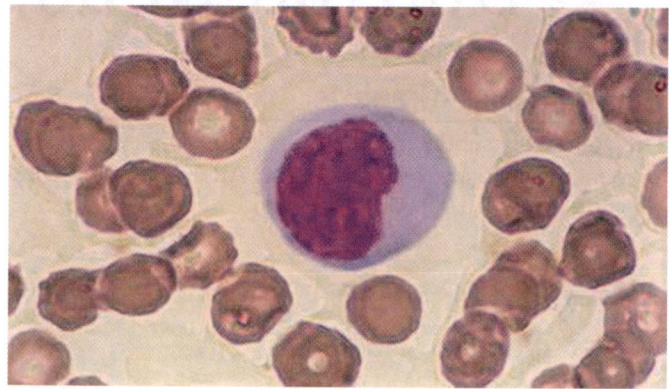

Questions

i. Identify the cell in the microscopic field and mention two important identifying features of this cell.
ii. Mention any two functions of this cell.
iii. Mention two conditions each in which there is an increase and decrease of this cell count.
iv. Name the stain that is routinely used in 1st MBBS practical for staining a blood smear for DLC and give the composition of the stain.
v. List the functions of any of the two components of the stain.

Answers

i. The cell that has been focused on is a **monocyte**. Usually, it has a kidney-shaped, spongy nucleus; its cytoplasm has a ground-glass appearance; and the nuclear–cytoplasmic ratio is 50:50.
ii. The primary function of the monocyte is **phagocytosis** (second line of defence). It participates in **immunity** (antigen presenting cell)
iii. Two such conditions of **monocytosis** (protozoan diseases like malaria/kala azar and ACTH therapy) and **monocytopenia** (aplastic anemia and septicemia).
iv. The composition of **Leishman stain** is: methylene blue, eosin, and acetone-free methyl alcohol.
v. Methylene blue stains the acidic part of the cell (nuclei–DNA, cytoplasm–RNA, and granules of basophils; methyl alcohol fixes the smear to the slide).

Spotter, Chart–Graph 5

Observe the cells in the microscopic field prepared for a differential leucocyte count (DLC), and answer the following questions:

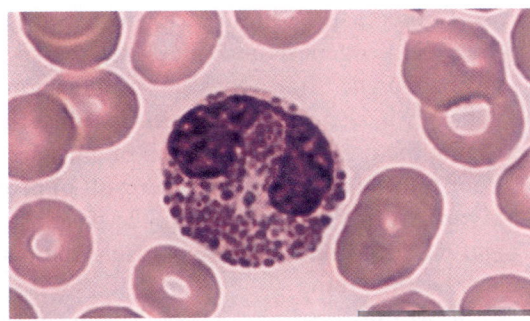

Questions

i. Identify the cell in the microscopic field and mention two important identifying features of this cell.
ii. Mention two main functions of this cell.
iii. Name two pathological conditions each in which there increase and decrease of this cell count.
iv. Mention one important cytokine that facilitates its development.
v. Name two major chemicals derived from its granules.

Answers

i. The cell under focus is an **eosinophil**. Usually, it has a bilobed nucleus; the nuclear lobes are connected by a thick strand, giving it the spectacular appearance; and its cytoplasm contains coarse, brick-red granules.
ii. The eosinophil participates in two important defence mechanisms: a) **allergy,** b) **helminthics infection**.
iii. Two conditions: **eosinophilia** (filariasis, ascariasis), **eosinopenia** (glucocorticoid therapy, Cushing's syndrome).
iv. The cytokine: **interleukin 5**.
v. Two major chemicals: a) **major basic protein** and b) **eosinophil cationic protein**.

Spotter, Chart–Graph 6

Observe the cells in the microscopic field prepared for a differential leucocyte count (DLC), and answer the following questions:

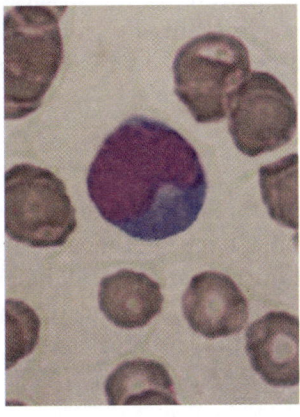

Questions

i. Identify the cell in the microscopic field and mention two important identifying features of this cell.
ii. Name the functional types of this cell and mention the main function of each type.
iii. Mention two conditions each of increase and decrease of this cell count.
iv. How is this cell developed in the bone marrow?
v. Name two important cytokines produced by this cell and give one function of each.

Answers

i. The cell focused on is a **large lymphocyte**. The nucleus is compact, occupying 80–90% of the cell; the cytoplasm is agranular; and the nuclear–cytoplasmic ratio is 80:20.
ii. Functional types and functions: **B cell**, mediates humoral immunity; **T cell**, mediates cellular immunity; **NK cell**, mediates innate and non-specific immunity and kill a variety of organisms and tumour cell.
iii. Two conditions of **lymphocytosis** (tuberculosis, infectious mononucleosis; **Lymphocytopenia:** Immunosuppressive therapy, ACTH therapy.
iv. **Development:** Lymphoid stem cell forms Pre-B cells and Pre-T cells that after further development in bone marrow and thymus respectively form B cell and T cell.
v. **B cells** secrete proinflammatory cytokines such as IL6, TNF-α, and IFN-γ, anti-inflammatory cytokines such as IL10, TGF-β; **T cell** secretes IL2, INF-γ and TGF-β.

Spotter, Chart–Graph 7

A schematic representation of a sarcotubular system of a skeletal muscle cell is given below:

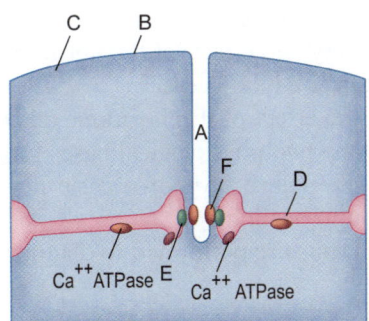

Questions

i. Identify the area labelled 'A'.
ii. Mention any two functions mediated by the area labelled 'A'.

iii. Identify the parts labelled 'D', 'E', and 'F'.

iv. Name two proteins involved in the uptake and binding of calcium by the structure labelled 'D'.

Answers

i. 'A' is the T tubule.

ii. It transfers the action potential from the surface of the muscle fibre to the interior, closer to the myofibrils. It connects ECF to interior of muscle cell for exchange of ions.

iii. **D**: sarcoplasmic reticulum, **E**: ryanodine receptor, and **F**: dihydropyridine receptor.

iv. a) SERCA (sarcoplasmic endoplasmic reticulum calcium ATPase)

b) Calsequestrin

Spotter, Chart–Graph 8

Observe the following schematic representation of a patient with a certain disease. Answer the following questions.

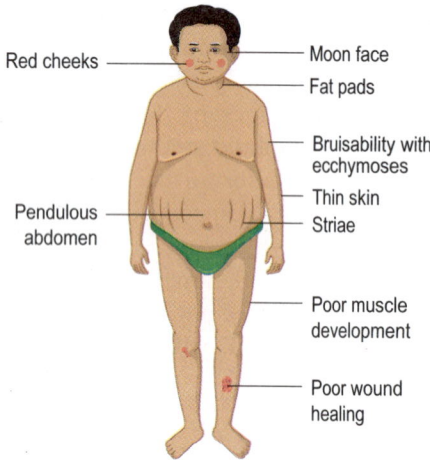

Questions

i. Identify the clinical condition depicted and state the cause of the disease.

ii. Mention any two effects of the hormone implicated in this disease on blood cells.

iii. What is the effect of this hormone on blood glucose? Provide any two physiological bases for it.

iv. What is the cause of poor muscle development and poor wound healing?

v. What lab tests are performed to diagnose the disease?

Answers

i. The disease is **Cushing's syndrome**, which occurs due to hypersecretion of glucocorticoids.

ii. **Lymphocytopenia, eosinopenia**, neutrophilia, and monocytosis.

iii. Cortisol **increases blood glucose** stimulates hepatic gluconeogenesis and increases the secretion of glycogenolytic hormones like glucagon and epinephrine; it also exerts an **anti-insulin effect** by decreasing the peripheral utilisation of glucose.

iv. a) **Poor muscle development is a result of proximal myopathy** due to proteolysis in the skeletal muscle and reduced bone mass. As a result, the patient's legs become thin.

b) **Poor wound healing**—hyperglycemia promotes the growth of organisms at the wound site. In addition, the state of decreased immunity also favours the growth of organisms.

v. **Laboratory tests:** Urine cortisol measurement, late-night salivary cortisol test, and dexamethasone suppression test.

Spotter, Chart–Graph 9

Observe the clinical sign given below and answer the following questions:

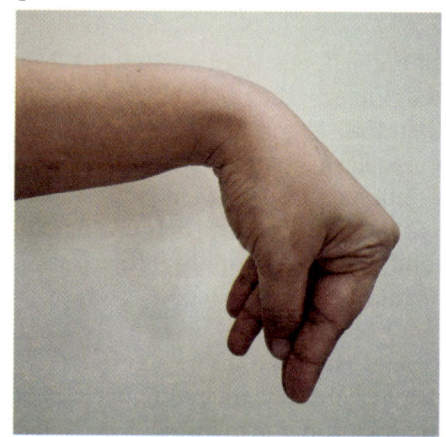

Questions

i. Name the clinical feature that you see in the picture.

ii. Name the condition in which this sign is seen and name the hormone deficiency that causes this disease.

iii. List two other features of this disease.

iv. Name three target organs for this hormone and mention the major effects of the hormone on these three organs.

Answers

i. The clinical feature in the picture is **Trousseau's sign**.

ii. The condition is hypocalcemic **tetany**. It is caused by **parathyroid hormone (PTH) deficiency**.

iii. Two other clinical features of this disease are Chvostek's sign and laryngeal spasm.

iv. a) **On the bone:** Resorption of bone

b) **On the GIT:** Increase in calcium and phosphate absorption (indirect)

c) **On the kidneys:** Increase in calcium reabsorption and decrease in phosphate reabsorption

Spotter, Chart–Graph 10

Observe the given picture of a patient and answer the following questions.

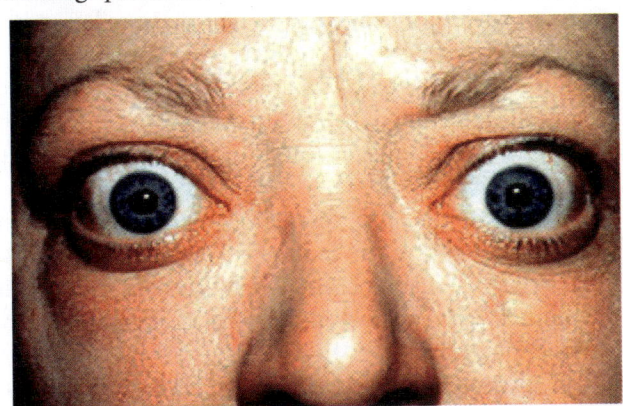

(*Courtesy:* Jonathan Trobe, M.D. - University of Michigan Kellogg Eye Center - The Eyes Have It, CC BY 3.0, https://commons. wikimedia.org/w/index.php?curid=16115992)

Questions

i.   What is the probable diagnosis?
ii. Name four important clinical features of this disease.
iii. Name two investigations for the diagnosis of this disease.
iv. Name the part of the cell where the receptor for the hormone (the hormone which is involved in this disease) is located.
v.   Name two groups of drugs for the treatment of this condition.

Answers

i.   The most probable diagnosis is hyperthyroidism.
ii. The important features are: heat intolerance, weight loss despite hyperphagia and increased BMR, exophthalmos, tachycardia, and palpitation.
iii. a) Estimation of TSH in plasma
     b) estimation of T_3 and T_4 in plasma
iv. The receptor is the nucleus of the cell.
v.   **a)** Thionamides/thioureas(propylthiouracil, carbimazole, methimazole, etc); and **b)** the anions (chlorate, perchlorate, pertechnetate, periodate, etc.).

Spotter, Chart–Graph 11

Observe the radiographic image shown below and answer the following questions.

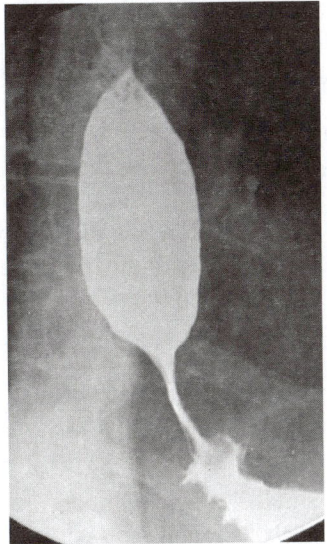

(*Courtesy:* Wikimedia Commons)

Questions

i.   Identify the disease from the X-ray findings and name the structure that is affected in the disease process.
ii. Name the sign this picture depicts. Name the nervous plexus that is defective in this condition.
iii. Name the two neurotransmitters that are defective in this condition.
iv. Name the drug that relieves this condition.

Answers

i.   The disease is achalasia cardia. The lower esophageal sphincter is affected.
ii. The sign is called **rat-tail sign**. The myenteric plexus is defective in this condition.
iii. Nitric oxide (NO) and vasoactive intestinal peptide (VIP) are defective.
iv. BOTOX (*Botulinum* toxin) is the treatment of choice.

Spotter, Chart–Graph 12

Observe the image below depicting an experimental set up for the assessment of gastric secretion, and answer the following questions:

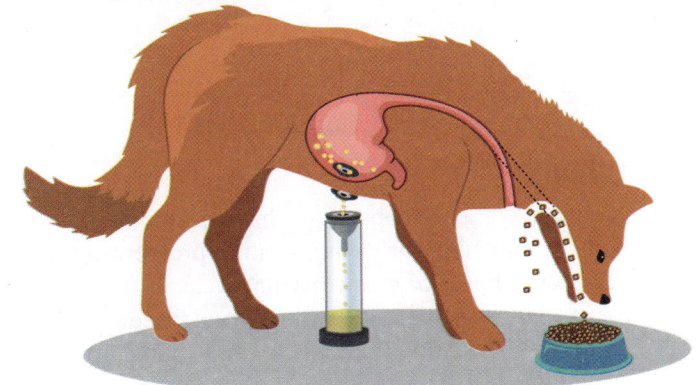

Questions

i.   Name the experimental set up illustrated.
ii. Name the phase of gastric secretion assessed by this experiment.
iii. List the stimuli that increase the secretion during this phase.
iv. Give the % of gastric secretion that occurs in this phase.
v.   Name two other phases of gastric secretion and the % of gastric juice secreted in each phase.

Answers

i.   This is a depiction of the sham feeding experiment.
ii. This experiment assesses the cephalic phase of gastric secretion.
iii. The sight, smell, thought of food, and taste of food increase gastric secretion.
iv. 40% of gastric secretion occurs in this phase.
v.   Other phases of gastric secretion: gastric phase (50–60%) and intestinal phase (about 10%).

Spotter, Chart–Graph 13

Observe the following chart depicting various changes in the menstrual cycle and answer the following questions:

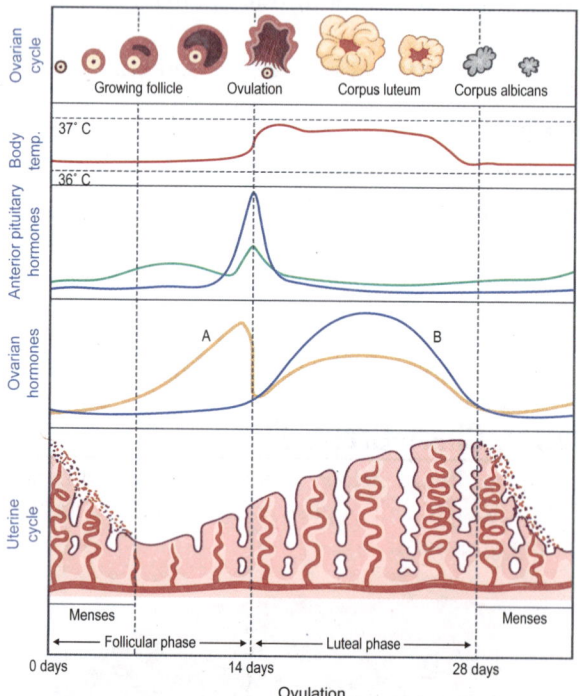

Questions

i.   Identify A and B depicting which hormones in the chart responsible for changes in the proliferative and secretory phases of the menstrual cycle.
ii. What causes menstruation (menstrual bleeding)?
iii. What is ovulation? Mention two indicators of ovulation.

iv. What is luteinisation? Mention two functions of the corpus luteum.

Answers

i.   a) Proliferative phase – estrogen
     b) Secretory phase – progesterone
ii. With the degeneration of the corpus luteum, the hormonal support to the endometrium is withdrawn; as a result, it becomes necrotic. The coiled arteries constrict and reduce the blood supply to endometrium. The foci of necrosis coalesce leading to confluent hemorrhage, which occurs along with sloughing of endometrium and results in menstrual bleeding.
iii. Ovulation is the process of the release of the ovum from the ovary. Indicators of ovulation: rise in basal body temperature, Mittelschmerz pain, Spinnbarkeit phenomenon, fern test, laparoscopy, and demonstration of LH surge.
iv. The process of formation of the corpus luteum from the corpus hemorrhagicum after ovulation is called leuteinisation. Functions of corpus luteum: Secretion of progesterone, providing the endocrinal environment for the implantation of the fertilised ovum, maintaining the early part of pregnancy by secreting progesterone until the placenta becomes functional.

Spotter, Chart–Graph 14

Identify the arrangement of the Sertoli cells with germ cells and answer the following questions:

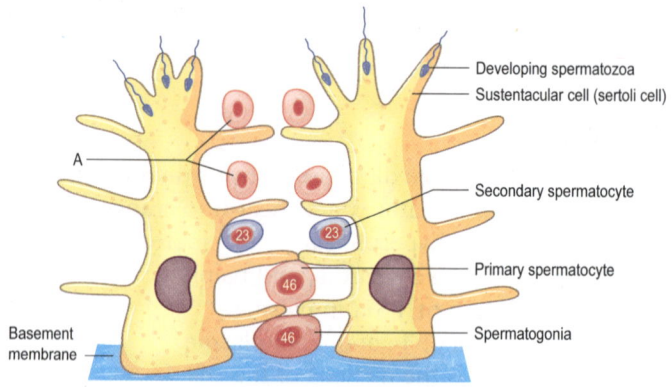

Questions

i.   Mention two important features of the arrangement of cells that govern their functions.
ii. Name the structures labelled as "A" in the diagram. Define spermiogenesis? Mention the normal sperm count.
iii. Name two main factors facilitating spermatogenesis.
iv. Write any two important functions of testosterone.

Answers

i. Two features of the arrangements of Sertoli cells governing their functions: (a) **a blood–testis barrier** for the seminiferous tubule is due to tight junctions between Sertoli cells; b) nourishment and growth of spermatids and **supporting spermiation.**

ii. Structures labeled as A in the picture are **spermatids.** Spermiogenesis is the process of development of spermatids into mature spermatozoa. Normal sperm count: ≥16 millions/ml of semen.

iii. a) Hormonal factors: Androgen, and gonadotrophins
   b) Environmental factors: Lower environmental temperature (30–35°C) facilitates spermatogenesis.

iv. Functions of testosterone: development of secondary sexual characteristics in males, b) stimulation of spermatogenesis, and c) anabolic effects – increase protein synthesis.

Spotter, Chart-Graph 15

Observe the image of the uterus below and answer the following questions:

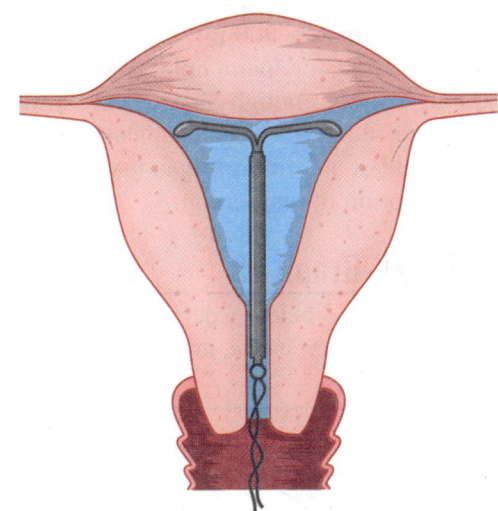

Questions

i. Name the contraceptive inserted into the uterus.
ii. Briefly explain the mechanism of IUCDs used for contraception.
iii. Mention two disadvantages of using IUCDs.
iv. Name two other temporary methods of contraception.

Answers

i. The device inserted into the uterus in this image is a copper – T.
ii. **Mechanism of action:** The presence of an IUCD interferes with the endometrial preparation for the acceptance of the blastocyst. Thus, implantation is

prevented. As a foreign body in the uterine cavity, an IUCD causes cellular and biochemical changes in the endometrium, impairing cervical mucus quality and sperm motility and viability.

iii. **Disadvantages:** Does not protect against sexually transmitted infections and can cause ectopic pregnancy.

iv. Two temporary methods of contraception: a) Barrier method and b) Oral contraceptive pills.

Spotter, Chart-Graph 16

Observe the structure of sperm below and answer the following questions:

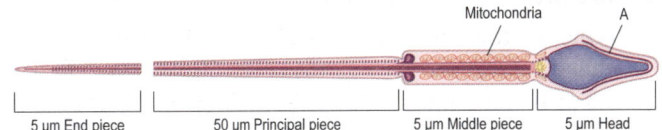

Questions

i. Which organelle represents the part 'A' labeled in the diagram of the sperm, and what is its function?
ii. What is the functional significance of the middle piece of the sperm containing mitochondria?
iii. What is capacitation?
iv. What is the role of the CatSper protein?
v. Mention two abnormalities identified in semen analysis.

Answers

i. The 'A' represents the acrosome, which is a lysosome rich in proteolytic enzymes. Acrosomal reaction promotes the penetration of sperm into the ovum.

ii. The middle piece contains numerous large mitochondria that supply energy (ATP) for sperm motility and metabolism.

iii. Capacitation is the process of final maturation that sperm undergo in the female genital tract, enabling them to fertilize the ovum.

iv. **Role of CatSper protein:** The principal piece of tail contains a protein called CatSper protein, which is a calcium channel. This allows cAMP-mediated calcium influx and facilitates sperm motility.

v. a) **Oligospermia** – sperm count <15 million/ml
   b) **Asthenozoospermia** – poor sperm motility
   c) **Teratozoospermia** – abnormal sperm morphology

Spotter, Chart-Graph 17

Observe the graph below depicting the relationship between intravesical volume and pressure. Answer the following questions related to the graph:

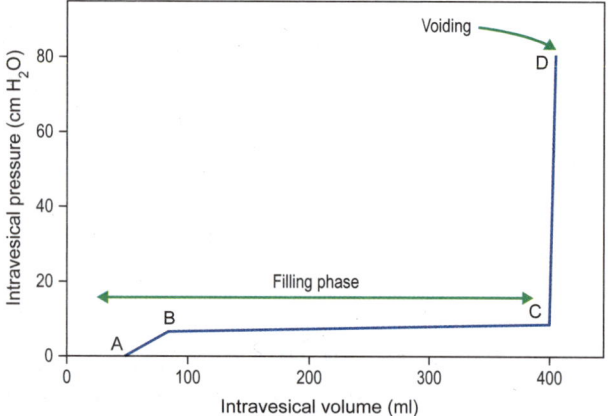

Questions

i.   What is the name of this graph and what are its phases?
ii. What is the name of the investigation used to obtain this graph?
iii. Explain Phase BC in the graph.
iv. At what age does cortical inhibition of micturition develop?

Answers

i.   a) **Name:** Cystometrogram
     b) **Phases:** Filling phase (ABC), pressure-rising phase (CD)
ii. **Cystometry** is the procedure to study the relationship between bladder volume and pressure.
iii. In Phase BC, the bladder fills without a significant rise in pressure until it exceeds 400 mL. This flat segment is due to the Law of Laplace, which states that pressure in a spherical viscus is equal to twice the wall tension divided by radius.
iv. Cortical control of micturition typically begins around age 2 and is fully developed by age 3.

Spotter, Chart–Graph 18

Observe the graph below representing lung volumes and capacities, and answer the following questions related to the graph:

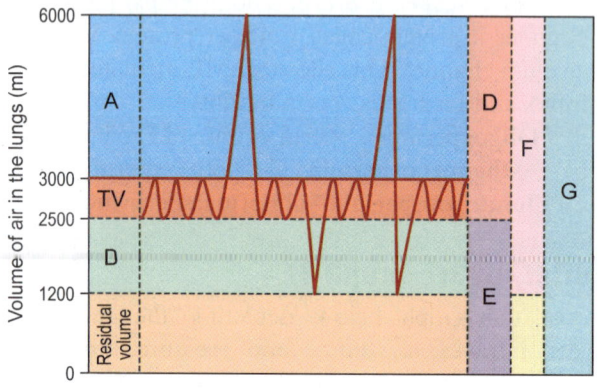

Questions

i.   Identify the lung volumes/capacities labeled 'A', 'B', 'D', 'E', and 'F'.
ii. Which lung volumes/capacities cannot be measured with a simple (student's) spirometer?
iii. Define tidal volume and mention its normal value.
iv. What is the physiological importance of the lung capacity marked 'E'?

Answers

i.   A – Inspiratory reserve volume (IRV)
     B – Expiratory reserve volume (ERV)
     D – Inspiratory capacity (IC)
     E – Functional residual capacity (FRC)
     F – Vital capacity (VC)
ii. The following cannot be measured by a simple (student's) spirometer:
     a) Functional residual capacity (FRC)
     b) Total lung capacity (TLC)
     c) Residual volume (RV)
iii. Tidal volume (TV) is the volume of air inspired or expired during normal quiet breathing. Its normal value is approximately 500 mL.
iv. FRC is important for maintaining stable gas tension in the lung so that enough air is always available for gas exchange along the alveolocapillary membrane. It prevents sudden alteration in gas tension due to any brief interruption of respiration.

Spotter, Chart–Graph 19

Observe the graph below depicting the oxygen–heemoglobin dissociation curve, and answer the following questions:

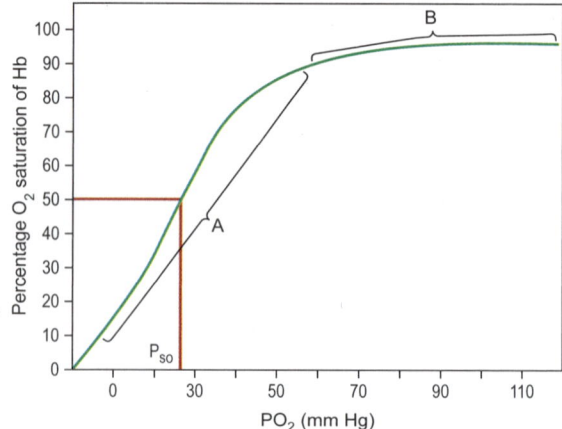

Questions

i.   Name the phases marked 'A' and 'B'.
ii. What is P_{50} and its clinical significance?
iii. What is the significance of high and low P_{50}?

iv. Name any two factors shifting the curve to right.
v.   Name any two factors shifting the curve to left.

Answers

i.   Phase A – Steep phase
     Phase B – Plateau phase

ii. P_{50} is the partial pressure of oxygen (PO_2) at which hemoglobin is 50% saturated. The normal P_{50} is approximately 27 mmHg at sea level. It indicates hemoglobin's affinity for oxygen.

iii. a) High P_{50} – reduced affinity of hemoglobin for oxygen (easier release to tissues)
     b) Low P_{50} – increased affinity of hemoglobin for oxygen (less release to tissues)

iv. **Right shift** – Increased temperature, decreased pH (acidosis), increased PCO_2, and increased 2,3-DPG

v.   **Left shift** – Decreased temperature, increased pH (alkalosis), decreased PCO_2, and decreased 2,3-DPG and carbon monoxide exposure

Spotter, Chart–Graph 20

Observe the schematic diagram of the respiratory membrane, and answer the following questions:

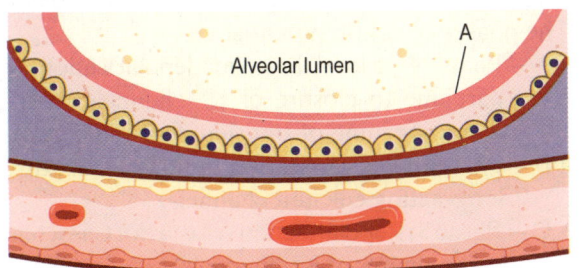

Questions

i.   What is the name of this membrane and what does 'A' represent in the diagram? List the layers of this membrane.

ii. List four factors affecting the diffusion of gases.

iii. State Fick's law. What is its relevance to this membrane?

Answers

i.   a) Alveolar-capillary membrane; A is surfactant layer.
     b) It has 10 layers: alveolar surfactant layer, layer of alveolar epithelial cells, basement membrane of alveolar epithelium, a thin layer of interstitial fluid, basement membrane of capillary endothelium, layer of capillary endothelial cells, plasma, red cell membrane, intra-erythrocyte fluid, and hemoglobin molecule.

ii. Factors affecting diffusion of gases:
     a) Difference in partial pressure of gas on both sides of the membrane
     b) Diffusing capacity of the membrane,

c)   Molecular weight of diffusing gases
d)   Solubility of gases
e)   Diffusion capacity of the membrane for the gases
f)   Surface area of the membrane

iii. Fick's law: The volume of gas diffusing per minute across a membrane is directly proportional to the membrane surface area, the diffusion coefficient of the gas, and the partial pressure difference of the gas, and is inversely proportional to membrane thickness.

Spotter, Chart–Graph 21

Observe the following graph of timed vital capacity (TVC) and answer the following questions:

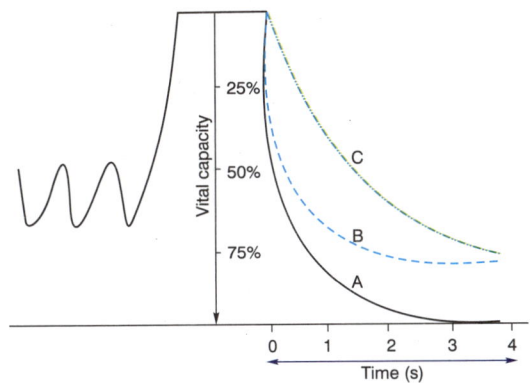

Questions

i.   What is FEV_1? What is its normal value?

ii. What does graph B represent? List four features of this abnormality.

iii. What does graph C represent? List four features of this abnormality.

Answers

i.   FEV1 is the fraction of the vital capacity expired in the 1st second. Its normal value is more than 80%, i.e., 80–85% of the forced vital capacity is expired in the 1st second.

ii. **Graph B depicts the restrictive pattern** of lung diseases. The main features of this pattern are decreased TLC, decreased VC, decreased RV, and normal preservation of FEV1 expressed in %.

iii. **Graph C depicts the obstructive pattern** of lung diseases. The main features of this pattern are: TLC is normal or elevated; RV is elevated due to trapping of air during expiration; ratio of RV/TLC is elevated, and FEV1 is less than 80% of TLC.

Spotter, Chart–Graph 22

Observe the graph below representing the alveolar and intrapleural pressure during respiration, and answer the following questions.

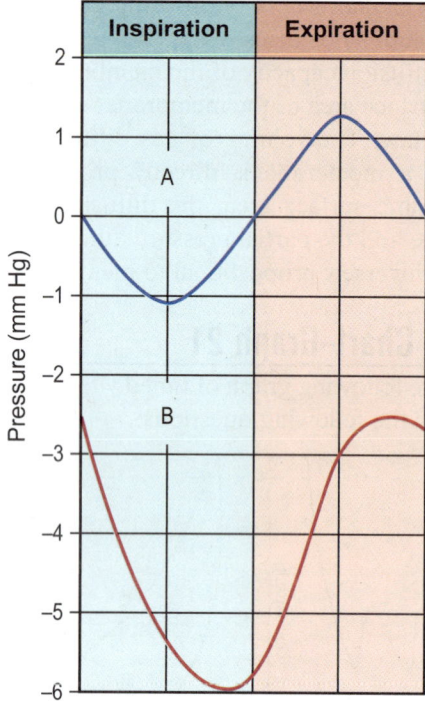

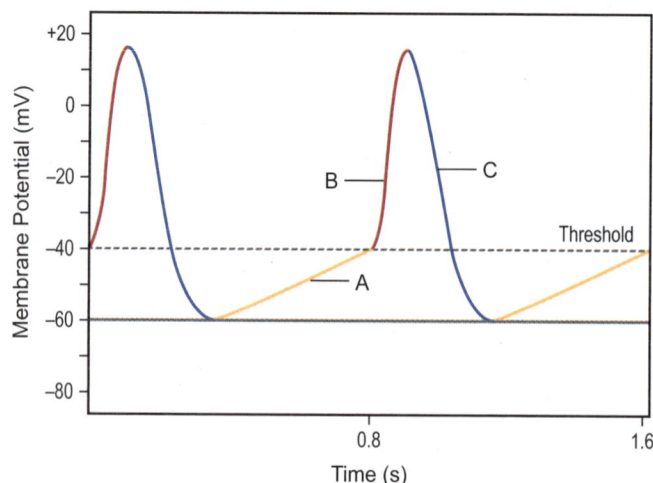

'A', 'B', and 'C', and mention the ionic basis for each of them.

iii. What is the specific name given to the potential marked as 'A' generated in the SA node?

iv. Describe the effects of sympathetic and parasympathetic stimulation on the phase marked as 'A'.

Questions

i.   What do 'A' and 'B' represent in this figure? What are the pressures of 'A' and 'B' as given in this picture during quiet inspiration and expiration?

ii.   Name one disease condition in which expiratory muscles are used against increased airway resistance.

iii. Name one condition each in which lung compliance is increased and decreased.

iv.   Name the condition where intrapleural pressure becomes equal to atmospheric pressure, leading to lung collapse and outward springing out of the chest wall.

Answers

i.   a) A represents intra-alveolar pressure: It is −1 mmHg during inspiration, +1 mmHg during expiration
      b) B represents intrapleural pressure: It is −6 mmHg during inspiration, −2.5 mmHg during expiration

ii.   Asthma

iii. Increased compliance – emphysema; decreased compliance – pulmonary fibrosis, atelectasis

iv.   Pneumothorax

Spotter, Chart–Graph 23

The graph below represents action potential recorded from a specific tissue of the heart. Answer the following questions related to this graph:

Questions

i.   Name the action potential that has been recorded.

ii.   Name the phases of the action potential marked as

Answers

i.   The slow response action potential has been recorded.

ii.   The phases of action potential are:
   • A – Phase 4: Slow diastolic depolarisation (early part due to closure of K^+ channels; later part due to opening of transient Ca^{2+} channels)
   • B – Phase 0: Depolarisation (influx of Ca^{2+} through long-acting calcium channels)
   • C – Phase 3: Repolarisation (closure of Ca^{2+} channels and opening of K^+ channels)

iii. The potential marked as 'A' generated in the SA node is called the **pacemaker potential or prepotential.**

iv.   a) Parasympathetic stimulation: The slope of 'A' (prepotential) is decreased, which decreases the heart rate.
      b) Sympathetic stimulation: The slope of 'A' (prepotential) becomes steeper, heart rate is increased.

Spotter, Chart–Graph 24

A schematic diagram of the conducting pathway of the heart is given blow. Answer the following questions related to the diagram:

Questions

i.   Label the parts marked 'A', 'B', 'C', and 'D'.

ii.   Which among 'A', 'B', 'C', and 'D' has the maximum and minimum impulse conduction velocity?

iii. What is the intrinsic rate of the structures marked 'A' and 'B' respectively?

iv.   What is the significance of 'AV nodal delay'?

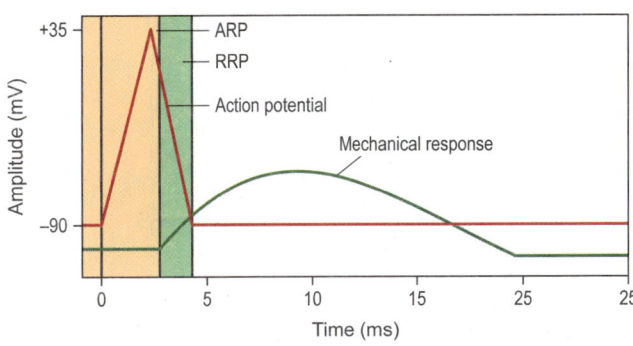

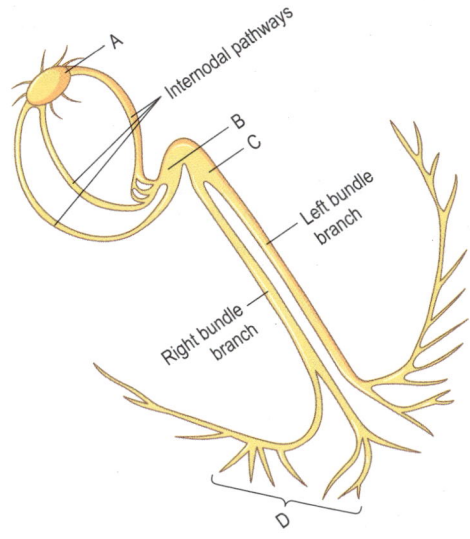

Answers

i. 'A' represents the SA node; 'B' represents the AV node; 'C' represents the AV bundle/bundle of His; and 'D' represents the Purkinje fibres.
ii. a) D – Purkinje fibres have the maximum conduction velocity; b) B – AV node has the minimum conduction velocity.
iii. A – SA node: 60 – 100/min; B – AV node: 40 – 60/min.
iv. a) Due to AV nodal delay, atrial depolarisation is completed much before ventricular depolarisation, which helps in ventricular filling and b) it maintains low ventricular rate in atrial fibrillation.

Spotter, Chart–Graph 25

Observe the graphs below depicting the schematic representation of action potential and mechanical response in skeletal and cardiac muscle. Answer the following questions related to the graphs:

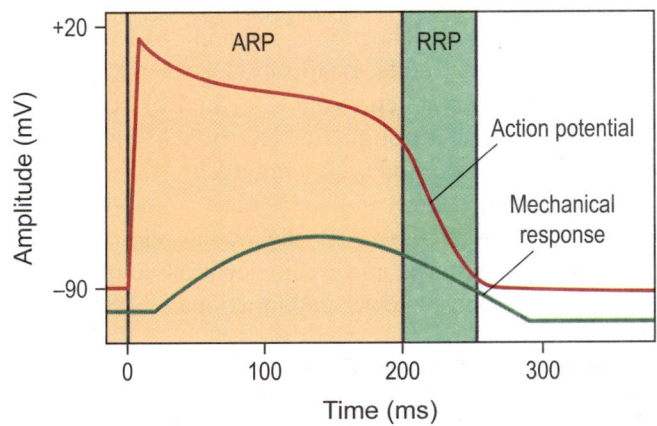

Questions

i. What are the full forms of ARP and RRP as depicted in the diagram? Compare the ARP of cardiac and skeletal muscle with the help of the diagrams given and briefly explain why the skeletal muscle can be tetanised, but not the cardiac muscle.
ii. What is tetanic contraction?
iii. What are the 2 types of action potentials occurring in heart? Where do they occur?
iv. Why does cardiac muscle action potential have a very long ARP?

Answers

i. ARP is the absolute refractory period and RRP is the relative refractory period. In the cardiac muscle, due to the long refractory period, a greater part of the mechanical response falls in ARP of the action potential (AP), whereas in the skeletal muscle, the mechanical response starts after the ARP. Therefore, cardiac muscle can't be tetanised.
ii. If the muscle is stimulated repeatedly at a very high frequency, continuous activation of the contractile mechanisms occurs without any relaxation, resulting in a sustained contraction known as tetanic contraction.
iii. a) Fast-response AP occurs in the atria, ventricular muscles, and Purkinje fibres and b) slow-response AP occurs in nodal tissues (SA node and AV node).
iv. Long ARP in cardiac muscle is due to the plateau phase (phase 2) of the action potential, the phase of sustained depolarisation that occurs due to the sustained increase in the permeability of the membrane to Ca^{++} ions.

Spotter, Chart–Graph 26

Observe the graphs given below depicting the electromechanical events that occur during the cardiac cycle. Answer the following questions related to these graphs:

Questions

i. What are the expansions of AP, LVP, LAP, LVEDV, and LVESV? What is the significance of LVEDV?

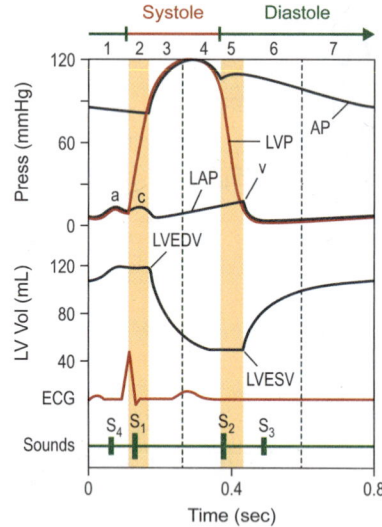

ii. Name the waves of the ECG in sequence, as depicted in the red colour graph.

iii. Define 'cardiac cycle'. What are the phases of systole and diastole in the cardiac cycle?

iv. What is the duration of cardiac cycle when HR is 75/min? What is the major impact on the cardiac cycle when the heart rate increases to 150/min?

v. What are the causes of the first heart sound (S_1)? To which ECG component and cardiac phase does it correspond?

Answers

i.   AP: Aortic pressure; LVP: Left ventricular pressure; LAP: Left atrial pressure; LVEDV: Left ventricular end-diastolic volume; LVESV: Left ventricular end-systolic volume. LVEDV determines the stroke volume by the Frank-Starling mechanism.

ii. P, Q, R, S, and T waves.

iii. Cardiac cycle is defined as the sequence of electrical and mechanical events occurring in the heart during a single beat. The phases of systole and diastole are: atrial systole and atrial diastole; ventricular systole, consisting of isovolumetric contraction, rapid ejection, and reduced ejection; and ventricular diastole, consisting of isovolumetric relaxation, rapid filling, and reduced filling.

iv. The duration of the cardiac cycle is 0.8 s when the heart rate is 75/min (systole: 0.3s and diastole: 0.5s). In tachycardia, the duration of diastole is reduced more than the duration of systole, hence the ventricular filling is compromised. This decreases stroke volume and cardiac output.

v.   a) S1 is due to sudden closure of the AV valves, rapid increase in tension in the ventricular muscles during

isometric contraction acting on filled ventricles, and turbulence created in the blood due to ventricular contraction. b) S1 corresponds to most part of QRS complex of ECG.

Spotter, Chart–Graph 27

Observe the graphs given below depicting two electrograms of heart. Answer the following questions related to these graphs:

Questions

i.   Identify the given graph.

ii.   What is the physiological significance and normal duration of the PA interval?

iii. What is the physiological significance and normal duration of the AH interval?

iv.   What is the physiological significance and normal duration of the HV interval?

v.   Explain the physiological basis behind AV nodal delay.

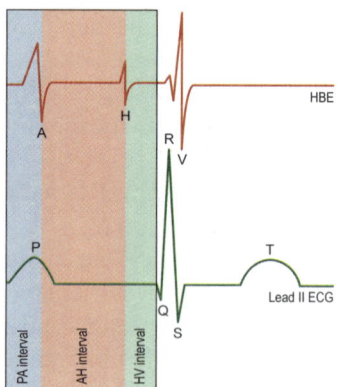

Answers

i.   The graph is a simultaneous recording of His bundle electrogram (HBE) and lead II ECG.

ii.   The PA interval represents the time of conduction from the SA node to the AV node. Its duration is 27 milliseconds.

iii. The AH interval is the time of conduction of an impulse through the AV node. Its duration is 92 milliseconds.

iv.   The HV interval represents the time of conduction of an impulse through the His bundle and bundle branches. Its duration is 43 milliseconds.

v.   Conduction velocity in the AV node is low (0.05m/s) due to the small size of the nodal cells and their branching patterns and weak electrical coupling as a result of relatively fewer gap junctions.

Spotter, Chart–Graph 28

Observe the graph below depicting the ECG waves, and answer the following questions:

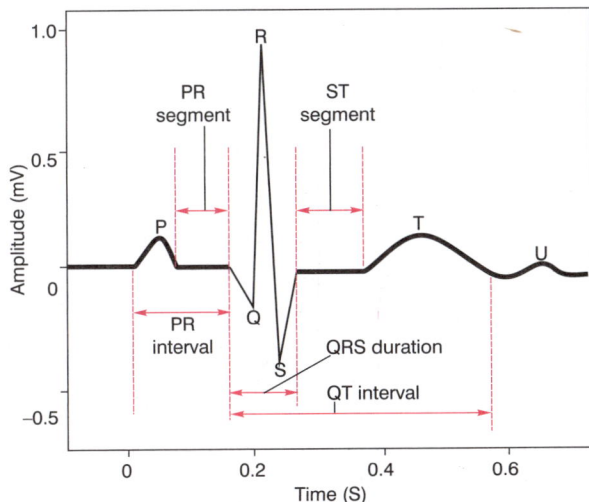

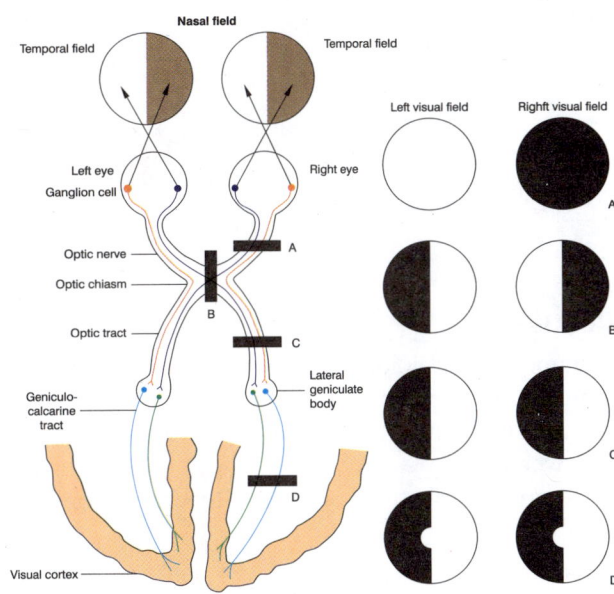

Questions

i. Calculate the approximate duration of the QT interval in this graph. What does the QT interval represent?
ii. Explain the basis of the P wave, QRS complex, and T wave.
iii. Write down the normal duration of the PR interval and name one condition in this interval that is prolonged.
iv. Name one condition each with the following features: a) tall T waves and b) inverted T waves.
v. Why is the limb lead II ECG considered to calculate the RR interval?

Answers

i. In this tracing, the QT interval is about 0.41 seconds. It represents ventricular depolarisation and repolarization. It essentially corresponds to the duration of their electrical systole.
ii. a) P wave: atrial depolarization; b) QRS complex: ventricular depolarization; and c) T wave: ventricular repolarization.
iii. The normal duration of the PR interval is 0.12–0.18 seconds. The PR interval is prolonged due to conduction blocks, digitalis, and rheumatic carditis.
iv. a) Tall T waves: hyperkalemia, acute MI; b) inverted T waves: myocardial ischemia, ventricular hypertrophy, bundle branch block, and digitalis effects.
v. The voltage in lead II is greater than the voltages in leads I and III because the heart vector generally extends in the same direction as the axis of lead II. Therefore, it is easy to calculate RR intervals in lead II.

Spotter, Chart–Graph 29

Observe the schematic diagram below of a neural pathway and answer the following questions:

Questions

i. Identify the neural pathway in this image and label the pathway components in sequence from top to bottom.
ii. Name the conditions resulting from lesions at the sites marked 'A', 'B', 'C', and 'D'.
iii. What is macular sparing? Briefly explain the physiological basis for it.

Answers

i. This is a diagram of the optic pathway. The components of this pathway are: optic nerve → optic chiasm → optic tract → lateral geniculate body → geniculo-calcrine tract → occipital or visual cortex.
ii. A – left-sided blindness (blindness in entire left eye visual field)*; B – heteronymous hemianopia (opposite sides of the visual fields, half blindness); C – homonymous hemianopia (same side of the visual field, half blindness); D – homonymous hemianopia with macular sparing.
iii. Macular sparing is the loss of peripheral field of vision with intact macular vision, which is seen in occipital lesions. This is because macular representation is separate from that of the peripheral fields and very large relative to that of the peripheral fields.

*Full marks will be given even if the side is mentioned.

Spotter, Chart–Graph 30

Observe the following schematic diagram depicting a physiological response in the eye, and answer the following questions:

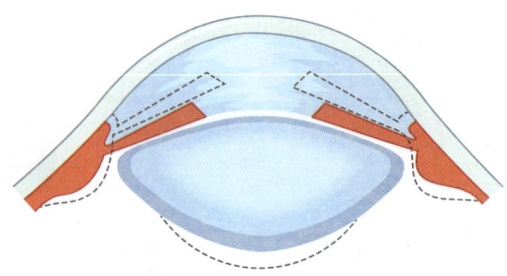

Questions

i.   Name the physiological response shown in the figure and mention its components.
ii. Trace the pathway of this response by making a flowchart.
iii. Describe the features of Argyll–Robertson pupil.

Answers

i.   This is the accommodation reflex. Its components are: increased anterior curvature of the lens, convergence of the eyeballs, and constriction of the pupils.
ii. Pathway:

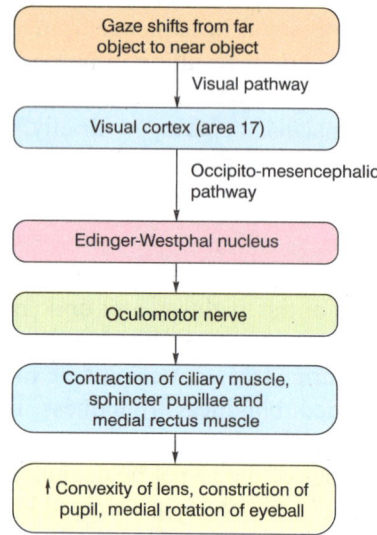

iii. The accommodation reflex is present and light reflex is absent.

Spotter, Chart–Graph 31

Observe the schematic diagram below of the gustatory pathway and answer the following questions:

Questions

i.   In the given diagram, what does the area labeled as 'A' represent and to which area of the sensory cortex does it project?

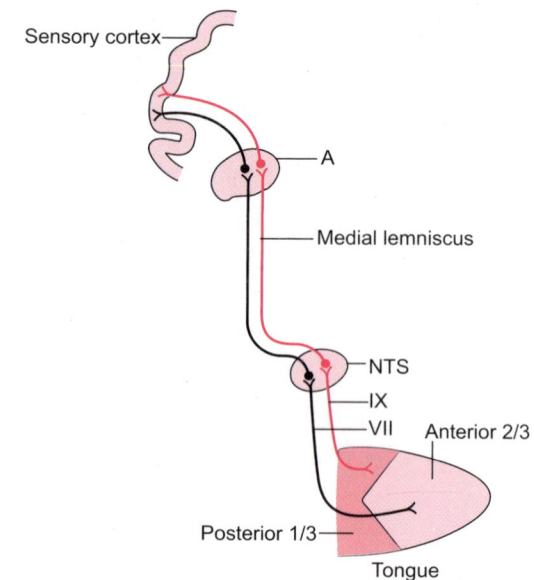

ii. Name the basic taste modalities and their preponderance in different parts of the tongue.
iii. Name the types of papillae and write their site of location on the tongue.
iv. List two special features of the gustatory pathway.

Answers

i.   The ventral postero-medial (VPM) nucleus of the thalamus, which in turn projects to the footplate of the post-central gyrus in the sensory cortex.
ii. Sweet (mainly at the tip of the tongue), salt (mainly in the centre of the dorsum of the tongue), bitter (mainly at the back of the tongue), sour (mainly on the lateral portion of the tongue), and umami.
iii. Circumvallate: back of the tongue; fungiform: near the tip of the tongue; and foliate: posterior edge of the tongue.
iv. Multiple cranial nerve afferents are involved, and they project to the ipsilateral gustatory (sensory) cortex.

Spotter, Chart–Graph 32

Observe the schematic diagram below of EEG recordings corresponding to different stages of sleep. Answer the questions given below:

Questions

i.   Mention the stages of sleep marked as 'B', 'E', and 'F', and name the EEG wave patterns in these stages.
ii. What do 'P', 'Q', and 'R' stand for?
iii. What is paradoxical sleep?
iv. List four differences between NREM and REM sleep.

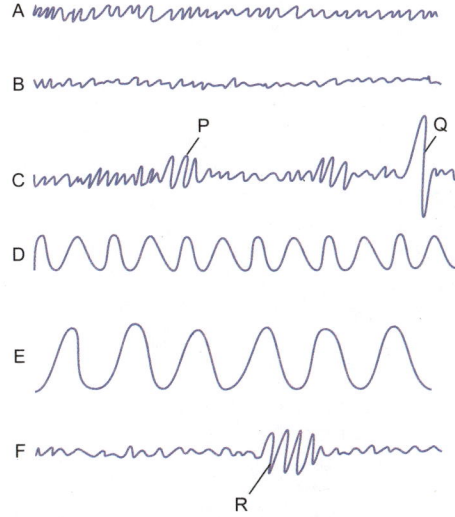

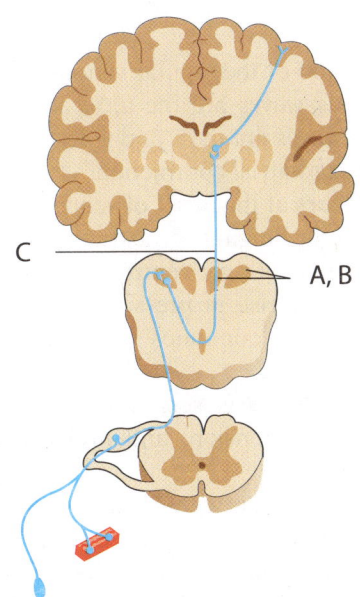

Answers

i. **B:** Stage I sleep, alpha wave; **E:** Stage IV sleep, delta wave; **F:** REM sleep, beta waves with PGO spikes.
ii. **P:** Sleep spindles; **Q:** K complex; **R:** PGO spikes.
iii. During REM sleep, the slow waves are replaced by rapid, low-voltage EEG activity. This is called paradoxical sleep because the EEG activity is very rapid, like the β rhythm seen in the awakened state, yet it is difficult to awaken the individual.
iv. Any four differences from the table given below:

Features	NREM	REM
Autonomic function	Sympathetic Inhibition	Sympathetic Activation
Eyeball movement	Absent	Present
Dreams	Not memorised	Memorised
Muscle tone	Inhibited	Profoundly depressed
EEG	Slow waves, high amplitude	High frequency, low voltage
Duration	75% of total sleep	25% of total sleep

Spotter, Chart–Graph 33

Observe the schematic diagram below of a particular sensory pathway, and answer the following questions:

Questions

i. Identify the structures labelled 'A', 'B', 'C'.
ii. List the sensations carried by this pathway.
iii. Name the cortical sensations.
iv. What is the Rhomberg sign?

Answers

i. **A:** Nucleus gracillis; **B:** Nucleus cuneatus; **C:** 2nd-order neuron/medial lemniscus

ii. The sensations carried by this pathway are: fine touch, vibration, proprioception, tactile localisation, two-point discrimination, and stereognosis.
iii. Cortical sensations: Tactile localisation, two-point discrimination, and stereognosis.
iv. **Romberg sign:** Inability to maintain a balanced standing position with feet together and eyes closed.

Spotter, Chart–Graph 34

Observe the graph given below, and answer the following questions:

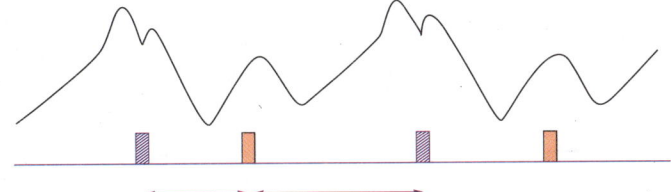

Questions

i.   Identify the given graph and name the waves (three upward waves and two downward waves).
ii. Write the mechanism of production of the three upward waves.
iii. Name three conditions in which the first wave in the graph becomes more prominent.
iv. What name is given to the first wave when it becomes a giant wave? Mention the mechanism of its genesis and the condition in which it is seen.
v.   Name two conditions in which the pressure represented by this graph is clinically observed to be increased.

Answers

i.   This is a graph of the jugular venous pressure (JVP). The upwards waves are the a, c, and v waves. The downward waves are the x and y descents.

ii. **a** wave: Due to atrial contraction.
     c wave: Occurs at the onset of ventricular systole and results from the bulging of the tricuspid valve ring into the right atrium as right ventricular pressure rises.
     v wave: Passive rise in pressure in the right atrium as venous return continues with the tricuspid valve closed.

iii. Prominent a wave is seen in pulmonary stenosis, pulmonary hypertension, and myxoma of the right atrium.

iv. It is called a cannon wave. It is seen when the right atrium contracts against a closed tricuspid valve. It is seen in cases of complete heart block, when atrial and ventricular systoles coincide.

v.   Two conditions: right ventricular failure and b) obstruction of the superior vena cava.

Spotter, Chart–Graph 35

Observe the ECG recording given below, and comment on the i. atrial rate, ii. ventricular rate, iii. PR interval, iv. QRS duration, and v. RR interval.

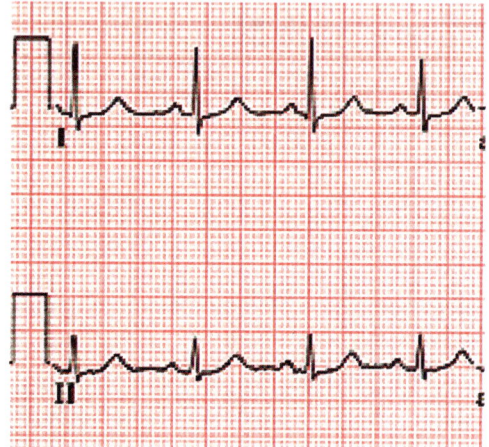

Answers:

i.   Atrial rate: 93/min
ii. Ventricular rate: 93/min
iii. PR interval: 0.16 second
iv. QRS Complex duration: 0.06 second
v.   RR interval: 0.64 second
     The ECG is within normal limits.

Spotter, Chart–Graph 36

Observe the given schematic diagram of the corticospinal tract (CST), and answer the following questions:

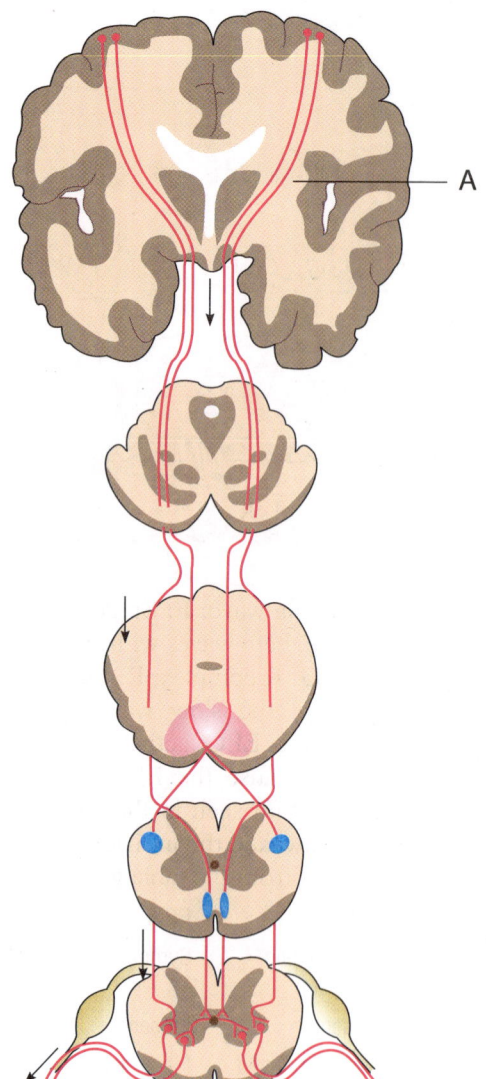

Questions

i.   Which corticospinal tract has a monosynaptic connection with lower motor neurons in the anterior horn of the spinal cord, and which muscle group does it influence?

ii. Which corticospinal tract is mainly involved in the regulation of posture, and to which system of descending pathways does it belong?

iii. The lesion marked as 'A' at this part of the CST in this diagram causes what kind of neurological deficit, and why?

iv. Hemorrhage of which artery causes a lesion at the part labeled 'A'? What is the specific name of this artery?

v.   List four major features of upper motor neuron (UMN) paralysis.

Answers

i.   a) Lateral CST and b) distal group of muscles.

ii.   a) Anterior CST and b) medial descending pathways.

iii. Labeling A is internal capsule. A lesion at the **internal capsule** causes maximum neurological deficit because fibres coming from different motor cortical areas pass through a narrow passage in the posterior limb of internal capsule. Therefore, lesion at internal capsule causes damage to the maximum number of descending fibres, including CST.

iv.   **The cortico-striate branch of the middle cerebral artery** is involved in the capsular lesion. The name of this artery is **Charcot's artery** or **artery of cerebral hemorrhage**.

v.   a) Atrophy of muscle is not seen; b) spastic paralysis with hypertonia of muscle occurs; c) deep tendon reflexes are exaggerated; and d) superficial reflexes are lost, and Babinski sign is positive (extensor planter response).

Spotter, Chart–Graph 37

Observe the schematic diagram given below, and answer the following questions:

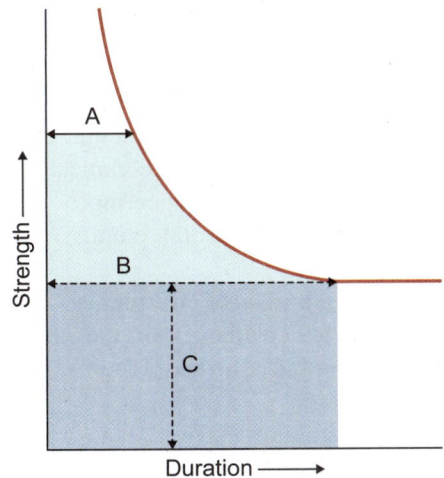

Questions

i.   What is the name of the curve and what does it depict?

ii.   What is curve A, and what does it represent?

iii. What is curve C, and what does it represent?

iv.   What is curve B, and what does it represent?

Answers

i.   This is strength duration Curve. Strength and duration are two important aspects of a stimulus. Both of them have a complimentary role in determining the excitability of a tissue. The relationship between the strength and duration of stimuli depicted in graph form is known as **strength-duration curve**.

ii.   **Level A is chronaxie.** Chronaxie is the *time required* for a stimulus of *double the rheobase strength* to produce an action potential. Usually, chronaxie gives

us a better idea about the excitability of a tissue. The lesser the chronaxie, the greater is the excitability. Nerves have a shorter chronaxie compared to muscles

iii. **Level C is rheobase.** To excite a tissue, the *lowest strength of current* required is termed as **rheobase**.

iv.   **Level B is utilization time.** The *minimum time* for which the rheobase must be applied to elicit an action potential is known as utilization time. A stimulus weaker than rheobase does not excite the tissue and a stimulus stronger than rheobase requires less time (less than utilization time) to elicit a response.

Spotter, Chart–Graph 38

Observe the given graph and answer the following questions:

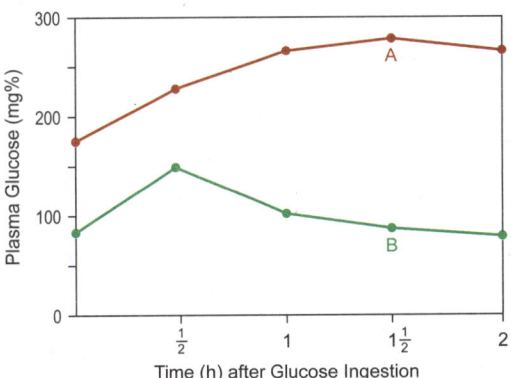

Questions

i.   Which investigation is represented by this graph and what is its purpose?

ii.   What do Graphs A and B represent? What are the key differences between them?

iii. Provide the fasting and postprandial blood glucose values for a normal, prediabetic, and diabetic individual.

iv.   List two categories of oral hypoglycemic agents used in type 2 diabetes mellitus (DM), along with their mechanisms of action.

v.   Mention two clinical symptoms of diabetes mellitus and explain the physiological basis of one.

Answers

i.   The investigation is oral glucose tolerance test. (OGTT). This is done for diagnosis of diabetes mellitus. It estimates the plasma glucose response to oral glucose tolerance.

ii.   'B' in normal GTT and 'A' is GTT of a diabetic patient. Note that the plasma glucose level remains always above the normal GTT value in diabetic patients and does not come back to normal range.

iii. The normal range of plasma glucose (70 to 99 mg%).

iv. Fasting and postprandial blood glucose values in mg%:

	Fasting	Postprandial
Normal and healthy	70–99	<140
Prediabetes	100–125	140–199
Diabetes	126 or more	200 or above

a) **Sulfonylureas** (e.g., Glipizide, Glyburide): Stimulate insulin secretion by binding to ATP-sensitive K$^+$ channels on pancreatic β-cells, causing depolarization and increased calcium influx.

b) **Biguanides** (e.g., Metformin): Inhibit hepatic gluconeogenesis, thereby reducing hepatic glucose output.

Spotter, Chart–Graph 39

Observe the following chart of recordings from an isolated nerve–muscle preparation, and answer the following questions:

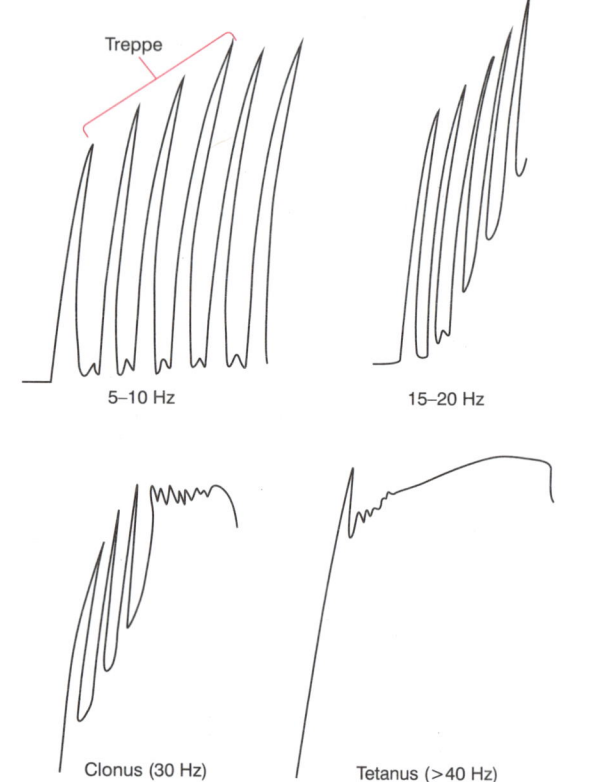

Questions

i. What physiological process is demonstrated in this chart? Provide a brief explanation.

ii. Define treppe and explain its physiological basis.

iii. Define clonus and describe its physiological application.

iv. What is the minimum tetanizing frequency (**MTF**)? List factors influencing MTF.

v. Define **tetanus** and state its clinical relevance.

Answers

i. The chart demonstrates the recordings of **genesis of tetanus in an isolated nerve–muscle preparation**. Tetanus refers to a state of sustained tonic contraction of the muscle (without relaxation) due to a rapidly repeated stimulation. If the rate of stimulation increases (higher frequency), tetanus ensues. When the muscle is stimulated below the tetanising frequency, incomplete tetanus (clonus) occurs.

ii. Treppe is also known as the **staircase phenomenon**; it is the progressive increase in the force of contraction for the first two to three contractions when a muscle is stimulated repeatedly. This occurs due to the **accumulation of calcium in the sarcoplasm** due to the application of repeated stimuli. Treppe is also seen in cardiac muscles. However, the cardiac muscle cannot be tetanised because of a longer refractory period.

iii. Clonus is a state of **partial tetanus** observed in experimental conditions (experimental clonus). This should not be confused with the clinical clonus, e.g., ankle clonus, seen in the upper motor neuron type of paralysis. In experimental clonus, relaxation is incomplete.

iv. The **minimal tetanisable frequency** (MTF) of a muscle can be calculated from the simple muscle curve (measuring the contraction period) by using the following formula:

MTF = 1/contraction period. For example, if the contraction period is 0.04 seconds, the MTF = 1/0.04 = 25 Hz. **Factors affecting MTF**: type of muscle, temperature in the environment, and the load acting on the muscle.

v. Tetanus is a **state of sustained contraction**. The muscle remains in a state of tonic contraction without relaxation. This occurs when a nerve–muscle preparation is stimulated at a high frequency. Rapid and repeated stimulation leads the stimuli to fall during the contraction phase so that the contractile processes are repeatedly activated. The muscle does not get time to relax. Therefore, with each stimulation, the muscle contracts without relaxation. Individual responses fuse to give a state of sustained contraction (tetanus). The muscles of our body, which are involved in the maintenance of posture, exhibit tetanic contraction (sustained contraction).

78 | Questions on Calculations

Questions on calculations provide students with an opportunity to demonstrate their understanding of the physical principles that govern the outputs of various physiological and clinical processes and determine the nature of pathophysiology or intensity of diseases. Often, these calculations are used as bedside methods to confirm or monitor the progress of diseases.

Usually, these questions appear as *'non-skill stations'* in the conduct of OSPE or as spotters. In theory exams, they can be part of clinical/applied questions. Most importantly, if students remember the simple formulas for the calculation, they secure full marks in questions on calculations, which helps them to get the best score in the practical examination. Therefore, calculations should be studied in detail and remembered vividly by students.

1. **Calculate the absolute counts of neutrophils, lymphocytes, and eosinophils from the data given below.**

   In a blood sample, the total leucocyte count was 6500/mm³; the neutrophil count was 60%; the lymphocyte count 30%; and the eosinophil count 5%.

Answer

- Absolute neutrophil count = 6500/100 × 60 = 3900/mm³
- Absolute lymphocyte count = 6500/100 × 30 = 1950/mm³
- Absolute eosinophil count = 6500/100 × 5 = 325/mm³

2. **Calculate the reticulocyte count from the data given below.**

   i. Number of RBCs in 100 oil-immersion fields = 4000
   ii. Number of reticulocytes in 100 oil-immersion fields = 40

Answer

In 4000 RBCs, the number of reticulocytes = 40
So, in 100 RBCs, the number of reticulocytes = 40/4000 × 100 = 1 reticulocyte
The reticulocyte count is 1% of red cells.

3. **Determine the mean corpuscular hemoglobin (MCH) from the data given below.**

   In a blood sample,
   i. RBC count = 4.8 million/mm³
   ii. Packed cell volume (PCV) = 42%
   iii. Hb level = 12 g/dL

Answer

$$MCH = \frac{Hb\,(g/dL)}{RBC\ count\,(million/mm^3)} \times 10$$

$$= \frac{12}{4.8} \times 10$$

$$= 25\ pg\,(25 \times 10^{-12}g)$$

4. **Determine the mean corpuscular hemoglobin concentration (MCHC) from the data given below.**

   In a blood sample,
   i. RBC count = 4.7 million/mm³
   ii. Packed cell volume (PCV) = 45%
   iii. Hb level = 14 g/dL

Answer

$$MCHC = \frac{Hb\,(g/dL)}{PCV\,(\%)} \times 100$$

$$= \frac{14}{45} \times 100$$

$$= 31.1\%$$

5. **Calculate the mean corpuscular volume (MCV) from the data given below.**

   In a blood sample,
   i. RBC count = 5 million/mm³
   ii. Packed cell volume (PCV) = 45%
   iii. Hb level = 14.6 g/dL

Answer

$$MCV = \frac{PCV\,(\%) \times 10}{RBC\ count\,(millions/mm^3)}$$

$$= \frac{45 \times 10}{5}$$

$$= 90\ fl\,(90 \times 10^{-15}l)$$

6. **Determine the colour index (CI) from the data given below.**

   In a blood sample,
   i. RBC count = 4.5 million/mm³
   ii. Packed cell volume (PCV) = 40%
   iii. Hb level = 12 g/dL

Answer

Normal 100 per cent RBC count = 5 million/mm³
Normal 100 per cent Hb concentration = 15 g/dL

$$CI = \frac{Hb \text{ per cent}}{RBC \text{ per cent}}$$

$$= \frac{\text{Estimated Hb} / \text{normal 100 per cent Hb}}{\text{Estimated RBC} / \text{normal 100 per cent RBC}}$$

$$= \frac{12/15}{4.5/5}$$

$$= \frac{0.8}{0.9}$$

$$= 0.88$$

The CI of the given sample is 0.88.

7. Calculate the nerve conduction velocity of the median nerve from the data given below.
   i.   Latent period with stimulation at the wrist = 3.45 ms
   ii. Latent period with stimulation at the elbow = 6.45 ms
   iii. Distance between the two stimulated points = 19.2 cm = 192 mm

Answer

Difference between two latencies = 6.45 ms – 3.45 ms = 3 ms

Distance travelled by the nerve impulses in 3 ms = 192 mm

Distance travelled by the nerve impulses in 1 ms = 192/3 = 64 mm

Distance travelled by the nerve impulses in 1000 ms = 64,000 mm

Or, the distance travelled by the nerve impulses in 1 s = 64 m

Therefore, the conduction velocity of the median nerve is 64 m/sec.

8. Calculate the work done by the gastrocnemius muscle of the frog from the following data:
   i.   Amplitude (height) of contraction recorded = 4 cm
   ii. Long arm of the lever from fulcrum to writing point (L) = 12 cm
   iii. Short arm of the lever from fulcrum to point of load (S) = 3 cm
   iv. Load (weight) lifted = 20 g

Answer

In the lever arrangement,

$$\text{magnification factor} = \frac{L}{S}$$

$$= \frac{12 \text{ cm}}{3 \text{ cm}}$$

$$= 4$$

$$\text{Actual height through which load was lifted} = \frac{\text{Amplitude of contraction}}{\text{Magnification factor}}$$

$$= \frac{4}{4} \text{ cm}$$

$$= 1 \text{ cm}$$

Work done = Load lifted × Actual height through which load was lifted
= 20 g × 1 cm
= 20 g cm

The work done is 20 g cm.

9. Find out the basal metabolic rate (BMR) of the subject from the data given below.
   i.   Oxygen consumption in 6 minutes = 1230 ml
   ii. Body surface area (BSA) of the subject = 1.5 m^2
   iii. Ideal BMR of the subject for the age and gender = 35 Cal/m^2 of BSA/hr

Answer

i.   Oxygen consumption in 6 minutes = 1230 ml
ii. Oxygen consumption in 60 min (1 hour) = 12300 ml = 12.30 litres
iii. Following consumption of 1 litre of oxygen, calories released = 4.8 Cal
iv. So, following consumption of 12.30 litres of oxygen, calories released = 4.8 × 12.30 = 59.04 Cal

$$BMR = \frac{\text{Calories consumed} / \text{hr}}{\text{BSA (per m}^2)}$$

$$= \frac{59.04}{1.5}$$

$$= 39 \text{ Cal} / \text{m}^2 \text{ BSA} / \text{hour}$$

The ideal BMR for the subject = 35 Cal/m^2 BSA/hour.
So, excess BMR = 39 – 35 = 4 Cal/m^2 BSA/hour.
So, BMR of the subject is in excess by 4 calories/m^2 BSA/ hour.

$$\text{Percentage excess} = \frac{\text{Excess BMR of the subject}}{\text{Ideal BMR of the subject for the age and gender}} \times 100$$

$$= \frac{4}{35} \times 100$$

$$= 11.42\%$$

Thus, the BMR of the subject is = +11.42% (normal range = ± 15%).

10. Calculate the inspiratory reserve volume (IRV), expiratory reserve volume (ERV), residual volume (RV), and functional residual capacity (FRC) from the given data.

i.   Tidal volume (TV) = 480 ml
ii. Inspiratory capacity (IC) = 3200 ml
iii. Vital capacity (VC) = 4200 ml
iv. Total lung capacity (TLC) = 5400 ml

Answer
IRV = IC – TV = 3200 – 480 = 2720 ml
ERV = VC – IC = 4200 – 3200 = 1000 ml
RV = TLC – VC = 5400 – 4200 = 1200 ml
FRC = ERV + RV = 1000 + 1200 = 2200 ml

11. **Determine the oxygen carrying capacity and oxygen content of arterial and venous blood samples from the data provided below.**
    i.   Percentage saturation of arterial blood with oxygen = 96%
    ii. Percentage saturation of venous blood with oxygen = 78%
    iii. Hemoglobin concentration = 12 g/100 ml

Answer
1 g of Hb carries 1.34 ml of oxygen
So, the oxygen carrying capacity of the given blood sample is 12 × 1.34 = 16.08 ml/100 ml of blood
Oxygen content of blood

$$= \frac{\text{Percentage saturation} \times \text{Oxygen carrying capacity}}{100}$$

Thus, oxygen content of arterial blood $= \dfrac{96 \times 16.08}{100}$

$$= 15.44 \, \text{ml} / 100 \, \text{ml}$$

Oxygen content of venous blood $= \dfrac{78 \times 16.08}{100}$

$$= 12.54 \, \text{ml} / 100 \, \text{ml}$$

Therefore, the oxygen carrying capacity of the given blood sample is 16.08 ml/100 ml; the oxygen content of arterial blood is 15.44 ml/100 ml and the oxygen content of venous blood 12.54 ml/100 ml.

12. **Find out the physiological dead space from the data given below.**
    i.   Tidal volume = 480 ml
    ii. Alveolar air PCO_2 = 42 mmHg
    iii. Expired air PCO_2 = 28 mmHg

Answer
Formula for physiological dead space

$$= \frac{\text{Alveolar air } PCO_2 - \text{Expired air } PCO_2}{\text{Alveolar air } PCO_2} \times \text{Tidal volume}$$

$$= \frac{42 - 28}{42} \times 480$$

$$= 160 \, \text{ml}$$

Therefore, the physiological dead space is 160 ml.

13. **Find out the breathing reserve and the dyspnea index from the data provided below.**
    i.   Respiratory rate = 15/min
    ii. Tidal volume = 400 ml
    iii. Maximal voluntary ventilation (MVV) = 120 litres

Answer
Respiratory minute
volume (MV) = Tidal volume × Respiratory rate
                   = 400 × 15
                   = 6000 ml
                   = 6 litres

Breathing reserve = MVV – MV
                   = 120 – 6 = 114 litres

$$\text{Dyspnea index} = \frac{\text{MVV} - \text{MV}}{\text{MVV}} \times 100$$

$$= \frac{114}{120} \times 100$$

$$= 95\%$$

Therefore, the breathing reserve is 114 litres and dyspnea index is 95%.

14. **Calculate the heart rate (HR) from the given ECG data.**
    i.   Total number of small squares between two R waves (RR interval) = 20
    ii. Speed of the paper = 25 mm/s

Answer

$$\text{One formula for HR} = \frac{1500}{\text{RR interval (in mm)}}$$

On the ECG paper, each small square is 1 mm.
So, the RR interval = 20 mm.

Thus, $HR = \dfrac{1500}{20}$

$= 75/\text{min}$

Another formula for $HR = \dfrac{60}{RR \text{ interval (in s)}}$

When the paper speed is 25mm/s, 1 mm = 0.04 s.
So, 20 mm (RR interval) will be 20×0.04 ms = 80 ms or 0.8 s.

Thus, $HR = \dfrac{60}{0.8}$

$= 75/\text{min}$

15. Calculate the stroke volume and cardiac output from the data given below.
   i.   Oxygen content of mixed venous blood = 14.5 ml/100 ml
   ii. Oxygen content of systemic arterial blood = 19.5 ml/100 ml
   iii. Heart rate = 72/min
   iv. Oxygen consumption = 250 ml/minute

Answer

$Cardiac\ output = \dfrac{Oxygen\ consumption\ per\ minute}{Arteriovenous\ oxygen\ difference} \times 100$

$= \dfrac{250}{19.5 - 14.5} \times 100$

$= \dfrac{250}{5} \times 100$

$= 5000$ ml / min or 5 litres / min

$Stroke\ volume = \dfrac{Cardiac\ output\ (ml / min)}{Heart\ rate\ (beats / min)}$

$= \dfrac{5000\ (ml / min)}{72\ (beats / min)}$

$= 69.44$ ml

Thus, the stroke volume is 69.44 ml and cardiac output is 5 litres/min.

16. Calculate the cardiac index from the data given below.
   i. Cardiac output = 4.5 litres/min
   ii. Body surface area (BSA) = 1.5 m^2

Answer

$Cardiac\ index = \dfrac{Cardiac\ output\ (litres / min)}{BSA\ (per\ m^2)}$

$= \dfrac{4.5}{1.5}$

$= 3$ litres / min / per m^2 BSA

So, the cardiac index is 3 litres/min/per m^2 BSA.

17. Determine the effective filtration pressure from the data given below.
   i.   Glomerular capillary hydrostatic pressure = 60 mmHg
   ii. Glomerular capillary oncotic pressure = 25 mmHg
   iii. Bowman's capsule hydrostatic pressure = 13 mmHg
   iv. Bowman's capsule oncotic pressure = 0 mmHg

Answer

Effective filtration pressure = (Glomerular capillary hydrostatic pressure + Bowman's capsule oncotic pressure) – (Glomerular capillary oncotic pressure + Bowman's capsule hydrostatic pressure)
Thus, the effective filtration
pressure $= (60 + 0) - (25 + 13)$
$= 60 - 38$
$= 22$ mmHg
So, the effective filtration pressure is 22 mmHg.

18. Determine the renal blood flow from the data given below.
   i.   Concentration of PAH in urine (U_{PAH}) = 12 mg/ml
   ii. Concentration of PAH in plasma (P_{PAH}) = 0.02 mg/ml
   iii. Rate of urine flow (V) = 1 ml/min
   iv. Hematocrit = 47%

Answer

$Plasma\ clearance\ of\ PAH = \dfrac{U_{PAH} \times V}{P_{PAH}}$

$= \dfrac{12 \times 1}{0.02}$

$= 600$ ml / min

Thus, the effective renal plasma flow (ERPF) is 600 ml/min.
Extraction ratio for PAH is 0.9, as about 90% of PAH in the arterial blood is removed during a single passage through the kidneys.

$So,\ the\ actual\ renal\ plasma\ flow\ (RPF) = \dfrac{ERPF}{Extraction\ ratio}$

$= \dfrac{600}{0.9}$

$= 667$ ml / min

$Renal\ blood\ flow = \dfrac{100}{100 - Hematocrit} \times RPF$

$= \dfrac{100}{100 - 47} \times 667$

$= 1258$ ml / min

So, the renal blood flow is 1258 ml/min.

19. Calculate the urea clearance from the given data.

   i.   Concentration of urea in blood (B_{Urea})
       = 30 mg/100 ml
   ii.   Concentration of urea in urine (U_{Urea}) = 15 mg/ml
   iii.   Rate of urine flow (V) = 1 ml/min

Answer

As the rate of urine flow is less than 2.0 ml/min, the formula of standard urea clearance is:

$$\frac{U_{Urea} \times \sqrt{V}}{B_{Urea}} \times 100$$

Thus, the urea clearance
of the given sample is

$$= \frac{15 \times \sqrt{1}}{30} \times 100$$

$$= 50 \text{ ml/min}$$

So, the urea clearance of the given sample is 50 ml/min.

20. Calculate glomerular filtration rate (GFR) from the given data.

   i.   Concentration of Inulin in plasma (P_{Inulin}) = 0.24 mg/100 ml
   ii.   Concentration of Inulin in urine (U_{Inulin}) = 28 mg/ ml
   iii.   Rate of urine flow (V) = 1.1 ml/min

Answer

$$\text{Plasma clearance of Inulin} = \frac{U_{Inulin} \times V}{P_{Inulin}}$$

$$= \frac{28 \times 1.1}{0.24}$$

$$= 128 \text{ ml / min}$$

Thus, the GFR is 128 ml/min.

79 | Problem-Solving Questions

Answers to problem-solving questions (PSQs) reveal the student's understanding of the deeper concepts and clinical applications of various topics. Usually, these questions are given as 'Non-Skill Stations' in the OSPE. In theory exams, they can be asked clinical/applied questions; they can also be asked during the viva.

1. **During hematological investigations, a patient's blood sample revealed a total leucocyte count (TLC) of 10,000/mm³ and 12% eosinophil in the differential leucocyte count (DLC).**

Questions

i. Calculate the absolute eosinophil count (AEC).
ii. What is the normal range of AEC?
iii. Mention two important functions of eosinophils.
iv. Name two important growth factors that regulate eosinophil development.
v. Name two diseases each associated with increased and decreased eosinophil counts.

Answers

i. AEC = DLC of eosinophil/100 x TLC
      = 12/100 x 10,000 = 1200/mm³ of blood.
ii. The normal range of AEC is 40 – 440 mm³ of blood.
iii. a) Eosinophils provide defence against parasitic infestations, especially in intestinal worm infestation and in filariasis, and b) are active in allergic conditions, in which they dampen the host's response by limiting antigen-induced release of mediators of inflammation.
iv. IL3 and IL5.
v. **Eosinophilia:** Filariasis and hookworm infestation; **eosinopenia:** Cushing syndrome and ACTH therapy

2. **The blood indices obtained from the hematological investigations of a patient admitted to your hospital are as shown below:**
   1. **PCV (hematocrit) = 35%**
   2. **RBC Count = 4 million cells/mm³**

Questions

i. Calculate the mean corpuscular volume (MCV) using the given data.
ii. State the normal value for MCV and interpret the observed result.
iii. What is the physiological significance of MCV?
iv. Name one condition each in which MCV is decreased and elevated.

Answers

i. MCV (fl) = Hematocrit (%) x 10 / RBC count in millions per mm³ of blood
      = 35 x 10 / 4 + 87 fl

ii. MCV defines the volume or size of an average RBC. It indicates whether the red cells are microcytic, normocytic, or macrocytic. Therefore, this test is very useful in the **morphological classification of anemia**: microcytic anemia, normocytic anemia, or macrocytic anemia.
iii. Normal value of MCV: 78 – 96 fl. The observed MCV is normal.
iv. Decreased MCV (**microcytosis**): Iron deficiency anemia; elevated MCV (**macrocytosis**): Megaloblastic anemia as seen in vitamin B_{12} deficiency.

3. **A patient in the medicine ward of the hospital, within the half an hour of starting a blood transfusion, developed shivering and fever, severe uneasiness, nausea and vomiting, shortness of breath, dark urine, chest and back pain, and tachycardia.**

Questions

i. What could be the cause of this patient's condition?
ii. What measures should be taken immediately?
iii. What is major cross-matching? What is its importance?
iv. Name four major complications of this kind of transfusion problem.
v. What is autologous blood transfusion?

Answers

i. **Mismatched blood transfusion** of ABO incompatibility, likely due to transfusion of the wrong blood type to the patient. It is possible that cross-matching was not performed before transfusing the blood.
ii. Immediately stop transfusion, start symptomatic treatment, and notify the blood bank to investigate the cause.
iii. In **major cross-matching**, the cells of the donor are directly matched against the plasma of the recipient. Since it is important to ensure that antibodies present in the recipient's plasma do not harm the donor's red cells, this is called major cross-matching. Major cross matching prevents mismatched blood transfusion.
iv. Four complications: a) **Acute hemolytic transfusion reactions:** Hemoglobinemia and **hemoglobinuria** and hemolytic jaundice; b) **acute renal failure** occurs due to Hb casts blocking the renal tubules and damaging the tubules; c) circulatory shock; and d) **hyperkalemia** (due to release of potassium ions from red cells) that can cause **cardiac arrest in diastole**.
v. **Autologous transfusion:** When the donor himself is the recipient, the blood collected is called autologous

donor blood and the transfusion is called autologous transfusion. This can be done prior to a planned surgery. Blood is collected every 72 hours three days prior to surgery or till the Hb level has not gone below 11 g%. Usually 2–4 units of blood of 250 mL each can be collected. Then, the same blood (recipient's own blood) is used during surgery.

4. **A 35-year-old woman presented to the OPD with h/o weakness in the extraocular muscles (ptosis) and muscles of the extremities. She mentions that she feels fine when she wakes up in the morning, but starts to feel the weakness soon after she becomes active; she also says that the condition is the worst in the evening. Her condition improves with rest. Her sensations appear normal.**

Questions
i. What is the probable diagnosis of the condition?
ii. What is the probable cause of this disease?
iii. Why does the condition worsen with activity and improve with rest?
iv. Name two treatment modalities.

Answers
i. The diagnosis **is myasthenia gravis.**
ii. Antibodies are produced against the nicotinic acetylcholine receptors at the neuromuscular junction (NMJ).
iii. During **rest and sleep**, acetylcholine (ACh) **accumulates at the NMJ**, improving muscle strength. With **activity**, ACh is used up faster than it is synthesized, leading to **worsening weakness**.
iv. a) Neostigmine (AChE inhibitors) and b) plasmapheresis (removes AChR antibodies).

5. **A 65-year-old obese male presented with a 3-month history of increased and excessive thirst. His blood reports revealed elevated fasting blood glucose levels.**

Questions
i. What is the likely diagnosis?
ii. What is the primary physiological mechanism of this disease?
iii. The concerned hormone binds to which receptor on the cell?
iv. Briefly explain the physiological basis of the above-mentioned symptoms.
v. List four hormones that increase blood glucose.

Answers
i. The diagnosis is **type 2 diabetes mellitus.**
ii. Insulin resistance is the primary mechanism.
iii. **Tyrosine kinase** is the enzyme.

iv. **Polyuria** (increased urination) occurs due to osmotic diuresis due to increased concentration of glucose in tubular fluid. **Polydipsia** (excessive thirst) occurs due to excessive urinary loss of water, which decreases plasma and ECF volume, which in turn stimulates the thirst centre.
v. Glucagon, epinephrine, glucocorticoid, and growth hormone.

6. **An adult with a chronic lung disease has a respiratory rate 30/minute and tidal volume of 200 ml.**

Questions
i. Calculate minute ventilation.
ii. Calculate alveolar ventilation.
iii. Comment on the data and results obtained from the given data.
iv. Mention how tidal volume can be increased physiologically.

Answers
i. Minute ventilation = Tidal volume (TV) × Respiratory rate (RR)
   = 200 × 30 = 6000 ml/min (or) 6 l/min.
ii. Alveolar ventilation = (TV – dead space volume) × RR
   = (200 – 150) × 30 = 1500 ml/min (or) 1.5 l/min
iii. The patient's tidal volume is significantly low (the normal value is about 500 mL). The respiratory rate is abnormally high (normal is about 12–18/min). Despite normal minute ventilation, alveolar ventilation is severely reduced due to high dead space proportion (150/200 mL). This impairs gaseous exchange, as only 50 mL per breath reaches alveoli.
iv. Tidal volume can be increased by practicing slow breathing exercises like *Anulom-Vilom pranayama*, which is known to increase alveolar ventilation.

7. **The following blood parameters were recorded while measuring the cardiac output of an individual.**
   • **The oxygen consumption of the body in one minute was 250 mL/min.**
   • **The arterial oxygen content (AO2) was 200 mL/L.**
   • **The venous oxygen content (VO2) was 150 mL/L.**

Questions
i. Name the method used for these estimations.
ii. Define cardiac output. State the normal value of cardiac output in adults.
iii. Calculate the cardiac output using the data given above (provide the formulae and steps involved in this calculation.)

iv. Mention two advantages and two disadvantages of this method of cardiac output measurement.

Answers

i. These estimations are made using **Fick's method.**
ii. **Cardiac output** is defined as the amount of blood ejected by each ventricle per minute. Cardiac output in adults is 5–6 litres/minutes.
iii. Cardiac output is calculated as:
iv. Output of left ventricle = Oxygen consumption of the body / $AO_2 - VO_2$
$$= 250/200-150 = 250/50$$
$$= 5 \text{ l/min.}$$
v. a) Advantages: accurate results, no chemical is injected; b) disadvantages: hospitalisation and expertise needed for catheterisation and simultaneous measurement of O_2 consumption makes the method practically difficult.

8. **A 60-year-old male presents to the casualty ward with acute onset of weakness in the right half of the body. On examination, hypertonia and spasticity were noted on the affected limb muscles, and there was no muscle atrophy. The left half of the body was normal.**

Questions

i. What is the probable diagnosis, and what is the most probable site of the lesion?
ii. What will be the planter reflex response on the right side?
iii. What will be the deep (tendon) reflexes on the right side? What is the physiological basis for these changes?
iv. Briefly explain why muscle tone is increased in this patient.

Answers

i. The probable diagnosis is right-sided hemiplegia and upper motor neuron (UMN) paralysis. The most probable site of the lesion is a left internal capsule.
ii. The **planter response** will be of the extensor type. Stroking the sole of the foot on the lateral aspect causes dorsiflexion of the big toe and fanning of the other toes (extensor plantar response; Babinski sign positive).
iii. **Deep (tendon) reflexes will be exaggerated:** Usually, the upper motor neurons are inhibitory to the lower motor neurons. In UMN paralysis, loss of these inhibitory influences increases the motor neuron discharge. The increased γ motor neuron discharge

increases the sensitivity of the muscle spindle to stretch. This results in increased deep tendon reflex.
iv. **Muscle hypertonia:** a) This occurs due to increased discharge of motor neurons and increased excitability of the motor neuron pool. b) Loss of inhibitory cortico-reticular influence makes the reticulospinal tract more facilitatory and increases gamma motor neuron discharge. Thus, muscle tone increases.

9. **A seven-year-old boy is brought to the Pediatric OPD by his father with complaints of crippling and pain in the right knee since infancy. History reveals that the boy bleeds for a long time even after a minor injury. On examination, it was found that the child has mild swelling, not only in the knee, but also in the ankle and wrist joints.**

Questions

i. What is the provisional diagnosis? What is the cause of the disease?
ii. What is the mode of transmission of the disease?
iii. How can the provisional diagnosis be confirmed?
iv. Briefly outline the physiological basis of the treatment of the disease.

Answers

i. The provisional diagnosis is **hemophilia A,** also known as classic hemophilia. This is a bleeding disorder that occurs due to the deficiency of factor VIII.
ii. It is an **X-linked recessive** hereditary disease. Women are carriers and generally do not suffer from the disease as they are protected by the second X chromosome, which is usually normal.
iii. **Assay of factor VIII in plasma** (which will be deficient) is diagnostic. Functional factor VIII coagulant activity can also be measured. Patients have prolonged APTT. PT and BT are normal.
iv. The treatment consists of the **transfusion of fresh blood** (as on storage factor VIII is rapidly lost) or transfusion of **factor VIII concentrate**. Fresh frozen plasma and cryoprecipitate both contain factor VIII. Attempts should be made to avoid aspirin, non-steroidal anti-inflammatory drugs, and other drugs that interfere with platelet aggregation.

10. **A 23-year-old male college student visited the medical OPD with complaints of leg pain, intermittent joint pain, and swelling in the hands and feet. These symptoms worsened when visiting higher altitudes (like hill stations), accompanied by pallor. A family history revealed similar complaints. Clinical examination revealed significant anemia without splenomegaly.**

Questions

i.   What is the provisional diagnosis and the probable cause of the disease?
ii. What is the mode of transmission and basic pathophysiology of the disease?
iii. How can the provisional diagnosis be confirmed?
iv. What is the cause of absence of splenomegaly in this disease?

Answers

i.   The provisional diagnosis is **sickle cell disease**. It occurs due to the presence of an abnormal hemoglobin called **HbS** in red cells.
ii. This is an autosomal recessive hereditary disorder in which red cells contain HbS. In HbS, glutamic acid is replaced by valine at the 6th position of beta chain. In deoxygenated states or less oxygenated states (e.g., at high altitudes), conformational changes induced by HbS make the cell more rigid and deformed to take the shape of a sickle. Therefore, cells undergo intravascular hemolysis. The anemia is usually *normochromic* and *normocytic*.
iii. The diagnosis is usually made by performing a **sickle test** (demonstrating sickling of red cells when the blood is mixed with a freshly prepared solution of a reducing agent like sodium metabisulphite), **hemoglobin solubility test** (relative insolubility of reduced HbS in phosphate buffer), and **hemoglobin electrophoresis**.
iv. Hyposplenism occurs due to repeated microinfarctions in the spleen, eventually leading to autosplenectomy. As a result, the spleen becomes fibrosed and non-palpable.

11. **A 25-year-old woman, in her second full-term pregnancy, delivered a baby with generalized edema. There was no history of complications during her first pregnancy. On clinical examination, the newborn had significant pallor and icterus. A peripheral blood smear showed numerous erythroblasts.**

Questions

i.   What is the provisional diagnosis, and what is the underlying pathophysiology? Why does it not usually occur during the first pregnancy but in subsequent pregnancies?
ii. What are the serious features indicating complications of the disease?
iii. What are the essential treatments?
iv. How can the disease be prevented?

Answers

i.   a) The provisional diagnosis is **erythroblastosis fetalis**. This is a hemolytic disease of the newborn, which occurs due to Rh incompatibility when an Rh-negative mother carries Rh-positive fetus during pregnancy.

     b) Usually, no reaction occurs in the first pregnancy. At the time of delivery during placental separation, a small amount of fetal blood leaks into the maternal circulation. This induces the formation of anti-Rh agglutinins in the mother. In subsequent pregnancies, the anti-Rh agglutinins from mother, which is predominantly IgG type crosses placenta to enter the fetal circulation and causes hemolysis. In third and subsequent pregnancies, the degree of hemolysis becomes more severe.

ii. a) Severe anemia from hemolysis; b) hemolytic jaundice (due to hemolysis) with serum bilirubin >25 mg%, c) hydrops fetalis—generalised fetal edema due to anemia and hypoproteinemia, and d) kernicterus—neurological damage from bilirubin crossing the immature blood-brain barrier and depositing in basal ganglia. As the blood–brain barrier (BBB) is not fully developed in fetuses, infants, and children, bilirubin enters the brain and gets deposited in the basal ganglia, causing kernicterus.

iii. **Treatment:** In about 50% of cases, the disease is limited to mild hemolysis and does not require treatment. In severe cases, major modalities of treatment are intrauterine fetal transfusion, exchange transfusion, and phototherapy.

     a.   **Intrauterine fetal transfusion:** If the disease is diagnosed during fetal life, fetal transfusion is carried out by the intraperitoneal route, which has replaced the direct intravascular fetal transfusion.

     b.   **Exchange transfusion:** This procedure removes sensitised red cells, bilirubin, and maternal antibody from the plasma. A double-volume exchange transfusion (2 x 80 ml/kg) replaces 90% of the infant's blood volume with antigen-negative red cells. Blood chosen for exchange should be ABO-negative, Rh-negative, and cross-matched against the mother's blood.

     c.   **Phototherapy:** Intensive phototherapy is very effective in reducing serum bilirubin levels.

iv. **Prevention:** Erythroblastosis fetalis is prevented by administering a single dose of anti-Rh antibodies in the form of **Rh immunoglobulin** during the postpartum period following the first delivery. The disease can also be prevented by **passive immunisation** of the mother with a small dose of Rh immunoglobulins during pregnancy.

12. **A 45-year-old male with a history of chronic cardiac disease was admitted to the medical emergency with features of severe breathlessness, which becomes more prominent at night and presents in paroxysms. On examination, pitting pedal edema was observed in the dependent areas.**

Questions

i.   What is your probable diagnosis, and what term is used for the nocturnal symptoms?
ii. Name two other clinical features of the disease, and mention which one is considered to be more clinically reliable.
iii. What investigation would you perform to confirm the diagnosis? What parameter will be defining?
iv. Name two separate categories of drugs that can be used for treatment and briefly mention the mechanism of one of them.

Answers

i.   The probable diagnosis is **congestive heart failure**. The night symptom is called **paroxysmal nocturnal dyspnea**.
ii. Two other clinical features are: tender hepatomegaly and increased JVP. Increased JVP is a more reliable sign of heart failure.
iii. **Echocardiography** is more useful for confirming heart failure. Decreased **ejection fraction** below 40% (40 to 50% is considered borderline) will confirm heart failure.
iv. Diuretics and digitalis are used for treatment. **Digitalis** improves heart function by **its positive inotropic effect**. It increases myocardial contractility and therefore, cardiac output. Digitalis acts by inhibiting the sodium–potassium pump's activity on the myocardial cells. Therefore, intracellular sodium increases, which is exchanged with extracellular calcium. This results in increased calcium concentration in the cell and increased myocardial contractility.

13. **A 40-year-old male presented with progressive darkening of the skin, especially over pressure points and sun-exposed areas over six months. On examination, the patient had low BP, and blood investigation revealed eosinophilia.**

Questions

i.   What will be the provisional diagnosis? What is the cause of the disease?

ii. Explain the mechanism of darkness of the skin in this patient.
iii. How will you confirm the disease?
iv. What important medical advice should be given and why?

Answers

i.   The likely diagnosis is **Addison's disease**. The atrophy of the adrenal cortex or adrenocortical insufficiency is usually due to an **autoimmune mechanism**. However, **tubercular infection** of the adrenal gland, secondary metastasis, amyloidosis, and cytomegalovirus infection affecting the gland could also produce the disease.
ii. Darkness of the skin reflects **hyperpigmentation**, especially marked over the pressure points, sun-exposed areas, and scar marks. This occurs due to the deficiency of plasma cortisol, which increases ACTH secretion by feedback mechanism. **ACTH has intrinsic MSH activity**, which causes hyperpigmentation.
iii. **Assay of plasma cortisol and ACTH:** Decreased plasma level of cortisol with increased ACTH is diagnostic.
iv. The patient should be advised **not to fast** and to avoid stressful situations. The patient develops rapid hypoglycemia on fasting. Stressful situations cause collapse.

14. **Following thyroid surgery, a patient was kept in the post-operative room. Next day, it was noted that the patient developed wrist muscle spasms. Investigation revealed a plasma calcium level of 4.2 mg%.**

Questions

i.   What is your provisional diagnosis? What is the cause of this condition?
ii. Name two other clinical signs of this condition.
iii. What are the effects of the hormone (which is deficient in this condition) on bone?
iv. How will you manage this condition?

Answers

i.   The provisional diagnosis is **hypocalcemic tetany**. During thyroid surgery, parathyroid glands have been removed by mistake along with thyroid tissue, and consequent acute deficiency of parathormone (PTH) results in lowering of plasma calcium concentration, which results in neuromuscular defects.
ii. a) **Chvostek's sign:** quick contraction of facial muscles of the same side upon tapping over the facial nerve at the angle of the jaw; b) **Trousseau's sign:** spasm of the muscles of the upper extremity that

causes the flexion of the wrist and thumb (i.e., flexion at metacarpophalangeal joints) with the extension of the fingers (i.e., extension of the interphalangeal joints).

iii. PTH acts on both osteoblasts and osteoclasts. It **stimulates osteoclastic activity** and osteocytic osteolysis, and at higher concentrations, inhibits the synthesis of collagen by osteoblasts. Thus, it activates both bone synthesis and resorption. The net effect is **increased bone resorption** and excess mobilisation of calcium and phosphates from the bones into the plasma.

iv. As this is a case of severe hypocalcemic tetany, immediate **calcium infusion** (intravenous calcium gluconate) is indicated for the management of acute hypocalcemia. However, for chronic hypocalcemia, the mainstay of treatment is **oral calcium and vitamin D supplements**.

15. A tall male has developed feminine features of gynecomastia. On examination, he was found to have female patterns of pubic hair, a small penis, and testicular atrophy.

Questions

i. What is the provisional diagnosis?
ii. What is the actual problem in this case?
iii. What test would you perform, and what results would you expect for diagnosis?
iv. What are the usual reproductive problems in this case? What will be the status of fertility of this person?

Answers

i. It is a case of **Klinefelter Syndrome.**
ii. Typically, it is characterised by the presence of feminine features in an apparent male with small testes. The patient is genetically female, but the presence of **an extra Y chromosome** causes the development of the testis.
iii. **Karyotyping** will confirm the diagnosis. The **karyotype is 47 XXY** (44 autosomes + XX sex chromosomes + one extra Y chromosome).
iv. The seminiferous tubules are not properly developed, and infertility results. Hence, the syndrome is otherwise called **seminiferous tubule dysgenesis.** The syndrome usually presents with **primary hypogonadism and infertility** in men.

16. Following a road traffic accident, a patient was admitted to the Neurosurgery department for neurological abnormalities. On special radiological investigations, it was found that half of the spinal cord on the right side was completely damaged by the injury (hemisection of the spinal cord).

Questions

i. What is the name of the syndrome that happens in hemisection of the spinal cord?
ii. What will be the pattern of sensory deficits in the side of the lesion and in the opposite side?
iii. What is the physiological basis of such a pattern of sensory deficits?
iv. What will be the motor deficits in this case?

Answers

i. This is called the **Brown-Séquard syndrome.** It occurs in hemisection of the spinal cord.
ii. On the **side of lesion,** the fine-touch sensation, proprioceptive sensations (sensations from tendons, muscles, joints, and vibration sense), and tactile discrimination are lost. **On the opposite side,** pain and thermal sensations are lost.
iii. This pattern of sensory deficits occurs because sensations of fine-touch, proprioception, and two-point discrimination ascend the dorsal column of the same side, whereas the sensations for pain and temperature ascend the anterolateral system on the opposite side of the spinal cord.
iv. **Motor deficit:** There is also **damage to the corticospinal tract** on the side of the hemisection of the spinal cord. This causes paresis (muscle weakness) and spasticity of muscles on the same side of the body.

17. A 56-year-old male patient presented to the Neurology OPD with complaints of slowness of movements for the last 2 years. On examination, there was akinesia, mask-like face, resting tremor, and lead-pipe rigidity of the limbs.

Questions

i. What is the provisional diagnosis and what is the cause of the disease?
ii. What type of gait is observed in these patients? Describe the gait.
iii. How will you confirm your diagnosis?
iv. Mention two latest modalities of treatment of this disorder.

Answers

i. The provisional diagnosis is **Parkinsonism.** Parkinson's disease results from the degeneration of nigrostriatal dopaminergic neurons in the basal ganglia.
ii. **Festinant gait:** The patient walks with an attitude, as if trying to catch the centre of gravity. He usually bends forward but does not fall; instead, he takes short, shuffling steps.

iii. The disease is diagnosed by functional dopaminergic imaging by SPECT, in which the uptake of the striatal dopaminergic marker, particularly in the posterior putamen, is reduced. Dopamine transporter (DaT) imaging by using radio-labeled ligand binding to dopaminergic terminals is performed to assess the nigrostriatal cell loss.

iv. a) **Transplantation of adrenal medulla** from one of the adrenal glands of the patient into his basal ganglia helps inregenerating the dopaminergic neurons and b) **transplantation of glomus cells** for treatment of parkinsonism; glomus cells from the carotid body are isolated and transplanted into the basal ganglia. The glomus cell releases dopamine locally and found to be encouraging.

18. **A 65-year-old male patient presented to the Neurology OPD with complaints of defects in coordination of movements for the last one year. On examination, there was a pendular knee jerk, muscle hypotonia, no paralysis, and no sensory deficit.**

Questions

i. What could possibly be the neurological disorder?
ii. Define the terminology used for incoordination of movement in this disorder. Name four specific features of this incoordination.
iii. Name two other bedside clinical tests to confirm your diagnosis.
iv. What is Charcot's triad? Name two diseases in which Charcot's triad is seen.

Answers

i. The provisional diagnosis is cerebellar disorder.
ii. a) **Ataxia**: Motor deficit in cerebellar disorder manifests mainly in the form of ataxia, which is defined as a defect in coordination due to errors in the rate, range, force, and direction of movement. b) Features of ataxia (any four):
   • Drunken gait
   • Scanning speech
   • Intention tremor
   • Adiadochokinesia
   • Rebound phenomenon
   • Decomposition of movement
iii. **Bedside function tests** are as follows: a) Tests for coordination:
   • Upper limbs: Finger-nose test, drawing circles in the air, etc.
   • Lower limbs: Heel–knee test, walking in a straight line, etc.
   b) Tests for postural stability: Ask the patient to stand erect with feet together and eyes open.

iv. **Charcot's triad** consists of nystagmus, intention tremor, and scanning speech (lalling speech like a baby) Seen in: a) cerebellar disorders and b) disseminated sclerosis that affects cerebellar functions.

19. **A 58-year-old male patient presented to the Neurology OPD with complaints of progressive** forgetfulness **for the last two years. On examination, there was dysnomia and paranomia.**

Questions

i. What are dysnomia and paranomia? What is the provisional diagnosis?
ii. What is the etiology of this disorder?
iii. Mention two important pathological diagnostic findings in this disease.
iv. How can this disease be prevented?

Answers

i. a) Dysnomia is a memory disorder marked by difficulty in recalling words, especially proper names or numbers. Paranomia is a verbal paraphasia where a person unintentionally uses a different word than he intended to say. b) Provisional diagnosis is Alzheimer's disease.
ii. Alzheimer's disease is due to the loss of cholinergic neurons projecting from the basal forebrain to the neocortex, amygdala, and hippocampus. Especially fibres from the nucleus basalis of Meynert are severely affected.
iii. Two pathologic features characteristic of the disease are: 1. Presence of neurofibrillary 'tangles' in the nerve cell cytoplasm is the cytopathologic hallmark of the disease. These tangles are fiber-like strands composed of a hyperphosphorylated form of the microtubular protein 'tau'. They appear like pairs of helical filaments. 2. The appearance of neuritic plaques scattered throughout the cerebral cortex. The plaques contain amyloid protein (amyloid β protein or Aβ protein) as the central core surrounded by degenerating nerve terminals.
iv. iv. Alzheimer's disease can be prevented by several lifestyle modifications such as healthy diet (fruits, vegetables, whole grain, olive oil, fish oil), regular exercise (moderate intensity aerobic exercise every day), mental stimulation (reading, puzzles, learning new skills, playing instrumental music), 7-8 hours of quality sleep, control of BP and blood sugar within the normal range, stress management, meditation, *pranayama* and *yogasana*.

20. **A 62-year-old male patient presented to the Ophthalmology OPD with ptosis (drooping of the upper eyelid), miosis (constricted pupil), and anhidrosis (loss of sweating) on the affected side of the face.**

Questions

i.   What is your provisional clinical diagnosis?

ii. What is the cause of this disease?

iii. What is the physiological basis of miosis, ptosis, and anhidrosis in this condition?

iv. Who described this syndrome? Mention two other medical terms associated with his name.

Answers

i.   The provisional diagnosis is Horner's syndrome.

ii. Horner's syndrome is due to oculosympathetic paralysis. It commonly occurs due to Pancoast tumour of the lung, cervical lymph node malignancy compressing the sympathetic chain. However, it may even be a congential problem.

iii. • Ptosis is due to paralysis of Müller's muscle (a part of the levator palpebrae superioris).

   • Miosis occurs due to paralysis of the dilator pupillae, allowing unopposed action of the sphincter pupillae.

   • Anhidrosis is due to loss of sympathetic innervation to sweat glands.

iv. Horner's syndrome was named after Johann Friedrich Horner (1831–1886), a 19th century Swiss ophthalmologist following his description of the condition in 1869. His name is also associated with: a)'Horner's muscle', the lacrimal portion of the orbicularis oculi muscle, also called as the tensor tarsi muscle and b) the 'Horner–Trantas spots', the small whitish-yellow chalky concretions of the conjunctiva around the corneal limbus.

80 | Normal Values

Normal physiological values are often asked in practical, viva, and theory examinations. They are often required as reference values for the diagnosis of diseases. Therefore, students should read and remember these values.

A. Blood

1. Hemogram

Total RBC count	
Men	4.5–6 million/mm³
Women	4–5.5 million/mm³
Hemoglobin	
Men	14–18 g/dl
Women	12–16 g/dl
Glycated Hb:	<5.7% (5.7 to 6.4% prediabetes)
Carboxy Hb:	Non-smokers: 0–2.3%, smokers: 2.1–4.2%
Packed cell volume (Hematocrit)	
Men	40–50%
Women	37–47%
Mean corpuscular volume (MCV)	78–96 fl
Mean corpuscular hemoglobin (MCH)	27–33 pg
Mean corpuscular Hb conc (MCHC)	30–37%
Colour index	0.85 0 1.10
Total leucocyte count	4000–11,000/mm³
Differential count	
Neutrophils	50–70%
Eosinophils	1–4%
Lymphocyte	20–40%
Monocyte	2–8%
Basophils	0–1%
Total platelet count	150,000–400,000/mm³
Reticulocyte count	0.5–1% of red cells
ESR	
Westergren method	
Men	3–5 mm at the end of 1 h
Women	5–12 mm at the end of 1 h
Wintrobe method)	
Men	0–9 mm at the end of 1 h
Women	0–20 mm at the end of 1 h
Osmotic fragility of red cells	Hemolysis begins at 0.45% of NaCl and completes at 0.35% of NaCl.

2. Coagulation studies

Bleeding time (Duke method)	1–5 min.
Clotting time (capillary tube method)	2–8 min.
Fibrinogen	200–400 mg%
Fibrin degradation product	10 mg/dl
Activated partial thromboplastin time (APTT)	25–36 sec.
Prothrombin time:	11–13.5 sec (INR: 0.3 to 1.3).
Thrombin time	12–19 sec.
Clot retraction time	50% by 1 h
Whole blood clot lysis time	> 24 h

3. Gases

PO_2	
Arterial blood (PaO_2)	80–100 mmHg
Venous blood	25–40 mmHg
PCO_2	
Arterial blood ($PaCO_2$)	35–45 mmHg
Venous blood	40–50 mmHg

4. pH
7.35–7.45

B. Serum

Bilirubin	
Adult	0.2–0.8 mg %
Newborn	0.5–5 mg %
At 3 days after birth	1–10 mg %
Creatinine	0.6-1.8 mg %
Calcium	9–11 mg/dl
Iron	50–150 mg/dl
Plasma glucose (fasting)	70–110 mg/dl (111–125 mg% is prediabetes)
Plasma glucose (postprandial, 2 hours)	< 140 mg%
Plasma glucose (random)	< 200 mg%
Electrolytes	
Sodium	136–145 meq/L

Potassium	3.5–5 meq/L	
Chlorides	96–106 meq/L	
Phosphorus (inorganic)	2.5–4.5 mg/dl	
Cholesterol	120–200 mg/dl	
Osmolality	280–295 mosm/kg of water	

C. Urine

Glucose	
Qualitative	Absent
Quantitative	16–300 mg/24 h
Protein	
Qualitative	Absent
Quantitative	10–150 mg/24 h
Bilirubin	Absent
Hemoglobin	Absent
Creatine	0–200 mg in 24 h
Creatinine	15–25 mg/kg body weight/day
Uric acid	250–750 mg/24 h
Urobilinogen	0.05–3.5 mg/24 h
Sodium	40–220 meq/24 h
Potassium	25–125 meq/24 h
Chloride	10–200 mmol/l
Calcium (normal diet)	100 – 300 mg/24 h
Osmolality	100–900 mosm/l
pH	4.6–8.0 (average 6)

D. Cerebrospinal fluid

Glucose	50–70 mg/dl
Protein	10–30 mg/dl
Bilirubin	Absent
Cells	0–5/mm³ (usually lymphocytes)
Chloride	110–125 mmol/l
Pressure	7–20 cm of water
pH	7.34–7.43

E. Semen

Liquefaction	Completes at 15 min.
Morphology	Minimum 4% normal

Motility	Minimum 42% motile
pH	7.2–8.0
Count	>16 million/ml
Volume	2–5 ml

F. Synovial fluid

Cells	200 cells/mm³
Glucose	Same as serum
Hyaluronic acid	2.5–4 g/dl
Proteins	2.5 g/dl
pH	7.32–7.64
Crystals	Absent

G. Stool

Fat	3–5 g/day
Nitrogen	2.2 g/24 h
Stercobilinogen	40–280 mg/24 h
Corpoporphyrin	15–500 mg/24 h

H. Cardiovascular parameters

Heart rate	: 60 to 100 per min.
Cardiac output	: 5 litres per min (each ventricle)
Cardiac Index	: 2.5–3.6 lit/min/sq mt BSA
Cardiac reserve	: 15–25 l/min (can be up to 40 l in athletes)
Systolic BP	: 100–119 mmHg (120–139 mmHg is prehypertension)
Diastolic BP	: 60–79 mmHg (80–89 mmHg is prehypertension)
Pulse pressure	: 20–50 mmHg
Stroke volume	: 60–80 ml
End-diastolic volume	: 130 ml
End-systolic volume	: 50 ml
Ejection fraction	: 50–70%

Bibliography

Hematology

Bain BJ, Bates I, Bates B, Laffan MA. 2021. *Dacie and Lewis Practical Hematology*; 12th edition. London: Churchill Livingstone.

Kaushansky K, Litchman MA, Prchal JT, Levi MM, Press OW, Burns LJ, Caliguri MA. 2020. *William's Hematology*; 9th edition. London: McGraw-Hill.

Pal GK and Pal P. 2003. *Textbook of Practical Physiology*; 2nd edition. Hyderabad, India: Orient Longman Publications.

Renu S, Pati HP, Mahapatra M (eds.). 2018. *de Gruchy's Clinical Hematology in Medical Practice*; 6th edition. London: Science.

Turgeon ML. 2019. *Linne and Ringsrud's Clinical Laboratory Science*; 8th edition. New York: Elsevier.

Human and Clinical Practicals

Bannister R and Mathews CJ (eds.). 2013. *Autonomic Failure: A Textbook of Clinical Disorders of the Autonomic Nervous System*; 5th edition. London: Oxford University Press.

Barett KE, Barman SM, Brooks HL and Yuan J (eds.). 2020. *Ganong's Review of Medical Physiology*; 26th edition. New York: McGraw-Hill.

Glynn M and Drake W (eds.), 2019. *Hutchison's Clinical Methods*; 23rd edition. London: WB Saunders.

Loscalzo J, Fauci AS, Kasper DL, Hauser SL, Longo DL, and Jameson JL (eds.). 2022. *Harrison's Principles of Internal Medicine*; 20th edition. New York: McGraw-Hill.

Johnson EW and Pease WS (eds.). 2015. *Practical Electromyography*; 3rd edition. London: Williams and Wilkins.

Kinirons M and Ellis H (eds.). 2011. *French's Index of Differential Diagnosis*; 15th edition. London: Butterworth-Heinemann.

Koeppen BM, Stanton BA. 2023. *Berne and Levy Physiology*; 8th edition. New York: Elsevier.

Mishra UK and Kalita J. 2019. *Clinical Neurophysiology*; 4th edition, New Delhi: Elsevier.

Narashiman C and Francis J (eds.). 2013. *An Introduction to Electrocardiography*; 8th edition. London: Wiley.

Ogilvie C. 1980. *Chamberlain's Symptoms and Signs in Clinical Medicine*; 10th edition. London: John Wright and Sons Ltd.

Pal GK, Pal P and Nanda N. 2025. *Comprehensive Textbook of Medical Physiology*; 4th edition, New Delhi: Jaypee Publications.

Pal GK, Pal P and Nanda N. 2025. *Textbook of Medical Physiology*; 5th edition. New Delhi: Elsevier (India) and Ahuja Publications.

Papadakis MA and Me Phee SJ (eds.). 2020. *Current Medical Diagnosis and Treatment*; 45th edition. New York: McGraw-Hill-Lange.

Sahu D. 1983. *Critical Approach to Clinical Medicine*. New Delhi: Vikas Publishing House Pvt Ltd.

Experimental Physiology

Bell GH. 1959. *Experimental Physiology*. London: Churchill Livingstone.

Ghosh MN. 2007. *Fundamentals of Experimental Pharmacology*; 3rd edition. Kolkata: Scientific Book Agency.

Levedahl BH, Barber AA and Grinnel A. 1971. *Laboratory Experiments in Physiology*; 8th edition. New York: CV Mosby Co.

Sharpey-Schafer EA. 2012. *Experimental Physiology*. London: Scholar Select Publication.

Tuttle WW and Schottelius BA. 1963. *Physiology Laboratory Manual*. New York: CV Mosby Co.

Index